Acute Stroke

NEUROLOGICAL DISEASE AND THERAPY

Acute Stroke

Bench to Bedside

edited by

Anish Bhardwaj
Oregon Health & Science University
Portland, Oregon, U.S.A.

Nabil J. Alkayed
Oregon Health & Science University
Portland, Oregon, U.S.A.

Jeffrey R. Kirsch
Oregon Health & Science University
Portland, Oregon, U.S.A.

Richard J. Traystman
Oregon Health & Science University
Portland, Oregon, U.S.A.

informa
healthcare

New York   London

Informa Healthcare USA, Inc.
270 Madison Avenue
New York, NY 10016

© 2007 by Informa Healthcare USA, Inc.
Informa Healthcare is an Informa business

No claim to original U.S. Government works
Printed in the United States of America on acid-free paper
10 9 8 7 6 5 4 3 2 1

International Standard Book Number-10: 0-8493-9870-3 (Hardcover)
International Standard Book Number-13: 978-0-8493-9870-4 (Hardcover)

Visit the Informa Web site at
www.informa.com

and the Informa Healthcare Web site at
www.informahealthcare.com

To our families.

Foreword

In the field of stroke, we are living in interesting—indeed, exhilarating—but also challenging times. One needs merely to consider the following:

- A sense of discouragement over the pitiable infrequency with which the only yet proven ameliorative therapy for acute ischemic stroke—intravenous tissue recombinant plasminogen activator—is actually being applied in clinical practice has begun to motivate stroke clinician-investigators to both develop strategies for widening the application of this therapy and validate other acute therapeutic approaches.
- Clinical-trial methodology as applied to stroke has improved greatly in both its sophistication and rigor, and many randomized clinical trials in stroke are currently ongoing, supported by the federal, pharmaceutical, and biotech sectors. (The superb website www.strokecenter.org provides a comprehensive status-report of completed and ongoing clinical trials in stroke.)
- Remarkable advances in clinical neuroimaging now permit us to observe the ongoing pathophysiology of ischemic and hemorrhagic stroke in real time and with dazzling clarity and spatial resolution. Diffusion- and perfusion-weighted magnetic resonance imaging and computed tomography perfusion and computed tomography angiography deserve particular mention.
- The field of neurointensive care has emerged as a key subspecialty of neurology, with much to offer in the management of acute stroke syndromes.
- Public awareness of the symptoms and signs of stroke and of the necessity for rapid intervention (the "therapeutic window") is slowly but surely growing. The laudable efforts of the American Heart Association (via its American Stroke Association) in this regard deserve particular recognition.
- In the laboratory, spectacular advances in molecular biology have shaped current directions in stroke research. It is now possible to investigate the effects of single-gene over- or underexpression on stroke pathophysiology by producing stroke in genetically altered murine strains and to survey the panoply of altered gene expression in stroke by the use of microarray technology. Intracellular molecular signaling mechanisms and their alterations in stroke are being extensively investigated. The potential of stem-cell approaches to recovery of brain function is also under current study.
- Animal models of ischemic and hemorrhagic stroke, which closely mimic relevant features of the human clinical disorders, are being studied with ever-increasing sophistication, and attention is being brought to bear on careful physiologic monitoring and a broad repertoire of tools for measuring functional and structural injury.
- Perhaps the most exciting recent development is the successful *translation* of laboratory advances to the bedside, particularly evident in ongoing clinical trials of neuroprotection that are being driven by the successful results emerging from studies in animal stroke models.

The guiding philosophy of the present volume, assembled under the wise editorship of Drs. Bhardwaj, Alkayed, Kirsch, and Traystman, is to emphasize *translationally* important topic areas in cerebrovascular disease, where advances at the bench lead to advances at the bedside. Both hemorrhage (subarachnoid and intracerebral) and ischemia (focal and global) are considered. In subarachnoid hemorrhage, despite sophisticated surgical and endovascular therapies, vexatious problems remain: prerupture aneurysmal growth and posttreatment vasospasm. In intracerebral hemorrhage, key issues include pharmacologic approaches to thwart hemorrhage expansion and to combat secondary-injury processes. In both focal and global ischemia, the challenge remains to translate laboratory successes in neuroprotection to the clinic. A potpourri of other key mechanistic, therapeutic, and stroke-management topics is also considered in this volume under the section "Dogmas, Controversies, and Future Directions." Taken together, the contributors to this timely volume offer the reader a rich menu to savor. Clinician-investigators will benefit from its breadth and depth.

Myron D. Ginsberg, MD
University of Miami, Miller School of Medicine,
Miami, Florida, U.S.A.

Preface

As the third leading cause of death in the United States, stroke constitutes a national health problem. Stroke accounts for 1 in every 15 deaths and is the major cause of disability in the country. Presently, in excess of 4 million Americans are stroke survivors. In the past, care for stroke patients had been mixed with an element of nihilism. However, over the last 2 decades, major advances have been made, and practices that were largely based on anecdotal experiences and physiologic inferences have evolved into more refined procedures and protocols in the management of this patient population.

Laboratory-based research in animal models has enhanced our understanding of pathophysiologic mechanisms of brain injury and provided important insights for possible therapeutic strategies and targets. Advances in neuroimaging and neurointerventional techniques have provided multiple avenues and improved approaches to early diagnosis and therapy in the acute phase of stroke. Clinical research with neuroprotective trials in focal ischemic stroke, though disappointing thus far, have further heightened the need for a multifaceted approach that concentrates equally on early recognition, diagnosis, and aggressive treatment. But stroke is more than just cerebral ischemia. Our understanding of the pathophysiology of brain injury following intracerebral and subarachnoid hemorrhage continues to grow from laboratory-based experimental work. Collaborative care by a specially trained team of neuro-intensivists, neurosurgeons, anesthesiologists, and nurses, and the advent of newer monitoring techniques in a dedicated neuro-intensive care unit have improved outcomes in patients with these subtypes of stroke.

While numerous textbooks on stroke are available, a large gap exists between basic science bench research and its translation into patient care in the field. The purpose of this book is to bridge this gap and present relevant bench research of "translational" significance, as well as its logical import, to the bedside. Each of the first 4 sections of the book begins with a chapter that covers research in the particular subarea, using appropriate animal models, and progresses through a continuum of the disease, from pathophysiology to clinical management to prognosis. The last section discusses controversies and future directions in stroke care, and it is hoped that the reader will be stimulated to investigate the many unanswered questions. Our intent with this book is to present a comprehensive review on the subject and provide clinicians, neuroscientists, and clinician scientists with a guide that will foster research of translational significance from bench to bedside and vice versa in this important area. We hope that we have achieved our goal.

We, the editors, are indebted to the authors for their valuable contributions. Special thanks are due to Tzipora Sofare, MA, for her efforts in editing this volume. Her close attention to detail and never-ending quest for accuracy and consistency have greatly contributed to its quality. We would also like to particularly express our thanks to the Johns Hopkins Clinician Scientist Program, the American Heart Association, the National Stroke Association, and the National Institutes of Health extramural programs, which have supported our investigative work and fellowship training programs in stroke and neurosciences critical care.

Anish Bhardwaj, MD, FAHA, FCCM
Nabil J. Alkayed, MD, PhD
Jeffrey R. Kirsch, MD
Richard J. Traystman, PhD, FCCM

Contents

Section V.   DOGMAS, CONTROVERSIES, AND FUTURE DIRECTIONS

Contributors

Andrei V. Alexandrov, MD, Director Stroke Research and Neurosonology Program, Barrow Neurological Institute, Phoenix, Arizona, USA

Nabil J. Alkayed, MD, PhD, Director[a], Associate Professor[b] [a]Core Molecular Laboratories and Training, [b]Department of Anesthesiology & Perioperative Medicine, Oregon Health & Science University, Portland, Oregon, USA

Yekaterina K. Axelrod, MD, Fellow Department of Neurosciences Critical Care, Washington University School of Medicine, St. Louis, Missouri, USA

Mona N. Bahouth, MSN, CRNP, Director Department of Neurology, University of Maryland School of Medicine, University of Maryland Medical Center, Baltimore, Maryland, USA

Kyra J. Becker, MD, Associate Professor Departments of Neurology and Neurological Surgery, Harborview Medical Center, University of Washington School of Medicine, Seattle, Washington, USA

Anish Bhardwaj, MD, FAHA, FCCM, Professor[a] and Director[b] [a]Departments of Neurology, Neurological Surgery, and Anethesiology & Perioperative Medicine, [b]Neurosciences Critical Care Program, Oregon Health & Science University, Portland, Oregon, USA

Thomas P. Bleck, MD, FCCM, Ruth Cain Ruggles Chairman[a], Vice Chairman[b], Professor[b] [a]Department of Neurology, Evanston Northwestern Healthcare, [b]Departments of Neurology, Neurosurgery, and Internal Medicine, Northwestern University Feinberg School of Medicine, Chicago, Illinois, USA

Cecil O. Borel, MD, Associate Professor Department of Anesthesiology, Duke University School of Medicine, Durham, North Carolina, USA

Ansgar M. Brambrink, MD, PhD, Associate Professor Department of Anesthesiology & Perioperative Medicine, Oregon Health & Science University, Portland, Oregon, USA

Gavin W. Britz, MD, MPH, Assistant Professor Department of Neurological Surgery, Harborview Medical Center, University of Washington, Seattle, Washington, USA

Thomas G. Brott, MD, Professor Department of Neurology, Mayo Clinic College of Medicine, Jacksonville, Florida, USA

Alastair M. Buchan, MD, Professor Acute Stroke Programme, John Radcliffe Hospital, University of Oxford, Headington, Oxford, UK

J. Ricardo Carhuapoma, MD, Assistant Professor Division of Neurosciences Critical Care, Departments of Neurology, Neurological Surgery, and Anesthesiology/Critical Care Medicine, Johns Hopkins University School of Medicine, Baltimore, Maryland, USA

Stephen Chang, MD, Resident Division of Interventional Neuroradiology, The Johns Hopkins Hospital, Baltimore, Maryland, USA

Michael Chopp, PhD, Professor and Director Department of Neurology, Henry Ford Health System, Wayne State University, Detroit, and Department of Physics, Oakland University, Rochester, Michigan, USA

Wayne M. Clark, MD, Professor[a] and Director[b] [a]Department of Neurology, [b]Stroke Program, Oregon Stroke Center, Oregon Health & Science University, Portland, Oregon, USA

Richard E. Clatterbuck, MD, PhD, Assistant Professor Departments of Neurosurgery and Neuroscience, Johns Hopkins University School of Medicine, Baltimore, Maryland, USA

Andrew M. Demchuk, MD, FRCPC, Associate Professor Department of Clinical Neurosciences, Calgary Stroke Program, Hotchkiss Brain Institute, University of Calgary, Calgary, Alberta, Canada

Michael N. Diringer, MD, Professor[a] and Director[b] [a]Departments of Neurology and Neurological Surgery, [b]Neurocritical Care Unit, Washington University School of Medicine, St. Louis, Missouri, USA

Christian Dohmen, MD Department of Neurology, Max-Planck Institute for Neurological Research, University of Cologne, Cologne, Germany

Aaron S. Dumont, MD, Fellow Department of Neurological Surgery, University of Virginia School of Medicine, Charlottesville, Virginia, USA

Mustapha A. Ezzeddine, MD, Assistant Professor Department of Neurology and Neurosciences, Zeenat Qureshi Stroke Research Center, University of Medicine and Dentistry of New Jersey (UMDNJ), Newark, New Jersey, USA

Christopher V. Fanale, MD, Associate Stroke Program Director Colorado Neurological Institute–Swedish Medical Center, Englewood, Colorado, USA

Donna M. Ferriero, MD, Professor Departments of Neurology and Pediatrics, University of California–San Francisco, San Francisco, California, USA

Madeline C. Fields, MD, Resident Department of Neurology, Mount Sinai School of Medicine, New York, New York, USA

Marc Fisher, MD, Professor Department of Neurology, University of Massachusetts Medical School, Worcester, Massachusetts, USA

Heather J. Fullerton, MD, MAS, Assistant Professor Departments of Neurology and Pediatrics, University of California–San Francisco, San Francisco, California, USA

Philippe Gailloud, MD, Associate Professor Division of Interventional Neuroradiology, The Johns Hopkins Hospital, Baltimore, Maryland, USA

Romergryko G. Geocadin, MD, Assistant Professor[a], Director[b], Associate Director[c] [a]Departments of Neurology, Anesthesiology/Critical Care Medicine, and Neurosurgery, Johns Hopkins University School of Medicine, [b]Neurosciences Critical Care Unit, Johns Hopkins Bayview Medical Center, and [c]Neurosciences Critical Care Division, The Johns Hopkins Medical Institutions, Baltimore, Maryland, USA

Rudolf Graf, PhD, Assistant Professor Department of Neurology, Max-Planck Institute for Neurological Research, University of Cologne, Cologne, Germany

Carmelo Graffagnino, MD, FRCPC, Associate Clinical Professor Department of Medicine/Neurology, Duke University Medical Center, Durham, North Carolina, USA

Wolf-Dieter Heiss, MD, Professor Department of Neurology, Max-Planck Institute for Neurological Research, University of Cologne, Cologne, Germany

Michael D. Hill, MD, MSc, FRCPC, Associate Professor[a] and Director[b] [a]Department of Clinical Neurosciences, Heart and Stroke Alberta Professorship in Stroke Research, [b]Foothills Medical Centre Stroke Unit, University of Calgary, Calgary, Alberta, Canada

Wesley Hsu, MD, Resident Department of Neurosurgery, Johns Hopkins University School of Medicine, Baltimore, Maryland, USA

Peter Hu, MS, CNE, Instructor Department of Anesthesiology, University of Maryland School of Medicine, University of Maryland Medical Center, Baltimore, Maryland, USA

Patricia D. Hurn, PhD, Professor and Vice Chairman of Research Department of Anesthesiology & Perioperative Medicine, Oregon Health & Science University, Portland, Oregon, USA

Jawad F. Kirmani, MD, Assistant Professor Department of Neurology and Neurosciences, Zeenat Qureshi Stroke Research Center, University of Medicine and Dentistry of New Jersey (UMDNJ), Newark, New Jersey, USA

Jeffrey R. Kirsch, MD, Professor and Chairman Department of Anesthesiology & Perioperative Medicine, Oregon Health & Science University, Portland, Oregon, USA

Raymond C. Koehler, PhD, Professor Department of Anesthesiology and Critical Care Medicine, Johns Hopkins University School of Medicine, Johns Hopkins Medical Institutions, Baltimore, Maryland, USA

Ines P. Koerner, MD, Fellow Department of Anesthesiology & Perioperative Medicine, Oregon Health & Science University, Portland, Oregon, USA

Julia Kofler, MD, Resident Department of Neuropathology, University of Pittsburgh School of Medicine, Pittsburgh, Pennsylvania, USA

Arthur M. Lam, MD, FRCPC, Professor, Anesthesiologist-in-Chief Departments of Anesthesiology and Neurological Surgery, Harborview Medical Center, University of Washington, Seattle, Washington, USA

Marian P. LaMonte, MD, MSN, Associate Professor Departments of Neurology and Emergency Medicine, University of Maryland School of Medicine, University of Maryland Medical Center, Baltimore, Maryland, USA

Steven R. Levine, MD, Professor The Stroke Center, Department of Neurology, Mount Sinai School of Medicine, New York, New York, USA

Fuhai Li, MD, Resident Department of Neurology, Duke University School of Medicine, Duke University Medical Center, Durham, North Carolina, USA

Yi Li, MD, Senior Staff Department of Neurology, Henry Ford Health System, Wayne State University, Detroit, Michigan, USA

Frederick W. Lombard, MBChB, FANZCA, Assistant Professor Department of Anesthesiology, Duke University School of Medicine, Durham, North Carolina, USA

Helmi L. Lutsep, MD, Associate Professor[a] and [b]Co-Director [a]Department of Neurology, [b]Stroke Program, Oregon Stroke Center, Oregon Health & Science University, Portland, Oregon, USA

Patrick D. Lyden, MD, FAAN, Professor[a] and Director[b] [a]Department of Neurosciences, University of California–San Diego, [b]UCSD Stroke Center, San Diego, California, USA

Colin Mackenzie, MBChB, Professor and Director Department of Anesthesiology, University of Maryland School of Medicine, University of Maryland Medical Center, Baltimore, Maryland, USA

Stephan A. Mayer, MD, Associate Clinical Professor[a] and Director[b] [a]Departments of Neurology and Neurosurgery, [b]Neurological Intensive Care Unit, Columbia University College of Physicians and Surgeons, Columbia University Medical Center, New York, New York, USA

Louise D. McCullough, MD, PhD, Assistant Professor and Director of Stroke Research Department of Neurology, University of Connecticut Health Center, Farmington, Connecticut, USA

José G. Merino, MD, MPhil, Staff Clinician Section on Stroke Diagnostics and Therapeutics, National Institute of Neurological Disorders and Stroke, Bethesda, Maryland, USA

Kieran Murphy, MD, FRCPC, Associate Professor Director of Interventional Neuroradiology, Department of Radiology, Johns Hopkins University School of Medicine, Baltimore, Maryland, USA

Neeraj S. Naval, MD, Instructor Division of Neurosciences Critical Care, Departments of Neurology, Neurological Surgery, and Anesthesiology/Critical Care Medicine, Johns Hopkins University School of Medicine, Baltimore, Maryland, USA

Alison J. Nohara, MD, Medical Director Interventional Neuroradiology, Eden Medical Center, Castro Valley, California, USA

Thaddeus S. Nowak, Jr., PhD, Professor Department of Neurology, University of Tennessee, Memphis, Tennessee, USA

Paul A. Nyquist, MD, MPH, Assistant Professor of Neurology Neurosciences Critical Care Division, Departments of Neurology, Neurological Surgery, Anesthesiology, and Critical Care Medicine, Johns Hopkins University School of Medicine, Baltimore, Maryland, USA

L. Creed Pettigrew, MD, MPH, Professor[a], Director[b] [a]Department of Neurology, [b]University of Kentucky Stroke Program, University of Kentucky Chandler Medical Center, Lexington, Kentucky, USA

Nader Pouratian, MD, PhD, Resident Department of Neurological Surgery, University of Virginia School of Medicine, Charlottesville, Virginia, USA

Gustavo Pradilla, MD, Resident Department of Neurosurgery, Johns Hopkins University School of Medicine, Johns Hopkins Medical Institutions, Baltimore, Maryland, USA

Adnan I. Qureshi, MD, Professor of Neurology and Radiology Department of Neurology and Neurosciences, Zeenat Qureshi Stroke Research Center, University of Medicine and Dentistry of New Jersey (UMDNJ), Newark, New Jersey, USA

Alejandro A. Rabinstein, MD, Associate Professor of Neurology[a], Consultant[b] [a]Mayo Clinic College of Medicine, [b]Neurological–Neurosurgical Intensive Care Unit, Saint Mary's Hospital, Rochester, Minnesota, USA

Marc Ribo, MD, Stroke Neurologist Unitat Neurovascular Hospital Vall d'Hebron, Universitat Autónoma de Barcelona, Barcelona, Spain

Daniele Rigamonti, MD, FACS, Vice-Chairman and Professor Department of Neurosurgery, Johns Hopkins University School of Medicine, Johns Hopkins Medical Institutions, Baltimore, Maryland, USA

Gustavo J. Rodríguez, MD, Vascular Neurology Fellow Department of Neurology and Neurosciences, Zeenat Qureshi Stroke Research Center, University of Medicine and Dentistry of New Jersey (UMDNJ), Newark, New Jersey, USA

Izabella Rozenfeld, MD, Resident Department of Neurology, Mount Sinai School of Medicine, New York, New York, USA

J. Michael Schmidt, PhD, Assistant Professor of Neuropsychology (in Neurology) Neurological Intensive Care Unit, Columbia University College of Physicians and Surgeons, Columbia University Medical Center, New York, New York, USA

Chandrasekaran Sivakumar, MD, Fellow Calgary Stroke Program, Foothills Medical Center, University of Calgary, Calgary, Alberta, Canada

Abhishek Srinivas, MD, Division of Interventional Neuroradiology, The Johns Hopkins Hospital, Baltimore, Maryland, USA

Suresh Subramaniam, MD, MSc Department of Clinical Neurosciences, University of Calgary, Calgary, Alberta, Canada

Rafael J. Tamargo, MD, FACS Walter E. Dandy Professor[a] and Director[b] [a]Departments of Neurosurgery, Otolaryngology, and Neck Surgery, [b]Department of Cerebrovascular Neurosurgery, Johns Hopkins University School of Medicine, Johns Hopkins Medical Institutions, Baltimore, Maryland , USA

Xian Nan Tang, MD, Fellow Department of Neurology, University of California–San Francisco, Veterans Affairs Medical Center, San Francisco, and Department of Anesthesia, Stanford University School of Medicine, Stanford, California, USA

Turgut Tatlisumak, MD, Associate Professor and Vice Chairman Department of Neurology, University of Helsinki, Helsinki University Central Hospital, Helsinki, Finland

Richard E. Temes, MD, Fellow Neurological Intensive Care Unit, Columbia University College of Physicians and Surgeons, Columbia University Medical Center, New York, New York, USA

Quoc-Anh Thai, MD, Assistant Chief of Service, Instructor Department of Neurosurgery, Johns Hopkins University School of Medicine, Johns Hopkins Medical Institutions, Baltimore, Maryland, USA

Richard J. Traystman, PhD, FCCM, Professor[a]**, Associate Vice President**[b]**, and Associate Dean**[c]
[a] Department of Anesthesiology & Perioperative Medicine, [b] Research Planning and Development, [c] Research School of Medicine, Oregon Health & Science University, Portland, Oregon, USA

Stanley Tuhrim, MD, Director[a]**, Professor**[b] [a] Division of Cerebrovascular Diseases, [b] Department of Neurology, Mount Sinai School of Medicine, New York, New York, USA

Kenneth R. Wagner, PhD, Research Associate Professor Department of Neurology, University of Cincinnati College of Medicine, and Veterans Affairs Medical Center, Medical Research Service, Cincinnati, Ohio, USA

Steven Warach, MD, PhD, Chief Section on Stroke Diagnostics and Therapeutics, National Institute of Neurological Disorders and Stroke, Bethesda, Maryland, USA

Eelco F. M. Wijdicks, MD, Professor of Neurology and Chair Division of Critical Care Neurology, Mayo Clinic College of Medicine, and Neurological–Neurosurgical Intensive Care Unit, Saint Mary's Hospital, Rochester, Minnesota, USA

Robert J. Wityk, MD, Director[a]**, Associate Professor**[b] [a] Cerebrovascular Division, [b] Department of Neurology, Johns Hopkins University School of Medicine, Baltimore, Maryland, USA

Yan Xiao, PhD, Associate Professor Department of Anesthesiology, University of Maryland School of Medicine, University of Maryland Medical Center, Baltimore, Maryland, USA

Midori A. Yenari, MD, Associate Professor Department of Neurology, University of California–San Francisco, Veterans Affairs Medical Center, San Francisco, and Department of Anesthesia, Stanford University School of Medicine, Stanford, California, USA

Zhen Zheng, MD, PhD, Fellow Department of Neurology, University of California–San Francisco, Veterans Affairs Medical Center, San Francisco, and Department of Anesthesia, Stanford University School of Medicine, Stanford, California, USA

Wendy C. Ziai, MD, Assistant Professor Departments of Neurology, Neurosurgery, and Anesthesia/Critical Care Medicine, Johns Hopkins University School of Medicine, Baltimore, Maryland, USA

1 | Animal Models of Subarachnoid Hemorrhage

Gustavo Pradilla, MD, Resident
Quoc-Anh Thai, MD, Assistant Chief of Service, Instructor
Department of Neurosurgery, Johns Hopkins University School of Medicine,
Johns Hopkins Medical Institutions, Baltimore, Maryland, USA

Rafael J. Tamargo, MD, FACS, Walter E. Dandy Professor[a] and Director[b]
[a] *Departments of Neurosurgery, Otolaryngology, and Neck Surgery,*
[b] *Department of Cerebrovascular Neurosurgery, Johns Hopkins University School of Medicine,*
Johns Hopkins Medical Institutions, Baltimore, Maryland, USA

INTRODUCTION

Cerebral vasospasm is the delayed narrowing of cerebral arteries exposed to blood. Although vasospasm typically occurs after subarachnoid hemorrhage (SAH) from rupture of a cerebral aneurysm, it can also develop after trauma (1,2) and infections (3). In humans, vasospasm presents as a biphasic phenomenon. Whereas acute vasospasm generally presents immediately after SAH and typically resolves within hours, chronic vasospasm occurs at 4 to 21 days and peaks 7 to 10 days after hemorrhage, with an overall angiographic incidence of 67% (4) and a clinical incidence of 37% (4). Chronic vasospasm causes delayed ischemic deficits, stroke, and death.

The etiology of vasospasm remains unclear. Current hypotheses include endothelial dysfunction secondary to inflammation of the arterial wall and transendothelial migration of macrophages and neutrophils (5,6), nitric oxide (NO) scavenging by such blood-degradation products as oxy-hemoglobin (7), depletion of NO secondary to NO synthase dysfunction (8), direct vasoconstriction due such to spasmogenic proteins as endothelin-1 (9), and dysregulation of electrolyte channels in the smooth muscle cell, such as K^+ (10) and Mg^{2+} (11).

In 1949, Robertson at the Royal Melbourne Hospital in Melbourne, Australia, was the first to describe delayed ischemia after SAH and to suggest that the ischemic changes could be related to temporary spasm of the supplying vessels (12). The first angiographic description of cerebral vasospasm after SAH was reported in 1951 (13). Since then, this condition has been studied extensively in experimental models.

Studies on the pathophysiology of cerebral vasospasm in humans have been attempted using postmortem specimens (14–18). Delayed postmortem artifacts, however, have prevented adequate analyses of genomic and proteomic variables, as well as testing of physiologic responses. To study cerebral vasospasm under more physiologic conditions, several experimental models have been developed. We present an overview of the different experimental models that have been used to date and comment on their technical and scientific characteristics.

IN VITRO MODELS OF VASOSPASM

In vitro models of vasospasm typically use an intracranial vessel that is harvested and either placed in a physiologic environment attached to a fixation device for recording of tension and other variables, or prepared for extraction of endothelial and smooth muscle cells for culture. The vessels can be harvested after exposure to blood *in vivo* or they can be harvested from a healthy animal for further experimental manipulation *in vitro*. Using these models, several pro-vasospastic agents have been characterized and some pharmacologic interventions have been proposed (19–24). Advantages of these in vitro models include a well-controlled environment, real-time observation of vascular tone and electrolyte changes, low cost, and an abundance of tissue for testing. Disadvantages include removal of the vessel from its natural environment, denervation of the arterial wall, absence of innate immunologic stimulus, and lack of prolonged injury and recovery periods. Due to these observations, the relevance of these models to human cerebral vasospasm has been questioned (25), and the injection and clot-placement models in animals remain more suitable alternatives.

IN VIVO MODELS OF VASOSPASM

Animal models of SAH have been used extensively to induce vasospasm and include multiple species and diverse techniques. Careful consideration must be given to the selection of the species, because factors—such as time course of vasospasm, manifestations of delayed ischemic deficits, responses to pharmacotherapy, anatomic composition of the arterial wall of cerebral vessels, and rates of clearing of subarachnoid blood, etc.—can differ from one species to another.

CREATION OF SAH AND INDUCTION OF VASOSPASM

Models of SAH should ideally consist of placement or injection of blood that surrounds a cerebral artery and results in consistent and reproducible, delayed vasospasm that lasts for several days, as confirmed by angiographic or morphometric analysis. These models should be reproducible and cost effective, and they should use species closest to humans. Whole blood is preferable to induce vasospasm, because erythrocyte hemolysate has been shown to be less capable of generating a delayed, sustained response (26,27). To induce vasospasm, a number of techniques have been used that lead to the development of delayed-onset, sustained arterial narrowing. These techniques can be grouped into 3 general categories: (i) puncture of an artery (endovascularly or under direct vision), (ii) surgical exposure of an artery and placement of an autologous blood clot obtained from another vessel, and (iii) injection of blood obtained from a peripheral vessel into the subarachnoid space. A disappointing feature common to all animal models of SAH and vasospasm is the lack of vasospasm-related ischemic, neurologic deficits (28), most likely secondary to an abundance of collateral blood flow in smaller vertebrates. However, in that most studies focus on the induction, prevention, and/or reversal of vessel constriction rather than on vasospasm-related ischemia, the absence of ischemic neurologic deficits in experimental animals has limited significance.

MONKEY MODELS

The first use of monkeys for the study of vasospasm was reported in 1965 (29). In this study, a transoral approach to the skull base was used to expose the basilar and vertebral arteries, vasospasm was induced through application of autologous blood, and measurements were taken by *in situ* photographic analyses of the vessel calibers.

Currently, the most popular technique is the one described in 1982 in cynomolgus monkeys (*Macaca fascicularis*) (30). In this model, a preoperative angiogram is obtained, a right frontotemporal craniectomy is performed, and the arachnoid cisterns encasing the internal carotid artery (ICA), anterior cerebral artery (ACA), and middle cerebral artery (MCA) are dissected. Arterial blood is withdrawn and allowed to clot, and the resulting clot is sectioned into fragments that are placed adjacent to the exposed vessels (Fig. 1). A repeat angiogram is obtained 7 days after surgery, and vasospasm is determined by comparison with the preoperative angiogram (Fig. 2). Angiographic vessel narrowing ranges from 31% to 100% and typically occurs in all animals (30). Severe vasospasm, defined as a reduction >50% in arterial caliber, was present in only approximately 25% of the animals. The mortality reported by the authors was 10% (30). In our laboratory, however, we have had no mortality attributable to the model (32,33).

Advantages of this model include a well-defined course of angiographic vasospasm, development of distal vessel narrowing, histopathologic modifications in the exposed vessels, loss of autoregulatory mechanisms, disruption of cerebral blood flow (CBF), presence of a contralateral control, and absence of pharmacologic responses to standard vasodilators. Disadvantages of the model include high costs and risk of contamination with simian herpes virus. This model has been extensively used as described, or with minor modifications, to test several experimental therapies (34–43) and to analyze proposed pathogenetic mechanisms (11,42,44–52).

(A) **(B)**

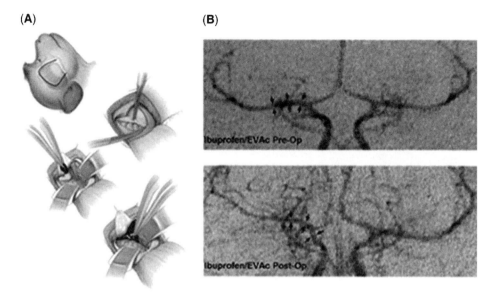

Figure 1 Monkey model of subarachnoid hemorrhage (SAH). (**A**) An artist's illustration of the surgical technique for induction of SAH in monkey. (**B**) Cerebral angiograms of a cynomolgus monkey before (*top*) and after (*bottom*) SAH.

Other popular techniques used to induce vasospasm in monkeys are based on blood injection into intracranial cisterns, a technique first described in 1968 that involves injection of 2 to 3 ml of blood into the cisterna magna (53) of African green monkeys. Modifications of this technique include injections into the subfrontal subarachnoid space (53) and prepontine cistern (via cervical laminectomy) (54). Standardization of blood volumes is critical to induce reproducible vasospasm with these methods. Disadvantages of this model, compared to clot placement techniques, include the lack of a contralateral control vessel and the high variability in the severity and course of the induced vasospasm. Models using rupture, puncture, or avulsion of the intracranial vessels were used in the past (55–58), but the high mortality rates and the limited reproducibility of vasospasm have been discouraging.

RABBIT MODELS

The first use of rabbits for the study of vasospasm was reported in 1969 (59). In this report, an occipital burr hole was placed and, under fluoroscopic guidance, a catheter was directed into the subarachnoid space close to the orbit and inserted into the right carotid artery. The goal of the study was to analyze the electrocardiographic changes that occur after SAH; vasospasm was not evaluated.

In the most common rabbit model used today, the atlanto-occipital membrane is surgically exposed, cerebrospinal fluid (CSF) is withdrawn, and 1.25 ml/kg of autologous arterial blood are injected into the surgically exposed cisterna magna, followed by placement of the animal head-down at 30° for 30 min to confine the blood to the intracranial cisterns (Fig. 2) (28,60). With this technique, peak vasospasm occurs 72 hr after SAH, and a 40% to 45% reduction in the diameter of the basilar artery is observed. A variation of this technique, using percutaneous injection of 1 ml/kg into the cisterna magna, produces similar results. A high correlation between angiographic and morphometric vasospasm has been observed in this model (61).

Advantages of this model include evaluation of an intracranial vessel, extensive histopathologic characterization, well-defined time course, and lower cost. Disadvantages include absence of reduction of CBF after single hemorrhage. Proponents of this model have used a double hemorrhage to induce more severe vasospasm (62,63). The need for double injection, however, has been questioned, because vasospasm is not significantly greater when compared to the single-injection technique (64).

(A)   **(B)**

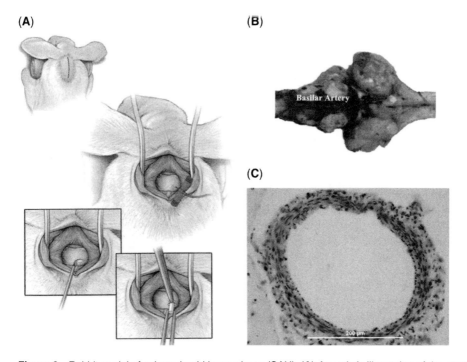

(C)

Figure 2   Rabbit model of subarachnoid hemorrhage (SAH). (**A**) An artist's illustration of the surgical technique for induction of SAH in the rabbit. (**B**) Photograph of a macroscopic specimen showing a blood clot around the basilar artery of a rabbit after induction of SAH. (**C**) Microphotograph of a cross-section of the basilar artery of rabbit after SAH. *Source*: From Ref. 31.

Numerous therapeutic agents have been tested, and those shown to prevent vasospasm include endothelin antagonists (65–67), calcium-channel blockers (68–70), nonsteroidal anti-inflammatory drugs (NSAIDs) (71), monoclonal antibodies against CD11/CD18 (72) and intercellular adhesion molecule 1 (ICAM-1) (73), and NO donors (31). Reversal of established vasospasm in this model has been achieved by intracardiac infusion of papaverine, sodium nitroprusside, and adenosine (74), by local delivery of diethyl-triamine nitric oxide (DETA-NO) (75), and by various other means.

To induce ischemia after posthemorrhagic vasospasm in rabbits, bilateral common carotid artery (CCA) ligations were performed 2 weeks prior to a double-injection SAH. This maneuver caused cerebral infarction in only 15% of animals (76). Other, less common techniques include transorbital blood injection into the chiasmatic cistern, rupture of the MCA (puncture via craniotomy), mechanical compression, puncture of the MCA and the superior sagittal sinus, blood injection into the interpeduncular cistern, and transclival puncture of the basilar artery.

An extracranial model using the CCA has also been reported in rabbits (77). In this model, the CCA is encased in polyvinyl chloride cuffs and autologous blood is injected. Vasospasm develops 24 to 48 hr after hemorrhage and persists for approximately 6 days. This model has been used to show eicosanoid production after SAH and induction of vasospasm with the injection of human blood. Therapeutic approaches tested in this model include prophylactic laser treatment and transluminal angioplasty.

DOG MODELS

The first dog model described for the study of vasospasm used a transoral/transclival approach to the chiasmatic cistern (78). In this study, only 42% of the animals experienced SAH after injection of 5 ml of arterial blood. Complications, such as intraventricular hemorrhages, meningitis, and subdural hematomas, developed, and the study showed that some of the animals developed symptomatic vasospasm. However, the authors did not perform lumen patency studies.

The next reported dog model used a craniotomy to implant a strain-measuring device around the ICA and a thread to later avulse the ICA and induce SAH (79). With this technique, acute and chronic vasospasm of the ICA were documented, with peak vasospasm (20% decrease in lumen patency) occurring 4 to 6 days after hemorrhage. This model demonstrated that serial intra-arterial injections of serotonin fail to induce chronic vasospasm. A modification of this technique was developed by avulsing the posterior communicating artery (PCoA) and measuring angiographic diameters (80). Vasospasm after avulsion of the PCoA was more severe than vasospasm after avulsion of the ICA and ranged from 25% to 40%. An acute phase developed 20 min after hemorrhage, followed by a delayed phase 24 hr later.

In the model that followed, 5 ml of blood was injected into the cisterna magna (81), which caused a decrease in the contractility of vasospastic arteries 7 days after hemorrhage. This model has been used to study several experimental treatments, including papaverine (82). Standardization of the angiographic technique and use of a Trendelenberg position for 15 min after injection to encase the subarachnoid clot within the intracranial cisterns improved the reproducibility of this method. The modified technique was reported to induce a 37% decrease in basilar artery vasospasm 30 min and 48 hr after hemorrhage (83,84). Experimental treatments tested in this fashion include Ca^{2+} channel blockers (85), NO donors (86), an angiotensin-converting enzyme inhibitor (87), and several NSAIDs (88). Further studies of a single injection of blood into the cisterna magna have shown, however, that this technique does not produce sustained severe vasospasm, and that histopathologic and pharmacologic changes are not consistently present (16,89).

To address this problem, the use of multiple injections of blood into the cisterna magna in dogs was proposed (16). This technique induced angiographic vasospasm; however, histopathologic or ultrastructural changes were not found. A modification of this technique led to the most popular model of SAH in dogs currently used. It consists of a standardized double injection of 4 ml of blood into the cisterna magna on the first and third days of the study. With this method, angiographic vasospasm of the basilar artery was reported in 82% of animals 5 days after the first injection (90,91). Further analyses showed histopathologic changes in the basilar artery that were associated with a decreased response to treatment with intra-arterial papaverine. Several experimental studies have been performed with this model. Advantages include a well-defined course of vasospasm that is comparable to that of humans, accessible percutaneous angiography, and histopathologic and pharmacologic changes. Disadvantages include limited monoclonal antibodies for analysis, elevated cost, and the need for a second injection.

CAT MODELS

SAH in cats was initially induced by electrical or mechanical stimulation, as well as by laceration of the basilar artery, and vasospasm was determined through diameter measurements under direct microscopic visualization (92–94) after a transclival approach. Vasospasm was also induced by lysed platelets, whole blood, hemolysate, serotonin, angiotensin, and norepinephrin (93,95,96) and was successfully prevented by treatment with chlorpromazine and papaverine (93,95). Whereas laceration of the basilar artery caused vasospasm that lasted for at least 100 min, mechanical spasm reverted within 15 min (93).

Blood injection into the cisterna magna causes angiographic vasospasm of the basilar artery at 4 hr and 1 to 7 days but fails to cause histopathologic changes in the smooth muscle cells (97). Nonetheless, this technique has been used to study CSF absorption after treatment with recombinant tissue plasminogen activator (98) to measure changes in intracranial pulse waves after SAH (99) and to study CBF post-SAH (100), despite reports of rapid clearing of blood from the subarachnoid space (101). Other techniques used include blood injection over the cerebral cortex (102), rupture of the MCA through puncture or incision (97,100), blood injection through a shunt from the abdominal aorta through the chiasmatic cistern (103), and avulsion of the MCA (104) or ICA (105). Cat models of vasospasm, however, have decreased in popularity in recent years due to the limited availability of biologic tools for protein analysis, scarce genetic information, and poor characterization of the onset and progression of vasospasm.

RAT MODELS

Although rats have been used extensively to reproduce vasospasm, a number of issues have limited the applicability of the obtained findings to the human disease, among them the lack of myointimal cells in intracranial vessels that might play a role in the intimal hyperplasia observed after vascular injury (106), high mortality rates, and early resolution of vasospasm.

Intracranial Models

The first intracranial model consisted of transclival exposure of the basilar artery for either puncture with a microelectrode or clot placement, followed by measurements of vessel diameter under direct vision (107). One study used this technique to measure electrolytic changes in the basilar artery and subarachnoid clot and had a mortality of 26%, with peak vasospasm occurring 1 hr after puncture and maximal delayed spasm of 15% at 48 hr (108). Puncture of the basilar artery, however, resulted in variable amounts of SAH, and direct measurement of the basilar artery suffered from significant interobserver variability.

The next model used transorbital blood injections into the chiasmatic cistern (109). A catheter was placed through a frontal burr hole and advanced around the hemisphere to the cistern to inject heparinized blood. This technique was used to test acute electrocardiographic changes, not vasospasm. Injection of heparinized blood could alter the development of vasospasm by preventing adequate clot formation, and the placement of a catheter "blindly" prevented localization of the SAH to one side and prevented the use of the contralateral side for control.

Models of blood injection into the cisterna magna used in other species were adapted for rats, following different methods. The first method described consisted of placing a burr hole in the parietal region and inserting a cannula into the cisterna magna to inject blood and induce vasospasm of the basilar artery. This model was injected with 0.3 ml of either fresh autologous arterial blood or mock CSF, and CBF was determined by tracking labeled microspheres for 1 hr after injection. Rats with experimental SAH showed a 40% decrease in CBF, whereas those that received saline injection showed only a 15% decrease (110). An increase in the volume of blood injected (0.6 ml) resulted in a decrease in CBF 3 hr after SAH that returned to normal values at 1, 2, 3, 7, and 14 days (111). In this model, variability of vasospasm was observed between Wistar and Sprague-Dawley rats. The second method consisted of a double injection, in which the posterior atlanto-occipital membrane was exposed, 0.1 ml of CSF was aspirated, mixed with 0.4 ml of venous blood, and 0.1 ml of the mixture was reinjected (112). In this model, corrosion casts of the cerebral arteries showed vasospasm that was not altered by nimodipine administration.

Endovascular perforation models were developed in rats and have become quite popular. These models are generally referred to as the "Sheffield model" because they were initially described by researchers using Wistar rats in 1995 at the Royal Hallamshire Hospital in Sheffield, UK (113). This technique has also been described in Sprague-Dawley rats (114). The technique consists of inserting a pointed 3-0 monofilament nylon suture into the ICA and advancing it until it perforates the ACA, which results in SAH in 89% of the animals and in intracerebral hemorrhage in the remaining 11%. This model has a reported mortality of approximately 50%, and the severity of vasospasm varies significantly; pharmacologic responses to delayed vasospasm and pathologic changes in the arterial wall do not occur (115). A study comparing injection into the cisterna magna with endovascular rupture through the ICA using a 3-0 or a 4-0 nylon suture showed that the 4-0 suture produced less SAH and resulted in lower peak intracranial pressure when compared to other groups and that CBF reductions were similar in all groups, with the injection group having a faster CBF recovery (116).

A more recent study was performed to compare the severity of vasospasm induced by either endovascular puncture with a 3-0 suture through the ICA, single injection of 0.3 ml of blood into the cisterna magna, or double injection of 0.3 ml (48-hr interval between injections) (117) in male Sprague-Dawley rats. Histopathologic examination and morphometric analysis were performed on the basilar artery and PCoA. The study showed that these techniques caused significant vasospasm, with the double-hemorrhage model inducing the most severe vasospasm. Double hemorrhage, however, caused the highest mortality rate (57%) and had significant variability in hemorrhage volumes when compared to the cisternal injection models. Whereas vasospasm after endovascular perforation or single hemorrhage was more pronounced in the PCoA, vasospasm after double hemorrhage was more pronounced in the basilar artery.

(A) **(B)**

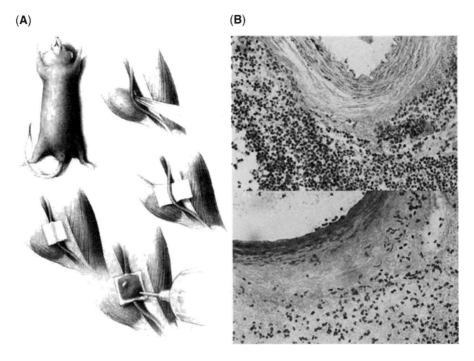

Figure 3 Rat femoral artery model of vasospasm. (**A**) Artist's illustration of the surgical technique for induction of vasospasm in the femoral artery of a rat. (**B**) Microphotograph of a cross-section of the femoral artery of a rat after peri-adventitial blood deposition. *Source*: From Ref. 119.

The authors concluded that the double-hemorrhage model was the most suitable alternative for studying mechanistic and therapeutic approaches for vasospasm.

Extracranial Models

Another currently popular model utilizes the rat femoral artery. This model consists of exposing the femoral artery, isolating it in a silicon cuff, and filling the cuff with blood or blood components (Fig. 3) (118). Peak morphometric vasospasm in this model occurs on day 7 and is accompanied by pathologic changes in the arterial wall. The major advantage of this model is the similarity of its course to that of human vasospasm. Other advantages are the availability of a contralateral control vessel and the controlled volume and localization of the hemorrhage. The main disadvantage of this model is the use of a systemic vessel, which excludes CSF clearance, changes in intracranial pressure, and central nervous system–specific inflammatory responses from the experimental variables. Several groups have shown that pharmacologic responses observed in this model correlate with those observed in other species (31,32,71,72,119–121) and that the pathologic changes observed are comparable to those seen after SAH in intracranial models and in humans.

MOUSE MODELS

Mouse models of vasospasm are similar to rat models and have been recently developed to take advantage of transgenic technology. The first model used endovascular perforation of the ACA (122). In this model, a 5-0 monofilament suture with a blunt end is advanced through the ICA up to the ACA until resistance is felt. The suture is advanced 5mm further to perforate the ACA and then withdrawn. Acute mortality with this model is 28%. To determine vasospasm, animals are perfused with 10% formalin, followed by carbon mixed with 10% gelatin. The diameter of the MCA is then measured under a microscope. Peak vasospasm in this model occurs on day 3 and results in an approximately 20% decrease in MCA diameter compared to

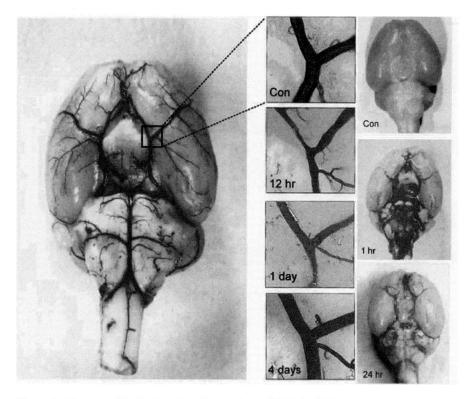

Figure 4   Mouse model of subarachnoid hemorrhage (SAH). (*Left*) Vasospasm determined after India ink injection. (*Right*) Evolution of the subarachnoid clot over time. *Source*: From Ref. 123.

controls. Studies performed with this model were designed to test the potential protective effect of overexpressed superoxide dismutase in transgenic mice.

Advantages of this model include a relatively low cost and the ability to use transgenic mice. Disadvantages include a high mortality rate, moderate vasospasm, lack of standardization of hemorrhagic volume, and interobserver variability when measuring MCA diameters.

A modified technique for intracisternal injection has been reported (123) in which the femoral artery is cannulated and 60 mL of blood is withdrawn and reinjected into the cisterna magna. This technique carries a mortality of approximately 3%; acute (6–12 hr) and chronic (1–3 days) vasospasm are observed after transthoracic perfusion with 10% gelatin and 10% India ink (Fig. 4). The diameters of the basilar artery, ACA, and MCA are measured using a digital camera and stereomicroscope. A histopathologic analysis of cross-sections of the analyzed vessels in the current study showed arterial wall changes consistent with those seen in other models. This model appears to be reproducible, accessible, and comparable to other murine models, and it has the advantage of lower mortality. Disadvantages include mild-to-moderate sustained vasospasm with peaks at 3 days in the ACA (21%) and at 1.5 days in the MCA (15%) and basilar artery (15%).

OTHER MODELS

Pig Models

A porcine model of vasospasm in pigs was developed that consists of placement of a catheter into the prepontine cistern, followed by two 12-ml injections of blood, with a 48-hr interval (124). Vasospasm was determined by angiography 48 hr after the first injection in 4 out of the 6 animals studied. Arterial injury was observed in specimens collected between 7 and 24 days after the initial hemorrhage. Pigs were selected due to their tendency to develop spontaneous atherosclerosis with age.

A model that followed a clot placement technique via frontotemporal craniotomy was developed to determine the ability of specific blood fractions that contain hemoglobin to induce morphometric vasospasm of the MCA 10 days after hemorrhage (125). In this study, the fractions that contained hemoglobin induced morphometric vasospasm and ultrastructural changes that were comparable to those observed in the MCA of animals exposed to whole blood.

Goat Models

Blood was injected into the basal cisterns of goats through a parietotemporal catheter to study the role of endothelin-1 in posthemorrhagic vasospasm and to test the ability of nicardipine to prevent SAH and endothelin-1–induced vasospasm (126). The authors reported a decrease of 28% in CBF at 3 days after hemorrhage that resolved by day 7.

CONCLUSIONS

Currently, *in vitro* models of vasospasm remain inferior to *in vivo* models, and their use is limited to specific goals, such as physiologic studies of electron channels and screening of potentially favorable treatments. Among animal models, small species, such as mice, rats, and rabbits, because of their availability and low cost, are ideal for screening for novel therapeutics and testing physiologic variables, but monkeys, which are phylogenetically closest to humans, should be studied before experimental treatments are applied to humans.

Most animal models used to study vasospasm employ either blood injection/blood clot placement techniques or vessel puncture/avulsion techniques to induce SAH and vasospasm. Injection/clot placement techniques are preferable. These techniques are easy to perform in most species, result in significant and consistent vessel narrowing, and are associated with decreased animal morbidity and mortality. Vessel puncture/avulsion techniques are less appealing due to high mortality rates. The selection of one technique over another must be made according to the experimental question to be addressed.

The use of extracranial arteries to study cerebral vasospasm remains controversial. Intracranial vessels are favored because blood breakdown products remain in the CSF for longer periods than they do in the soft tissues, neural regulation of arterial tone differs between intracranial and extracranial vessels, and immunologic responses in the brain are modulated through central nervous system–specific pathways.

The most common endpoint in animal models of vasospasm is vessel narrowing, determined by either morphometric or angiographic vessel diameter. Among all animal models, the rabbit and monkey models are currently the best models of SAH and vasospasm.

REFERENCES

1. Zubkov AY, Lewis AI, Raila FA, Zhang J, Parent AD. Risk factors for the development of post-traumatic cerebral vasospasm. Surg Neurol 2000; 53:126–130.
2. Zubkov AY, Pilkington AS, Bernanke DH, Parent AD, Zhang J. Posttraumatic cerebral vasospasm: clinical and morphological presentations. J Neurotrauma 1999; 16:763–770.
3. Yamashima T, Kashihara K, Ikeda K, Kubota T, Yamamoto S. Three phases of cerebral arteriopathy in meningitis: vasospasm and vasodilatation followed by organic stenosis. Neurosurgery 1985; 16:546–553.
4. Dorsch NW. Cerebral arterial spasm—a clinical review. Br J Neurosurg 1995; 9:403–412.
5. Dumont AS, Dumont RJ, Chow MM, et al. Cerebral vasospasm after subarachnoid hemorrhage: putative role of inflammation. Neurosurgery 2003; 53:123–133.
6. Sercombe R, Dinh YR, Gomis P. Cerebrovascular inflammation following subarachnoid hemorrhage. Jpn J Pharmacol 2002; 88:227–249.
7. Macdonald RL, Weir BK. A review of hemoglobin and the pathogenesis of cerebral vasospasm. Stroke 1991; 22:971–982.
8. Pluta RM. Delayed cerebral vasospasm and nitric oxide: review, new hypothesis, and proposed treatment. Pharmacol Ther 2005; 105:23–56.
9. Chow M, Dumont AS, Kassell NF. Endothelin receptor antagonists and cerebral vasospasm: an update. Neurosurgery 2002; 51:1333–1341; discussion 1342.

10. Aihara Y, Jahromi BS, Yassari R, Nikitina E, Agbaje-Williams M, Macdonald RL. Molecular profile of vascular ion channels after experimental subarachnoid hemorrhage. J Cereb Blood Flow Metab 2004; 24:75–83.

11. Macdonald RL, Curry DJ, Aihara Y, Zhang ZD, Jahromi BS, Yassari R. Magnesium and experimental vasospasm. J Neurosurg 2004; 100:106–110.

12. Robertson EG. Cerebral lesions due to intracranial aneurysms. Brain 1949; 72:150–185.

13. Ecker A, Riemenschneider PA. Arteriographic demonstration of spasm of the intracranial arteries with special reference to saccular arterial aneurysms. J Neurosurg 1951; 8:660–667.

14. Conway LW, McDonald LW. Structural changes of the intradural arteries following subarachnoid hemorrhage. J Neurosurg 1972; 37:715–723.

15. Crompton MR. The pathogenesis of cerebral infarction following the rupture of cerebral berry aneurysms. Brain 1964; 87:491–510.

16. Eldevik OP, Kristiansen K, Torvik A. Subarachnoid hemorrhage and cerebrovascular spasm. Morphological study of intracranial arteries based on animal experiments and human autopsies. J Neurosurg 1981; 55:869–876.

17. Hughes JT, Schianchi PM. Cerebral artery spasm. A histological study at necropsy of the blood vessels in cases of subarachnoid hemorrhage. J Neurosurg 1978; 48:515–525.

18. Smith RR, Clower BR, Grotendorst GM, Yabuno N, Cruse JM. Arterial wall changes in early human vasospasm. Neurosurgery 1985; 16:171–176.

19. Wilkins RH, Wilkins GK, Gunnells JC, Odom GL. Experimental studies of intracranial arterial spasm using aortic strip assays. J Neurosurg 1967; 27:490–500.

20. Sundt TM Jr., Winkelmann RK. Humoral responses of smooth muscle from rabbit subarachnoid artery compared to kidney, mesentery, lung, heart, and skin vascular smooth muscle. Stroke 1972; 3:717–725.

21. Allen GS, Henderson LM, Chou SN, French LA. Cerebral arterial spasm. 1. In vitro contractile activity of vasoactive agents on canine basilar and middle cerebral arteries. J Neurosurg 1974; 40:433–441.

22. Boullin DJ, Mohan J, Grahame-Smith DG. Evidence for the presence of a vasoactive substance (possibly involved in the aetiology of cerebral arterial spasm) in cerebrospinal fluid from patients with subarachnoid haemorrhage. J Neurol Neurosurg Psychiatr 1976; 39:756–766.

23. Okwuasaba FK, Weir BK, Cook DA, Krueger CA. Effects of various intracranial fluids on smooth muscle. Neurosurgery 1981; 9:402–406.

24. Brandt L, Ljunggren B, Anderson KE, Hindfelt B, Teasdale G. Vasoconstrictive effects of human post-hemorrhagic cerebrospinal fluid on cat pial arterioles in situ. J Neurosurg 1981; 54:351–356.

25. Wellum GR, Peterson JW, Zervas NT. The relevance of in vitro smooth muscle experiments to cerebral vasospasm. Stroke 1985; 16:573–581.

26. Kuroki M, Kanamaru K, Suzuki H, Waga S, Semba R. Effect of vasospasm on heme oxygenases in a rat model of subarachnoid hemorrhage. Stroke 1998; 29:683–688; discussion 688–689.

27. Macdonald RL, Weir BK, Grace MG, Martin TP, Doi M, Cook DA. Morphometric analysis of monkey cerebral arteries exposed in vivo to whole blood, oxyhemoglobin, methemoglobin, and bilirubin. Blood Vessels 1991; 28:498–510.

28. Nakagomi T, Kassell NF, Sasaki T, et al. Effect of subarachnoid hemorrhage on endothelium-dependent vasodilation. J Neurosurg 1987; 66:915–923.

29. Echlin FA. Spasm of basilar and vertebral arteries caused by experimental subarachnoid hemorrhage. J Neurosurg 1965; 23:1–11.

30. Espinosa F, Weir B, Boisvert D, Overton T, Castor W. Chronic cerebral vasospasm after large subarachnoid hemorrhage in monkeys. J Neurosurg 1982; 57:224–232.

31. Gabikian P, Clatterbuck RE, Eberhart CG, Tyler BM, Tierney TS, Tamargo RJ. Prevention of experimental cerebral vasospasm by intracranial delivery of a nitric oxide donor from a controlled-release polymer: toxicity and efficacy studies in rabbits and rats. Stroke 2002; 33:2681–2686.

32. Clatterbuck RE, Gailloud P, Ogata L, et al. Prevention of cerebral vasospasm by a humanized anti-CD11/CD18 monoclonal antibody administered after experimental subarachnoid hemorrhage in nonhuman primates. J Neurosurg 2003; 99:376–382.

33. Pradilla G, Thai QA, Legnani FG, et al. Local delivery of ibuprofen via controlled-release polymers prevents angiographic vasospasm in a monkey model of subarachnoid hemorrhage. Neurosurgery 2005; 57 (1 suppl):184–190.

34. Afshar JK, Pluta RM, Boock RJ, Thompson BG, Oldfield EH. Effect of intracarotid nitric oxide on primate cerebral vasospasm after subarachnoid hemorrhage. J Neurosurg 1995; 83:118–122.

35. Findlay JM, Weir BK, Steinke, D, Tanabe T, Gordon P, Grace M. Effect of intrathecal thrombolytic therapy on subarachnoid clot and chronic vasospasm in a primate model of SAH. J Neurosurg 1988; 69:723–735.

36. Findlay JM, Weir BK, Gordon P, Grace M, Baughman R. Safety and efficacy of intrathecal thrombolytic therapy in a primate model of cerebral vasospasm. Neurosurgery 1989; 24:491–498.

37. Inoue T, Shimizu H, Kaminuma T, Tajima M, Watabe K, Yoshimoto T. Prevention of cerebral vasospasm by calcitonin gene-related peptide slow-release tablet after subarachnoid hemorrhage in monkeys. Neurosurgery 1996; 39:984–990.

38. Nosko M, Weir BK, Lunt A, Grace M, Allen P, Mielke B. Effect of clot removal at 24 hours on chronic vasospasm after SAH in the primate model. J Neurosurg 1987; 66:416–422.

39. Handa Y, Weir BK, Nosko M, Mosewich R, Tsuji T, Grace M. The effect of timing of clot removal on chronic vasospasm in a primate model. J Neurosurg 1987; 67:558–564.

40. Steinke DE, Weir BK, Findlay JM, Tanabe T, Grace M, Krushelnycky BW. A trial of the 21-aminosteroid U74006F in a primate model of chronic cerebral vasospasm. Neurosurgery 1989; 24:179–186.

41. Hino A, Weir BK, Macdonald RL, Thisted RA, Kim CJ, Johns LM. Prospective, randomized, double-blind trial of BQ-123 and bosentan for prevention of vasospasm following subarachnoid hemorrhage in monkeys. J Neurosurg 1995; 83:503–509.

42. Pluta RM, Oldfield EH, Boock RJ. Reversal and prevention of cerebral vasospasm by intracarotid infusions of nitric oxide donors in a primate model of subarachnoid hemorrhage. J Neurosurg 1997; 87:746–751.

43. Horky LL, Pluta RM, Boock RJ, Oldfield EH. Role of ferrous iron chelator 2,2'-dipyridyl in preventing delayed vasospasm in a primate model of subarachnoid hemorrhage. J Neurosurg 1998; 88:298–303.

44. Findlay JM, Weir BK, Kanamaru K, Espinosa F. Arterial wall changes in cerebral vasospasm. Neurosurgery 1989; 25:736–745; discussion 745–736.

45. Macdonald RL, Weir BK, Runzer TD, et al. Etiology of cerebral vasospasm in primates. J Neurosurg 1991; 75:415–424.

46. Pluta RM, Deka-Starosta A, Zauner A, Morgan JK, Muraszko KM, Oldfield EH. Neuropeptide Y in the primate model of subarachnoid hemorrhage. J Neurosurg 1992; 77:417–423.

47. Pluta RM, Zauner A, Morgan JK, Muraszko KM, Oldfield EH. Is vasospasm related to proliferative arteriopathy? J Neurosurg 1992; 77:740–748.

48. Macdonald RL, Weir BK, Runzer TD, Grace MG, Poznansky MJ. Effect of intrathecal superoxide dismutase and catalase on oxyhemoglobin-induced vasospasm in monkeys. Neurosurgery 1992; 30:529–539.

49. Macdonald RL, Weir BK, Young JD, Grace MG. Cytoskeletal and extracellular matrix proteins in cerebral arteries following subarachnoid hemorrhage in monkeys. J Neurosurg 1992; 76:81–90.

50. Handa Y, Kabuto M, Kobayashi H, Kawano H, Takeuchi H, Hayashi M. The correlation between immunological reaction in the arterial wall and the time course of the development of cerebral vasospasm in a primate model. Neurosurgery 1991; 28:542–549.

51. Handa Y, Hayashi M, Takeuchi H, Kobayashi H, Kawano H, Kabuto M. Effect of cyclosporine on the development of cerebral vasospasm in a primate model. Neurosurgery 1991; 28:380–385; discussion 385–386.

52. Pluta RM, Boock RJ, Afshar JK, et al. Source and cause of endothelin-1 release into cerebrospinal fluid after subarachnoid hemorrhage. J Neurosurg 1997; 87:287–293.

53. Landau B, Ransohoff J. Prolonged cerebral vasospasm in experimental subarachnoid hemorrhage. Neurology 1968; 18:1056–1065.

54. Alksne JF, Branson PJ. Prevention of experimental subarachnoid hemorrhage-induced intracranial arterial vasonecrosis with phosphodiesterase inhibitor phthalazinol (EG-626). Stroke 1979; 10:638–644.

55. Clower BR, Smith RR, Haining JL, Lockard J. Constrictive endarteropathy following experimental subarachnoid hemorrhage. Stroke 1981; 12:501–508.

56. Boisvert DP, Pickard JD, Graham DI, Fitch W. Delayed effects of subarachnoid hemorrhage on cerebral metabolism and the cerebrovascular response to hypercapnia in the primate. J Neurol Neurosurg Psychiatry 1979; 42:892–898.

57. Fitch W, Pickard JD, Tamura A, Graham DI. Effects of hypotension induced with sodium nitroprusside on the cerebral circulation before, and one week after, the subarachnoid injection of blood. J Neurol Neurosurg Psychiatr 1988; 51:88–93.

58. Pickard JD, Boisvert DP, Graham DI, Fitch W. Late effects of subarachnoid haemorrhage on the response of the primate cerebral circulation to drug-induced changes in arterial blood pressure. J Neurol Neurosurg Psychiatr 1979; 42:899–903.

59. Offerhaus L, van Gool J. Electrocardiographic changes and tissue catecholamines in experimental subarachnoid haemorrhage. Cardiovasc Res 1969; 3:433–440.

60. Chan RC, Durity FA, Thompson GB, Nugent RA, Kendall M. The role of the prostacyclin-thromboxane system in cerebral vasospasm following induced subarachnoid hemorrhage in the rabbit. J Neurosurg 1984; 61:1120–1128.

61. Lehman RM, Kassell NF, Nazar GB, et al. Morphometric methods in the study of vasospasm. In: Wilkins RH, ed. Cerebral Vasospasm. New York: Raven Press, 1988:13–117.

62. Zuccarello M, Soattin GB, Lewis AI, Breu V, Hallak H, Rapoport RM. Prevention of subarachnoid hemorrhage-induced cerebral vasospasm by oral administration of endothelin receptor antagonists. J Neurosurg 1996; 84:503–507.

63. Ono S, Date I, Onoda K, et al. Decoy administration of NF-kappaB into the subarachnoid space for cerebral angiopathy. Hum Gene Ther 1998; 9:1003–1011.

64. Spallone A, Pastore FS. Cerebral vasospasm in a double-injection model in rabbit. Surg Neurol 1989; 32:408–417.

65. Foley PL, Caner HH, Kassell NF, Lee KS. Reversal of subarachnoid hemorrhage-induced vasoconstriction with an endothelin receptor antagonist. Neurosurgery 1994; 34:108–112; discussion 112–103.

66. Roux S, Loffler BM, Gray GA, Sprecher U, Clozel M, Clozel JP. The role of endothelin in experimental cerebral vasospasm. Neurosurgery 1995; 37:78–85; discussion 85–76.

67. Wanebo JE, Arthur AS, Louis HG, et al. Systemic administration of the endothelin-A receptor antagonist TBC 11251 attenuates cerebral vasospasm after experimental subarachnoid hemorrhage: dose study and review of endothelin-based therapies in the literature on cerebral vasospasm. Neurosurgery 1998; 43:1409–1417; discussion 1417–1408.

68. Takahashi S, Kassell NF, Toshima M, Dougherty DA, Foley PL, Lee KS. Effect of U88999E on experimental cerebral vasospasm in rabbits. Neurosurgery 1993; 32:281–288; discussion 288.

69. Pasqualin A, Vollmer DG, Marron JA, Tsukahara T, Kassell NF, Torner JC. The effect of nicardipine on vasospasm in rabbit basilar artery after subarachnoid hemorrhage. Neurosurgery 1991; 29:183–188.

70. Vorkapic P, Bevan RD, Bevan JA. Pharmacologic irreversible narrowing in chronic cerebrovasospasm in rabbits is associated with functional damage. Stroke 1990; 21:1478–1484.

71. Frazier JL, Pradilla G, Wang PP, Tamargo RJ. Inhibition of cerebral vasospasm by intracranial delivery of ibuprofen from a controlled-release polymer in a rabbit model of subarachnoid hemorrhage. J Neurosurg 2004; 101:93–98.

72. Pradilla G, Wang PP, Legnani FG, Ogata L, Dietsch GN, Tamargo RJ. Prevention of vasospasm by anti-CD11/CD18 monoclonal antibody therapy following subarachnoid hemorrhage in rabbits. J Neurosurg 2004; 101:88–92.

73. Bavbek M, Polin R, Kwan AL. Monoclonal antibodies against ICAM-1 and CD 18 attenuate cerebral vasospasm after experimental subarachnoid hemorrhage in rabbits. Stroke 1998; 29:1930–1936.

74. Nakagomi T, Kassell NF, Hongo K, Sasaki T. Pharmacological reversibility of experimental cerebral vasospasm. Neurosurgery 1990; 27:582–586.

75. Pradilla G, Thai QA, Legnani FG, et al. Delayed intracranial delivery of a nitric oxide donor from a controlled-release polymer prevents experimental cerebral vasospasm in rabbits. Neurosurgery 2004; 55:1393–1400.

76. Endo S, Branson PJ, Alksne JF. Experimental model of symptomatic vasospasm in rabbits. Stroke 1988; 19:1420–1425.

77. Pickard JD, Walker V, Vile J, Perry S, Smythe PJ, Hunt R. Oral nimodipine reduces prostaglandin and thromboxane production by arteries chronically exposed to a periarterial haematoma and the antifibrinolytic agent tranexamic acid. J Neurol Neurosurg Psychiatr 1987; 50:727–731.

78. Lougheed WM, Tom M. A method of introducing blood into the subarachnoid space in the region of the circle of Willis in dogs. Can J Surg 1961; 4:329–337.

79. Brawley BW, Strandness DE Jr. Continuous recording of the intracranial internal carotid artery size in the dog. J Surg Res 1967; 7:250–253.

80. Nagai H, Suzuki Y, Sugiura M, Noda S, Mabe H. Experimental cerebral vasospasm. 1: Factors contributing to early spasm. J Neurosurg 1974; 41:285–292.

81. Toda N, Ozaki T, Ohta T. Cerebrovascular sensitivity to vasoconstricting agents induced by subarachnoid hemorrhage and vasospasm in dogs. J Neurosurg 1977; 46:296–303.

82. Nagai H, Noda S, Mabe H. Experimental cerebral vasospasm. Part 2: Effects of vasoactive drugs and sympathectomy on early and late spasm. J Neurosurg 1975; 42:420–428.

83. Allen GS, Bahr AL. Cerebral arterial spasm: part 10. Reversal of acute and chronic spasm in dogs with orally administered nifedipine. Neurosurgery 1979; 4:43–47.

84. Kistler JP, Lees RS, Candia G, Zervas NT, Crowell RM, Ojemann RG. Intravenous nitroglycerin in experimental cerebral vasospasm. A preliminary report. Stroke 1979; 10:26–29.

85. Gioia AE, White RP, Bakhtian B, Robertson JT. Evaluation of the efficacy of intrathecal nimodipine in canine models of chronic cerebral vasospasm. J Neurosurg 1985; 62:721–728.

86. Kawasaki S. Sequential ultrastructural changes of experimental cerebral vasospasm in dogs (author's transl). Neurol Med Chir (Tokyo) 1980; 20:237–245.

87. Gavras H, Andrews P, Papadakis N. Reversal of experimental delayed cerebral vasospasm by angiotensin-converting enzyme inhibition. J Neurosurg 1981; 55:884–888.

88. White RP, Robertson JT. Comparison of piroxicam, meclofenamate, ibuprofen, aspirin, and prostacyclin efficacy in a chronic model of cerebral vasospasm. Neurosurgery 1983; 12:40–46.

89. Nagasawa S, Handa H, Naruo Y, Moritake K, Hayashi K. Experimental cerebral vasospasm arterial wall mechanics and connective tissue composition. Stroke 1982; 13:595–600.

90. Liszczak TM, Varsos VG, Black PM, Kistler JP, Zervas NT. Cerebral arterial constriction after experimental subarachnoid hemorrhage is associated with blood components within the arterial wall. J Neurosurg 1983; 58:18–26.

91. Liszczak TM, Black PM, Tzouras A, Foley L, Zervas NT. Morphological changes of the basilar artery, ventricles, and choroid plexus after experimental SAH. J Neurosurg 1984; 61:486–493.

92. Kapp J, Mahaley MS Jr., Odom GL. Cerebral arterial spasm. 1. Evaluation of experimental variables affecting the diameter of the exposed basilar artery. J Neurosurg 1968; 29:331–338.

93. Kapp J, Mahaley MS Jr., Odom GL. Cerebral arterial spasm. 2. Experimental evaluation of mechanical and humoral factors in pathogenesis. J Neurosurg 1968; 29:339–349.

94. Kapp J, Mahaley MS Jr., Odom GL. Cerebral arterial spasm. 3. Partial purification and characterization of a spasmogenic substance in feline platelets. J Neurosurg 1968; 29:350–356.

95. Blaumanis OR, Grady PA. Experimental cerebral vasospasm: resolution by chlorpromazine. Surg Neurol 1982; 17:263–268.

96. Flamm ES, Kim J, Lin J, Ransohoff J. Phosphodiesterase inhibitors and cerebral vasospasm. Arch Neurol 1975; 32:569–571.

97. Mayberg MR, Houser OW, Sundt TM Jr. Ultrastructural changes in feline arterial endothelium following subarachnoid hemorrhage. J Neurosurg 1978; 48:49–57.

98. Brinker T, Seifert V, Stolke D. Effect of intrathecal fibrinolysis on cerebrospinal fluid absorption after experimental subarachnoid hemorrhage. J Neurosurg 1991; 74:789–793.

99. Cardoso ER, Reddy K, Bose D. Effect of subarachnoid hemorrhage on intracranial pulse waves in cats. J Neurosurg 1988; 69:712–718.

100. Umansky F, Kaspi T, Shalit MN. Regional cerebral blood flow in the acute stage of experimentally induced subarachnoid hemorrhage. J Neurosurg 1983; 58:210–216.

101. Simmonds WJ. The absorption of blood from the cerebrospinal fluid in animals. Aust J Exp Biol Med Sci 1952; 30:261–270.

102. Levitt P, Wilson WP, Wilkins RH. The effects of subarachnoid blood on the electrocorticogram of the cat. J Neurosurg 1971; 35:185–191.

103. Trojanowski T. Experimental subarachnoid haemorrhage. Part II: extravasation volume and dynamics of subarachnoid arterial bleeding in cats. Acta Neurochir (Wien) 1982; 64:103–108.

104. Kapp JP, Clower BR, Azar FM, Yabuno N, Smith RR. Heparin reduces proliferative angiopathy following subarachnoid hemorrhage in cats. J Neurosurg 1985; 62:570–575.

105. Shigeno T, Fritschka E, Brock M, Schramm J, Shigeno S, Cervos-Navarro J. Cerebral edema following experimental subarachnoid hemorrhage. Stroke 1982; 13:368–379.

106. Schwartz SM, deBlois D, O'Brien ER. The intima. Soil for atherosclerosis and restenosis. Circ Res 1995; 77:445–465.

107. Barry KJ, Gogjian MA, Stein BM. Small animal model for investigation of subarachnoid hemorrhage and cerebral vasospasm. Stroke 1979; 10:538–541.

108. Shiguma M. Change in the ionic environment of cerebral arteries after subarachnoid hemorrhage. Especially of potassium ion concentration in subarachnoid hematoma and its role in cerebral vasospasm. Neurol Med Chir (Tokyo) 1982; 22:805–812.

109. Lacy PS, Earle AM. A small animal model for electrocardiographic abnormalities observed after an experimental subarachnoid hemorrhage. Stroke 1983; 14:371–377.

110. Solomon RA, Antunes JL, Chen RY, Bland L, Chien S. Decrease in cerebral blood flow in rats after experimental subarachnoid hemorrhage: a new animal model. Stroke 1985; 16:58–64.

111. Swift DM, Solomon RA. Subarachnoid hemorrhage fails to produce vasculopathy or chronic blood flow changes in rats. Stroke 1988; 19:878–882.

112. Rickels E, Zumkeller M. Vasospasm after experimentally induced subarachnoid haemorrhage and treatment with nimodipine. Neurochirurgia (Stuttg) 1992; 35:99–102.

113. Veelken JA, Laing RJ, Jakubowski J. The Sheffield model of subarachnoid hemorrhage in rats. Stroke 1995; 26:1279–1283; discussion 1284.

114. Bederson JB, Germano IM, Guarino L. Cortical blood flow and cerebral perfusion pressure in a new noncraniotomy model of subarachnoid hemorrhage in the rat. Stroke 1995; 26:1086–1091; discussion 1091–1082.

115. Marshman LA, Morice AH, Thompson JS. Increased efficacy of sodium nitroprusside in middle cerebral arteries following acute subarachnoid hemorrhage: indications for its use after rupture. J Neurosurg Anesthesiol 1998; 10:171–177.

116. Schwartz AY, Masago A, Sehba FA, Bederson JB. Experimental models of subarachnoid hemorrhage in the rat: a refinement of the endovascular filament model. J Neurosci Methods 2000; 96:161–167.

117. Gules I, Satoh M, Clower BR, Nanda A, Zhang JH. Comparison of three rat models of cerebral vasospasm. Am J Physiol Heart Circ Physiol 2002; 283:H2551–H2559.

118. Okada T, Harada T, Bark DH, Mayberg MR. A rat femoral artery model for vasospasm. Neurosurgery 1990; 27:349–356.

119. Thai QA, Oshiro EM, Tamargo RJ. Inhibition of experimental vasospasm in rats with the periadventitial administration of ibuprofen using controlled-release polymers. Stroke 1999; 30:140–147.
120. Tierney TS, Clatterbuck RE, Lawson C, Thai QA, Rhines LD, Tamargo RJ. Prevention and reversal of experimental posthemorrhagic vasospasm by the periadventitial administration of nitric oxide from a controlled-release polymer. Neurosurgery 2001; 49:945–951; discussion 951–943.
121. Clatterbuck RE, Oshiro EM, Hoffman PA, Dietsch GN, Pardoll DM, Tamargo RJ. Inhibition of vasospasm with lymphocyte function-associated antigen-1 monoclonal antibody in a femoral artery model in rats. J Neurosurg 2002; 97:676–682.
122. Kamii H, Kato I, Kinouchi H, et al. Amelioration of vasospasm after subarachnoid hemorrhage in transgenic mice overexpressing CuZn-superoxide dismutase. Stroke 1999; 30:867–871; discussion 872.
123. Lin CL, Calisaneller T, Ukita N, Dumont AS, Kassell NF, Lee KS. A murine model of subarachnoid hemorrhage-induced cerebral vasospasm. J Neurosci Methods 2003; 123:89–97.
124. Takemae T, Branson PJ, Alksne JF. Intimal proliferation of cerebral arteries after subarachnoid blood injection in pigs. J Neurosurg 1984; 61:494–500.
125. Mayberg MR, Okada T, Bark DH. The role of hemoglobin in arterial narrowing after subarachnoid hemorrhage. J Neurosurg 1990; 72:634–640.
126. Alabadi JA, Salom JB, Torregrosa G, Miranda FJ, Jover T, Alborch E. Changes in the cerebrovascular effects of endothelin-1 and nicardipine after experimental subarachnoid hemorrhage. Neurosurgery 1993; 33:707–714; discussion 714–705.

2 | Pathogenesis of Cerebral Aneurysm Growth and Rupture

Wesley Hsu, MD, Resident
Department of Neurosurgery, Johns Hopkins University School of Medicine, Baltimore, Maryland, USA

Richard E. Clatterbuck, MD, PhD, Assistant Professor
Departments of Neurosurgery and Neuroscience, Johns Hopkins University School of Medicine, Baltimore, Maryland, USA

INTRODUCTION

Each year, approximately 35,000 people in the United States suffer a subarachnoid hemorrhage (SAH) secondary to a ruptured intracerebral aneurysm. It is estimated that 3.6% to 6% of the general population harbor one or more intracerebral aneurysms, although the exact prevalence is unknown (1). In patients with known unruptured aneurysms, the annual risk of rupture is approximately 1.3% (2). Despite progress in the diagnosis and treatment of cerebral aneurysms, 25% to 50% of aneurysmal SAH (aSAH) patients do not survive (3). Of survivors, only 20% are fully independent after six months (4). Clinicians have considerable interest in advancing the ability to diagnose and treat aneurysms. A sophisticated understanding of the pathogenesis of aneurysmal formation remains elusive. Intracranial saccular aneurysms are focal dilatations of the arterial wall that typically develop at the apex of a bifurcation in or near the Circle of Willis. Although the prevalence of intracranial aneurysms is unknown, it is estimated that 5% to 8% of the general population harbor these aneurysms, and 15% to 30% of this group have multiple lesions (5–9).

HISTOLOGY

An understanding of normal cerebral artery architecture is essential to the understanding of aneurysmal formation and progression. Cerebral arteries are composed of three primary layers: the inner tunica intima, tunica media (muscularis), and outer tunica externa (adventitia) (Fig. 1). The collagenous intima is covered by a layer of endothelial cells. The media is comprised of elastic fibers and smooth muscle cells that secrete many of the growth factors and cytokines essential for vascular remodeling. Separating the intima and media is the internal elastic lamina (IEL), which is essentially a longitudinal arrangement of fibers composed of an elastin core. This core is composed of tropoelastin molecules cross-linked by lysyl oxidase. The adventitia is composed of fibroblasts and collagen. Contrary to prevailing misconceptions, intracranial arteries have vasa vasorum (10). Unlike most systemic arteries, however, intracranial arteries lack an external elastic lamina, which might make them vulnerable to hemodynamic stress and aneurysmal formation (11). In normal cerebral arteries, these layers are generally intact. However, it is common for gaps to exist in the medial layer of intracranial arteries. Described by Forbus in 1930, these "medial defects of Forbus" are found most commonly at the apex of a bifurcation, but they also frequently exist at the lateral angles of arterial bifurcations (12). These medial defects were once believed to be congenital defects and were considered the *locus minoris resistentiae* (place of least resistance) of the arterial bifurcation. As we will discuss, however, our understanding of these defects has changed.

The extracellular matrix of cerebral arteries is composed of a collagen and elastin scaffold embedded in a collection of glycoproteins and proteoglycans (13). The tensile strength of

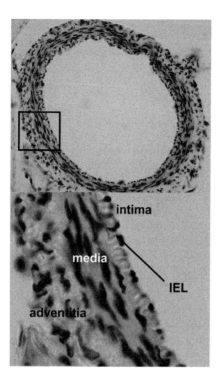

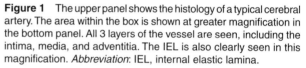

Figure 1   The upper panel shows the histology of a typical cerebral artery. The area within the box is shown at greater magnification in the bottom panel. All 3 layers of the vessel are seen, including the intima, media, and adventitia. The IEL is also clearly seen in this magnification. *Abbreviation*: IEL, internal elastic lamina.

a vessel is governed primarily by its elastin and collagen content (14). Elastin fibers are critical for vessel wall tension at low systolic pressures. As the elastic fibers become taut at higher pressures, the load is transferred to collagen fibers. The collagen fibers mediate resistance to vessel wall deformation at physiologic pressures (14). Collagen is also critical for vessel wall integrity, because vessels treated with collagenase are prone to rupture (15). The extracellular collagen network is composed primarily of Type I and Type III collagen. After production of procollagen by smooth muscles and fibroblasts, posttranslational processing leads to the formation of triple helix strands of collagen alpha chains. These chains provide the framework for vessel strength during exposure to high intraluminal pressure (16).

PATHOLOGY

Saccular aneurysms (Fig. 2) are usually located at the vascular bifurcations within the Circle of Willis. At the bifurcation, the aneurysm most commonly originates at the apex. The wall of an aneurysm consists primarily of collagen, with some smooth muscle cells and only isolated fragments of elastic lamina (17,18). At the level of the neck, the IEL almost completely disappears. Furthermore, the intima becomes thickened near the neck, and atheroma is frequently present (19). The endothelial layer is generally preserved along the wall of the entire aneurysm. It is thin along the aneurysmal wall and becomes thicker at the aneurysmal neck. Larger aneurysms might contain layers of thrombus and occasionally become partially or completely thrombosed. The vasa vasorum might contain evidence of atherosclerosis and partial occlusion (19). Aneurysms are not uncommonly multiloculated (>1 discrete dome). In an autopsy review of ruptured and unruptured aneurysms, 57% of ruptured aneurysms and 26% of unruptured aneurysms >4 mm in size were found to be multiloculated (20).

Three types of early aneurysmal changes typically found at arterial bifurcations have been described: funnel-shaped dilations, areas of thinning, and microscopic evaginations (21). Funnel-shaped dilations, most commonly appearing at the posterior communicating artery/internal carotid artery junction, have attenuated walls and a complete loss of the elastic lamina (21,22). Areas of thinning occur at the apex and/or tissue adjacent to the apex. These areas

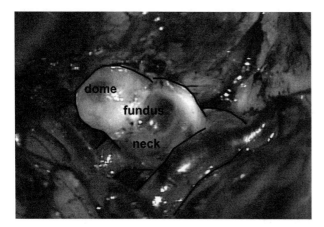

Figure 2 This intraoperative photograph shows an aneurysm at the middle cerebral artery bifurcation. The distal middle cerebral branches can be seen on each side of the body or fundus of the aneurysm. A secondary bleb (or loculation) is arising from the fundus of this lesion, creating a new dome. The neck of the aneurysm lies at the base of the fundus and can be clearly seen in this image.

are extremely thin and can be nearly transparent. Microscopic evaginations often involve a medial defect of the apex. Interestingly, these evaginations can incorporate a portion, if not the entirety, of the medial defect, but they generally do not originate from the defect itself (21). At the apex of the aneurysm, the fibrous wall is usually its thinnest and is the site most likely to rupture. In a review of 289 autopsy specimens of patients who died from intracerebral hemorrhage, the site of rupture of the aneurysm was evaluated. In 227 cases, the rupture occurred along the fundus, and only 6 ruptured along the neck (23).

THEORIES OF SACCULAR ANEURYSM ETIOLOGY

Controversy continues over the etiology of intracranial saccular aneurysms. The leading theories can be divided into 2 groups. The first group argues that congenital or early developmental factors are responsible for aneurysmal formation. The second favors acquired, or postnatal, changes in the intracerebral vasculature. These views are certainly not mutually exclusive, and it is likely that multiple factors are responsible for aneurysmal formation.

One of the earliest theories of congenital origin of aneurysms is known as the medial defect theory, which states that congenital defects of the vascular media (defects of Forbus) are the starting points for the formation of aneurysms. Studies by Forbus demonstrated that the media at the apex of cerebral arterial bifurcations is often absent (12). However, autopsy studies suggested that such bifurcation medial defects are common and can occur in 80% of the population, including those without aneurysms (24). It was argued that these areas are relatively weak and are susceptible to the hemodynamic stress of blood flow. Forbus likens aneurysmal formation to the formation of "false diverticulum" in areas of inherent weakness in intestinal walls (areas where large vessels enter). Just as false diverticula develop over time with peristaltic intestinal movements, cerebral aneurysms form over time at medial defects under the effects of blood pulsation. Without the media for support, the IEL is easily damaged and becomes the nidus for aneurysmal growth.

However, some observations argue against congenital medial defects as the origin of aneurysms. Medial defects increase in frequency with age (24), which indicates that these defects are not all congenital. They are more common in the posterior circulation, which does not coincide with the most common locations of saccular aneurysms (25). They are also located in extracranial arteries, where aneurysms are uncommon (21,26). Medial defects are common at the lateral angles of bifurcations, yet saccular aneurysms do not typically form there (17,20,26,27). Interestingly, studies of early aneurysmal formation suggest that the initial mural thinning or microevagination often occurs adjacent to the apical raphe and not at the raphe itself (21,28,29).

Stehbens disputes the idea that the medial defect is a defect at all and argues instead for a functional role (30). The term "medial defect" suggests that some sort of deficiency exists. He suggests that a better term would be "medial raphe" to emphasize the possible functional role of the lack of media at the apical bifurcation. He argues that the media of adjoining walls will pull in opposite directions during vasoconstriction and suggests that the apex acts as an anchor for the muscle. In support of this theory, it has been shown that the apex is composed of collagen fibrils that anchor the smooth muscle of the media and provide more stability for the vessel wall (31). Thus, the apex of the bifurcation might not be an area of weakness, even without media. Furthermore, animal models of cerebral aneurysms and autopsy studies both suggest that the early development of aneurysms occurs at sites other than medial defects (32,33).

The medial defect theory is not the only congenital theory that has been proposed. In 1933, Drennan proposed that aneurysms originate from remnants of embryonic vessels. If they existed, such remnants would certainly be an inherent weakness in the vessel wall, which would be susceptible to hemodynamic stress (34). However, no evidence of such remnants has been revealed, despite multiple studies of the histology of normal arterial bifurcations (28). Bremer hypothesized that vessels of the primitive capillary plexus might have failed to atrophy, providing a focus for vessel wall dilatation and aneurysmal formation (35). However, vessels do not commonly exit from the apex of an aneurysm.

CONNECTIVE TISSUE DISORDERS AND ANEURYSMAL FORMATION

Evidence suggests that certain inherited diseases, specifically diseases that might cause an inherent weakness in all vessel walls, including cerebral vessels, predispose individuals to aneurysmal formation. The disease most strongly linked to aneurysmal formation is autosomal dominant (adult) polycystic kidney disease (APKD), a common hereditary disorder that affects 1 in every 400 to 1000 live births. This systemic disease leads to formation of cysts in ductal organs, such as the kidney and liver (36). The two most common genes associated with this disorder are PKD1 and PKD2. PKD1, located on chromosome 16p13.3, encodes the polycystin 1 protein (37) and accounts for approximately 85% of cases (38). This protein has a large extracellular region and might participate in cell–cell and cell–matrix interactions. PKD2, located on chromosome 4q13–23, encodes the polycystin 2 protein and is present in approximately 10% of affected families. Polycystin 2 might interact with polycystin 1 to transduce signals from extracellular ligands (39). Although the exact function of these proteins remains unclear, they might be involved in vessel wall integrity (40). Three prospective studies using noninvasive imaging techniques (i.e., magnetic resonance angiography) estimate the prevalence of cerebral aneurysms in APKD to be 8% (41–44). However, another prospective study failed to show a significant difference between the prevalence of cerebral aneurysms in patients with APKD compared to the normal population (41).

Ehlers-Danlos syndrome (EDS) is a heterogeneous group of disorders characterized by joint laxity, easy bruising, and hyperelastic skin. The most lethal is EDS Type IV, also known as vascular Ehlers-Danlos. It is an autosomal dominant disorder of the COL3A1 gene, which encodes Type III procollagen. Type III collagen is a major component of distensible tissues, including arteries and veins (45,46). The cause of death in patients with EDS is typically a vascular accident of medium-sized vessels (47–49). The prevalence of aneurysms in EDS patients is not known, although one study suggests that those with EDS Type IV are at a higher risk of developing a carotid-cavernous fistula and intracranial aneurysms (50).

Interestingly, a subset of patients without EDS with aneurysms might have a decrease in the ratio of Type III to Type I collagen (51–53), although this data has been challenged (54). Others have found that some patients with cerebral aneurysms exhibited a deficiency in Type III collagen production (55,56) and that a specific allele of the COL3A1 might be associated with intracerebral aneurysms (57).

Other diseases have traditionally been associated with an increased risk of intracranial aneurysms, although the relationship is a matter of debate. For example, multiple case reports have led some to believe that neurofibromatosis Type 1 (NF1) is associated with an increased risk of aneurysmal formation (58–61). NF1 is a hereditary neurocutaneous disorder of the NF1 gene that encodes the tumor suppressor protein neurofibromin and might be involved in the development of vascular connective tissue (62). However, more recent studies suggest that NF1 patients are at no greater risk of developing aneurysms than is the general population (63,64).

Likewise, Marfan's syndrome is commonly believed to be a risk factor for developing intracranial aneurysms. Mutations of the fibrillin gene on chromosome 15q21 lead to a connective tissue disorder that affects the cardiovascular, skeletal, pulmonary, ocular, and central nervous systems. Fibrillin is an important structural component of the extracellular matrix (65,66). Multiple case reports document intracranial aneurysms in patients with Marfan's syndrome (67–71). Although an autopsy study of 7 patients with Marfan's syndrome revealed 2 cases of intracranial aneurysms (72), a larger autopsy series of 25 patients revealed only 1 case of an intracranial aneurysm (10).

FAMILIAL ANEURYSMAL FORMATION

At least some role for congenital factors in the development of aneurysms is evidenced by studies that show a higher prevalence of cerebral aneurysms among family members of affected cohorts. Some studies suggest that the prevalence of familial cerebral aneurysms (defined as at least 2 affected first-degree relatives in the same family) ranges from 6% to 10% (73–78). One study found a 20% prevalence rate, and this was true for Caucasian, African American, and Hispanic patients (73). Another study found inheritance patterns suggestive of multiple modes of inheritance, with patterns suggestive of, but not definitive for, autosomal dominant, autosomal dominant with incomplete penetrance, and autosomal recessive inheritance (79).

Patients with familial intracranial aneurysms experience SAH at an earlier age, compared to those with nonfamilial aneurysms (76,77,80–83), although the severity of hemorrhage is no different between familial and nonfamilial aSAH (76,84). In some families with multiple affected generations, latter generations experience aSAH at a younger age, a pattern of genetic disease known as *anticipation* that can be associated with expanding triplet repeats (80,85). Definitive evidence that genetic anticipation plays a role in familial intracranial aneurysms remains to be demonstrated (83).

Genetics might play a role in aneurysmal formation, even in the absence of Mendelian inheritance. Recently, single nucleotide polymorphisms of collagen Type 1–alpha 2 (COL1A2) have been associated with familial as well as with nonfamilial cerebral aneurysms (86). Interestingly, one of these polymorphisms leads to an amino acid substitution at the location for keratin sulfate proteoglycan binding.

MECHANICAL FACTORS IN ANEURYSMAL FORMATION

Initiation

The apex of the intracerebral arterial bifurcation is the most common site for aneurysms, perhaps due to several factors, including the properties of fluid flow in an arterial bifurcation. Because blood flowing along the walls of a vessel is slowed by viscous drag, the actual flow occurs in several concentric layers of increasing velocity from the periphery to the center. Blood flowing in the center of the vessel and, thus, least hindered by viscous drag is called the *axial stream*. The axial stream is directed at the apex of the bifurcation, resulting in hemodynamic stress unique to this location. Increases in the angle of the bifurcation, blood flow, and blood pressure all increase the stress directed into the arterial apex. Thus, shear stress is much greater at the apex than it is at other areas of the bifurcation. Acute increases in shear stress at the apical blood–vascular interface might lead to endothelial damage and exposure of underlying basement membrane (87) and/or fragmentation of the IEL (30,88), perhaps the initial insult that leads to aneurysmal formation. Furthermore, the kinetic energy of the axial stream is converted to pressure energy (stagnation pressure) as it decelerates at the apex, thus adding another unique stressor to this area of the bifurcation (12).

Although the apex is the site of unique hemodynamic stress and, therefore, the site most susceptible to aneurysmal formation, the reason why certain individuals develop aneurysms and others do not remains elusive. A simple explanation would be that certain individuals are susceptible to aneurysmal formation due to a congenital weakness specific to the apex, such as a medial defect of Forbus. However, as discussed above, the historical view—that the arrangement of the medial layer at bifurcations is a congenital defect—is currently debated.

Alterations in the flow of blood through the intracranial vessels might lead to increased wall stress and subsequent aneurysmal formation. Aneurysmal formation after iatrogenic manipulation of vascular flow (i.e., extracranial–intracranial bypass) has been demonstrated (89). Alterations in blood flow that develop as a result of increased arterial flow to an arteriovenous malformation can lead to aneurysmal formation (90,91). Indeed, it is estimated that 10% of saccular aneurysms occur on the arterial vessels that feed arteriovenous malformations (92). Interestingly, it has been shown that removal of an arteriovenous malformation can lead to reduction in the size of an aneurysm on the afferent arterial vessel when the aneurysm is adjacent to the nidus (93).

Certain patterns of the cerebral vasculature lead to altered patterns of hemodynamic stress. For example, multiple case studies demonstrate anterior communicating artery aneurysms in the setting of a size imbalance of the proximal segments of the anterior cerebral arteries (33,94–97). Those in favor of the congenital theory argue that such anatomic variation is secondary to an unidentified congenital defect ανδ; therefore, aneurysms that are associated with these variations must also be secondary to congenital issues. However, no evidence suggests that variations in the Circle of Willis are actually congenital abnormalities. Furthermore, anatomic variations of the cerebral vasculature are no more likely to occur in patients with aneurysms (33).

Growth and Rupture

Multiple factors participate in aneurysmal initiation, growth, and eventual rupture, including mechanical factors. It is logical to assume that increases in aneurysmal wall stress increase the risk of aneurysmal rupture. Wall stress is defined by Laplace's law:

$$S = p \cdot r / 2t$$

where S is the wall stress, p the intraluminal pressure, r the aneurysmal radius, and t the aneurysmal wall thickness. Because an aneurysmal wall is composed primarily of collagen, it has been hypothesized that it should rupture if stress exceeds 10^9 dynes/cm^2 (the breaking strength of collagen) (98).

Increases in intraluminal pressure and/or increases in the size of an aneurysm increase wall stress and, therefore, the susceptibility to rupture. Intraluminal pressure is also caused by multiple factors, among them, systolic blood pressure (25). Thus, any increases in systemic blood pressure will be reflected in intraluminal pressure. Because of the decreased distensibility of the aneurysmal wall relative to the normal cerebral vasculature due to the high collagen content, the wall experiences a greater degree of stress for a given pressure. Evidence suggests that an aneurysmal wall might experience 10 times the amount of stress seen by a normal cerebral artery at a given pressure (25), which is consistent with the idea that systemic hypertension has a role in aneurysmal growth and rupture. Further, aneurysms might be susceptible to rupture during times of increased systemic pressure, such as during a Valsalva maneuver, heavy lifting, coitus, and trauma (99). One computer model of a Valsalva maneuver suggests that enough pressure can be developed in such situations to lead to aneurysmal rupture (100). However, clinical series fail to demonstrate a preponderance of patients undertaking physical exertion at the time of rupture.

It is believed that turbulence of blood flow promotes the enlargement and rupture of cerebral aneurysms. Turbulent flow is characterized by the random and volatile fluctuation of pressure and velocity of fluid particles, in contrast to the stable pressure and velocity characterized by laminar flow. Turbulence in arterial vessels occurs when blood flow exceeds a critical velocity, described by the Reynold's number, as defined by the following equation:

$$Re = \rho V \cdot D / \eta$$

where ρ is the fluid density, V is the average fluid velocity, D is the vessel radius, and η is the fluid viscosity. In a long straight tube using a Newtonian fluid, turbulence first appears at a Reynolds number of 2000.

Blood flow at a cerebral bifurcation has been modeled by Ferguson using glass tubes (101). He showed that the Reynold's number for bifurcations in the Circle of Willis *without* an aneurysm is between 600 and 750, while a value of approximately 400 was derived for models of bifurcations *with* aneurysms. His work led him to propose that, although the Reynolds number was low enough for turbulence to develop at a bifurcation with an aneurysm, it was unlikely that normal bifurcations would have significant turbulent blood flow. Thus, it is unlikely that turbulence is an *initiating* factor in aneurysmal formation but might have a causal role in the *growth and eventual rupture* of aneurysms. Using glass models of aneurysms, it was shown that turbulent flow occurs within the aneurysmal sac at low flow rates, which is in line with visualizing turbulence within the sacs of animal models (102). Further evidence of turbulent flow is provided by intraoperative measurement of bruits emanating from the aneurysmal sac (101). Despite intentional induction of hypotension during aneurysmal clipping, the investigators discovered evidence of bruits originating from the aneurysmal sac in 10 out of 17 cases, with an average frequency of 460 Hz. Using a thin-shell assumption applied to a hypothetical spherical model, Hung and Botwin argue that the frequency of these bruits falls within the natural frequency of many aneurysms (103). If the frequency of the bruit is the same as the natural frequency of an aneurysm, the resulting resonance could lead to structural weakness, aneurysm enlargement, and eventual rupture. However, Doppler recordings in patients undergoing craniotomy for aneurysmal clipping detected periodic flow fluctuations of only 7–16 Hz (104). These flow fluctuations are lower than the natural frequency of a fluid-filled aneurysmal sac, which is estimated to exceed 100 Hz. These lower frequency vibrations would not lead to aneurysmal propagation.

A computer simulation of pulsatile blood flow in and around saccular aneurysms has clarified our understanding of how hemodynamics might lead to aneurysmal wall stress (105). The model suggests that during the acceleration phase of systole, blood moves into the aneurysm along the proximal wall and exits at the distal wall. Interestingly, during both the deceleration phase of systole and the diastolic phase, blood flow through the aneurysm might actually reverse by entering along the distal wall of the aneurysm and leaving by the proximal wall. This pattern of flow oscillation leads to considerable amounts of wall shear stress, particularly at the distal wall of the aneurysm. It is hypothesized that the endothelial cells at the distal wall undergo continuous injury. Perhaps individuals who are capable of maintaining vascular homeostasis are able to heal these microinjuries and avoid aneurysmal growth, and those who are unable to respond adequately can develop dilation of the aneurysmal neck and aneurysmal growth. If this hypothesis is true, growth would likely originate from the distal wall, and not from the aneurysmal dome. This would explain the importance of obliterating the neck of the aneurysm during clipping or coiling procedures (106), because any aneurysmal neck tissue from the distal wall would be subject to hemodynamic stress and future aneurysmal growth as a consequence.

It is unclear why some intracranial aneurysms rupture and others do not. Certain aneurysms develop significant amounts of thrombus within the sac, which might serve to dampen fluctuations in pressure and, therefore, decrease wall stress and damage to the endothelium. This thrombus might develop in situations of significant turbulence (107) or if flow stasis (98) is within the sac. Multiple computer simulations of blood flow within an aneurysm suggest that vortex formation occurs within aneurysms during the cardiac cycle, thereby creating a nidus for thrombus formation (105,108).

HYPERTENSION

Studies support a correlation between systemic hypertension and intracranial aneurysms. In a review of 16 clinical and 8 autopsy studies of 26,125 patients with intracranial aneurysms, 43.5% had a history of hypertension (109). Currently, an estimated 30% of the US population has hypertension (110).

Data also suggest that hypertension is a risk factor for aneurysmal rupture. In a review of 20,767 Medicare patients with unruptured aneurysms, not only was the prevalence of hypertension significantly higher in the aneurysm group (43.2% vs. 34.4%), but follow-up data showed that hypertension was a significant risk factor for subsequent SAH (111). In a review of the literature for longitudinal and case–control studies that evaluated risk factors for SAH, in addition to smoking and alcohol consumption, hypertension was found to be a significant risk factor (112).

Hypertension has also been associated with multiple aneurysms (7,113,114). One study showed that a higher systolic pressure was associated with an increased number of aneurysms in females. Other studies find that hypertension is a significant risk factor for multiple aneurysms in men and women (7,114). Although a 1998 study did not find a significant correlation between hypertension and multiple aneurysms, it was acknowledged that noncorrelation might have been due to a higher level of antihypertensive medication use in the population sample (8). Furthermore, a study investigating the characteristics of Japanese intracerebral aneurysm patients between the ages of 20 and 39 found that these patients did not have a significantly higher rate of hypertension compared to the normal Japanese population of the same age (115).

Animal models support a role for hypertension in the formation of cerebral aneurysms (5,116–121). These models involve the creation of saccular cerebral aneurysms in rats, using a combination of experimental hypertension (deoxycortisone acetate injections or renal infarction), ligation of the carotid artery, and oral B-aminopropionitrile (BAPN). BAPN, which is a lathyrogen, weakens connective tissue and, therefore, leads to vessel wall weakness. In these animal models, experimental hypertension and ligation of the carotid artery was sufficient for induction of aneurysmal formation, although the addition of BAPN increased the frequency of formation.

If hypertension does play a role in aneurysmal formation, the mechanism of action is not entirely clear. Hypertension might initiate vascular endothelial injury through shear stress (87). Intimal thickening might result from chronic hypertension (122), which has been hypothesized to limit the diffusion of nutrients into the intima and media (109). Chronic hypertension might have a deleterious effect on arterial wound healing by enhancing arterial myointimal thickening (123,124), and it might decrease the reticular fibers in the arterial wall (122), thus weakening the vessel and making it more susceptible to insult. It has been hypothesized that hypertension might lead to occlusion of the vasa vasorum, supplying intracranial vessels, thus leading to medial necrosis and weakening of the vessel walls (109).

VESSEL WALL HOMEOSTASIS AND ANEURYSMAL FORMATION

Changes in the normal flow of blood through cerebral arteries, as in hypertension or increased efferent flow to an arteriovenous malformation, might initiate a cascade of molecular events designed to maintain cellular homeostasis of the vessel wall during regulation of cerebrovascular tone and repair of vasculature microinjury. It has been suggested that alterations in the ability to regulate this homeostasis might predispose some individuals to aneurysmal formation (125,126). For example, the regulation of Type IV collagen could possibly be impaired in certain individuals due to an overactivity of Type IV collagenase [also known as matrix metalloproteinase 9 (MMP-9)]. It has been demonstrated that a polymorphism of the promoter for MMP-9 might be associated with the development of aneurysms (127). Thus, under situations that challenge normal cerebrovascular wall homeostasis, dysregulation of normal molecular responses that lead to enzymatic destruction of Type IV collagen by Type IV collagenase might predispose to weakening of the vessel wall and aneurysmal formation. This hypothesis is consistent with ultrastructural studies that show that, in aneurysmal walls, collagen fibers are structurally normal but often arranged in a disorganized fashion (21), perhaps suggesting an abnormal increase in collagen degradation rather than impaired collagen synthesis (125).

A study was conducted of mRNA expression of 6 different genes that encode proteins believed to be important for modulating arterial flow (prostacyclin stimulating factor) and vascular repair [peanut (PNUT), secreted protein acidic and rich in cysteine/osteonectin/BM-40 (SPARC), and retinoic acid induced (RAI)]. Also studied were key components of the extracellular matrix (fibronectin and Type III collagen). Results showed no significant difference in gene expression between unruptured aneurysmal domes and samples of the superficial temporal and occipital artery of patients without intracranial aneurysms (127). This lack of a difference might be secondary to the use of an extracranial artery as a control, in that an intracranial artery cannot be justifiably sampled from control patients. However, this study design certainly lays the groundwork for the evaluation of other proteins critical for vessel wall homeostasis.

Elastase plays an important role in vessel wall homeostasis, and its potential role in the formation of aneurysms has been investigated (128). Elastase is a versatile enzyme that is capable of degrading multiple proteins, including collagen Types I to IV, laminin, proteoglycans, and fibronectin (129–132). It is regulated primarily by two inhibitors: alpha-1 antitrypsin and alpha-2 macroglobulin (133,134). Intracerebral vessel integrity depends on the homeostatic deconstruction and reconstruction of the vessel wall, and elastase plays an important role in this aspect of vessel wall homeostasis (135). It has been demonstrated that patients with aneurysms, whether ruptured or unruptured, might have elevated levels of plasma elastase (136,137). In these studies, the elevation in elastase was unrelated to its role as an acute-phase reactant, because no significant difference was observed in elastase levels between patients with unruptured and those with early-ruptured aneurysms, and elevated plasma elastase levels were unrelated to a decrease in the level of alpha-1 antitrypsin (136,137). In contrast to these findings, others do not find an increase in plasma elastase in patients with unruptured aneurysms. Plasma elastase was shown to be elevated only after aneurysmal rupture in the context of post-SAH leukocytosis (138). Interestingly, elastase has been used in an animal model to create intracerebral and carotid aneurysms (139–141). These models depend on local, as opposed to systemic, delivery of elastase, which suggests that any role of elastase in the development of aneurysms depends on its local activity at the site of formation. The relevance of such models to *de novo* aneurysmal formation is unclear, because elastase-mediated breakdown of the IEL does not result in the typical changes seen in cerebral aneurysms, such as transversely oriented tears and fragmentation of the IEL (17,142).

TRAUMATIC INTRACRANIAL ANEURYSMS

Traumatic intracranial aneurysms are rare lesions that result from direct injury to the vessel wall. Much of our knowledge of such injuries has been derived from clinical experiences during wartime (143,144). Bullet and shrapnel penetrating the cranial vault are known to result in aneurysm formation, whether immediate or delayed. Injuries caused by lower-velocity foreign objects, such as knife wounds, as well as iatrogenic injury to intracranial vessels, have also been reported to result in aneurysmal formation (145–148). Even blunt head trauma can result in intracranial aneurysmal formation (149,150). Although it has been reported that approximately 20% of traumatic aneurysms resolve on their own (151), aggressive surgical management of these lesions is indicated.

INFECTIOUS ANEURYSM

Originally called "mycotic" aneurysms by Osler at a time when infectious processes were labeled as such, infectious aneurysms are actually more commonly caused by bacterial rather than fungal infections. They comprise approximately 5% of intracranial aneurysms. It is common for multiple infected aneurysms to occur simultaneously, and they more commonly occur in distal branches of the middle cerebral artery. Formation of infectious aneurysms occurs via multiple pathways, but the process is believed to begin in the adventitia and progress toward the lumen (152). Septic emboli, often from bacterial endocarditis, become lodged in the vasa vasorum, followed by inflammation and destruction of the vessel wall.

CONCLUSIONS

Despite significant research and investment in resources, the pathogenesis of cerebral aneurysms remains to be completely elucidated. Early investigators argued in favor of a congenital etiology of aneurysmal formation, including hypotheses involving the medial defects of Forbus and other possible sources of weakness inherent to vessel walls at birth. Subsequent researchers focused on developmental factors in aneurysmal formation, including such mechanical factors as hypertension, turbulence, and resonance. Interestingly, current research has refocused on a congenital etiology, namely genetic factors, that might predispose some individuals to aneurysmal formation. It is likely that a combination of congenital and developmental factors participates in aneurysmal formation and rupture, and it is hoped that further efforts to understand these factors will lead to improved treatment and diagnostic modalities to improve the morbidity and mortality of patients with intracerebral aneurysms.

REFERENCES

1. Rinkel GJ, Djibuti M, Algra A, van Gijn J. Prevalence and risk of rupture of intracranial aneurysms: a systematic review. Stroke 1998; 29:251–256.
2. Juvela S, Porras M, Poussa K. Natural history of unruptured intracranial aneurysms: probability of and risk factors for aneurysm rupture. J Neurosurg 2000; 93(3):379–387.
3. Sacco RL, Mayer SA. Epidemiology of intracerebral hemorrhage. In: Feldmann E, ed. Intracerebral Hemorrhage. Armonk, New York: Futura Publishing Co., 1994:3–23.
4. Broderick JP, Adams HP Jr., Barsan W, et al. Guidelines for the management of spontaneous intracerebral hemorrhage: a statement for healthcare professionals from a special writing group of the Stroke Council, American Heart Association. Stroke 1999; 30(4):905–915.
5. Hashimoto N, Handa H. The fate of untreated symptomatic cerebral aneurysms: analysis of 26 patients with clinical course of more than five years. Surg Neurol 1982; 18(1):21–26.
6. Kassell N, Torner JC. Size of intracranial aneurysms. Neurosurgery 1983; 12(3):291–297.
7. Ostergaard JR, Hog E. Incidence of multiple intracranial aneurysms. Influence of arterial hypertension and gender. J Neurosurg 1985; 63(1):49–55.
8. Qureshi AI, Suarez JI, Parekh PD, et al. Risk factors for multiple intracranial aneurysms. Neurosurgery 1998; 43(1):22–26.
9. Sekhar LN, Heros RC. Origin, growth, and rupture of saccular aneurysms: a review. Neurosurgery 1981; 8(2):248–260.
10. Conway JE, Hutchins GM, Tamargo RJ. Marfan syndrome is not associated with intracranial aneurysms. Stroke 1999; 30(8):1632–1636.
11. Ostergaard JR. Risk factors in intracranial saccular aneurysms. Aspects on the formation and rupture of aneurysms, and development of cerebral vasospasm. Acta Neurol Scand 1989; 80(2):81–98.
12. Forbus WD. On the origin of miliary aneurysms of superficial cerebral arteries. Bull Johns Hopkins Hosp 1930; 47:239–284.
13. Mayne R. Collagenous proteins of blood vessels. Arteriosclerosis 1986; 6:585–593.
14. Roach MR, Burton AC. The reason for the shape of the distensibility curves of arteries. Can J Biochem Physiol 1957; 35(8):681–690.
15. Dobrin PB, Baker WH, Gley WC. Elastolytic and collagenolytic studies of arteries. Implications for the mechanical properties of aneurysms. Arch Surg 1984; 119(4):405–409.
16. Hayashi K. Fundamental and applied studies of mechanical properties of cardiovascular tissues. Biorheology 1982; 19(3):425–436.
17. Hassler O. Morphological studies on the large cerebral arteries, with reference to the aetiology of subarachnoid haemorrhage. Acta Psychiatr Scand Suppl 1961; 154:1–145.
18. Lang ER, Kidd M. Electron microscopy of human cerebral aneurysms. J Neurosurg 1965; 22(6):554–562.
19. Scanarini M, Mingrino S, Giordano R, Baroni A. Histological and ultrastructural study of intracranial saccular aneurysmal wall. Acta Neurochir (Wien) 1978; 43(3–4):171–182.
20. Crompton MR. Mechanism of growth and rupture in cerebral berry aneurysms. Br Med J 1966; 5496:1138–1142.
21. Stehbens WE. Histopathology of cerebral aneurysms. Arch Neurol 1963; 8:272–285.
22. Hassler O, Saltzman GF. Histologic changes in infundibular widening of the posterior communicating artery. A preliminary report. Acta Pathol Microbiol Scand 1959; 46:305–312.
23. Crompton MR. The pathogenesis of cerebral aneurysms. Brain 1966; 89(4):797–814.
24. Glynn LE. Medial defects in the circle of Willis and their relation to aneurysm formation. J Pathol Bacteriol 1940; 51:213–222.
25. Ferguson GG. Direct measurement of mean and pulsatile blood pressure at operation in human intracranial saccular aneurysms. J Neurosurg 1981; 36(5):560–563.
26. Stehbens WE. Medial defects of the cerebral arteries of man. J Pathol Bacteriol 1959; 78:179–185.
27. Sahs AL. Observations on the pathology of saccular aneurysms. J Neurosurg 1966; 24(4):792–806.
28. Stehbens WE. Pathology of the Cerebral Blood Vessels. St. Louis, Missouri: CV Mosby, 1972.
29. Stehbens WE. Aetiology of cerebral aneurysms. Lancet 1981; 2:524–525.
30. Stehbens WE. Etiology of intracranial berry aneurysms. J Neurosurg 1989; 70:823–831.
31. Finlay HM, Whittaker P, Canham PB. Collagen organization in the branching region of human brain arteries. Stroke 1998; 29(8):1595–1601.
32. Futami K, Yamashita J, Higashi S. Do cerebral aneurysms originate at the site of medial defects? Microscopic examinations of experimental aneurysms at the fenestration of the anterior cerebral artery in rats. Surg Neurol 1998; 50(2):141–146.
33. Stehbens WE. Aneurysms and anatomical variation of cerebral arteries. Arch Pathol 1963; 75:45–64.
34. Drennan AM. Discussion. Edinb Med J 1933; 40:234–235.
35. Bremer JL. Congenital aneurysms of the cerebral arteries. Arch Pathol 1943; 35:819–831.
36. Gabow PA. Autosomal dominant polycystic kidney disease. N Engl J Med 1993; 329(5):332–342.

37. Hughes J, Ward CJ, Peral B, et al. The polycystic kidney disease 1 (PKD1) gene encodes a novel protein with multiple cell recognition domains. Nat Genet 1995; 10(2):151–160.
38. Pieke SA, Kimberling WJ, Kenyon JB, Gabow P. Genetic heterogeneity of polycystic kidney disease: an estimate of the proportion of families unlinked to chromosome 16. Am J Hum Genet Suppl 1989; 45:A58.
39. Qian F, Germino FJ, Cai Y, Zhang X, Somlo S, Germino GG. PKD1 interacts with PKD2 through a probable coiled-coil domain. Nat Genet 1997; 16:179–183.
40. Arnaout MA. The vasculopathy of autosomal dominant polycystic kidney disease: insights from animal models. Kidney Int 2000; 58:2599–2610.
41. Chapman AB, Rubinstein D, Hughes R, et al. Intracranial aneurysms in autosomal dominant polycystic kidney disease. N Engl J Med 1992; 327(13):916–920.
42. Huston J, Torres VE, Sulivan PP, Offord KP, Wiebers DO. Value of magnetic resonance angiography for the detection of intracranial aneurysms in autosomal dominant polycystic kidney disease. J Am Soc Nephrol 1993; 3:1871–1877.
43. Pirson Y, Chauveau D. Intracranial aneurysms in autosomal dominant polycystic kidney disease. In: Watson M, Torres V, eds. Polycystic Kidney Disease. Oxford: Oxford University Press, 1996:530–547.
44. Ruggieri PM, Poulos N, Masaryk TJ, et al. Occult intracranial aneurysms in polycystic kidney disease: screening with MR angiography. Radiology 1994; 191:33–39.
45. Beighton P. The Ehlers-Danlos syndromes. In: Beighton P, ed. McKusick's Heritable Disorders of Connective Tissue. 5th ed. St. Louis, Missouri: Mosby, 1993:189–251.
46. Steinmann B, Royce PM, Superti-Furga A. The Ehlers-Danlos syndromes. In: Royce PM, Steinmann B, eds. Connective Tissue and Its Heritable Disorders: Molecular, Genetic, and Medical Aspects. New York, New York: Wiley-Liss, 1993:351–407.
47. Cikrit DF, Miles JH, Silver D. Spontaneous arterial perforation: the Ehlers-Danlos specter. J Vasc Surg 1987; 5(2):248–255.
48. Germain DP. Clinical and genetic features of vascular Ehlers-Danlos syndrome. Ann Vasc Surg 2002; 16(3):391–397.
49. Lauwers G, Nevelsteen A, Daenen G, Lacroix H, Suy R, Frijns JP. Ehlers-Danlos syndrome Type IV: a heterogeneous disease. Ann Vasc Surg 1997; 11(2):178–182.
50. North KN, Whiteman DAH, Pepin MG, Byers PH. Cerebrovascular complications in Ehlers-Danlos syndrome Type IV. Ann Neurol 1995; 38:960–964.
51. de Paepe A, van Landegem W, de Keyser F, de Reuck J. Association of multiple intracranial aneurysms and collagen type III deficiency. Clin Neurol Neurosurg 1988; 90(1):53–56.
52. Neil-Dwyer G, Bartlett JR, Nicholls AC, Narcisi P, Pope FM. Collagen deficiency and ruptured cerebral aneurysms. A clinical and biochemical study. J Neurosurg 1983; 59(1):16–20.
53. Oxlund H. Relationships between the biomechanical properties, composition and molecular structure of connective tissues. Connect Tissue Res 1986; 15(1–2):65–72.
54. Leblanc R, Lozano AM, van der Rest M, Guttmann RD. Absence of collagen deficiency in familial cerebral aneurysms. J Neurosurg 1989; 70(6):837–840.
55. Ostergaard JR, Oxlund H. Collagen type III deficiency in patients with rupture of intracranial saccular aneurysms. J Neurosurg 1987; 67(5):690–696.
56. Pope FM, Nicholls AC, Narcisi P, Bartlett J, Neil-Dwyer G, Doshi B. Some patients with cerebral aneurysms are deficient in type III collagen. Lancet 1981; 1(8227):973–975.
57. Brega KE, Seltzer WK, Munro LG, Breeze RE. Genotypic variations of type III collagen in patients with cerebral aneurysms. Surg Neurol 1996; 46(3):253–256.
58. Benatar MG. Intracranial fusiform aneurysms in von Recklinghausen's disease: case report and literature review. J Neurol Neurosurg Psychiatr 1994; 57:1279–1280.
59. Frank E, Brown BM, Wilson DF. Asymptomatic fusiform aneurysm of the petrous carotid artery in a patient with von Recklinghausen's neurofibromatosis. Surg Neurol 1989; 32:75–78.
60. Muhonen MG, Godersky JC, VanGilder JC. Cerebral aneurysms associated with neurofibromatosis. Surg Neurol 1991; 36:470–475.
61. Zhao JZ, Han XD. Cerebral aneurysm associated with von Recklinghausen's neurofibromatosis: a case report. Surg Neurol 1998; 50(6):592–596.
62. Gregory PE, Gutmann DH, Mitchell A, et al. Neurofibromatosis Type 1 gene product (neurofibromin) associates with microtubules. Somat Cell Mol Genet 1993; 19:265–274.
63. Conway JE, Hutchins GM, Tamargo RJ. Lack of evidence for an association between neurofibromatosis type I and intracranial aneurysms: autopsy study and review of the literature. Stroke 2001; 32(11):2481–2485.
64. Riccardi VM. Neurofibromatosis: Phenotype, Natural History, and Pathogenesis. 2nd ed. Baltimore, Maryland: Johns Hopkins University Press, 1992.
65. Dietz HC, Pyeritz RE. Mutations in the human gene for fibrillin-1 (FBN1) in the Marfan syndrome and related disorders. Hum Mol Genet 1995; 4:1799–1809.

66. Sakai LY, Keene DR, Engvall E. Fibrillin, a new 350-kD glycoprotein, is a component of extracellular microfibrils. J Cell Biol 1986; 103:2499–2509.

67. Croisile B, Deruty R, Pialat J, Chazot G, Jourdan C. Aneurysme de a carotide supra-clinoidienne et mega-dolicho-arteres cervicales dans un syndrome de Marfan. Neurochirugie 1988; 34:342–347.

68. Ohtsuki H, Sugiura M, Iwaki K, Nishikawa M, Yasuno M. A case of Marfan's syndrome with ruptured distal middle cerebral aneurysm. No Shinkei Geka 1984; 12:983–985.

69. Resende LA, Asseis EA, Da Silva Costa L, Gallina RA. Sindrome de Marfan e aneurismas intracraniolos gigantes. Arq Neuropsiquiatr 1984; 42:294–297.

70. Rose BS, Pretorius DL. Dissecting basilar artery aneurysm in Marfan syndrome: case report. AJNR Am J Neuroradiol 1991; 12:503–504.

71. Speciali JG, Lison MP, Junqueira GL. Aneurismo intracraniano na sindroe de Marfan. Arq Neuropsiquiatr 1971; 29:453–457.

72. Schievink WI, Parisi JE, Piepgras DG, Michels VV. Intracranial aneurysms in Marfan syndrome: an autopsy study. Neurosurgery 1997; 41:866–870.

73. Kim DH, Van Ginhoven G, Milewicz DM. Incidence of familial intracranial aneurysms in 200 patients: comparison among Caucasian, African-American, and Hispanic populations. Neurosurgery 2003; 53(2):302–308.

74. Kojima M, Nagasawa S, Lee YE, Takeichi Y, Tsuda E, Mabuchi N. Asymptomatic familial cerebral aneurysms. Neurosurgery 1998; 43(4):776–781.

75. Raaymakers TW, Rinkel GJ, Ramos LM. Initial and follow-up screening for aneurysms in families with familial subarachnoid hemorrhage. Neurology 1998; 51(4):1125–1130.

76. Ronkainen A, Hernesniemi J, Ryynanen M. Familial subarachnoid hemorrhage in East Finland 1977–1990. Neurosurgery 1993; 33:787–797.

77. Schievink WI, Schaid DJ, Michels VV, Piepgras DG. Familial aneurysmal subarachnoid hemorrhage: a community-based study. J Neurosurg 1995; 83:426–429.

78. Wang PS, Longstreth WT, Koepsell TD. Subarachnoid hemorrhage and family history: a population-based case-control study. Arch Neurol 1995; 52:202–204.

79. Wills S, Ronkainen A, van der Voet M, et al. Familial intracranial aneurysms: an analysis of 346 multiplex Finnish families. Stroke 2003; 34(6):1370–1374.

80. Bromberg JEC, Rinkel GJE, Algra A, et al. Familial subarachnoid hemorrhage: distinctive features and patterns of inheritance. Ann Neurol 1995; 38:929–934.

81. Leblanc R, Melanson D, Tampieri D, Guttmann RD. Familial cerebral aneurysms: a study of 13 families. Neurosurgery 1995; 37:633–639.

82. Lozano AM, Leblanc R. Familial intracranial aneurysms. J Neurosurg 1987; 66:522–528.

83. Ruigrok YM, Rinkel GJ, Wijmenga C, Van Gijn J. Anticipation and phenotype in familial intracranial aneurysms. J Neurol Neurosurg Psychiatr 2004; 75(10):1436–1442.

84. Bromberg JEC, Rinkel GJE, Algra A, Limburg M, van Gijn J. Outcome in familial subarachnoid hemorrhage. Stroke 1995; 26:961–963.

85. Bailey IC. Familial subarachnoid haemorrhage. Ulster Med J 1993; 62:119–126.

86. Yoneyama T, Kasuya H, Onda H, et al. Collagen type I alpha2 (COL1A2) is the susceptible gene for intracranial aneurysms. Stroke 2004; 35(2):443–448.

87. Fry DL. Acute vascular endothelial changes associated with increased blood velocity gradients. Circ Res 1968; 22(2):165–197.

88. Kim C, Kikuchi H, Hashimoto N, Kojima M, Kang Y, Hazama F. Involvement of internal elastic lamina in development of induced cerebral aneurysms in rats. Stroke 1988; 19(4):507–511.

89. Fein JM. Bypass induced cerebral aneurysm. Neurol Res 1985; 7(1):46–52.

90. Miyasaka K, Wolpert SM, Prager RJ. The association of cerebral aneurysms, infundibula, and intracranial arteriovenous malformations. Stroke 1982; 13(2):196–203.

91. Okamoto S, Handa H, Hashimoto N. Location of intracranial aneurysms associated with cerebral arteriovenous malformation: statistical analysis. Surg Neurol 1984; 22(4):335–340.

92. Batjer H, Suss RA, Samson D. Intracranial arteriovenous malformations associated with aneurysms. Neurosurgery 1986; 18(1):29–35.

93. Shenkin HA, Jenkins F, Kim K. Arteriovenous anomaly of the brain associated with cerebral aneurysm. Case report. J Neurosurg 1971; 34:225–228.

94. Jacques L. Aneurysm and anomaly of the circle of Willis. Arch Pathol 1926; 1:213–220.

95. Kayembe KN, Sasahara M, Hazama F. Cerebral aneurysms and variations in the circle of Willis. Stroke 1984; 15(5):846–850.

96. Kirgis HD, Fisher WL, Llewellyn RC, Peebles EM. Aneurysms of the anterior communicating artery and gross anomalies of the circle of Willis. J Neurosurg 1966; 25(1):73–78.

97. Wilson G, Riggs HE, Rupp C. The pathologic anatomy of ruptured cerebral aneurysms. J Neurosurg 1954; 11:128–134.

98. Roach MR. A model study of why some intracranial aneurysms thrombose but others rupture. Stroke 1978; 9(6):583–587.

99. Komatsu S, Seki H, Uneoka K, Takaku A, Suzuki J. Rupturing factors of intracranial aneurysm: season, weather and psychosomatic strain. In: Suzuki J, ed. Cerebral Aneurysms: Experience with 1000 Directly Operated Cases. Tokyo: Neuron Publishing Co., 1979:25–31.
100. Duros J, Clark ME, Kufahl RH, Nadvornik P. On the rupture of an aneurysm. Neurol Res 1991; 13(4):217–223.
101. Ferguson GG. Turbulence in human intracranial saccular aneurysms. J Neurosurg 1970; 33:485–487.
102. Kikut RP. Experimental studies of intraaneurysmal blood flow. Vop Neurokhir 1966; 2:17–21.
103. Hung EJ, Botwin MR. Mechanics of rupture of cerebral saccular aneurysms. J Biomech 1975; 8(6):385–392.
104. Steiger HJ. Pathophysiology of development and rupture of cerebral aneurysms. Acta Neurochir Suppl (Wien) 1990; 48:1–57.
105. Gonzalez CF, Cho YI, Ortega HV, Moret J. Intracranial aneurysms: flow analysis of their origin and progression. AJNR Am J Neuroradiol 1992; 13(1):181–188.
106. Drake CG, Vanderlinden RG. The late consequences of incomplete surgical treatment of cerebral aneurysms. J Neurosurg 1967; 27(3):226–238.
107. Smith RL, Blick EF, Coalson J, Stein PD. Thrombus production by turbulence. J Appl Physiol 1972; 32(2):261–264.
108. Wille SO. Pulsatile pressure and flow in an arterial aneurysm simulated in a mathematical model. J Biomed Eng 1981; 3(2):153–158.
109. Inci S, Spetzler RF. Intracranial aneurysms and arterial hypertension: a review and hypothesis. Surg Neurol 2000; 53(6):530–540.
110. National Center for Health Statistics. Health, United States, 2004 with Chartbook on Trends in the Health of Americans. Hyattsville, Maryland: National Center for Health Statistics, 2004.
111. Taylor CL, Yuan Z, Selman WR, Ratcheson RA, Rimm AA. Cerebral arterial aneurysm formation and rupture in 20,767 elderly patients: hypertension and other risk factors. J Neurosurg 1995; 83(5):812–819.
112. Teunissen LL, Rinkel GJ, Algra A, van Gijn J. Risk factors for subarachnoid hemorrhage: a systematic review. Stroke 1996; 27(3):544–549.
113. Andrews RJ, Spiegel PK. Intracranial aneurysms. Age, sex, blood pressure, and multiplicity in an unselected series of patients. J Neurosurg 1979; 51(1):27–32.
114. Rinne J, Hernesniemi J, Puranen M, Saari T. Multiple intracranial aneurysms in a defined population: prospective angiographic and clinical study. Neurosurgery 1994; 35(5):803–808.
115. Kamitani H, Masuzawa H, Kanazawa I, Kubo T. Saccular cerebral aneurysms in young adults. Surg Neurol 2000; 54(1):59–66.
116. Handa H, Hashimoto N, Nagata I, Hazama F. Saccular cerebral aneurysms in rats: a newly developed animal model of the disease. Stroke 1983; 14(6):857–866.
117. Hashimoto N, Handa H, Hazama F. Experimentally induced cerebral aneurysms in rats. Surg Neurol 1978; 10(1):3–8.
118. Hashimoto N, Handa H, Hazama F. Experimentally induced cerebral aneurysms in rats: Part II. Surg Neurol 1979; 11:243–246.
119. Hashimoto N, Handa H, Hazama F. Experimentally induced cerebral aneurysms in rats: Part III. Surg Neurol 1979; 11:299–304.
120. Kondo S, Hashimoto N, Kikuchi H, Hazama F, Nagata I, Kataoka H. Cerebral aneurysms arising at nonbranching sites. An experimental study. Stroke 1997; 28(2):398–403.
121. Nagata I, Handa H, Hashimoto N, Hazama F. Experimentally induced cerebral aneurysms in rats: Part VI. Hypertension. Surg Neurol 1980; 14(6):477–479.
122. Hegedus K. The effects of hypertension on the wall of the large intracranial arteries with special reference to the changes of some connective tissue elements. Acta Morphol Hung 1988; 36(3–4):227–234.
123. Clowes AW, Clowes MM. Influence of chronic hypertension on injured and uninjured arteries in spontaneously hypertensive rats. Lab Invest 1980; 43(6):535–541.
124. Clowes AW, Clowes MM. The influence of hypertension on injury-induced myointimal thickening. Surgery 1980; 88(2):254–259.
125. Kassam A, Horowitz M, Chang YF, Peters D. Altered arterial homeostasis and cerebral aneurysms: a review of the literature and justification for a search of molecular biomarkers. Neurosurgery 2004; 54(5):1199–1111.
126. Peters DG, Kassam AB, Feingold E, et al. Molecular anatomy of an intracranial aneurysm: coordinated expression of genes involved in wound healing and tissue remodeling. Stroke 2001; 32(4):1036–1042.
127. Kassam AB, Horowitz M, Chang YF, Peters D. Altered arterial homeostasis and cerebral aneurysms: a molecular epidemiology study. Neurosurgery 2004; 54(6):1450–1460.
128. Cohen JR, Mandell C, Margolis I, Chang J, Wise L. Altered aortic protease and antiprotease activity in patients with ruptured abdominal aortic aneurysms. Surg Gynecol Obstet 1987; 164(4):355–358.
129. Janoff A, Feinstein G, Malemud CJ, Elias JM. Degradation of cartilage proteoglycan by human leukocyte granule neutral proteases—a model of joint injury. I. Penetration of enzyme into rabbit articular cartilage and release of 35SO4-labeled material from the tissue. J Clin Invest 1976; 57(3):615–624.

130. McDonald JA, Kelley DG. Degradation of fibronectin by human leukocyte elastase. Release of biologically active fragments. J Biol Chem 1980; 255(18):8848–8858.
131. Watanabe H, Hattori S, Katsuda S, Nakanishi I, Nagai Y. Human neutrophil elastase: degradation of basement membrane components and immunolocalization in the tissue. J Biochem (Tokyo) 1990; 108(5):753–759.
132. Werb Z, Banda MJ, McKerrow JH, Sandhaus RA. Elastases and elastin degradation. J Invest Dermatol 1982; 79:154–159.
133. Janoff A. Elastase in tissue injury. Annu Rev Med 1985; 36:207–216.
134. Ohlsson K, Olsson I. The neutral proteases of human granulocytes. Isolation and partial characterization of granulocyte elastases. Eur J Biochem 1974; 42(2):519–527.
135. Cohen JR, Mandell C, Wise L. Characterization of human aortic elastase found in patients with abdominal aortic aneurysms. Surg Gynecol Obstet 1987; 165(4):301–304.
136. Baker CJ, Fiore A, Connolly ES Jr., Baker KZ, Solomon RA. Serum elastase and alpha-1-antitrypsin levels in patients with ruptured and unruptured cerebral aneurysms. Neurosurgery 1995; 37(1):56–61.
137. Connolly ES Jr., Huang J, Goldman JE, Holtzman RN. Immunohistochemical detection of intracranial vasa vasorum: a human autopsy study. Neurosurgery 1996; 38(4):789–793.
138. Sakai N, Nakayama K, Tanabe Y, Izumiya Y, Nishizawa S, Uemuara K. Absence of plasma protease-antiprotease imbalance in the formation of saccular cerebral aneurysms. Neurosurgery 1999; 45(1):34–38.
139. Altes TA, Cloft HJ, Short JG, et al. 1999 ARRS Executive Council Award. Creation of saccular aneurysms in the rabbit: a model suitable for testing endovascular devices. American Roentgen Ray Society. Am J Roentgenol 2000; 174(2):349–354.
140. Hoh BL, Rabinov JD, Pryor JC, Ogilvy CS. A modified technique for using elastase to create saccular aneurysms in animals that histologically and hemodynamically resemble aneurysms in human. Acta Neurochir (Wien) 2004; 146(7):705–711.
141. Miskolczi L, Guterman LR, Flaherty JD, Hopkins LN. Saccular aneurysm induction by elastase digestion of the arterial wall: a new animal model. Neurosurgery 1998; 43(3):595–600.
142. Marshman LA. Elastin degradation in the superficial temporal arteries of patients with intracranial aneurysms reflects changes in plasma elastase. Neurosurgery 1998; 43(4):982.
143. Aarabi B. Traumatic aneurysms of brain due to high velocity missile head wounds. Neurosurgery 1988; 22:1056–1063.
144. Haddad FS, Haddad GF, Taha J. Traumatic intracranial aneurysms caused by missiles: their presentation and management. Neurosurgery 1991; 28(1):1–7.
145. du Trevou MD, van Dellen JR. Penetrating stab wounds to the brain: the timing of angiography in patients presenting with the weapon already removed. Neurosurgery 1992; 31(5):905–911.
146. Cosgrove GR, Villemure JG, Melancon D. Traumatic intracranial aneurysm due to arterial injury at surgery. Case report. J Neurosurg 1983; 58(2):291–294.
147. Dolenc VV, Lipovsek M, Slokan S. Traumatic aneurysm and carotid-cavernous fistula following transsphenoidal approach to a pituitary adenoma: treatment by transcranial operation. Br J Neurosurg 1999; 13(2):185–188.
148. Quattrocchi KB, Nielsen SL, Poirier V, Wagner FC Jr. Traumatic aneurysm of the superior cerebellar artery: case report and review of the literature. Neurosurgery 1990; 27(3):476–479.
149. Voelker JL, Ortiz O. Delayed deterioration after head trauma due to traumatic aneurysm. W V Med J 1997; 93(6):317–319.
150. Yazbak PA, McComb JG, Raffel C. Pediatric traumatic intracranial aneurysms. Pediatr Neurosurg 1995; 22(1):15–19.
151. Amirjamshidi A, Rahmat H, Abbassioun K. Traumatic aneurysms and arteriovenous fistulas of intracranial vessels associated with penetrating head injuries occurring during war: principles and pitfalls in diagnosis and management. A survey of 31 cases and review of the literature. J Neurosurg 1996; 84(5):769–780.
152. Bohmfalk GL, Story JL, Wissinger JP, Brown WE Jr. Bacterial intracranial aneurysm. J Neurosurg 1978; 48(3):369–382.

3 | Pathogenesis of Cerebral Vasospasm

Frederick W. Lombard, MBChB, FANZCA, Assistant Professor
Cecil O. Borel, MD, Associate Professor
Department of Anesthesiology, Duke University School of Medicine,
Durham, North Carolina, USA

INTRODUCTION

Cerebral vasospasm can be defined in terms of angiographic findings or clinical signs. Ecker and Riemenschneider first described angiographic vasospasm in 1951 (1). Angiographic vasospasm can be detected in up to 70% of patients following subarachnoid hemorrhage (SAH) (2). Clinically, cerebral vasospasm usually starts 3 to 5 days following SAH, exhibits maximal narrowing between days 5 and 14, and gradually resolves over 2 to 4 weeks (3). Clinical cerebral vasospasm, or neurologic deterioration due to cerebral ischemia, is less common and develops in 20% to 30% of patients with SAH.

Because the time course of clinical cerebral vasospasm parallels that of angiographic vasospasm and clinical symptoms often improve following intra-arterial injections of vasodilators or balloon angioplasty, clinical vasospasm is thought to be the result of persistent narrowing of the arterial lumen of the major extraparenchymal arteries. The extent of angiographic vasospasm in the proximal cerebral circulation, therefore, has been used as the most important outcome measure in animal models of the disease. However, infarctions on CT scans of patients with vasospasm typically occur in multiple territories, and the correlation between the severity of angiographic narrowing and clinical vasospasm is not entirely clear. Mounting evidence suggests that vascular proliferation may play an important additional role in the development of delayed cerebral ischemia through altered cerebral vascular compliance and cerebral autoregulation changes (4–7).

The volume of the subarachnoid clot is the only consistently demonstrated risk factor for vasospasm, and it is widely accepted that the pathogenic stimuli responsible for vasospasm are released from the blood clot (8). However, less agreement exists regarding the exact nature of these factors and the signaling pathways and mechanisms involved in the pathogenesis of vasospasm. Current evidence suggests that vasospasm is probably the result of prolonged pathologic arterial constriction of sensitized vessels. With time, arteries that are exposed to subarachnoid blood become less compliant and less responsive to vasodilator therapy. These changes coincide with progressive structural changes within all of the layers of the vessel wall, closely resembling the vascular remodeling response to injury in other disease states. In common with other forms of vascular remodeling, proposed mechanisms include inflammation, free radicals and oxidative stress, and endothelial dysfunction, resulting in intracellular signaling perturbations of the protein kinase, nitric oxide (NO), and, possibly, other pathways. Endothelial dysfunction and injury may alter the normal balance between vasoconstrictor and vasodilatory mechanisms. Once disturbed, the contraction mechanism of the vessels may be sensitized or upregulated, resulting in exaggerated or even paradoxical vasoconstriction. Furthermore, vascular injury may result in abnormal vessel wall thickening due to accelerated smooth muscle cell proliferation and collagen deposition. The summation of these events may result in decreased regional cerebral oxygen delivery and ischemic deficits.

Vessels are comprised of living tissues with complex, biochemical functions. Smooth muscle cells (SMCs), which reside in the medial layer, not only provide a motor to control vessel tone but also fulfill a host of other functions: proliferation, chemotaxis, adhesion, secretion, and various metabolic functions (9). In addition, great redundancy and overlap exist in signaling pathways that control these functions. Therefore, both the actions of vasoconstrictors (e.g., endothelin, angiotensin, and catecholamines) and the consequences of inhibiting endogenous vasodilators (e.g., NO) include vascular proliferation. Likewise, the effects of vasodilator therapy, such as calcium channel blockade, which has been shown to improve outcome without reducing

Table 1 Therapies that Prevent Vasospasm

Therapy	Pathway	Effects
Endothelin blockade (10)	MAPK dephosphorylation	Smooth muscle cell growth arrest
Nitric oxide donors (11)	Increased cGMP	
Thrombin inhibition (12)	MAPK dephosphorylation	
Calcium channel blockade (13)	Decreased MAPK translocation	
MAPK antisense (14)	Decreased MAPK proteins	Smooth muscle cell and fibroblast growth arrest
Serine protease inhibitors (15)	Decreased platelet-derived growth factors	

Abbreviations: MAPK, mitogen-activated protein kinase; cGMP, cyclic guanosine monophosphate.

the incidence of angiographic vasospasm, include the inhibition of vascular proliferation. In fact, a number of other diverse therapies that ameliorate vasospasm all share this feature (Table 1). The overall control of SMC function and the regulation of its responses to changing environmental cues are extremely complex activities that are just beginning to be understood.

ETIOLOGY OF VASOSPASM

Potential Pathogens

The principal cause of vasospasm is the periarterial subarachnoid blood clot. Several substances that have been implicated in vasospasm are gradually released from the blood clot (Table 2). Of these, the most extensively studied is oxyhemoglobin, which is widely believed to be the principal pathogen of vasospasm (17). However, it is likely that the cascade of events that eventually lead to irreversible vasoconstriction is modulated by many other factors. Studies designed to examine the importance of the different fractions of the breakdown products of whole blood have predominantly focused on the ability of these substances to cause cerebral arteries to contract, as well as the timeframe within which these substances can be measured in the cerebrospinal fluid (CSF). As we begin to unravel the intracellular events that follow SAH, we might be able to better appreciate the importance of these substances.

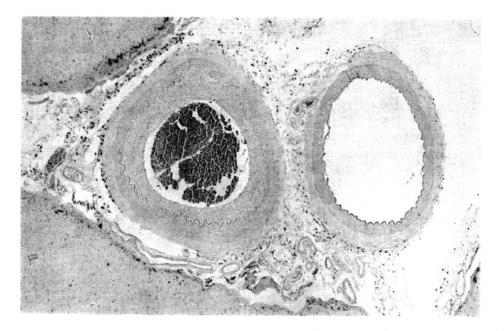

Figure 1 Two branches of the right middle cerebral artery in a patient 12 months after subarachnoid hemorrhage. Cerebral blood vessel (*left*) shows marked intimal proliferation, compared to normal (*right*). *Source*: From Ref. 21.

Table 2 Potential Spasmogens Released After Subarachnoid Hemorrhage and Their Possible Role in Vasospasm

Spasmogen or process	Possible role
Erythrocytes and contents	
Oxyhemoglobin and breakdown products, such as hemin, iron, bilirubin, and globin chains	Vasoconstriction, promotion of free radical reactions, blockage of NO vasodilatation, increase in endothelin release, blockage of perivascular nerve effects, and alteration of eicosanoid release
Products of free radical reactions stimulated by hemoglobin oxidation	Possible vasoconstriction
Adenosine nucleotides	Vasoconstriction
Cytosolic proteins	Unknown
Erythrocyte membranes	Lipid peroxidation
Platelet contents	
Serotonin	Possible vasoconstriction early after SAH
Adenosine	Vasoconstriction
Growth factors	Vasoconstriction
Leukocytes and inflammatory mediators	
Leukocytes	Vasoconstriction
Eicosanoids	Increased vasoconstriction by prostaglandins and thromboxanes, decreased vasodilatation by decreased PGI_2
Cytokines (interferons, tumor necrosis factor, interleukins, macrophage-derived cytokines, growth factors, chemokines, monokines)	Increased inflammation, possible vasoactive effects
Products of the coagulation cascade	
Fibrin degradation products	Increased vasoconstriction due to other spasmogens
Fibrinogen	Unknown
Thrombin	Unknown
Other serum proteins	Unknown

Abbreviations: SAH, subarachnoid hemorrhage; NO, nitric oxide.
Source: Adapted from Ref. 16.

Morphologic Manifestations of Vascular Injury

Most researchers agree that severe structural damage occurs in the arterial wall following SAH (18–28). Subendothelial edema develops, the endothelial layer and internal lamina are disrupted, and vascular SMCs (VSMCs) infiltrate the endothelium. Endothelial cell vacuolization and desquamation can be observed, followed by progressive intimal fibrosis and proliferation (Fig. 1) (21). The medial layer also exhibits SMC proliferation, vacuolization, and a generalized loss of myofilaments (phenotypic modulation). Cell necrosis and an increase in collagen in the extracellular matrix are well described. These structural changes are progressive, correlate with the development of angiographic vasospasm, and clearly represent a significant injury or vascular response to injury (24,27,29).

The importance of these arterial morphologic changes in the pathogenesis of clinical vasospasm is not clear, however. Some authors argue that structural changes, in particular intimal proliferation, generally tend to follow the angiographic phase of vasospasm (30,31). Nevertheless, although some microscopic manifestations of arterial injury might not be evident during the early phases of vasospasm, precursor events, such as subtle phenotypic modulation of VSMCs, including calcium sensitization and switching of contractile VSMC to a noncontractile state, might occur (32,33).

The mechanism of injury is not entirely clear either but is almost certainly multifactorial. The extent of the injury is related to the size of the blood clot, and reducing the clot size by either irrigation or fibrinolytic therapy reduces the severity of vasospasm (34–36). The adventitial layer of the cerebral arteries is thin and lacks an external elastic lamina and vasavasorum. Cerebral arteries probably receive their nourishment from the CSF, which penetrates the adventitia through pores (37), leaving the cerebral arteries extremely vulnerable to the toxic milieu that develops following SAH.

An "Inflammatory Soup"

Immediately following SAH, complex series of biochemical cascades associated with coagulation, complement activation, inflammation, and processes of phagocytosis and repair, such as the release and synthesis of growth factors, are activated. These systems are in place to promote wound healing. However, given the large amount of blood that remains trapped in the sub-arachnoid space and the unusual vulnerability of the cerebral arteries, these triggered responses may cause more harm than benefit.

Additionally, the gradual breakdown of erythrocytes results in high concentrations of free hemoglobin. It is uncertain how hemoglobin causes vasospasm. Proposed mechanisms include direct action on VSMCs, scavenging of NO, and increased production of endothelin, free radicals, lipid peroxidases, and eicosanoids (17). However, pure hemoglobin does not readily increase intracellular calcium levels and is not particularly toxic to VSMCs, suggesting that the indirect effects of hemoglobin are probably more important (38).

ENDOTHELIAL DYSFUNCTION

The intact endothelium produces endothelium-derived relaxing factors, such as NO, prostacyclin, and endothelium-derived hyperpolarizing factor (39), and endothelium-derived constricting factors (40), such as endothelin, angiotensin II, and thromboxanes. The presence of a normal endothelium maintains appropriate vasodilation, inhibits platelet activity, and suppresses growth of intimal cells and VSMCs. Disturbances of the metabolic and regulatory functions of the endothelium contribute to the pathophysiology of many vascular disease states, resulting in vasospasm and VSMC phenotypic modulation. Endothelial dysfunction and structural damage are well-documented features of cerebral vasospasm.

Disruption of NO pathways

NO, a potent dilator of cerebral blood vessels, plays a major role in the regulation of cerebral vascular tone (39). Three sources of NO are found in the brain: endothelial NO synthetase (eNOS) and neuronal NO synthetase (nNOS), which are expressed in a constitutive manner, and inducible NO synthetase, which is not expressed under normal conditions in most cells but can be expressed in all major cell types (endothelium, vascular smooth muscle, neurons, and glia) in response to a variety of stimuli (primarily proinflammatory stimuli) (41).

NO, released from endothelial cells, diffuses to adjacent SMCs and activates soluble guanylate cyclase (sGC). Cyclic guanosine monophosphate (cGMP) is generated, which leads to activation of protein kinase G (PKG) (42). This kinase phosphorylates various intracellular proteins, including the myosin light chain regulatory subunit, and activates intracellular pumps, sequestering free Ca^{2+} into intracellular stores, thereby relaxing SMCs (43).

In addition to promoting vasodilation, NO plays several other important roles in vascular homeostasis. It inhibits platelet aggregation by the same cGMP/PKG-dependent mechanism that causes vasodilation in SMCs (44), it inhibits SMC growth, and it is a potent antagonist of inflammation by mechanisms unrelated to cGMP (45,46).

Impaired endothelium-dependent relaxation, or endothelial dysfunction, has been shown to be present after experimental SAH in animal and human cerebral arteries (47–50). Mechanisms that have been proposed for this well-documented finding include scavenging of NO and destruction of NO-releasing neurons by oxyhemoglobin (51). In addition, metabolites of hemoglobin, such as bilirubin-oxidized fragments, increase levels of the arginine metabolite asymmetric dimethylarginine, an endogenous inhibitor of eNOS (51). An alternative and even more intriguing hypothesis involves the reaction of NO with superoxide, which is formed during the spontaneous oxidation of oxyhemoglobin to methemoglobin (52). Superoxide reacts with NO at near diffusion-limited rates to form another potent free radical, peroxynitrite, which in turn oxidizes tetrahydrobiopterin, an essential coenzyme of NOS (53). Tetrahydrobiopterin deficiency has been shown to uncouple NOS, thereby switching the vascular protective NO-producing enzyme to an enzyme that may initiate, or even accelerate, vascular injury by producing superoxide (54,55).

Reduced expression of sGC may also be related to the impairment of endothelium-dependent vasodilation in vasospasm (56). However, other studies have indicated that the responses to nitrovasodilators are normal after SAH, suggesting that the activity of sGC is unaltered (40,57,58). Further, CSF levels of nitrite, a direct metabolite of NO, are decreased after SAH and during vasospasm, suggesting a decreased availability of NO, due to either increased consumption or decreased production by nNOS and/or eNOS (51,59).

Endothelin

In addition to impaired endothelial production of NO, endothelial production of endothelin may be a major mechanism that contributes to vasospasm after SAH. Endothelin, the most powerful vasoconstrictor yet identified in biologic systems, as well as being a potent constrictor of cerebral arteries, may also participate in the pathogenesis of vascular injury. Although not well studied in the cerebral circulation, endothelin induces vascular inflammatory response and remodeling. It exercises proliferative actions on VSMCs, promotes the production of fibroblasts, modulates the synthesis of the extracellular matrix, and affects vascular permeability (60–64).

After SAH, levels of ET-1 are increased in the basilar artery and in CSF (65–67). Stimuli that cause endothelin gene expression after SAH are not well defined, but endothelin gene expression is inhibited by NO and cGMP and can be enhanced by several factors, including hemoglobin, thrombin, reactive oxygen species (ROS), transforming growth factor-β, and tumor necrosis factor-α (68–73).

Two subtypes of endothelin receptors have been identified, endothelin-A (ET A) and endothelin-B (ET B) receptors. In general, ET A receptors are expressed in vascular muscle and mediate contraction (Fig. 2) (74). The response to activation of ET B receptors depends on localization of the receptor. ET B receptors are expressed in SMCs in some blood vessels and mediate contraction. In contrast, activation of endothelial ET B receptors produces relaxation of blood vessels through the release of prostacyclin or NO (73,74).

Both ET A and ET B receptors are coupled to phospholipase C (PLC) via a guanosine triphosphate (GTP)-binding protein (76). Activation of PLC causes phosphatidylinositol hydrolysis, rapid formation of 1,4,5-inositol triphosphate (IP 3), and accumulation of

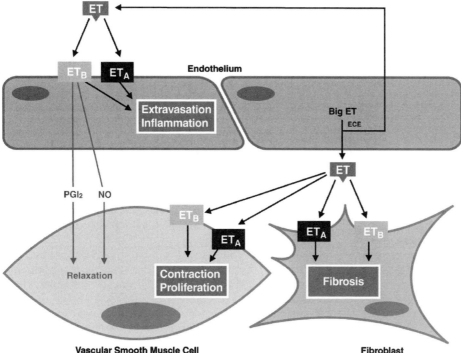

Figure 2 Endothelin mechanism of action. Normal pathways of endothelin on endothelium and vascular smooth muscle cells. *Source*: From Ref. 75.

1,2-diacylglycerol. IP 3 stimulates the release of Ca^{2+} from intracellular stores, including endoplasmic reticulum. This initial transient increase in intracellular Ca^{2+} concentration is followed by a sustained increase, probably due to an influx of extracellular Ca^{2+} through dihydropyridine-sensitive, voltage-dependent, L-type Ca^{2+} channels, or receptor-operated cation channels, leading to sustained VSMC contraction (62). Furthermore, endothelin-1 also activates rhoA/rho kinase (77). The rhoA/rho kinase pathway plays a very important role in Ca^{2+} sensitization in cerebral arteries (78). Ca^{2+} activates myosin light chain kinase (MLCK) to increase myosin light chain (MLC) phosphorylation. Activated rhoA appears to inhibit MLC phosphatase activity via rho kinase and to increase the level of MLC phosphorylation.

In addition to vasoconstriction, endothelin-1 also has mitogenic properties, causing proliferation and hypertrophy of SMCs and fibroblasts. Intracellular kinase cascades, including the sequential activation of raf-1, mitogen-activated protein kinase (MAPK), and S6 kinase II, are activated (62).

Several studies in experimental animals, including nonhuman primates, suggest that vasospasm after experimental SAH can be significantly attenuated by antagonists of ET A receptors, such as BQ-123, or combined ET A/ET B receptor antagonists (79–82). Endothelin-1 is produced from its precursor, big ET-1, by endothelin-converting enzyme (ECE). Activity of ECE in the basilar artery increases 3-fold after SAH, which may also contribute to vasospasm (81). Phosphoramidon and CGS-26303, inhibitors of ECE, attenuate vasospasm after SAH (83). Antisense oligonucleotides for prepro-ET-1 mRNA inhibit contraction of the basilar artery in response to hemolysate (84).

Free Radicals

ROS, although initially regarded primarily as potentially damaging by-products of oxidative cell metabolism, appear to be key mediators of cellular signaling and important modulators of cerebral vascular tone, particularly in endothelium-dependent responses (85). Under normal physiologic conditions, the rate and magnitude of oxidant formation is balanced by the rate of oxidant elimination. However, when ROS production is enhanced, the overproduction of oxidants overwhelms the cellular antioxidant capacity, resulting in oxidative stress and dysregulation of physiologic processes. Free radicals may also react with and damage cell lipids, proteins, and nucleic acids. Increasing evidence suggests that an elevation of oxidative stress and associated oxidative damage are mediators of vascular injury in various cardiovascular pathologies. Several studies indicate a pathophysiologic role of oxidative stress in cerebral vasospasm (55).

A number of sources produce free radicals after SAH, but the principal process in vasospasm is probably the spontaneous oxidation of oxyhemoglobin to methemoglobin, leading to the production of superoxide ($\bullet O_2^-$) and hydroxyl ($\bullet OH$) radicals (Fig. 3) (52). The iron in hemoglobin also catalyzes the formation of hydroxyl from hydrogen peroxide within the cerebral arterial wall via the Fenton and Haber–Weiss reactions. Additionally, the antioxidant capacity of the CSF is very limited, rendering the vulnerable cerebral arteries highly susceptible to free radical attack.

As discussed earlier, superoxide and other radicals react extremely efficiently with NO, resulting in loss of NO bioavailability and endothelial dysfunction. In addition to impairing NO-mediated responses, oxidative stress impairs neurovascular coupling and potassium channel–mediated vasodilation (86,87). Vasoconstrictor mechanisms may also be enhanced by oxidative stress. Rho kinase may predispose vessels to vasoconstriction or vasospasm through effects on calcium sensitization. Rho kinase activity may be increased as a consequence of loss of inhibitory effects of NO on rho kinase activity or by direct effects of ROS to promote the activity of rho kinase (88).

However, the effects of ROS signaling extend beyond the regulation of vascular tone. ROS play an essential role in propagating the signals of several growth factors, peptide hormones, and cytokines, such as platelet-derived growth factor, endothelin, angiotensin II, interleukin-1, and tumor necrosis factor (89). Evidence is emerging that redox processes markedly influence the balance of the activities between the various MAPK systems that appear to regulate vascular force generation, proliferation, and adaptive responses to injury (90,91).

The integrity of the blood–brain barrier can also be threatened by exposure of the endothelial cells to ROS-induced activation of matrix metalloproteinase-9 (MMP-9)(92). The development of cerebral vasospasm after SAH is preceded by increases in serum MMP-9 and vascular endothelial growth factor levels (93). Cell membrane lipid peroxidation and oxidative damage

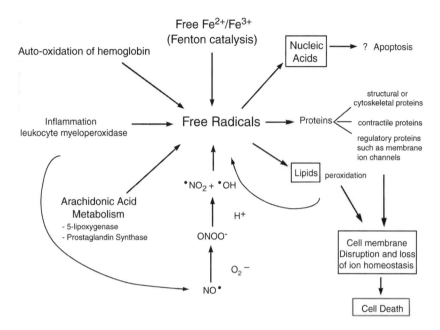

Figure 3 Diagram of pathways for free radical generation after subarachnoid hemorrhage. *Source*: From Ref. 16.

of DNA and mitochondria are other consequences of oxidative stress that have been implicated in the etiology of cerebral vasospasm after SAH (94). Lipid peroxidation, in particular, brings about the activation of membrane phospholipase A2, release of arachidonic acid (AA), intercellular accumulation of diacylglycerol, and activation of protein kinase C (95,96).

Potassium Channels

Four types of potassium channels are expressed in the cell membranes of VSMCs in cerebral vessels, each with a different profile of functional characteristics and stimuli for activation (97). In general, activation, or opening, of potassium channels in VSMCs results in the efflux of potassium ions, membrane hyperpolarization, and, ultimately, vascular relaxation due to closure of voltage-gated calcium channels and reduced intracellular calcium concentration (39). Endothelium-derived hyperpolarizing factor, an important factor in endothelium-mediated vasodilation, produces relaxation by activating potassium channels (39). Further, vasoconstrictors, such as epinephrine, norepinephrine, angiotensin II, endothelin, and thromboxane A2 depolarize the muscle membrane and have been shown to inhibit K channels (98).

Decreased potassium conductance may contribute to vasospasm after SAH. Cerebral vascular muscle is depolarized after SAH, and this depolarization probably contributes to vasospasm (99,100). Moreover, depolarization is most likely due to reduced activity of potassium channels in VSMCs (100–102). Potassium channels normally conduct an outward hyperpolarizing current and may play an important role in maintaining resting membrane potential. Consistent with this, hemolysate induces both depolarization and contraction of cerebral arteries, and depolarization can be significantly enhanced when potassium channels are blocked (100,103).

The 4 types of K$^+$ channels that have been described in cerebral blood vessels are (i) adenosine triphosphate (ATP)–sensitive (K$_{ATP}$), (ii) calcium-activated (K$_{Ca}$), (iii) voltage-dependent (K$_v$, also called delayed rectifier), and (iv) inwardly rectifying (K$_{IR}$).

Potassium channels, in general, play a major role in cerebrovascular autoregulation. ATP- sensitive (K$_{ATP}$) channels, in particular, respond to changes in intracellular metabolism and are defined based on sensitivity to intracellular ATP, which inhibits activity of the channel. Dissociation of ATP from the channel or reductions in PO$_2$ or pH result in channel opening and hyperpolarization and produce vasorelaxation. These channels are also subject to a variety of vasodilator and vasoconstrictor agents that operate through cyclic adenosine monophosphate (cAMP) or protein kinase A (PKA) and protein kinase C (PKC), respectively (104).

Vasoconstrictors, such as norepinephrine, endothelin, vasopressin, and 5-HT, trigger the release of PLC and diacylglycerol (DAG) and ultimately elevate PKC, which closes K_{ATP} channels, depolarizes the membrane, and causes vasoconstriction. The K_{ATP} channel activator chromakalimand calcitonin gene–related peptide, which hyperpolarize vessels, are very effective vasodilators of spastic arteries following SAH (99,105).

Calcium-activated (K_{Ca}) channels are thought to be the most abundant in vascular smooth muscle, with up to 10^4 channels estimated to be present per cell (98). They are defined based on their activation by increases in the concentration of intracellular calcium. Activity of K_{Ca} channels increases with membrane depolarization, and they play an important role in the control of myogenic tone in cerebral arteries. They can also be affected by other vasoactive stimuli. Cerebral microvessels can produce 20-hydroxyeicosatetraenoic acid (20-HETE) from AA via a P450 enzyme. 20-HETE is a potent vasoconstrictor that may produce this effect, at least in part, by inhibition of activity of K_{Ca} channels in cerebral vascular muscle. Vasoconstrictors that activate PLC, such as norepinephrine and endothelin, may increase levels of AA and CYP metabolites of AA.

Voltage-dependent (K_v) channels, also called delayed rectifier potassium channels, increase their activity with membrane depolarization and are important regulators of VSMC membrane potential in response to depolarizing stimuli. Relatively little is known about the physiologic importance of these potassium channels in the cerebral circulation.

In contrast to calcium-dependent and voltage-dependent potassium channels, inward-rectifier potassium (K_{IR}) channels are opened by membrane hyperpolarization (98). These potassium channels normally conduct an outward hyperpolarizing current and may play an important role in maintaining resting membrane potential. Western blotting and immuno-histochemistry performed on vasospastic VSMCs showed an increase in the expression of K_{IR} channels in dogs (100). The significance of this finding is not clear, but it might represent a compensatory mechanism-opposing vasospasm. Alternatively, this might be a manifestation of VSMC phenotypic change. Dramatic alterations in the expression and activity of K^+ channels, causing marked changes in the cell's electrical properties, accompany VSMC proliferation. However, the mechanisms by which changes in K^+ channel activity influence cellular growth pathways are poorly understood (106).

The Role of Eicosanoids

Arachidonic acid comprises part of the membrane phospholipid pool and is released in a single-step reaction by activated phospholipase A_2 (PLA_2). PLA_2 can be activated by various agonists, such as norepinephrine, angiotensin II, cytokines, and free radicals (107,108). Activated PLC and phospholipase D are also able to release free AA but not directly. Rather, they generate lipid products that contain AA (diacylglycerol and phosphatidic acid, respectively), which can be released subsequently by monoacylglycerol- and diacylglycerol-lipases. Once released, free AA has 3 possible fates: reincorporation into phospholipids, diffusion outside the cell, and metabolism. Metabolism is carried out by 3 distinct enzyme pathways: cyclooxygenase, lipoxygenases, and CYP. Metabolism of free AA by cyclooxygenases and lipoxygenases leads to the formation of prostaglandins, thromboxanes, and leukotrienes, with important roles in the regulation of vascular tone and inflammation (109). Cyclooxygenase- and lipoxygenase-catalyzed AA metabolism is well characterized, and both these pathways are targets of approved drugs. In contrast, our knowledge of metabolism of AA by CYP enzymes is more limited, although recent efforts in this area hold the promise that new drug targets will also emerge from this pathway.

Cerebral blood vessels synthesize vasoconstrictive prostaglandins (prostaglandin F2α, E2, A1, and B2, and the powerful vasodilator prostacyclin PGI_2). In addition, cerebral vessels are constricted by thromboxane A2 and B2. Some evidence suggests that prostaglandin synthesis is significantly altered after SAH, in that production of vasoconstricting prostaglandins and thromboxanes is increased and synthesis of PGI_2 is decreased (110,111). However, prostaglandin synthesis inhibitors, such as aspirin, are not very effective in reversing vasospasm, and indomethacin might even exacerbate vasospasm (112,113). These agents typically have multiple actions, which might include the inhibition of vasodilator pathways.

Leukotrienes, the products of the lipoxygenase pathway, are synthesized only in very small amounts in experimental models of vasospasm, and no changes are detectable in CSF leukotriene-levels post-SAH (114). Additionally, even in large concentrations, leukotrienes are only weak vasoconstrictors and are, therefore, unlikely to play an important role in vasospasm (115).

Recent studies have drawn attention to the role of 20-HETE in the development of cerebral vasospasm and demonstrated that 20-HETE plays an important role in both the acute and delayed phases of experimental cerebral vasospasm (116,117). 20-HETE is a potent cerebral vasoconstrictor that is produced by the metabolism of AA by CYP4A enzymes in cerebral arteries (118). 20-HETE activates PKC, Ras, tyrosine kinase, MAPK, and rho/rho kinase pathways, promotes calcium entry by depolarizing cerebral arteries secondary to blockade of K_{Ca} channels, and increases Ca^{2+} influx by activating L-type Ca^{2+} channels in the cerebral vasculature (117). Furthermore, 20-HETE contributes to the vasoconstrictor responses to endothelin, angiotensin II, serotonin, vasopressin, and norepinephrine (117). The concentration of 20-HETE in CSF increases markedly after SAH, and inhibitors of the synthesis or actions of 20-HETE prevent the acute fall in cerebral blood flow after SAH and fully reverse delayed vasospasm in the rat (116,117). It is, therefore, possible that elevated production of 20-HETE might represent the final common pathway that leads to cerebral vasospasm, if such a pathway indeed exists.

VASCULAR REMODELING FOLLOWING SAH

In some ways, the term "vasospasm" is a misnomer, because it implies a reactive vascular tone that increases with a secondary vessel narrowing. There may be a critical difference between arterial vasospasm and cerebral vasospasm following SAH, because cerebral vessels lose their reactivity to most agents that act directly on vessel walls. For example, NO and nitroprusside normally act directly to dilate smooth muscle in vessel walls but have little effect in treating ischemic deficits due to cerebral vasospasm (49,58). An active tone increase implies a significant decrease in elasticity due to the contraction, yet the vessel wall actually becomes softer and more "putty-like" with cerebral vasospasm. It is unclear why the onset of delayed ischemic deficits due to cerebral vasospasm occurs several days after the initial SAH, when arterial spasm of cerebral blood vessels is often present on early arteriograms.

Arterial remodeling is a concept that was used in the past to describe any change in vessel wall structure. More recently, however, it has been used specifically to refer to a change in vessel cross-sectional area within the external elastic lamina (119). Cerebral vasospasm following SAH fits both these descriptions. Remodeling is an active process of structural alteration that involves changes in at least 4 cellular processes—cell growth, cell death, cell migration, and production or degradation of extracellular matrix (120). It is usually an adaptive response to long-term changes in hemodynamic conditions but may also result from vascular injury and contribute to the pathophysiology of vascular diseases. Inward remodeling denotes a reduction in vessel size. In low-flow states, or following endothelial or adventitial injury, accentuated production of mitogenic and fibrogenic growth factors mediates inward modeling by increasing SMC proliferation and collagen deposition and cross-linking (120). Some of the factors that regulate the growth of vascular cells in the pathogenesis of cerebral vasospasm are listed in Table 3.

Cerebral VSMC turnover begins rapidly after SAH (121). However, the SMCs may require a more potent stimulus to begin mitotic activity, such as the later combination of relative ischemia and the mix of growth factors available from the blood that coats the outer wall.

Table 3 Mediators of Vascular Remodeling Associated with Cerebral Vasospasm

Growth promoters	Growth inhibitors
Platelet-derived growth factors (121)	Nitric oxide (11)
Vascular endothelial growth factor (121)	Heparin sulfate (122)
Transforming growth factor (123)	Prostacyclines (PGI$_2$) (110)
Basic fibroblast growth factor (124)	
Endothelin (125)	
Inflammatory cytokines: CD-18	
(126, 127), IL-1β,IL-6, and TNF-α (128)	
Thromboxane (129)	

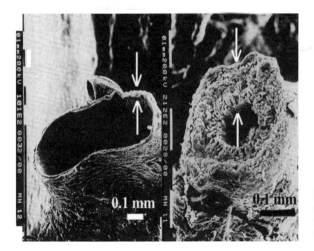

Figure 4 Scanning electron micrograph of a cerebral blood vessel in spasm (*right*) compared to a normal contralateral cerebral artery (*left*) in a nonhuman primate. *Source*: From Ref. 130.

The vessel thickening would then correspond to a combination of (i) vessel necrosis of SMCs in the media and (ii) mitosis and hypertrophy of an underlying population of cells, which would lead to smooth muscle renewal and proliferation. The SMC proliferation would presumably then proceed over days to a few weeks, leading to a repopulation of the media and to resumption of normal vessel reactivity and caliber (Fig. 4).

Thus, the time course of delayed ischemic deficits due to cerebral vasospasm may be delayed due to the slow onset of smooth muscle necrosis over several days, which, together with the combination of mitotic activity and hypertrophy of remaining cells, markedly increases the width of the media, leading to shrinkage of the vessel lumen. The 5-day period may be an unfortunate superimposition of these 2 processes of necrosis with associated cell swelling and the secondary hypertrophy and mitotic activity of SMC turnover. This time period is compounded by the slow lysis of blood products by CSF and a correspondingly slow resumption of adequate vessel nutrition, presumably, as CSF adventitial pores are reopened or reconstituted.

CEREBRAL BLOOD FLOW

Many investigators have studied the changes that occur in the cerebral hemodynamics during vasospasm, but results are conflicting, probably because of heterogeneous study populations, different treatments, and nonstandardized measurement techniques. A number of positron emission tomography studies have indicated that soon after SAH, prior to developing delayed cerebral metabolic rate of oxygen, and cerebral blood flow are decreased and cerebral blood volume (CBV) is increased (131–133). In patients who do develop arteriographic vasospasm, though, regional CBV is reduced in spite of an increase in regional oxygen extraction fraction, which is usually associated with compensatory distal arteriolar vasodilation and increases in regional CBV (134). A potential explanation for this finding could be spastic parenchymal vessels losing the ability to vasodilate in response to tissue hypoxia. This adds further evidence to support the theory of microvascular involvement in cerebral vasospasm.

Unless complicated by hydrocephalus or intracerebral hemorrhage, autoregulation of cerebral blood flow in response to changes in cerebral perfusion pressure is preserved during the early period. However, widespread dysautoregulation, which could persist for more than 3 weeks, soon sets in (135–138). For this reason, hypotension is particularly poorly tolerated and is one of the single most important factors to avoid in the management of these patients. The vasoconstrictor response to hypocapnia is well preserved in all vessels, but affected vessels fail to vasodilate in response to hypercapnia (139).

Infarction following SAH is typically diffuse and multiterritorial, unlike other causes of cerebral infarction, such as embolic events or intravascular thrombosis. It is thought to occur in areas of relative hypoperfusion, resembling the ischemic penumbra.

CONCLUSIONS AND FUTURE DIRECTIONS

The pathophysiology of cerebral vasospasm is a complex and poorly understood phenomenon. Spasmogens released from the subarachnoid clot activate multiple overlapping pathways that result in abnormal vasoconstriction and SMC proliferation. Other factors released from the clot result in endothelial dysfunction and injury, further disrupting the delicate balance between cerebral vasodilatation and constriction. Changes in VSMC growth, death, and migration, and in cellular matrix result in vascular remodeling, altering vessel lumen and compliance. Cerebral oxygen delivery is ultimately compromised regionally or globally. New therapeutic approaches to the prevention and treatment of cerebral vasospasm will evolve as our understanding of the underlying pathophysiologic mechanisms improves.

REFERENCES

1. Ecker A, Riemenschneider PA. Arteriographic demonstration of spasm of the intracranial arteries, with special reference to saccular arterial aneurysms. J Neurosurg 1951; 8:660–667.
2. Kassell NF, Sasaki T, Colohan AR, Nazar G. Cerebral vasospasm following aneurysmal subarachnoid hemorrhage. Stroke 1985; 16:562–572.
3. Mayberg MR, Batjer HH, Dacey R, et al. Guidelines for the management of aneurysmal subarachnoid hemorrhage. A statement for healthcare professionals from a special writing group of the Stroke Council, American Heart Association. Circulation 1994; 90:2592–2605.
4. Ohkuma H, Suzuki S, Kudo K, et al. Cortical blood flow during cerebral vasospasm after aneurysmal subarachnoid hemorrhage: three-dimensional N-isopropyl-p-[(123)I] iodoamphetamine single photon emission CT findings. AJNR Am J Neuroradiol 2003; 24:444–450.
5. Ohkuma H, Suzuki S. Histological dissociation between intra- and extraparenchymal portion of perforating small arteries after experimental subarachnoid hemorrhage in dogs. Acta Neuropathol (Berl) 1999; 98:374–382.
6. Ohkuma H, Itoh K, Shibata S, Suzuki S. Morphological changes of intraparenchymal arterioles after experimental subarachnoid hemorrhage in dogs. Neurosurgery 1997; 41:230–235; discussion 235–236.
7. Ohkuma H, Manabe H, Tanaka M, Suzuki S. Impact of cerebral microcirculatory changes on cerebral blood flow during cerebral vasospasm after aneurysmal subarachnoid hemorrhage. Stroke 2000; 31:1621–1627.
8. Fisher CM, Kistler JP, Davis JM. Relation of cerebral vasospasm to subarachnoid hemorrhage visualized by computerized tomographic scanning. Neurosurgery 1980; 6:1–9.
9. Owens GK, Kumar MS, Wamhoff BR. Molecular regulation of vascular smooth muscle cell differentiation in development and disease. Physiol Rev 2004; 84:767–801.
10. Zimmermann M, Seifert V. Endothelin and subarachnoid hemorrhage: an overview. Neurosurgery 1998; 43:863–875; discussion 875–876.
11. Thomas JE, McGinnis G. Safety of intraventricular sodium nitroprusside and thiosulfate for the treatment of cerebral vasospasm in the intensive care unit setting. Stroke 2002; 33:486–492.
12. Kudo A, Suzuki M, Yoshitaka K, et al. Intrathecal administration of thrombin inhibitor ameliorates cerebral vasospasm. Cerbrovasc Dis 2000; 10:424–430.
13. Kasuya H, Onda H, Takeshita M, et al. Efficacy and safety of nicardipine prolonged-release implants for preventing vasospasm in humans. Stroke 2002; 33:1011–1015.
14. Satoh M, Parent AD, Zhang JH. Inhibitory effect with antisense mitogen-activated protein kinase oligodeoxynucleotide against cerebral vasospasm in rats. Stroke 2002; 33:775–781.
15. Zhang Z, Nagata I, Kikuchi H, et al. Broad-spectrum and selective serine protease inhibitors prevent expression of platelet-derived growth factor-BB and cerebral vasospasm after subarachnoid hemorrhage: vasospasm caused by cisternal injection of recombinant platelet-derived growth factor-BB. Stroke 2001; 32:1665–1672.
16. Weir B, Macdonald RL, Stoodley M. Etiology of cerebral vasospasm. Acta Neurochir Suppl 1999; 72:27–46.
17. Macdonald RL, Weir BK. A review of hemoglobin and the pathogenesis of cerebral vasospasm. Stroke 1991; 22:971–982.
18. Crompton MR. The pathogenesis of cerebral infarction following the rupture of cerebral berry aneurysms. Brain 1964; 87:491–510.
19. Eldevik OP, Kristiansen K, Torvik A. Subarachnoid hemorrhage and cerebrovascular spasm. Morphological study of intracranial arteries based on animal experiments and human autopsies. J Neurosurg 1981; 55:869–876.
20. Alksne JF, Branson PJ. A comparison of intimal proliferation in experimental subarachnoid hemorrhage and atherosclerosis. Angiology 1976; 27:712–720.

21. Conway LW, McDonald LW. Structural changes of the intradural arteries following subarachnoid hemorrhage. J Neurosurg 1972; 37:715–723.
22. Hughes JT, Schianchi PM. Cerebral artery spasm. A histological study at necropsy of the blood vessels in cases of subarachnoid hemorrhage. J Neurosurg 1978; 48:515–525.
23. Kapp JP, Clower BR, Azar FM, et al. Heparin reduces proliferative angiopathy following subarachnoid hemorrhage in cats. J Neurosurg 1985; 62:570–575.
24. Mayberg MR, Okada T, Bark DH. Morphologic changes in cerebral arteries after subarachnoid hemorrhage. Neurosurg Clin N Am 1990; 1:417–432.
25. Takemae T, Branson PJ, Alksne JF. Intimal proliferation of cerebral arteries after subarachnoid blood injection in pigs. J Neurosurg 1984; 61:494–500.
26. Mizukami M, Kin H, Araki G, et al. Is angiographic spasm real spasm? Acta Neurochir (Wien) 1976; 34:247–259.
27. Fein JM, Flor WJ, Cohan SL, Parkhurst J. Sequential changes of vascular ultrastructure in experimental cerebral vasospasm. Myonecrosis of subarachnoid arteries. J Neurosurg 1974; 41:49–58.
28. Espinosa F, Weir B, Shnitka T, et al. A randomized placebo-controlled double-blind trial of nimodipine after SAH in monkeys. Part 2: Pathological findings. J Neurosurg 1984; 60:1176–1185.
29. Mayberg MR, Okada T, Bark DH. The significance of morphological changes in cerebral arteries after subarachnoid hemorrhage. J Neurosurg 1990; 72:626–633.
30. Macdonald RL, Weir BK, Young JD, Grace MG. Cytoskeletal and extracellular matrix proteins in cerebral arteries following subarachnoid hemorrhage in monkeys. J Neurosurg 1992; 76:81–90.
31. Findlay JM, Weir BK, Kanamaru K, Espinosa F. Arterial wall changes in cerebral vasospasm. Neurosurgery 1989; 25:736–745; discussion 745–746.
32. Somlyo AP, Somlyo AV. Ca^{2+} sensitivity of smooth muscle and nonmuscle myosin II: modulated by G proteins, kinases, and myosin phosphatase. Physiol Rev 2003; 83:1325–1358.
33. Koide M, Nishizawa S, Ohta S, et al. Chronological changes of the contractile mechanism in prolonged vasospasm after subarachnoid hemorrhage: from protein kinase C to protein tyrosine kinase. Neurosurgery 2002; 51:1468–1474; discussion 1474–1476.
34. Findlay JM, Weir BK, Steinke D, et al. Effect of intrathecal thrombolytic therapy on subarachnoid clot and chronic vasospasm in a primate model of SAH. J Neurosurg 1988; 69:723–735.
35. Inagawa T, Kamiya K, Matsuda Y. Effect of continuous cisternal drainage on cerebral vasospasm. Acta Neurochir (Wien) 1991; 112:28–36.
36. Alksne JF, Branson PJ, Bailey M. Modification of experimental post-subarachnoid hemorrhage vasculopathy with intracisternal plasmin. Neurosurgery 1988; 23:335–337.
37. Zervas NT, Liszczak TM, Mayberg MR, Black PM. Cerebrospinal fluid may nourish cerebral vessels through pathways in the adventitia that may be analogous to systemic vasa vasorum. J Neurosurg 1982; 56:475–481.
38. Marton LS, Wang X, Kowalczuk A, et al. Effects of hemoglobin on heme oxygenase gene expression and viability of cultured smooth muscle cells. Am J Physiol Heart Circ Physiol 2000; 279:H2405–H2413.
39. Faraci FM, Heistad DD. Regulation of the cerebral circulation: role of endothelium and potassium channels. Physiol Rev 1998; 78:53–97.
40. Katusic ZS, Milde JH, Cosentino F, Mitrovic BS. Subarachnoid hemorrhage and endothelial L-arginine pathway in small Brain stem arteries in dogs. Stroke 1993; 24:392–399.
41. Faraci FM, Brian JE Jr. Nitric oxide and the cerebral circulation. Stroke 1994; 25:692–703.
42. Lincoln TM, Dey N, Sellak H. Invited review: cGMP-dependent protein kinase signaling mechanisms in smooth muscle: from the regulation of tone to gene expression. J Appl Physiol 2001; 91:1421–1430.
43. Ignarro LJ. Biosynthesis and metabolism of endothelium-derived nitric oxide. Annu Rev Pharmacol Toxicol 1990; 30:535–560.
44. Radomski MW, Palmer RM, Moncada S. The role of nitric oxide and cGMP in platelet adhesion to vascular endothelium. Biochem Biophys Res Commun 1987; 148:1482–1489.
45. Bouchie JL, Hansen H, Feener EP. Natriuretic factors and nitric oxide suppress plasminogen activator inhibitor-1 expression in vascular smooth muscle cells. Role of cGMP in the regulation of the plasminogen system. Arterioscler Thromb Vasc Biol 1998; 18:1771–1779.
46. Garg UC, Hassid A. Nitric oxide-generating vasodilators and 8-bromo-cyclic guanosine monophosphate inhibit mitogenesis and proliferation of cultured rat vascular smooth muscle cells. J Clin Invest 1989; 83:1774–1777.
47. Edwards DH, Byrne JV, Griffith TM. The effect of chronic subarachnoid hemorrhage on basal endothelium-derived relaxing factor activity in intrathecal cerebral arteries. J Neurosurg 1992; 76:830–837.
48. Hongo K, Ogawa H, Kassell NF, et al. Comparison of intraluminal and extraluminal inhibitory effects of hemoglobin on endothelium-dependent relaxation of rabbit basilar artery. Stroke 1988; 19:1550–1555.
49. Onoue H, Kaito N, Akiyama M, et al. Altered reactivity of human cerebral arteries after subarachnoid hemorrhage. J Neurosurg 1995; 83:510–515.

50. Iuliano BA, Pluta RM, Jung C, Oldfield EH. Endothelial dysfunction in a primate model of cerebral vasospasm. J Neurosurg 2004; 100:287–294.
51. Pluta RM. Delayed cerebral vasospasm and nitric oxide: review, new hypothesis, and proposed treatment. Pharmacol Ther 2005; 105:23–56.
52. Misra HP, Fridovich I. The generation of superoxide radical during the autoxidation of hemoglobin. J Biol Chem 1972; 247:6960–6962.
53. Landmesser U, Dikalov S, Price SR, et al. Oxidation of tetrahydrobiopterin leads to uncoupling of endothelial cell nitric oxide synthase in hypertension. J Clin Invest 2003; 111:1201–1209.
54. Werner ER, Gorren AC, Heller R, et al. Tetrahydrobiopterin and nitric oxide: mechanistic and pharmacological aspects. Exp Biol Med (Maywood) 2003; 228:1291–1302.
55. Faraci FM. Oxidative stress: the curse that underlies cerebral vascular dysfunction? Stroke 2005; 36:186–188.
56. Kasuya H, Weir BK, Nakane M, et al. Nitric oxide synthase and guanylate cyclase levels in canine basilar artery after subarachnoid hemorrhage. J Neurosurg 1995; 82:250–255.
57. Kanamaru K, Weir BK, Findlay JM, et al. Pharmacological studies on relaxation of spastic primate cerebral arteries in subarachnoid hemorrhage. J Neurosurg 1989; 71:909–915.
58. Hatake K, Wakabayashi I, Kakishita E, Hishida S. Impairment of endothelium-dependent relaxation in human basilar artery after subarachnoid hemorrhage. Stroke 1992; 23:1111–1116; discussion 1116–1117.
59. Pluta RM, Thompson BG, Dawson TM, et al. Loss of nitric oxide synthase immunoreactivity in cerebral vasospasm. J Neurosurg 1996; 84:648–654.
60. Schiffrin EL. Vascular endothelin in hypertension. Vascul Pharmacol 2005; 43:19–29.
61. Li L, Fink GD, Watts SW, et al. Endothelin-1 increases vascular superoxide via endothelin(A)-NADPH oxidase pathway in low-renin hypertension. Circulation 2003; 107:1053–1058.
62. Miyauchi T, Masaki T. Pathophysiology of endothelin in the cardiovascular system. Annu Rev Physiol 1999; 61:391–415.
63. Duerrschmidt N, Wippich N, Goettsch W, et al. Endothelin-1 induces NAD(P)H oxidase in human endothelial cells. Biochem Biophys Res Commun 2000; 269:713–717.
64. Browatzki M, Schmidt J, Kubler W, Kranzhofer R. Endothelin-1 induces interleukin-6 release via activation of the transcription factor NF-kappaB in human vascular smooth muscle cells. Basic Res Cardiol 2000; 95:98–105.
65. Hirose H, Ide K, Sasaki T, et al. The role of endothelin and nitric oxide in modulation of normal and spastic cerebral vascular tone in the dog. Eur J Pharmacol 1995; 277:77–87.
66. Kobayashi H, Hayashi M, Kobayashi S, et al. Cerebral vasospasm and vasoconstriction caused by endothelin. Neurosurgery 1991; 28:673–678; discussion 678–679.
67. Kraus GE, Bucholz RD, Yoon KW, et al. Cerebrospinal fluid endothelin-1 and endothelin-3 levels in normal and neurosurgical patients: a clinical study and literature review. Surg Neurol 1991; 35:20–29.
68. Durieu-Trautmann O, Federici C, Creminon C, et al. Nitric oxide and endothelin secretion by brain microvessel endothelial cells: regulation by cyclic nucleotides. J Cell Physiol 1993; 155:104–111.
69. Boulanger C, Luscher TF. Release of endothelin from the porcine aorta. Inhibition by endothelium-derived nitric oxide. J Clin Invest 1990; 85:587–590.
70. Goto K, Hama H, Kasuya Y. Molecular pharmacology and pathophysiological significance of endothelin. Jpn J Pharmacol 1996; 72:261–290.
71. Estrada C, Gomez C, Martin C. Effects of TNF-alpha on the production of vasoactive substances by cerebral endothelial and smooth muscle cells in culture. J Cereb Blood Flow Metab 1995; 15:920–928.
72. Ohlstein EH, Storer BL. Oxyhemoglobin stimulation of endothelin production in cultured endothelial cells. J Neurosurg 1992; 77:274–278.
73. Rubanyi GM, Polokoff MA. Endothelins: molecular biology, biochemistry, pharmacology, physiology, and pathophysiology. Pharmacol Rev 1994; 46:325–415.
74. Gray GA, Webb DJ. The endothelin system and its potential as a therapeutic target in cardiovascular disease. Pharmacol Ther 1996; 72:109–148.
75. Actlion Pharmaceuticals US Inc. (www.endothelinscience.com).
76. Simonson MS, Dunn MJ. Cellular signaling by peptides of the endothelin gene family. Faseb J 1990; 4:2989–3000.
77. Mi ao L, Dai Y, Zhang J. Mechanism of RhoA/Rho kinase activation in endothelin-1-induced contraction in rabbit basilar artery. Am J Physiol Heart Circ Physiol 2002; 283:H983–H989.
78. Nakayama K, Obara K, Tanabe Y, et al. Interactive role of tyrosine kinase, protein kinase C, and Rho/Rho kinase systems in the mechanotransduction of vascular smooth muscles. Biorheology 2003; 40:307–314.
79. Foley PL, Caner HH, Kassell NF, Lee KS. Reversal of subarachnoid hemorrhage-induced vasoconstriction with an endothelin receptor antagonist. Neurosurgery 1994; 34:108–112; discussion 112–113.

80. Hino A, Weir BK, Macdonald RL, et al. Prospective, randomized, double-blind trial of BQ-123 and bosentan for prevention of vasospasm following subarachnoid hemorrhage in monkeys. J Neurosurg 1995; 83:503–509.

81. Roux S, Loffler BM, Gray GA, et al. The role of endothelin in experimental cerebral vasospasm. Neurosurgery 1995; 37:78–85; discussion 86.

82. Shigeno T, Clozel M, Sakai S, et al. The effect of bosentan, a new potent endothelin receptor antagonist, on the pathogenesis of cerebral vasospasm. Neurosurgery 1995; 37:87–90; discussion 91.

83. Caner HH, Kwan AL, Arthur A, et al. Systemic administration of an inhibitor of endothelin-converting enzyme for attenuation of cerebral vasospasm following experimental subarachnoid hemorrhage. J Neurosurg 1996; 85:917–922.

84. Onoda K, Ono S, Ogihara K, et al. Inhibition of vascular contraction by intracisternal administration of preproendothelin-1 mRNA antisense oligoDNA in a rat experimental vasospasm model. J Neurosurg 1996; 85:846–852.

85. Paravicini TM, Sobey CG. Cerebral vascular effects of reactive oxygen species: recent evidence for a role of NADPH-oxidase. Clin Exp Pharmacol Physiol 2003; 30:855–859.

86. Kazama K, Anrather J, Zhou P, et al. Angiotensin II impairs neurovascular coupling in neocortex through–NADPH oxidase-derived radicals. Circ Res 2004; 95:1019–1026.

87. Erdos B, Simandle SA, Snipes JA, et al. Potassium channel dysfunction in cerebral arteries of insulin-resistant rats is mediated by reactive oxygen species. Stroke 2004; 35:964–969.

88. Didion SP, Lynch CM, Baumbach GL, Faraci FM. Impaired endothelium-dependent responses and enhanced influence of Rho-kinase in cerebral arterioles in type II diabetes. Stroke 2005; 36:342–347.

89. Daou GB, Srivastava AK. Reactive oxygen species mediate Endothelin-1-induced activation of ERK1/2, PKB, and Pyk2 signaling, as well as protein synthesis, in vascular smooth muscle cells. Free Radic Biol Med 2004; 37:208–215.

90. Jin N, Rhoades RA. Activation of tyrosine kinases in H_2O_2-induced contraction in pulmonary artery. Am J Physiol 1997; 272:H2686–H2692.

91. Kunsch C, Medford RM. Oxidative stress as a regulator of gene expression in the vasculature. Circ Res 1999; 85:753–766.

92. Kim GW, Gasche Y, Grzeschik S, et al. Neurodegeneration in striatum induced by the mitochondrial toxin 3-nitropropionic acid: role of matrix metalloproteinase-9 in early blood-Brain barrier disruption? J Neurosci 2003; 23:8733–8742.

93. McGirt MJ, Lynch JR., Blessing R, et al. Serum von Willebrand factor, matrix metalloproteinase-9, and vascular endothelial growth factor levels predict the onset of cerebral vasospasm after aneurysmal subarachnoid hemorrhage. Neurosurgery 2002; 51:1128–1134; discussion 1134–1135.

94. Mori T, Nagata K, Town T, et al. Intracisternal increase of superoxide anion production in a canine subarachnoid hemorrhage model. Stroke 2001; 32:636–642.

95. Tyler DD. Role of superoxide radicals in the lipid peroxidation of intracellular membranes. FEBS Lett 1975; 51:180–183.

96. Takuwa Y, Matsui T, Abe Y, et al. Alterations in protein kinase C activity and membrane lipid metabolism in cerebral vasospasm after subarachnoid hemorrhage. J Cereb Blood Flow Metab 1993; 13:409–415.

97. Faraci FM, Sobey CG. Role of potassium channels in regulation of cerebral vascular tone. J Cereb Blood Flow Metab 1998; 18:1047–1063.

98. Nelson MT, Quayle JM. Physiological roles and properties of potassium channels in arterial smooth muscle. Am J Physiol 1995; 268:C799–C822.

99. Zuccarello M, Bonasso CL, Lewis AI, et al. Relaxation of subarachnoid hemorrhage-induced spasm of rabbit basilar artery by the K+ channel activator cromakalim. Stroke 1996; 27:311–316.

100. Weyer GW, Jahromi BS, Aihara Y, et al. Expression and function of inwardly rectifying potassium channels after experimental subarachnoid hemorrhage. J Cereb Blood Flow Metab 2005; 26:382-391.

101. Quan L, Sobey CG. Selective effects of subarachnoid hemorrhage on cerebral vascular responses to 4-aminopyridine in rats. Stroke 2000; 31:2460–2465.

102. Aihara Y, Jahromi BS, Yassari R, et al. Molecular profile of vascular ion channels after experimental subarachnoid hemorrhage. J Cereb Blood Flow Metab 2004; 24:75–83.

103. Fujiwara S, Kuriyama H. Hemolysate-induced contraction in smooth muscle cells of the guinea pig basilar artery. Stroke 1984; 15:503–510.

104. Quayle JM, Nelson MT, Standen NB. ATP-sensitive and inwardly rectifying potassium channels in smooth muscle. Physiol Rev 1997; 77:1165–1232.

105. Ahmad I, Imaizumi S, Shimizu H, et al. Development of calcitonin gene-related peptide slow-release tablet implanted in CSF space for prevention of cerebral vasospasm after experimental subarachnoid haemorrhage. Acta Neurochir (Wien) 1996; 138:1230–1240.

106. Neylon CB. Potassium channels and vascular proliferation. Vascul Pharmacol 2002; 38:35–41.

107. Mukherjee AB, Miele L, Pattabiraman N. Phospholipase A2 enzymes: regulation and physiological role. Biochem Pharmacol 1994; 48:1–10.

108. Guidarelli A, Cantoni O. Pivotal role of superoxides generated in the mitochondrial respiratory chain in peroxynitrite-dependent activation of phospholipase A2. Biochem J 2002; 366:307–314.

109. Funk CD. Prostaglandins and leukotrienes: advances in eicosanoid biology. Science 2001; 294: 1871–1875.

110. Sasaki T, Murota SI, Wakai S, et al. Evaluation of prostaglandin biosynthetic activity in canine basilar artery following subarachnoid injection of blood. J Neurosurg 1981; 55:771–778.

111. Maeda Y, Tani E, Miyamoto T. Prostaglandin metabolism in experimental cerebral vasospasm. J Neurosurg 1981; 55:779–785.

112. White RP, Hagen AA, Robertson JT. Effect of nonsteroid anti-inflammatory drugs on subarachnoid hemorrhage in dogs. J Neurosurg 1979; 51:164–171.

113. Brandt L, Andersson KE, Edvinsson L, Ljunggren B. Effects of extracellular calcium and of calcium antagonists on the contractile responses of isolated human pial and mesenteric arteries. J Cereb Blood Flow Metab 1981; 1:339–347.

114. Yokota M, Tani E, Maeda Y. Biosynthesis of leukotrienes in canine cerebral vasospasm. Stroke 1989; 20:527–533.

115. Cook DA. Mechanisms of cerebral vasospasm in subarachnoid haemorrhage. Pharmacol Ther 1995; 66:259–284.

116. Takeuchi K, Miyata N, Renic M, et al. Hemoglobin, NO and 20-HETE interactions in mediating cerebral vasoconstriction following SAH. Am J Physiol Regul Integr Comp Physiol 2006; 290:R84-89.

117. Takeuchi K, Renic M, Bohman QC, et al. Reversal of delayed vasospasm by an inhibitor of the synthesis of 20-HETE. Am J Physiol Heart Circ Physiol 2005; 289:H2203-2211.

118. Gebremedhin D, Lange AR, Narayanan J, et al. Cat cerebral arterial smooth muscle cells express cytochrome P450 4A2 enzyme and produce the vasoconstrictor 20-HETE which enhances L-type Ca^{2+} current. J Physiol 1998; 507(Pt 3):771–781.

119. Ward MR, Pasterkamp G, Yeung AC, Borst C. Arterial remodeling. Mechanisms and clinical implications. Circulation 2000; 102:1186–1191.

120. Gibbons GH, Dzau VJ. The emerging concept of vascular remodeling. N Engl J Med 1994; 330: 1431–1438.

121. Borel CO, McKee A, Parra A, et al. Possible role for vascular cell proliferation in cerebral vasospasm after subarachnoid hemorrhage. Stroke 2003; 34:427–433.

122. Tekkok IH, Tekkok S, Ozcan OE, et al. Preventive effect of intracisternal heparin for proliferative angiopathy after experimental subarachnoid haemorrhage in rats. Acta Neurochir (Wien) 1994 127:112–117.

123. Kitazawa K, Tada T. Elevation of transforming growth factor-beta 1 level in cerebrospinal fluid of patients with communicating hydrocephalus after subarachnoid hemorrhage. Stroke 1994; 25: 1400–1404.

124. Ogane K, Wolf EW, Robertson JH. Role of basic fibroblast growth factor in the course of cerebral vasospasm in an experimental model of subarachnoid hemorrhage. Neurol Res 2002; 24:365–372.

125. Zuccarello M. Endothelin: the "prime suspect" in cerebral vasospasm. Acta Neurochir Suppl 2001; 77:61–65.

126. Bavbek M, Polin R, Kwan AL, et al. Monoclonal antibodies against ICAM-1 and CD18 attenuate cerebral vasospasm after experimental subarachnoid hemorrhage in rabbits. Stroke 1998; 29:1930–1935; discussion 1935–1936.

127. Clatterbuck RE, Gailloud P, Ogata L, et al. Prevention of cerebral vasospasm by a humanized anti-CD11/CD18 monoclonal antibody administered after experimental subarachnoid hemorrhage in nonhuman primates. J Neurosurg 2003; 99:376–382.

128. Fassbender K, Hodapp B, Rossol S, et al. Inflammatory cytokines in subarachnoid haemorrhage: association with abnormal blood flow velocities in basal cerebral arteries. J Neurol Neurosurg Psychiatr 2001; 70:534–537.

129. Suzuki S, Sobata E, Iwabuchi T. Prevention of cerebral ischemic symptoms in cerebral vasospasm with trapidil, an antagonist and selective synthesis inhibitor of thromboxane A2. Neurosurgery 1981; 9:679–685.

130. Nosko M, Weir B, Krueger C, et al. Nimodipine and chronic vasospasm in monkeys: Part 1. Clinical and radiological findings. Neurosurgery 1985; 16:129–136.

131. Kawamura S, Sayama I, Yasui N, Uemura K. Sequential changes in cerebral blood flow and metabolism in patients with subarachnoid haemorrhage. Acta Neurochir (Wien) 1992; 114:12–15.

132. Hino A, Mizukawa N, Tenjin H, et al. Postoperative hemodynamic and metabolic changes in patients with subarachnoid hemorrhage. Stroke 1989; 20:1504–1510.

133. Grubb RL Jr., Raichle ME, Eichling JO, Gado MH. Effects of subarachnoid hemorrhage on cerebral blood volume, blood flow, and oxygen utilization in humans. J Neurosurg 1977; 46:446–453.

134. Yundt KD, Grubb RL Jr., Diringer MN, Powers WJ. Autoregulatory vasodilation of parenchymal vessels is impaired during cerebral vasospasm. J Cereb Blood Flow Metab 1998; 18:419–424.

135. Voldby B, Enevoldsen EM, Jensen FT. Cerebrovascular reactivity in patients with ruptured intracranial aneurysms. J Neurosurg 1985; 62:59–67.

136. Darby JM, Yonas H, Marks EC, et al. Acute cerebral blood flow response to dopamine-induced hypertension after subarachnoid hemorrhage. J Neurosurg 1994; 80:857–864.
137. Touho H, Karasawa J, Ohnishi H, et al. Evaluation of therapeutically induced hypertension in patients with delayed cerebral vasospasm by xenon-enhanced computed tomography. Neurol Med Chir (Tokyo) 1992; 32:671–678.
138. Nornes H, Knutzen HB, Wikeby P. Cerebral arterial blood flow and aneurysm surgery. Part 2: Induced hypotension and autoregulatory capacity. J Neurosurg 1977; 47:819–827.
139. Hassler W, Chioffi F. CO2 reactivity of cerebral vasospasm after aneurysmal subarachnoid haemorrhage. Acta Neurochir (Wien) 1989; 98:167–175.

4 | Surgical Management of Aneurysmal Subarachnoid Hemorrhage

Quoc-Anh Thai, MD, Assistant Chief of Service, Instructor
Gustavo Pradilla, MD, Resident
Daniele Rigamonti, MD, FACS, Vice-Chairman and Professor
Department of Neurosurgery, Johns Hopkins University School of Medicine, Johns Hopkins Medical Institutions, Baltimore, Maryland, USA

INTRODUCTION

Aneurysmal subarachnoid hemorrhage (aSAH) is caused by the rupture of intracranial aneurysms. Although it represents a small proportion of cerebrovascular accidents, aSAH leads to a disproportionately high morbidity and mortality. Twenty-five percent of cerebrovascular mortality is due to aSAH (1), which represents only 3% of all strokes (2). The case-fatality rate is reported to be between 25% and 67% (1,3). Of those who survive, 50% have a disability requiring aid in performing activities of daily living (1,4). Refinements of diagnostic tools, such as computed tomography angiography (CTA) and magnetic resonance angiography (MRA), as well as the advent of therapeutic options in the field of endovascular interventional neuroradiology, have facilitated treatment for these patients, but they have also presented new challenges in management decisions for health care professionals. In this chapter, we will focus on the surgical management of aSAH and briefly discuss the presentation, diagnosis, and grading of SAH, as well as the prognostic factors and treatment options.

CLINICAL PRESENTATION OF aSAH

Chapter 7 contains a detailed review of the clinical presentation of aSAH. In brief, the classic clinical presentation is the sudden onset of a severe headache, often described as the "worst headache of my life." Approximately 50% of patients with SAH report an instantaneous onset, and the other half describe its onset in seconds or minutes (5). Signs of meningismus, with complaints of nuchal discomfort or changes in mental status, often follow the headache in patients with a ruptured aneurysm. The blood can also cause irritation of the meninges and result in photophobia, neck soreness/stiffness, Brudzinski's sign, Kernig's sign, and even a low-grade fever that occurs within 6 to 24 hr after an aSAH (6). As a result of the thick blood clots in the basal cisterns, a communicating hydrocephalus can develop, and, in cases with intraventricular hemorrhages (IVHs), a noncommunicating hydrocephalus can occur from blockage of the foramina of Magendie and Luschka, resulting in the characteristic dilatation of all 4 ventricles (7).

DIAGNOSIS OF SUBARACHNOID HEMORRHAGE AND ANEURYSMS

The first diagnostic test for a suspected aSAH is a noncontrast head CT (Fig. 1). The sensitivity of detecting an aSAH within the first 24 hr of hemorrhage is 92% and decreases by about 7% each 24 hr thereafter (8). A false positive may occur in the rare case of generalized brain edema that causes venous congestion in the subarachnoid space, mimicking an aSAH (9). The Fisher Scale (Table 1) assigns a numeric rating of the hemorrhage and facilitates prediction of the risk for vasospasm by grading the amount of blood on initial presentation.

In suspected aSAH cases, if the head CT is not diagnostic, a lumbar puncture is mandatory. The lumbar puncture remains the most sensitive test for aSAH. Once a hemorrhage occurs in the subarachnoid space and blood becomes mixed in the cerebrospinal fluid (CSF), sufficient lysis of the red blood cells and formation of bilirubin and oxyhemoglobin form within 6 to 12 hr

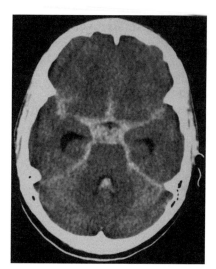

Figure 1 Noncontrast head computed tomography showing aneurysmal subarachnoid hemorrhage. Acute blood in the subarachnoid space appears as diffuse hyperintensities in the chiasmatic, Sylvian, and interhemispheric cisterns. Also note intraventricular hemorrhage in the fourth ventricle associated with hydrocephalus (enlarged temporal horns).

(9), giving the CSF a yellow tinge, or xanthochromia, after centrifugation. Therefore, in addition to routine CSF labs, CSF bilirubin should be checked.

The gold standard in the diagnosis of aneurysms is intra-arterial (IA) digital subtraction angiography. This enables visualization of the aneurysm in relation to its parent vessel, definition of the collateral circulation, and assessment for vasospasm. To assess all of these characteristics thoroughly, it is imperative that the angiogram includes contrast injection of both carotid arteries and both vertebral arteries a 4-vessel angiogram), with multiple views (anteroposterior, lateral, and oblique) of each injection. The risk of such a study in qualified centers is very low. One meta-analysis reported a transient or permanent neurologic complication risk of 1.8% in patients with aSAH and 0.3% in patients without aSAH (10). The risk of permanent neurologic damage is as low as 0.09% (11).

Procedural risks are eliminated in MRA or CTA, but their detection rate is lower. They are especially useful in planning for surgery when definition of the surrounding anatomy is necessary, as three-dimensional reconstruction with interactive manipulation of the views is possible. However, they remain inadequate replacements for IA angiography in the diagnosis of aneurysms at this time. Direct comparisons of CTA and MRA with IA angiograms showed that the accuracy of CTA/MRA is approximately 90% and is improving (12). CTA sensitivity and specificity are 91% and 95%, respectively (13). In the period prior to 1995, CTA accuracy was 84%, and in the period subsequent to that, it was 93% (12). MRA sensitivity and specificity have been reported at 83% and 97%, respectively (14). However, the detection rate decreases dramatically with smaller aneurysms and becomes negligible for sizes less than 3 mm. MRA accuracy is reported at 90% and has not changed significantly. Although further improvements are expected for these noninvasive tests, IA angiograms remain the gold standard for detection of intracranial aneurysms. Therefore, it is crucial that patients with suspected aSAH have the following tests in this order: 1) noncontrast head CT, 2) lumbar puncture if head CT is nondiagnostic, and 3) IA angiography in cases with confirmed aSAH.

Table 1 The Fisher Scale Grades the Amount of Hemorrhage on a Diagnostic Head Computed Tomography, Which Then Can Be Used to Assess for Risk of Vasospasm

Fisher grade	Blood on computed tomography (direct measurement, no calibration to actual thickness)
1	No subarachnoid blood detected
2	Diffuse or vertical layers <1 mm thick
3	Localized clot and/or vertical layer <1 mm thick
4	Intracerebral or intraventricular clot with diffuse or no aSAH

Abbreviation: aSAH, aneurysmal subarachnoid hemorrhage.

Table 2 The Glasgow Coma Scale Assesses Patient's Mental State on Arrival

Points	Best eye	Best verbal	Best motor
6	N/A	N/A	Obeys
5	N/A	Oriented	Localizes pain
4	Spontaneous	Confused	Withdraws to pain
3	To speech	Inappropriate	Flexor (decorticate)
2	To pain	Incomprehensible	Extensor (decerebrate)
1	None	None	None

GRADING AND PROGNOSIS OF aSAH

The single most important predictor of outcome after an aSAH is the presenting level of consciousness. The mental status and consciousness level seen during triage are routinely quantified by health care personnel using the Glasgow Coma Scale (GCS) (Table 2). The assessments of eye opening, verbal responses, and motor commands contribute to the initial assessment and reflect the sum of the other prognostic factors associated with SAH, such as extent of hemorrhage, injury to the brain, size of ruptured aneurysm, patient's age, contributing medical illnesses, and others (15). Proper assessment of all these factors provides an accurate probability of outcome. The accuracy of assessment of all these factors greatly influences the accuracy of predicting outcome and, therefore, greatly influences patient management decisions.

The Hunt and Hess SAH scale (16) (Table 3) was introduced to quantify the severity of SAH and includes the signs of SAH, such as nuchal rigidity, cranial nerve palsy, hemiparesis, and others. The scale also relied on the patients' subjective report of their headache. Although these integrated assessments result in a strong predictive factor, the subjective components of the scale are vulnerable to variances in interpretation between different examiners and examinees. For example, "mild" versus "moderate" headaches reported by the patient could change the rating of SAH severity. The reported high interobserver disagreement (15) makes the scale less reliable.

The World Federation of Neurological Surgeons (WFNS) scale (Table 4) eliminates the subjective aspects of the Hunt and Hess scale and incorporates the GCS score as the basis for grading SAH. It effectively uses the objective criteria of the GCS to yield a WFNS SAH scale. Although this scale is easier to memorize and use, its categories have not been validated clinically.

The GCS for grading SAH (17) remains the simplest scale to use, with the highest predictive value for discharge GCS and lowest interobserver variability. The GCS SAH scale incorporates the clinically validated GCS as the objective criteria for grading aSAH (Table 5), utilizing a known scoring system and eliminating any subjective aspects. The GCS SAH Grade I is equivalent to a GCS of 15. Thereafter, the GCS SAH grade increases by 1 for decremental changes of 3 points on the GCS. For example, GCS SAH Grade II equals GCS of 14, 13, or 12, and GCS SAH Grade III equals GCS of 11, 10, or 9, etc. This facilitates memorization, but even if the initial care providers do not know the GCS SAH scale, their record of the GCS, itself, is documentation of the SAH scale. The validity of the GCS SAH scale is clear in direct comparison with the Hunt and Hess and WFNS scales (17). In our opinion, the high predictive value, low interobserver variability, and ease of use make the GCS SAH scale a preferred scale.

COMPLICATIONS AFTER aSAH

The major initial complications after an aSAH associated with high morbidity and mortality are hydrocephalus and rebleeding. Hydrocephalus is present radiographically in 15% to 20%

Table 3 Hunt and Hess Subarachnoid Hemorrhage Scale

Grade	Clinical assessment
I	Asymptomatic or mild headache
II	Moderate to severe headache, nuchal rigidity, cranial nerve palsy
III	Lethargy, confusion, mild focal deficit
IV	Stupor, moderate to severe hemiparesis, early decerebrate rigidity
V	Deep coma, decerebrate rigidity, moribund

Table 4 World Federation of Neurological Surgeons Subarachnoid Hemorrhage Scale

Grade	GCS and clinical assessment
I	15
II	13–14, without focal deficit
III	13–14, with focal deficit
IV	7–12
V	3–6

Abbreviation: GCS, Glasgow Coma Scale.

of patients with aSAH on admission (18), and an additional 3% develop hydrocephalus within 1 week after aSAH (19), resulting in shunt-dependent hydrocephalus in more than 20% of all aSAH patients (20–23). When associated with IVH, CSF outflow is blocked at the foramina of Magendie and Luschka, resulting in a noncommunicating 4-ventricle dilation hydrocephalus (7). However, approximately 50% of patients with hydrocephalus do not have radiographically evident IVH (18). When decreasing mental status is in the setting of hydrocephalus, the standard of care is insertion of an intraventricular catheter for external CSF drainage, which can be done under standard sterility at the bedside and improves the level of consciousness in 78% of patients (19). However, rebleeding rate is reported to increase to 43% with intraventricular drainage, versus 15% in patients without drainage (19). To prevent this dreadful complication, it is recommended to set the initial pop-off pressure at ≥20 mmHg to prevent the creation of a pressure gradient that could cause re-rupture of the aneurysm.

Rebleeding increases morbidity and mortality significantly. One study reported a mortality rate for rebleeding of 80%, compared to 41% in patients without rebleeding (24). Rebleeding is a major risk in all patients with aSAH within the first 24 hr and remains high during the first 2 weeks. The actual rate is unknown but has been reported to be as high as 15% (25) in the initial hours. Afterward, the rate of rebleeding drops to 1.5% per day and continues to decline over the next 2 weeks. The total risk of rebleeding for the first 2 weeks has been reported at 19% (25). Considering the high mortality associated with rebleeding and the incidence of early rebleeding, prompt medical and surgical management is critical in the setting of an aSAH.

SURGICAL INTERVENTION

The high risks of rebleeding, poor medical management options for treating vasospasm in the setting of an unsecured aneurysm, and time course of vasospasm are all factors that make prompt, definitive surgical intervention the best therapy. Neurosurgical treatment of aneurysms began in 1937, when Walter Dandy surgically treated the first aneurysm patient at Johns Hopkins Hospital. Modern microsurgical treatment of aneurysm evolved in the 1960s and 1970s under the innovative leadership of Charles Drake and Gazi Yasargil, who incorporated the use of the operating microscope for clipping of aneurysms. Since then, the techniques of microneurosurgery and skull-base surgery have reached maturity, and aneurysm clips are routinely used to occlude the neck of the aneurysm and exclude the weak saccular portion from the cerebral circulation.

Table 5 Glasgow Coma Scale for Aneurysmal Subarachnoid Hemorrhage

Grade	GCS score
I	15
II	14–12
III	11–9
IV	8–6
V	5–3

Abbreviation: GCS, Glasgow Coma Scale.

Timing of surgery is essential in achieving optimal outcome, and the time course of vasospasm is the major consideration. "Early surgery" has been advocated for several obvious practical reasons. Prompt clipping of an aneurysm eliminates the risk of rebleeding, which is theoretically associated with increased morbidity and mortality. Also, once an aneurysm is secured, treatment of vasospasm is facilitated with the use of triple-H therapy (hypertension, hypervolemia, and hemodilution), an option that is dangerous in an unsecured aneurysm. Vasospasm and edema may complicate surgery that is delayed from 7 to 10 days after aSAH, when vasospasm is at its peak. Another surgical option is that of "late surgery," in which clipping is accomplished after 12 to 14 days, when vasospasm has resolved and edema has subsided. The Cooperative Study on the Timing of Aneurysm Surgery showed that the results of early surgery were equivalent to those of late surgery (26,27). This was a prospective observational study involving 3521 patients from 60 centers collected over a period of 2.5 years. Comparably good outcomes were reported for surgery that was performed on days 0 to 3 (63%) and days 4 to 6 (60%) post-aSAH. Delayed surgery on days 11 to 14 post-aSAH also yielded similar results (62%), as did late surgery on days 15 to 32 (63%). Surgery during days 7 to 10 after aSAH had the worst outcome, and this period coincides with the peak of vasospasm.

The intraoperative dissection technique is crucial for aneurysm clipping. Using an operating microscope, dissection should focus on sharply separating arachnoid tissues to facilitate separation of vascular structures from the parenchyma. The first goal of the dissection is to gain proximal control. Prior to attempting dissection near the aneurysm, the surgeon must be able to emergently occlude the vessel that supplies the aneurysm in the case of an intraoperative rupture. In cases in which intracranial proximal control is not an option (e.g., ophthalmic artery aneurysms), an extracranial neck dissection for proximal control is required prior to the craniotomy. Blunt dissection should be avoided, especially near the aneurysm due to the high risk of tearing the frail dome. Also, a blunt tear is much more difficult to repair than a punctate tear made using sharp dissection techniques. Once the aneurysm is reached, meticulous dissection of the aneurysm neck is required, to ensure optimal clip placement and to reduce iatrogenic rupture of the aneurysm.

Temporary arterial occlusion is a useful option to aid in the surgical dissection and, ultimately, in the clipping of aneurysms. This technique, when used properly, can reduce the risk of intraoperative rupture when dissecting near the aneurysm, can facilitate optimal placement of the permanent clip, and is indicated in cases where more involved neck dissection is required and those in which extensive adhesions are located near the aneurysm. Prior to applying temporary clips, hemodynamic status must be stable and the patient's intravascular volume and systemic blood pressure should be normalized (higher blood pressure should be maintained for hypertensive patients). The patient should be anesthetized to electroencephalographic burst suppression. The temporary arterial occlusion should be applied with a "temporary clip" that has a closing pressure approximately half that of a permanent clip. This will decrease the risk of intimal damage to the vessel. Although the exact placement of the temporary clip is case specific, the general guideline is that it should allow maximal aneurysm exposure while minimizing the risk of infarction.

The technique used in treating the aneurysm is as important as the dissection and application of the clip. Clip selection is crucial in excluding the aneurysm from the systemic circulation. Careful measurement of the aneurysm on the angiogram should be correlated with the intraoperative findings. The clip size should be at least 1.53× the diameter of the aneurysm, as application of the clip will lead to collapse and elongation of the neck of the aneurysm. In certain circumstances, application of a clip is not possible due to the anatomy or shape of the aneurysm. An alternative maneuver is wrapping the aneurysm, although the outcome of this technique is debatable. In another technique, called "trapping," clips are placed proximal and distal to the aneurysm to interrupt flow. Depending upon the anatomic location, this procedure can be associated with ischemic sequelae.

Post-clipping protocol is as important as pre-clipping protocol. Once the clip is in place, careful visual inspection must be made to ensure that optimal placement has occurred and no other vessels are compromised, especially in cases where the clip is placed too close to the parent vessel, decreasing its diameter. Papaverine is applied to all exposed and manipulated arteries to facilitate redilatation to premanipulation diameters. Then, intraoperative angiography is performed to ensure proper clip placement. Improper clip placement that requires reexploration and clip adjustment was seen on intraoperative angiography in 11% of the cases in one study (28).

Endovascular intervention for aneurysms is a more recent technique and is a promising minimally invasive option for the treatment of aneurysms. Endovascular interventional neuroradiology began in the 1970s, when Fedor Serbinenko used detachable latex balloons to occlude the supplying artery of the aneurysm or to occlude the aneurysm sac itself (29). Modern endovascular treatment of aneurysms started in 1991, when Guido Guglielmi introduced an electrolytic detachable platinum coil (Guglielmi detachable coils) (30,31). These coils are inserted through a femoral artery cannula via a microcatheter that can be threaded to the location of the aneurysm. The coils are then packed into the saccular portion and separated from the microcatheter by electrolysis, thus excluding the aneurysmal sac from cerebral circulation.

The use of endovascular coiling for the treatment of aneurysms is rapidly increasing worldwide, which is a reflection of improved coil design and refinements of techniques, as more centers subspecialize in this area. A few centers are reserving surgery as a back-up option when coiling is deemed unsuitable. It is estimated that approximately 1500 patients worldwide per month are being treated by endovascular coiling, and more than 100,000 patients with aneurysms have been treated with endovascular coiling (32).

The level of expertise at the neurosurgical center is a crucial determinant of outcome in patients who undergo surgical treatment of aneurysms, especially clipping. Microsurgical techniques of aneurysmal clipping are technically demanding and usually are not employed for most neurosurgical cases. The neurosurgical centers that treat the average patient population without a referral bias would typically not encounter a high volume of aneurysm patients, thus limiting the experience of the surgeons. A study on the effects of patient volume on the outcome of craniotomy and aneurysmal clipping showed that institutions that performed more than 30 craniotomies per year had a 43% reduction in mortality rates. Also, centers that performed more than 30 aneurysm clippings per year had a 43% reduction in mortality rates (33). Similar results have been noted in other studies, suggesting that patients with aSAH will have improved outcome if their surgery is performed at a high-volume institution.

CONCLUSION

aSAH remains a devastating problem, with high morbidity and mortality. Improvements in CTA and MRA have aided in the detection of aneurysms and have facilitated planning for intervention. Although their sensitivity and accuracy of detecting aneurysms (which have improved during the past decade) exceed 90%, the IA digital subtraction angiogram remains the gold standard for diagnosing aneurysms. Currently, aneurysm treatment should ideally be referred to specialized centers of excellence that have subspecialists in both cerebrovascular neurosurgery and endovascular interventional neuroradiology who perform a high volume of cases. The deciding factor for a good outcome is not necessarily the type of intervention, but the volume of procedures that have been performed at a particular center; center expertise can reduce mortality by 43% (33).

REFERENCES

1. Wardlaw JM, White PM. The detection and management of unruptured intracranial aneurysms. Brain 2000; 123(Pt 2):205–221.
2. Sudlow CL, Warlow CP. Comparable studies of the incidence of stroke and its pathological types: results from an international collaboration. International Stroke Incidence Collaboration. Stroke 1997; 28:491–499.
3. Hop JW, Rinkel GJ, Algra A, van Gijn J. Case-fatality rates and functional outcome after subarachnoid hemorrhage: a systematic review. Stroke 1997; 28:660–664.
4. Hijdra A, Braakman R, van Gijn J, Vermeulen M, van Crevel H. Aneurysmal subarachnoid hemorrhage. Complications and outcome in a hospital population. Stroke 1987; 18:1061–1067.
5. Linn FH, Rinkel GJ, Algra A, van Gijn J. Headache characteristics in subarachnoid haemorrhage and benign thunderclap headache. J Neurol Neurosurg Psychiatr 1998; 65:791–793.
6. Greenberg M. Handbook of Neurosurgery. Vol. 2. Lakeland: Greenberg Graphics, 1997.
7. Komotar RJ, Olivi A, Rigamonti D, Tamargo RJ. Microsurgical fenestration of the lamina terminalis reduces the incidence of shunt-dependent hydrocephalus after aneurysmal subarachnoid hemorrhage. Neurosurgery 2002; 51:1403–1412; discussion 1412–1413.
8. Osborn, Anne G. Diagnostic Neuroaudiology. St Louis, MI: Mosby; 1994.

9. van Gijn J, Rinkel GJ. Subarachnoid haemorrhage: diagnosis, causes, and management. Brain 2001; 124:249–278.

10. Cloft HJ, Joseph GJ, Dion JE. Risk of cerebral angiography in patients with subarachnoid hemorrhage, cerebral aneurysm, and arteriovenous malformation: a meta-analysis. Stroke 1999; 30:317–320.

11. Crzyska U, Freitag J, Zeumer H. Selective cerebral intraarterial DSA. Complication rate and control of risk factors. Neuroradiology 1990; 32:296–299.

12. White PM, Wardlaw JM, Easton V. Can noninvasive imaging accurately depict intracranial aneurysms? A systematic review. Radiology 2000; 217:361–370.

13. Pedersen HK, Bakke SJ, Hald JK, et al. CTA in patients with acute subarachnoid haemorrhage. A comparative study with selective, digital angiography and blinded, independent review. Acta Radiol 2001; 42:43–49.

14. Raaymakers TW, Buys PC, Verbeeten B Jr., et al. MR angiography as a screening tool for intracranial aneurysms: feasibility, test characteristics, and interobserver agreement. Am J Roentgenol 1999; 173:1469–1475.

15. Tamargo RJ, Walter KA, Oshiro EM. Aneurysmal subarachnoid hemorrhage: prognostic features and outcomes. New Horiz 1997; 5:364–375.

16. Hunt WE, Hess RM. Surgical risk as related to time of intervention in the repair of intracranial aneurysms. J Neurosurg 1968; 28:14–20.

17. Oshiro EM, Walter KA, Piantadosi S, Witham TF, Tamargo RJ. A new subarachnoid hemorrhage grading system based on the Glasgow Coma Scale: a comparison with the Hunt and Hess and World Federation of Neurological Surgeons Scales in a clinical series. Neurosurgery 1997; 41:140–147; discussion 147–148.

18. Suarez-Rivera O. Acute hydrocephalus after subarachnoid hemorrhage. Surg Neurol 1998; 49:563–565.

19. Hasan D, Vermeulen M, Wijdicks EF, Hijdra A, van Gijn J. Management problems in acute hydrocephalus after subarachnoid hemorrhage. Stroke 1989; 20:747–753.

20. Auer LM, Mokry M. Disturbed cerebrospinal fluid circulation after subarachnoid hemorrhage and acute aneurysm surgery. Neurosurgery 1990; 26:804–808; discussion 808–809.

21. Gjerris F, Borgesen SE, Sorensen PS, et al. Resistance to cerebrospinal fluid outflow and intracranial pressure in patients with hydrocephalus after subarachnoid haemorrhage. Acta Neurochir (Wien) 1987; 88:79–86.

22. Grant JA, McLone DG. Third ventriculostomy: a review. Surg Neurol 1997; 47:210–212.

23. Joakimsen O, Mathiesen EB, Monstad P, Selseth B. CSF hydrodynamics after subarachnoid hemorrhage. Acta Neurol Scand 1987; 75:319–327.

24. Rosenorn J, Eskesen V, Schmidt K, Ronde F. The risk of rebleeding from ruptured intracranial aneurysms. J Neurosurg 1987; 67:329–332.

25. Kassell NF, Torner JC. Aneurysmal rebleeding: a preliminary report from the Cooperative Aneurysm Study. Neurosurgery 1983; 13:479–481.

26. Kassell NF, Torner JC, Haley EC Jr., Jane JA, Adams HP, Kongable GL. The International Cooperative Study on the Timing of Aneurysm Surgery. Part 1: Overall management results. Neurosurg 1990; 73:18–36.

27. Kassell NF, Torner JC, Jane JA, Haley EC Jr., Adams HP. The International Cooperative Study on the Timing of Aneurysm Surgery. Part 2: Surgical results. J Neurosurg 1990; 73:37–47.

28. Chiang VL, Gailloud P, Murphy KJ, Rigamonti D, Tamargo RJ. Routine intraoperative angiography during aneurysm surgery. J Neurosurg 2002; 96:988–992.

29. Serbinenko FA. Balloon catheterization and occlusion of major cerebral vessels. J Neurosurg 1974; 41:125–145.

30. Guglielmi G, Vinuela F, Dion J, Duckwiler G. Electrothrombosis of saccular aneurysms via endovascular approach. Part 2: Preliminary clinical experience. J Neurosurg 1991; 75:8–14.

31. Guglielmi G, Vinuela F, Sepetka I, Macellari V. Electrothrombosis of saccular aneurysms via endovascular approach. Part 1: Electrochemical basis, technique, and experimental results. J Neurosurg 1991; 75:1–7.

32. Hopkins LN, Lanzino G, Guterman LR. Treating complex nervous system vascular disorders through a "needle stick": origins, evolution, and future of neuroendovascular therapy. Neurosurgery 2001; 48:463–475.

33. Solomon RA, Mayer SA, Tarmey JJ. Relationship between the volume of craniotomies for cerebral aneurysm performed at New York state hospitals and in-hospital mortality. Stroke 1996; 27:13–17.

5 | Endovascular Management of a Patient After Subarachnoid Hemorrhage

Stephen Chang, MD, Resident
Abhishek Srinivas, MD, Fellow
Division of Interventional Neuroradiology, The Johns Hopkins Hospital, Baltimore, Maryland, USA

Kieran Murphy, MD, FRCPC, Associate Professor
Director of Interventional Neuroradiology, Department of Radiology,
Johns Hopkins University School of Medicine, Baltimore, Maryland, USA

INTRODUCTION

Just as Darwin introduced the concept of evolution as occurring by quantum leaps, so the endovascular management of intracranial aneurysms represents medical quantum evolution. We are used to physicians moving jobs but not losing or changing jobs. Image-guided therapy is, in Business Language lingo, a "destructive" technology that is redistributing the care of patients with intracranial aneurysms amongst new tribes of physicians called "endovascular neurosurgeons" or "neurointerventional radiologists." Our job is to best inform the patient of their therapeutic options and ensure that they are equally safe in all hands. A discussion of these options follows.

Aneurysmal subarachnoid hemorrhage (aSAH) represents the most common nontraumatic etiology of subarachnoid hemorrhage (SAH). CT scan is 95% (1) sensitive in detecting SAH (2). In approximately 94% of patients with a spontaneous SAH, angiography will detect a causal lesion, principally, an aneurysm (3). In 6% of cases, no cause will be identified; these are considered angionegative SAH. Current management strategies include repeating cerebral angiography after 7 to 10 days, during which a number of patients will rebleed. One study found that, in 15% of patients with spontaneous SAH, the source of bleeding could not be determined despite repeat angiography; most of these patients will have a very typical perimesencephalic distribution of SAH (4). It has been suggested that magnetic resonance angiography (MRA), in conjunction with CT results, be performed in patients with SAH of unknown etiology before catheter angiography is repeated (3). Patients with angiographically negative SAH have a better course, with better neurologic status, fewer complications, and better outcomes, than patients with positive findings on angiogram; therefore, it has been suggested that repeat angiograms be performed only on patients with atypical blood distribution for angionegative SAH (5). Repeat angiography plays an important role in defining the site of an initially occult aneurysm, particularly if the initial angiogram was compromised by vasospasm or if one part of the vascular tree was not optimally visualized (6).

TEAM- AND CONSENSUS-BASED APPROACH TO ANEURYSM CARE

Recent studies have shown that the presence of both endovascular and surgical treatment options creates better patient outcomes (7,8). A combined team approach of direct surgery and endovascular coiling has been shown to lead to good outcomes in the treatment for paraclinoid aneurysms, where patients with higher-risk lesions were offered the option of endovascular treatment (9), an approach supported by many other groups.

ENDOVASCULAR MANAGEMENT FOLLOWING aSAH

Treatment of acute aSAH consists of occluding the aneurysm to prevent rebleed, attempting to prevent vasospasm, and maintaining blood flow to the brain through vessels in vasospasm. Endovascular treatment has been shown to be as safe as, or safer than, surgical clipping for patients with aSAH. A comparison of surgical clipping and endovascular treatment in 109 patients with acute aSAH found comparable survival rates, recovery rates, and neuropsychologic test scores among recovered patients from both groups and a statistically significant increase in superficial brain retraction injury and ischemic lesion among surgical patients (10). Another study demonstrated endovascular coiling of aSAH to cause less structural damage than surgery, but cognitive outcome was primarily determined by resulting complications (11).

COILING

In patients with whom both techniques are possible, several studies have found that endovascular therapy is preferable to surgery, because it carries a lower risk of adverse outcomes and in-hospital death, shorter length of hospital stay, and decreased hospital charges (12). A study that compared surgical clipping with endovascular coil embolization in the treatment of unruptured cerebral aneurysms reported statistically significant increases in adverse outcomes, length of stay, and hospital charges for surgical clipping (13). In-hospital mortality was also increased, but the difference was not statistically significant. In another study, surgical patients were more likely than coiled patients to experience symptoms, disability, and longer recovery rates (14). Further, Guglielmi detachable coil (GDC)–treated intracranial aneurysms resulted in only a 2.5% rate of rupture and a 1% rate of treatment-related death (15), whereas another group had a 0% rate of aneurysmal rupture and mortality (16).

DEVELOPMENTS

Surgical clipping had been the established modality of treatment for ruptured and unruptured cerebral aneurysms until 1991, when GDC embolization was introduced as an alternative method for treating selected aneurysm patients. Endovascular treatment has since evolved based on enhanced clinical experience and technologic improvements. Selection of aneurysms appropriate for coiling has improved, and over the last decade, the range of coils was increased, with the availability of multidimensional coils that allow safer initial coil placement and the development of softer coils (17).

Endovascular therapy is now a well-established treatment modality for a variety of cerebrovascular central nervous system disorders. Dramatic improvements in the field of neuroendovascular surgery have been made, including the development of techniques that provide treatment options for conditions previously thought to be untreatable.

Over the past 15 years, flexible microcatheters have been developed, which allow navigation to the distal intracranial and spinal circulation by percutaneous cannulation of the femoral artery or vein. Techniques to embolize aneurysms, including occlusion of parent arteries and endosaccular packing, have evolved to treat previously inoperable aneurysms. Advances in coil technology have also focused on coating applications that modify the biologic reaction to the coil surface. Recent advances have been made in gene therapy, which might allow for the enhancement of direct gene transfer *in situ* by coated coils (18). Ongoing device developments and technologic advances and refinements continue to revolutionize the field of neuroendovascular therapy. Combined with a better clinical understanding of disease pathophysiology, minimally invasive neuroendovascular techniques are rapidly providing treatment options for a wide spectrum of neurologic diseases (19).

SKILL ACQUISITION

Several studies have shown that procedural outcomes are better at high-volume institutions, because of either greater physician experience or methods of practice. Hospitals with low volumes of aSAH cases were found to have 40% greater odds of patient death in-hospital, compared to hospitals with high case volumes (20). Evidence suggests that the perfecting of endovascular procedures involves a learning curve. In a study that showed that the risk of complications with coil embolization of unruptured aneurysms decreased dramatically with physician experience (21), complications occurred in 53% of the first 5 cases that each of 3 physicians treated, and in only 10% of later cases. Similarly, a second study concluded that 90% of complications occurred in the first half of procedures involving an endoluminal graft, demonstrating a clear learning and development curve (22). Yet another study reported a steep learning curve associated with GDC use in treating aneurysms, finding operator experience critical in achieving optimal therapeutic results (23).

STENT ASSISTANCE

Wide-necked and fusiform aneurysms present distinct challenges for interventional neuroradiologists and neurosurgeons, because the aneurysms can involve entire vessels or be irregular in shape. Coils might migrate after deployment, with a potential to occlude the vessel or to embolize. In these circumstances, stent-assisted coiling has proven its utility. In a study of stent-assisted endovascular coil occlusion of wide-necked saccular intracranial aneurysms, it was found that 100% of patients achieved 95% occlusion or better with the aid of a self-expanding microstent (24). The long-term durability of endovascular occlusion of wide-necked cerebral aneurysms has been improved with stent-assisted coiling, resulting in improved aneurysmal occlusion and fewer cases of parent-vessel occlusion (25,26).

Stent-assisted coiling has also been documented in the treatment of wide-necked bifurcation aneurysms, a finding that might have implications for the management of basilar apex and other bifurcation aneurysms (27,28). Successful coiling of a wide-necked basilar bifurcation aneurysm with the use of self-expanding stents in a Y-configuration, double-stent-assisted technique has been reported (27). Furthermore, intracranial vertebral artery dissection has been successfully treated by intravascular stent and endosaccular GDC coils, skirting the hemodynamic complications of the usual technique of balloon occlusion of the vertebral artery (VA). The stenting–coiling association option appears to preserve arterial flow and maintain selective occlusion of the aneurysmal pouch (29). A combination of endovascular stenting and coil packing holds promise as a favorable alternative for the treatment of intracranial aneurysms that are otherwise unsuitable for surgical clipping or coil embolization.

However, despite the promise of stent-assisted coiling, several potential complications must be addressed. Cases of stent malposition within large aneurysms, including dislodgement during microcatheterization, stent movement after deployment, stent movement during coiling, and vasospasm during stenting, have been reported in the literature (26,30,31). In particular, early versions of the Neuroform stent were difficult to pass through tortuous vessels and presented the risk of migration because of their softness (31). Additionally, stent deployment has been documented to result in immediate rupture of the artery (32).

BALLOON ASSISTANCE

In addition to stent-assisted coiling, balloon-assisted coiling is a possible technique for the management of broad-necked cerebral aneurysms. Balloons are currently used to temporarily occlude parent vessels of aneurysms to determine adequacy of collateral flow, as in treatment of carotid ophthalmic artery aneurysms (33). Recently, several studies have demonstrated the efficacy and safety of balloon-assisted GDC (BAGDC) therapy for wide-necked aneurysms or aneurysms with a neck-to-body ratio close to 1 (34–36). GDC therapy presents challenges for interventional radiologists because of the risk of coil migration or coil protrusion into the parent vessel. By using a microcatheter-mounted nondetachable balloon to provide a temporary barrier across the aneurysmal neck, GDCs were deployed safely within a variety of aneurysms, resulting in a 90.9% rate of good-to-excellent clinical outcomes (34). A 100% rate of 95% to 100% aneurysm embolization of wide-necked intracranial aneurysms was reported in another study, with 96% of patients remaining at their preprocedure neurologic baseline (37). It was found that balloon assistance helps by forcing the coil to assume the 3D shape of the aneurysm without impinging on the parent artery, while also stabilizing the microcatheter in the aneurysm during coil delivery (37). BAGDC also allows more-dense intra-aneurysmal coil packing without parent-artery compromise than does the use of GDCs alone (38).

As with stent assistance, balloon assistance is associated with several complications that must be resolved. aSAH-induced vasospasm followed by hemorrhagic infarction, as well as several cases of intra-arterial thrombus, has been reported at the site of balloon deployment (37), and thromboembolic complication rates of up to 18% have been reported (35). This technique also occasionally results in subtotal or incomplete aneurysmal occlusion, with a correlation between aneurysm size and occlusion rate (36). BAGDC also produces a temporary rise in intra-aneurysmal pressure, a sudden change that might contribute to rupture (39). Furthermore, the technique increases technical complexity, due to the manipulation of a second microcatheter and an inflatable balloon (34).

MATRIX OR PGA/PGLA COATINGS ON COILS

Acceleration of intra-aneurysmal clot organization and fibrosis might help prevent aneurysmal recanalization after endovascular treatment. Matrix coils are platinum coils coated with an absorbable polyglycolic-polylactic acid (PGLA) copolymer. Approximately 70% of the coil volume comprises PGLA coating, which is typically absorbed by the body within 90 days. Although the amount of platinum per coil is the same in GDC-10 coils and Matrix coils, the additional biodegradable copolymer coating contributes to a larger diameter. The manufacturer claims that this attribute offers several advantages over bare platinum coils, such as increased packing density and an accelerated conversion of thrombus. However, because the polymer coating is not radio-opaque, radiolucent gaps appear between adjacent coils, which might lead to a false sense of assurance for the neurointerventional radiologist when attempting a dense, tightly packed coil.

A comparison of the efficacy of packing with Matrix versus GDC coils revealed that, 14 days postprocedure, the angiographic measurement of neointimal thickness at aneurysmal neck level showed statistically significant differences between Matrix- and GDC-treated aneurysms (0.41 mm for Matrix vs. 0.25 mm for GDC), whereas 3-month angiograms revealed that aneurysms treated with Matrix coils were 18% smaller than baseline, but GDC-treated aneurysms remained essentially unchanged (40). However, although neck tissue thickness was higher in Matrix-treated aneurysms up to 3 months later, no difference was seen at 6 months. It was concluded that Matrix coils accelerated aneurysm fibrosis and neointima formation without parent-artery stenosis (40).

DETACHMENT SYSTEMS

Some research has been conducted recently in new detachment systems. The mainstay of detachable coiling systems, GDC, uses an electric current to facilitate detachment. Although this method is effective, it takes several minutes to fully detach (41), and the time required for electrolytic detachment becomes progressively prolonged as more coils are placed. One study found that laser-activated, detachable coil devices, while effective in embolizing aneurysms, allow for detachment within a matter of seconds (42). In addition, innovative mechanically detachable systems, such as the Detach-18 Coil System (DCS), show great promise. DCS uses a J-shaped coil, which is suitable for use in giant aneurysms (43). A study comparing DCS to GDC found the DCS system to detach faster, within a mean time of 21 sec, and using a combination of GDC and DCS was found to optimize cost and operating time (44). A general drawback of mechanically detachable designs is their preclusion of the ability to retract the coil, once it has been completely advanced beyond the catheter tip. An evaluation of a microcatheter-based retrievable platinum coil detachment system that does not have this limitation found premature detachment in only 1 out of 229 coils (45).

CAP AND ONYX FOR ANEURYSMAL FILLING

Cellulose acetate polymer (CAP) solution is a new Japanese liquid embolic material dissolved in DMSO that has been used clinically for the thrombosis of cerebral aneurysms (46) and has been shown to be a safe and useful embolic agent for arteriovenous malformations (AVMs) (47). Longer-term follow-up studies are required to better evaluate the clinical safety and effectiveness of this solution. CAP was associated with complications, including aneurysmal rupture and parent-artery stenosis, as well as strong chemical corrosion, which led to acute chemical damage of the aneurysmal wall and inflammatory cell infiltration (48).

Onyx, another liquid embolic polymer based on CAP, has been proposed as an alternative treatment for aneurysms and AVMs. It is a biocompatible, nonadhesive liquid polymer that, upon contact with blood, precipitates and solidifies to form a soft and spongy embolus. One study achieved complete aneurysmal occlusion in 79% of cases and subtotal occlusion in 13%. Aneurysmal occlusion rates were concluded to be superior to those for coil occlusion, and treatment morbidity rates were comparable to those for coil occlusion (49). Another study reported good results in the treatment of 23 patients with AVMs (50).

Like CAP, Onyx is not without its drawbacks. An important limitation is the poor control of migration of Onyx into the parent artery. The use of assistance devices, such as microcoils, microstents, and balloons, help to achieve faster and more complete filling of the aneurysm with Onyx but do not completely preclude intractable migration of Onyx into the parent artery (51). Cases of transient and permanent neurologic deficits, SAH, massive reflux of Onyx into the afferent artery peduncle (52), and incomplete filling of the aneurysmal sac (52,53) have also been reported. Additionally, imaging of Onyx on MR and CT presented some challenges. Onyx appears hypointense on MR images, interferes with MRA in patients with stents, and creates artifacts that hinder CT evaluation (53). These disadvantages must be overcome before Onyx can play a greater role in endovascular treatment.

VESSEL OCCLUSION AS A METHOD OF TREATING ANEURYSMS

Vessel occlusion is a viable treatment technique for several types of aneurysms, including those that are difficult to access surgically, wide-necked, or large. An evaluation of the stability of intracranial berry aneurysmal occlusion with detachable coils found only a 14% recurrence rate of completely occluded aneurysms and a 0% rate of rebleeding (54). In a study in which 3 patients with peripheral cerebellar artery aneurysms were treated by parent-vessel occlusion, good or excellent clinical recovery was achieved by all patients, and parent-vessel occlusion was demonstrated to be feasible, safe, and effective (55). It has been suggested that parent-vessel occlusion be considered the first option for treatment of VA-dissecting pseudoaneurysms in patients who will tolerate sacrifice of the parent vessel along its diseased segment (56). Permanent occlusion of the VA for vertebrobasilar fusiform and dissecting aneurysms has also been proven as a useful therapeutic endovascular technique with good long-term outcomes (57). For large cavernous sinus aneurysms, proximal occlusion of the internal carotid artery (ICA) is the treatment of choice. Long-term follow-up of patients treated by proximal occlusion of the carotid artery by Silverstone clamping revealed neurologic improvement and no aneurysm rupture in 8 of 11 patients, although several complications were reported (58). The authors of the study suggested that therapeutic carotid artery occlusion be preceded by strict test ICA occlusion. Currently, Food and Drug Administration (FDA)-approved detachable silicon balloons are not available in the United States, a situation that is hampering clinical care.

BTO AND PREPROCEDURE ECIC BYPASS

Balloon test occlusion (BTO) is performed prior to vessel sacrifice to assess adequacy of collateral blood flow and cerebrovascular reserve. Claimed to be safe, reliable, and simple to perform, it has been used to evaluate a multitude of vessels, including the ICA (59), straight sinus (60), and ophthalmic artery (33). However, it has been found that test occlusion of the ICA still misses a significant number of patients with inadequate cerebrovascular reserve (61). Combination with a hypotensive challenge, whereby hypotension was induced to two-thirds of mean arterial blood pressure for 20 min or until a deficit was perceived, greatly increased the sensitivity of BTO, and the predictive value of a negative test was high (62). It is also recommended that patients who have undergone artery sacrifice be monitored in an intensive care unit for 48 hr to decrease the incidence of hypotension and resultant cerebrovascular ischemia (61).

In cases where BTO is positive, a preprocedure extracranial–intracranial (ECIC) arterial bypass is sometimes performed to improve cerebrovascular reserve. Although a key 1985 study found no benefit in the treatment of patients with extensive cerebrovascular disease by ECIC bypass, several more recent studies have demonstrated the procedure to be more promising, finding that it increases total brain blood supply and allows for the restoration of local perfusion in hemodynamically compromised brain tissue (63). Additionally, a retrospective study found that, following ECIC bypass, signs and symptoms were improved and risk for future cerebrovascular events was reduced (64). Angiography is the established means of assessing bypass patency, but MRA (65) and multislice CTA (66) appear to be effective imaging modalities as well. This adjunct is not fail-proof, however, as in the reported case of a patient who suffered a hemodynamic stroke despite ECIC bypass prior to permanent balloon occlusion (PBO); the consequent suggestion was to consider ECIC bypass before PBO in the event of reduction of more than 50% mean blood flow velocity on BTO (67).

VERTEBRAL DISSECTING ANEURYSMS

The natural history of dissecting vertebral artery aneurysms (DVAA) is not well described; however, once the artery is ruptured with SAH, high morbidity and mortality rates have been reported (68). DVAA are often caused by a shearing injury at the origin of the meningeal branch of the VA. Indeed, one study reported that 69% of patients rebled before they reached therapy; of these, 57% rebled within 24 hr, with a mortality rate of 46.7% (69). Other investigators have shown SAH with isolated vertebrobasilar dissection to have a rebleed rate of 30% to 70% within hours to weeks, including a fatality rate of approximately 50% (70–77). A recent study of endovascular management of vertebrobasilar dissecting aneurysms found the mortality rates in a treated group to be approximately 20% and, in the untreated group, approximately 50% (78). Thus, although these lesions are complicated and often treacherous, their high rebleed mortality rate warrants urgent aggressive management. These lesions can be complicated, requiring collaborative, often creative and innovative strategies, integrating the talents of the entire neuroscience team.

The first step in DVAA evaluation is a careful, selective 4-vessel cervicocerebral angiography to confirm abnormalities, including irregular and tapered luminal narrowing (secondary to the hematoma) with dilated segments, fusiform dilatation, ripple "wavy" dilations, delayed contrast flow/occlusion, and retention of contrast in the vessel wall or intimal flap (79). Importantly, associated multivessel dissections of the carotid or contralateral VA are found in up to two-thirds of VA dissections (80). Correlation of findings with CT and/or magnetic resonance imaging is mandatory to identify associated signs of brain stem infarct (lateral medullary syndrome), focal hematoma adjacent to the basilar artery in the prepontine cistern, or other posterior fossa abnormalities.

It is useful to review the histopathology of DVAA, because it helps to explain why aSAH can result from two different patterns of VA dissection, i.e., those isolated to the intradural V4 segment and those originating in the extradural cervical segment, extending into the intradural segment (79). The wall of the intradural V4 segment shows thin adventitial and muscular layers, absence of external elastic lamina and thicker internal elastic lamina, as compared to the extradural cervical segment of the VA (69,75,80–83). Thus, a subadvential dissection of the cervical VA is the culprit when VA dissection is associated with localized posterior fossa aSAH.

Surgical repair of these lesions is now rarely performed. Endovascular therapy depends on the location of the lesion. Most often, this requires a deconstructive trapping procedure, sacrificing the parent vessel of the aneurysm. However, the decision to use this procedure depends upon the lesion location, configuration, dominant VA, collateral circulation, adjacent branch involvement [posterior inferior cerebellar artery (PICA), anterior inferior cerebellar artery (AICA)], anterior spinal artery, or basilar artery), time of presentation, and, if possible, results of a BTO prior to permanent occlusion of the injured vessel to simulate the effects of permanent occlusion (78). Typically, if the disrupted segment is proximal to the origin of the PICA, the VA can be occluded proximal to PICA, such that flow is maintained to PICA from the contralateral VA via retrograde filling of the distal VA. If the disrupted segment is distal to the origin of the PICA, the VA is occluded distal to the PICA, and flow is maintained to the PICA from the ipsilateral VA.

Reconstructive procedures in DVAA are rarely indicated, but parent-vessel sparing has been safely performed, with variable success, combining stents and coils (56,84–89), stent-within-a-stent (90–92), and stent-grafts (93,94).

It is difficult to angiographically determine the dissected length of the injured VA. In fact, postmortem histology of the distal intracranial segment of an acute DVAA shows the wall to be primarily composed of clot (95). Thus, if reconstruction is attempted, it is important to remember that the healing process of the intradural VA is unpredictable, in part, because of the previously described normal histologic fragmentation of this segment. Furthermore, it is unknown if normal structural integrity will return. Thus, frequent imaging is warranted to monitor for interval regrowth or contained disruption (56).

VASOSPASM AFTER aSAH

For those who survive the initial event of aneurysmal rupture, the leading cause of morbidity and mortality has changed over the past 25 years. Previously, early rebleeding was the main culprit, but this has been minimized by early surgical repair (96). Today, cerebral vasospasm is the greatest threat to functional brain recovery and life. In fact, 7% of patients die of vasospasm (97), 7% have severe neurologic deficits associated with vasospasm (98), and another 20% have delayed ischemic neurologic deficits secondary to vasospasm (98). Although CT/CTA perfusion techniques are increasingly utilized (99,100), symptomatic vasospasm refractory to medical management therapy must be evaluated with 4-vessel cerebral angiography. Invariably, an angiographic vasospasm pattern is evident in most SAH patients on days 4 through 12. Balloon and chemical angioplasty with selective intra-arterial bolus injection of vasodilators are the options. The clinician guides the decision to treat. If the severe vasospasm involves the ICA, A1, or M1 segments, angioplasty has been shown to be technically feasible, with durable results and significant clinical improvement. If more distal cerebral artery involvement is detected, selective intra-arterial infusion of vasodilators has been shown to improve parenchymal perfusion by reducing the degree of vasospasm and, thus, improve outcome scores.

Papaverine is the only FDA-approved intra-arterial vasodilator. It is short lived but not without risk. Reported complications include rapid increases in intracranial pressure (which typically return to normal with discontinuance of papaverine infusion) (101), transient neurologic deficits (including mydriasis) (102), brain stem depression (103,104), monocular blindness (105), seizures (105,106), thrombocytopenia (107), precipitation of embolic crystals (108), and paradoxic exacerbation of vasospasm that leads to cerebral infarction (109). In fact, at higher concentrations, papaverine can precipitate in blood, which can also be embolic.

These issues have led clinical investigators to try other vasodilatory agents, with most interest centered around calcium entry blockers, such as nimodipine (110), nicardipine (111), and verapamil (112), which have shown promise in small numbers of patients. Duration of their effects is not known; however, because the drugs are infused locally, some believe their molecular nature causes deep penetration into the brain tissue, resulting in the desired prolonged effects. Best results might be obtained when treatment is begun within 2 hr of the onset of symptoms (113), but positive results might be seen up to 24 hr after onset (114,115).

GDC COILING AND INTRAVENTRICULAR rtPA AFTER ANEURYSM

Intraventricular hemorrhage and clotting is considered a predictor of poor outcome after SAH, leading to poor neurologic grade and acute hydrocephalus. Two patients who had ruptured cerebral aneurysms and extensive casting of their ventricular systems with blood were treated with GDC coiling and intraventricular recombinant tissue plasminogen activator (rtPA), after which clot resolution was demonstrated radiographically, and both had marked improvement in neurologic status (116). According to one study, patients treated with rtPA had a shorter length of stay, decreased mortality, and better Glasgow Outcome Scale and modified Rankin Scale scores at discharge, and they needed fewer interventions for hydrocephaly (117). However, some studies have reported hemorrhagic complications, such as epidural hematomas and hemorrhage extension, with intraventricular fibrinolysis (118). In addition, excessive amounts of intraventricular rtPA can cause additional brain tissue injury by way of intraventricular leukocytosis and edema of periventricular tissues and choroid plexus (119). One group hypothesized that these complications would be minimized with a lower dose of rtPA and found that intraventricular fibrinolysis was effective at a lower dose than previously reported in the literature (120).

INTRAOPERATIVE ANGIOGRAPHY AND OUTCOME OF CLIP POSITION IN THE OPERATING ROOM

Most surgeons prefer to avoid a second surgical attempt to treat residual or recurrent aneurysms after surgical clipping. Intraoperative angiography provides the benefit of visualizing residual aneurysm or unintended occlusion of parent vessels, thus allowing adjustment of the clip during the same operation. Although 88% of aneurysms treated by surgical clipping achieved complete aneurysmal closure in a study of patients with ruptured and unruptured aneurysms, ruptured, posterior circulation, and large/giant aneurysms were prone to incomplete clipping (121). The authors suggested that these aneurysms should receive either postoperative or intraoperative angiographic evaluation. At the same time, unexpected failures have been associated with clipping of numerous anterior circulation aneurysms, implying that intraoperative angiography could be beneficial (121). Findings on intraoperative angiography prompted reexploration and clip readjustment in 11% of clipped aneurysms in one study (122). False-negative and false-positive results were found in 12.5% of intraoperative angiograms, although only 2.6% of patients suffered complications (123). The benefits of intraoperative angiography must be weighed against the complications associated with repeated angiography and prolonged vascular access, in addition to possible false negatives and positives, but it appears that routine intraoperative angiography is safe and helpful in a significant number of cases.

POSTCOIL FOLLOW-UP—COIL COMPRESSION AND RECANALIZATION

Recurrent hemorrhage in the case of incompletely treated aneurysms is well known. A study of occlusion stability and long-term efficacy versus rebleeding in aSAH patients who were initially successfully treated with coil embolization discovered rebleeding in 7.9% of patients with recurrent aneurysms, and one case (0.4%) of rebleeding in patients who were stable by angiography, demonstrating the need for periodic follow-up angiography in order to identify patients with aneurysmal recurrence and high risk of rebleeding (124).

Despite posttreatment angiography, which demonstrates total aneurysmal occlusion, rebleeding is still a very real possibility. Recurrent aneurysms can be due to coil compaction, migration, or dislocation. Seven patients, 4 of whom received coiling, experienced recurrent aneurysmal ruptures, with a mean latency of 9.5 months from initial treatment (125). Several other cases have been reported in which rerupture of aneurysms occurred months to years after embolization—in some cases, despite angiographic occlusion on immediate postprocedural and 6-month angiographies (126). Reperfusion of the aneurysmal neck after coiling is not a rare complication and often necessitates renewed intervention (127). One study found major aneurysmal recurrences in 20.7% of coiled patients that appeared at a mean of 16.49 months after treatment, a small percentage of whom bled at a mean of 31.32 months after treatment (128). Because additional coiling of previously coiled aneurysms has a low procedural complication rate and decreases the risk of rebleeding (129), long-term monitoring of patients treated by endosaccular coiling is important to ensure optimal patient care.

NEW ANEURYSMS AND THE NEED FOR FOLLOW-UP

After adjustment for age and hypertension, female sex and cigarette smoking have been found to be independent risk factors for aneurysmal formation and growth (130). New formation of aneurysms at different sites have been reported up to 17 years after initial treatment for aneurysmal occlusion, implying a need for long-term follow-up by periodical cerebral angiography (58). In addition, 2 cases have been reported of *de novo* intracranial aneurysmal formation that developed quickly (131). One patient developed 2 new aneurysms within a 6-month period, whereas the other developed 2 new aneurysms within a 22-month period. Short screening intervals might be necessary in patients at high risk for new aneurysmal formation, including patients who are young, are female, are cigarette smokers, have a history of arterial hypertension, have first-degree relatives with intracranial aneurysms, or who have been previously treated for an intracranial aneurysm.

ACUTE VS. CHRONIC ANEURYSMS (COCAINE-RELATED BLEED SITES)

The exact mechanism by which berry aneurysms form remains undetermined, but research indicates that propagation and rupture of the aneurysm are aggravated by hypertension and tachycardia (132). The drug most often associated with acute cerebrovascular events is cocaine. Intracerebral hemorrhages or SAHs are the most frequently observed cerebrovascular complications of this drug (123). Several mechanisms might be responsible for the cerebrovascular complications. Traditional teaching is that hypertension is the likely precursive factor in cocaine-induced aneurysmal rupture, and a sudden rise in systemic arterial pressure might cause hemorrhages, frequently in association with an underlying aneurysm or AVM. Recent reports have indicated that these patients might have underlying vascular malformations (133,134). Rupture of aneurysms and AVMs has been detected in up to half of the patients with hemorrhagic stroke due to cocaine abuse. In addition to stroke, cocaine seems to provoke vascular headache (135). Cocaine abuse appears to be a significant negative factor in the natural history of cerebral aneurysms, especially in young adults (136). Cocaine use predisposed aneurysmal rupture at a significantly earlier age and in much smaller aneurysms, particularly of those located in the anterior circulation (137,138).

OUR PHILOSOPHY ON ANEURYSMS

The current treatment methods for aSAH include surgical clipping and endovascular coiling. Coiling has been popular in Europe for more than a decade and is now the method of treatment for 60% to 70% of aneurysms; however, it is less popular in the United States. Despite many recent studies that have shown coiling to be more effective than surgical clipping in terms of cost, recovery time, and morbidity and mortality reduction, only approximately 30% of aneurysms are coiled (8,12–16). Currently, only approximately 300 hospitals out of United States' 3000 offer coiling as an option to clipping. We believe that patients should have an informed choice on whether to receive treatment by coiling or clipping. More neurosurgeons, neurologists, and neuroradiologists should be trained in this technique so that the choice is available to greater numbers of people. The insurance reimbursement system might also need to be reevaluated and changed in a way that discourages turf battles over which technique, surgical or endovascular, is performed, so that the patients are evaluated in an unbiased manner that determines which treatment is best for them. Additionally, we recognize the need for more studies to evaluate the long-term efficacy and safety of coiling.

It is clear that endovascular coiling is one of the most important developments in the treatment of intracranial aneurysms within the last decade. Although surgical therapy of aneurysms over the past 32 years has reduced the mortality associated with aSAH from 35% to 17.8%, it is also apparent that not all aneurysms can be optimally treated with surgery. Aneurysms are complex lesions that are best approached by complementary, not competing, therapies. We believe that the current challenge is not to prove whether endovascular coiling or surgical clipping is "better," but, instead, to define which types of aneurysm are best approached surgically, endovascularly, or by a combination of the 2 techniques (139).

REFERENCES

1. U-King-Im JM, Koo B, Trivedi RA, et al. Current diagnostic approaches to subarachnoid haemorrhage. Eur Radiol 2005; 15(6):1135–1147.
2. Rohde V, Mayfrank L, Bertalanffy H, Mull M, Gilsbach JM. Aneurysmal subarachnoid hemorrhage: role of computerized tomography for correct prediction of the ruptured aneurysm site. Zentralbl Neurochir 2003; 64(3):116–22.
3. Vassilouthis J, Chrysikopoulos CH, Seferis CH. Magnetic resonance angiography demonstration of an angiographically occult anterior communicating artery aneurysm. Br J Neurosurg 1997; 11(5):448–51.
4. Jafar JJ, Weiner HL. Surgery for angiographically occult cerebral aneurysms. J Neurosurg 1993; 79(5):674–9.
5. Vaitkevicius G, Lukosevicius S, Gvazdaitis AR. Diagnosis of angiographically negative spontaneous subarachnoid hemorrhage. Medicina (Kaunas) 2002; 38(2):147–50.

6. Kaim A, Proske M, Kirsch E, von Weymarn A, Radu EW, Steinbrich W. Value of repeat-angiography in cases of unexplained subarachnoid hemorrhage (SAH). Acta Neurol Scand 1996; 93(5):366–73.

7. Johnston SC. Effect of endovascular services and hospital volume on cerebral aneurysm treatment outcomes. Stroke 2000; 31(1):111–117.

8. Molyneux A, Kerr R, Stratton I, Sandercock P, Clarke M, Shrimpton J, Holman R. International Subarachnoid Aneurysm Trial (ISAT) Collaborative Group. International

9. Hoh BL, Carter BS, Budzik RF, Putman CM, Ogilvy CS. Results after surgical and endovascular treatment of paraclinoid aneurysms by a combined neurovascular team. Neurosurgery 2001; 48(1):78–89.

10. Koivisto T, Vanninen R, Hurskainen H, Saari T, Hernesniemi J, Vapalahti M. Outcomes of early endovascular versus surgical treatment of ruptured cerebral aneurysms. A prospective randomized study. Stroke 2000; 31(10):2369–2377.

11. Hadjivassiliou M, Tooth CL, Romanowski CA, et al. Aneurysmal SAH: cognitive outcome and structural damage after clipping or coiling. Neurology 2001; 56(12):1672–1677.

12. Johnston SC, Zhao S, Dudley RA, Berman MF, Gress DR. Treatment of unruptured cerebral aneurysms in California. Stroke 2001; 32(3):597–605.

13. Johnston SC, Dudley RA, Gress DR, Ono L. Surgical and endovascular treatment of unruptured cerebral aneurysms at university hospitals. Neurology 1999; 52(9):1799–1805.

14. Johnston SC, Wilson CB, Halbach VV, et al. Endovascular and surgical treatment of unruptured cerebral aneurysms: comparison of risks. Ann Neurol 2000; 48(1):11–19.

15. Sluzewski M, Bosch JA, van Rooij WJ, Nijssen PC, Wijnalda D. Rupture of intracranial aneurysms during treatment with Guglielmi detachable coils: incidence, outcome, and risk factors. J Neurosurg 2001; 94(2):238–240.

16. Roy D, Milot G, Raymond J. Endovascular treatment of unruptured aneurysms. Stroke 2001; 32(9):1998–2004.

17. Dovey Z, Misra M, Thornton J, Charbel FT, Debrun GM, Ausman JI. Guglielmi detachable coiling for intracranial aneurysms: the story so far. Arch Neurol 2001; 58(4):559–564.

18. Ribourtout E, Raymond J. Gene therapy and endovascular treatment of intracranial aneurysms. Stroke 2004; 35(3):786–793.

19. Patel AB, Johnson DM. Endovascular treatment of neurovascular disorders. Mt Sinai J Med 2004; 71(1):29–41.

20. Cross DT 3rd, Tirschwell DL, Clark MA, et al. Mortality rates after subarachnoid hemorrhage: variations according to hospital case volume in 18 states. J Neurosurg 2003; 99(5):810–817.

21. Singh V, Gress DR, Higashida RT, Dowd CF, Halbach VV, Johnston SC. The learning curve for coil embolization of unruptured intracranial aneurysms. AJNR Am J Neuroradiol 2002; 23(5):768–771.

22. Gordon MK, Lawrence-Brown MM, Hartley D, et al. A self-expanding endoluminal graft for treatment of aneurysms: results through the development phase. Aust N Z J Surg 1996; 66(9):621–625.

23. Turjman F, Massoud TF, Sayre J, Vinuela F. Predictors of aneurysmal occlusion in the period immediately after endovascular treatment with detachable coils: a multivariate analysis. AJNR Am J Neuroradiol 1998; 19(9):1645–1651.

24. Henkes H, Bose A, Felber S, et al. Endovascular coil occlusion of intracranial aneurysms assisted by a novel self-expandable nitinol microstent (Neuroform). Interv Neuroradiol 2002; 8(2):107–119.

25. Benitez RP, Silva MT, Klem J, Veznedaroglu E, Rosenwasser RH. Endovascular occlusion of wide-necked aneurysms with a new intracranial microstent (Neuroform) and detachable coils. Neurosurgery 2004; 54(6):1359–1367.

26. Liu JM, Huang QH, Xu Y, Hong B, Zhang L, Zhang X. Combined stent and coil in endovascular treatment of intracranial wide-necked and fusiform aneurysms. Chin Med J (Engl) 2004; 117(1):54–57.

27. Chow MM, Woo HH, Masaryk TJ, Rasmussen PA. A novel endovascular treatment of a wide-necked basilar apex aneurysm by using a Y-configuration, double-stent technique. AJNR Am J Neuroradiol 2004; 25(3):509–512.

28. Perez-Arjona E, Fessler RD. Basilar artery to bilateral posterior cerebral artery 'Y stenting' for endovascular reconstruction of wide-necked basilar apex aneurysms: report of three cases. Neurol Res 2004; 26(3):276–281.

29. Meder JF, Bracard S, Arquizan C, Trystram D, Fredy D. Endovascular treatment using endoprosthesis and metallic stents for aneurysmal dissection of the intracranial vertebral artery. J Neuroradiol 2001; 28(3):166–175.

30. Broadbent LP, Moran CJ, Cross DT 3rd, Derdeyn CP. Management of neuroform stent dislodgement and misplacement. AJNR Am J Neuroradiol 2003; 24(9):1819–1822.

31. Li YX, Li XF, Wu SC, Liu W. Application of Neuroform stent in the treatment of intracranial aneurysm. Zhongguo Yi Xue Ke Xue Yuan Xue Bao 2004; 26(6):647–650.

32. Wada H, Piotin M, Boissonnet H, Spelle L, Mounayer C, Moret J. Carotid rupture during stent-assisted aneurysm treatment. AJNR Am J Neuroradiol 2004; 25(5):827–829.

33. Shaibani A, Khawar S, Bendok B, Walker M, Russell EJ, Batjer HH. Temporary balloon occlusion to test adequacy of collateral flow to the retina and tolerance for endovascular aneurysmal coiling. AJNR Am J Neuroradiol 2004; 25(8):1384–1386.

34. Nelson PK, Levy DI. Balloon-assisted coil embolization of wide-necked aneurysms of the internal carotid artery: medium-term angiographic and clinical follow-up in 22 patients. AJNR Am J Neuroradiol 2001; 22(1):19–26.

35. Moret J, Ross IB, Weill A, Piotin M. The retrograde approach: a consideration for the endovascular treatment of aneurysms. Am J Neuroradiol 2000; 21(2):262–268.

36. Cottier JP, Pasco A, Gallas S, et al. Utility of balloon-assisted Guglielmi detachable coiling in the treatment of 49 cerebral aneurysms: a retrospective, multicenter study. AJNR Am J Neuroradiol 2001; 22(2):345–351.

37. Lefkowitz MA, Gobin YP, Akiba Y, et al. Balloon-assisted Guglielmi detachable coiling of wide-necked aneurysma: Part II—clinical results. Neurosurgery 1999; 45(3):531–537.

38. Mericle RA, Wakhloo AK, Rodriguez R, Guterman LR, Hopkins LN. Temporary balloon protection as an adjunct to endosaccular coiling of wide-necked cerebral aneurysms: technical note. Neurosurgery 1997; 41(4):975–8.

39. Akiba Y, Murayama Y, Vinuela F, Lefkowitz MA, Duckwiler GR, Gobin YP. Balloon-assisted Guglielmi detachable coiling of wide-necked aneurysms: Part I—experimental evaluation. Neurosurgery 1999; 45(3):519–27.

40. Murayama Y, Tateshima S, Gonzalez NR, Vinuela F. Matrix and bioabsorbable polymeric coils accelerate healing of intracranial aneurysms: long-term experimental study. Stroke 2003; 34(8):2031–2037.

41. Guglielmi G, Vinuela F, Dion J, Duckwiler G. Electrothrombosis of saccular aneurysms via endovascular approach. Part 2: Preliminary clinical experience. J Neurosurg 1991; 75(1):8–14.

42. Geremia G, Haklin M. Embolization of experimentally created aneurysms with a laser-activated detachable coil device. AJNR Am J Neuroradiol 1998; 19(3):566–569.

43. Yang XJ, Song DL, Wu ZX, et al. Embolization of intracranial aneurysms with new mechanically detachable coils. Zhongguo Yi Xue Ke Xue Yuan Xue Bao 2002; 24(5):527–529.

44. Sugiu K, Katsumata A, Kusaka N, et al. Combined use of electrolytically and mechanically detachable platinum coils for endovascular treatment of cerebral aneurysms—technical note. Neurol Med Chir (Tokyo) 2004; 44(5):269–73.

45. Murphy KJ, Mandai S, Gailloud P, et al. Neurovascular embolization: in vitro evaluation of a mechanical detachable platinum coil system. Radiology 2000; 217(3):904–906.

46. Hirotsune N, Kinugasa K, Mandai S, et al. Combined use of cellulose acetate polymer and retrievable platinum coils for the thrombosis of cervical carotid aneurysms. Acta Med Okayama 2000; 54(4):153–164.

47. Tokunaga K, Kinugasa K, Kawada S, et al. Embolization of cerebral arteriovenous malformations with cellulose acetate polymer: a clinical, radiological, and histological study. Neurosurgery 1999; 44(5):981–989.

48. Yang X, Wu Z, Li Y, Sun Y, Yin K. Comparison of cellulose acetate polymer and electrolytic detachable coils for treatment of canine aneurysmal models. Chin Med Sci J 2002; 17(1):47–51.

49. Molyneux AJ, Cekirge S, Saatci I, Gal G. Cerebral Aneurysm Multicenter European Onyx (CAMEO) trial: results of a prospective observational study in 20 European centers. AJNR Am J Neuroradiol 2004; 25(1):39–51.

50. Jahan R, Murayama Y, Gobin YP, Duckwiler GR, Vinters HV, Vinuela F. Embolization of arteriovenous malformations with Onyx: clinicopathological experience in 23 patients. Neurosurgery 2001; 48(5):984–995.

51. Murayama Y, Vinuela F, Tateshima S, Vinuela F Jr., Akiba Y. Endovascular treatment of experimental aneurysms by use of a combination of liquid embolic agents and protective devices. AJNR Am J Neuroradiol 2000; 21(9):1726–1735.

52. Florio F, Lauriola W, Nardella M, Strizzi V, Vallone S, Trossello MP. Endovascular treatment of intracranial arterio-venous malformations with Onyx embolization: preliminary experience. Radiol Med (Torino) 2003; 106(5–6):512–520.

53. Saatci I, Cekirge HS, Ciceri EF, Mawad ME, Pamuk AG, Besim A. CT and MR imaging findings and their implications in the follow-up of patients with intracranial aneurysms treated with endosaccular occlusion with onyx. AJNR Am J Neuroradiol 2003; 24(4):567–578.

54. Cognard C, Weill A, Spelle L, Piotin M, Castaings L, Rey A, Moret J. Long-term angiographic follow-up of 169 intracranial berry aneurysms occluded with detachable coils. Radiology 1999; 212(2):348–356.

55. Lubicz B, Leclerc X, Gauvrit JY, Lejeune JP, Pruvo JP. Endovascular treatment of peripheral cerebellar artery aneurysms. AJNR Am J Neuroradiol 2003; 24(6):1208–1213.

56. MacKay CI, Han PP, Albuquerque FC, McDougall CG. Recurrence of a vertebral artery dissecting pseudoaneurysm after successful stent-supported coil embolization: case report. Neurosurgery 2003; 53(3):754–759.

57. Leibowitz R, Do HM, Marcellus ML, Chang SD, Steinberg GK, Marks MP. Parent vessel occlusion for vertebrobasilar fusiform and dissecting aneurysms. AJNR Am J Neuroradiol 2003; 24(5):902–907.

58. Niiro M, Shimozuru T, Nakamura K, Kadota K, Kuratsu J. Long-term follow-up study of patients with cavernous sinus aneurysm treated by proximal occlusion. Neurol Med Chir (Tokyo) 2000; 40(2):88–96.

59. Sudhakar KV, Sawlani V, Phadke RV, Kumar S, Ahmed S, Gujral RB. Temporary balloon occlusion of internal carotid artery: a simple and reliable clinical test. Neurol India 2000; 48(2):140–143.

60. Houdart E, Saint-Maurice JP, Boissonnet H, Bonnin P. Clinical and hemodynamic responses to balloon test occlusion of the straight sinus: technical case report. Neurosurgery 2002; 51(1):254–256.

61. McIvor NP, Willinsky RA, TerBrugge KG, Rutka JA, Freeman JL. Validity of test occlusion studies prior to internal carotid artery sacrifice. Head Neck 1994; 16(1):11–16.

62. Standard SC, Ahuja A, Guterman LR, et al. Balloon test occlusion of the internal carotid artery with hypotensive challenge. AJNR Am J Neuroradiol 1995; 16(7):1453–1458.

63. Neff KW, Horn P, Dinter D, Vajkoczy P, Schmiedek P, Duber C. Extracranial-intracranial arterial bypass surgery improves total brain blood supply in selected symptomatic patients with unilateral internal carotid artery occlusion and insufficient collateralization. Neuroradiology 2004; 46(9):730–737.

64. Mendelowitsch A, Taussky P, Rem JA, Gratzl O. Clinical outcome of standard extracranial-intracranial bypass surgery in patients with symptomatic atherosclerotic occlusion of the internal carotid artery. Acta Neurochir (Wien) 2004; 146(2):95–101.

65. Horn P, Vajkoczy P, Schmiedek P, Neff W. Evaluation of extracranial-intracranial arterial bypass function with magnetic resonance angiography. Neuroradiology 2004; 46(9):723–729.

66. Teksam M, McKinney A, Truwit CL. Multi-slice CT angiography in evaluation of extracranial-intracranial bypass. Eur J Radiol 2004; 52(3):217–220.

67. Eckert B, Thie A, Carvajal M, Groden C, Zeumer H. Predicting hemodynamic ischemia by transcranial Doppler monitoring during therapeutic balloon occlusion of the internal carotid artery. AJNR Am J Neuroradiol 1998; 19(3):577–582.

68. Nakagawa K, Touho H, Morisako T, et al. Long-term follow-up study of unruptured vertebral artery dissection: clinical outcomes and serial angiographic findings. J Neurosurg 2000; 93(1):19–25.

69. Mizutani T, Aruga T, Kirino T, Miki Y, Saito I, Tsuchida T. Recurrent subarachnoid hemorrhage from untreated ruptured vertebrobasilar dissecting aneurysms. Neurosurgery 1995; 36(5):905–911.

70. Caplan LR, Baquis GD, Pessin MS, et al. Dissection of the intracranial vertebral artery. Neurology 1988; 38(6):868–877.

71. Kawamata T, Tanikawa T, Takeshita M, Onda H, Takakura K, Toyoda C. Rebleeding of intracranial dissecting aneurysm in the vertebral artery following proximal clipping. Neurol Res 1994; 16(2):141–144.

72. Yamada M, Kitahara T, Kurata A, Fujii K, Miyasaka Y. Intracranial vertebral artery dissection with subarachnoid hemorrhage: clinical characteristics and outcomes in conservatively treated patients. J Neurosurg 2004; 101(1):25–30.

73. Kurata A, Ohmomo T, Miyasaka Y, Fujii K, Kan S, Kitahara T. Coil embolization for the treatment of ruptured dissecting vertebral aneurysms. AJNR Am J Neuroradiol 2001; 22(1):11–18.

74. Ono J, Yamaura A, Kobayashi S, et al. Long-term outcome in patients with intracranial arterial dissection and subarachnoid hemorrhage: analysis of 25 consecutive managed patients in vertebrobasilar system. Surg Cereb Stroke 2001; 29:183–188.

75. Yamaura A, Watanabe Y, Saeki N. Dissecting aneurysms of the intracranial vertebral artery. J Neurosurg 1990; 72(2):183–188.

76. Aoki N, Sakai T. Rebleeding from intracranial dissecting aneurysm in the vertebral artery. Stroke 1990; 21(11):1628–1631.

77. Kamiyama H, Nomura M, Abe H. Diagnosis for the intracranial dissecting aneurysms. Surg Cereb Stroke 1990; 18:50–56.

78. Rabinov JD, Hellinger FR, Morris PP, Ogilvy CS, Putman CM. Endovascular management of vertebrobasilar dissecting aneurysms. AJNR Am J Neuroradiol 2003; 24(7):1421–1428.

79. Shin JH, Suh DC, Choi CG, Leei HK. Vertebral artery dissection: spectrum of imaging findings with emphasis on angiography and correlation with clinical presentation. Radiographics 2000; 20(6):1687–1696.

80. Mokri B, Houser OW, Sandok BA, Piepgras DG. Spontaneous dissections of the vertebral arteries. Neurology 1988; 38(6):880–885.

81. Wilkinson IM. The vertebral artery. Extracranial and intracranial structure. Arch Neurol 1972; 27(5):392–396.

82. Clower BR, Sullivan DM, Smith RR. Intracranial vessels lack vasa vasorum. J Neurosurg 1984; 61(1):44–48.

83. Sasaki O, Ogawa H, Koike T, Koizumi T, Tanaka R. A clinicopathological study of dissecting aneurysms of the intracranial vertebral artery. J Neurosurg 1991; 75(6):874–882.

84. Lylyk P, Cohen JE, Ceratto R, Ferrario A, Miranda C. Combined endovascular treatment of dissecting vertebral artery aneurysms by using stents and coils. J Neurosurg 2001; 94(3):427–432.

85. Lylyk P, Ceratto R, Hurvitz D, Basso A. Treatment of a vertebral dissecting aneurysm with stents and coils: technical case report. Neurosurgery 1998; 43(2):385–388.

86. Han PP, Albuquerque FC, Ponce FA, et al. Percutaneous intracranial stent placement for aneurysms. J Neurosurg 2003; 99(1):23–30.

87. Sugiu K, Takahashi K, Muneta K, Ohmoto T. Rebleeding of a vertebral artery dissecting aneurysm during stent-assisted coil embolization: a pitfall of the "stent and coil" technique. Surg Neurol 2004; 61(4):365–370.

88. Lanzino G, Wakhloo AK, Fessler RD, Hartney ML, Guterman LR, Hopkins LN. Efficacy and current limitations of intravascular stents for intracranial internal carotid, vertebral, and basilar artery aneurysms. J Neurosurg 1999; 91(4):538–546.

89. Phatouros CC, Sasaki TY, Higashida RT, et al. Stent-supported coil embolization: the treatment of fusiform and wide-neck aneurysms and pseudoaneurysms. Neurosurgery 2000; 47(1):107–113.

90. Mehta B, Burke T, Kole M, Bydon A, Seyfried D, Malik G. Stent-within-a-stent technique for the treatment of dissecting vertebral artery aneurysms. AJNR Am J Neuroradiol 2003; 24(9):1814–1818.

91. Benndorf G, Herbon U, Sollmann WP, Campi A. Treatment of a ruptured dissecting vertebral artery aneurysm with double stent placement: case report. AJNR Am J Neuroradiol 2001; 22(10):1844–1848.

92. Benndorf G, Campi A, Schneider GH, Wellnhofer E, Unterberg A. Overlapping stents for treatment of a dissecting carotid artery aneurysm. J Endovasc Ther 2001; 8(6):566–570.

93. Felber S, Henkes H, Weber W, Miloslavski E, Brew S, Kuhne D. Treatment of extracranial and intracranial aneurysms and arteriovenous fistulae using stent grafts. Neurosurgery 2004; 55(3):631–638.

94. Chiaradio JC, Guzman L, Padilla L, Chiaradio MP. Intravascular graft stent treatment of a ruptured fusiform dissecting aneurysm of the intracranial vertebral artery: technical case report. Neurosurgery 2002; 50(1):213–216.

95. Mizutani T, Kojima H, Asamoto S, Miki Y. Pathological mechanism and three-dimensional structure of cerebral dissecting aneurysms. J Neurosurg 2001; 94(5):712–717.

96. Kassell NF, Torner JC, Jane JA, Haley EC Jr., Adams HP. The International Cooperative Study on the Timing of Aneurysm Surgery. Part 2: Surgical results. J Neurosurg 1990; 73(1):37–47.

97. Pickard JD, Murray GD, Illingworth R, et al. Effect of oral nimodipine on cerebral infarction and outcome after subarachnoid haemorrhage: British aneurysm nimodipine trial. BMJ 1989; 298(6674):636–642.

98. Kassell NF, Torner JC, Haley EC Jr., Jane JA, Adams HP, Kongable GL. The International Cooperative Study on the Timing of Aneurysm Surgery. Part 1: Overall management results. J Neurosurg 1990; 73(1):18–36.

99. Hoeffner EG, Case I, Jain R, et al. Cerebral perfusion CT: technique and clinical applications. Radiology 2004; 231(3):632–44.

100. Goldsher D, Shreiber R, Shik V, Tavor Y, Soustiel JF. Role of multisection CT angiography in the evaluation of vertebrobasilar vasospasm in patients with subarachnoid hemorrhage. AJNR Am J Neuroradiol 2004; 25(9):1493–1498.

101. McAuliffe W, Townsend M, Eskridge JM, Newell DW, Grady MS, Winn HR. Intracranial pressure changes induced during papaverine infusion for treatment of vasospasm. J Neurosurg 1995; 83(3):430–434.

102. Hendrix LE, Dion JE, Jensen ME, Phillips CD, Newman SA. Papaverine-induced mydriasis. AJNR Am J Neuroradiol 1994; 15(4):716–718.

103. Barr JD, Mathis JM, Horton JA. Transient severe brain stem depression during intraarterial papaverine infusion for cerebral vasospasm. AJNR Am J Neuroradiol 1994; 15(4):719–723.

104. Mathis JM, DeNardo A, Jensen ME, Scott J, Dion JE. Transient neurologic events associated with intraarterial papaverine infusion for subarachnoid hemorrhage-induced vasospasm. AJNR Am J Neuroradiol 1994; 15(9):1671–1674.

105. Clouston JE, Numaguchi Y, Zoarski GH, Aldrich EF, Simard JM, Zitnay KM. Intraarterial papaverine infusion for cerebral vasospasm after subarachnoid hemorrhage. AJNR Am J Neuroradiol 1995; 16(1):27–38.

106. Marks MP, Steinberg GK, Lane B. Intraarterial papaverine for the treatment of vasospasm. AJNR Am J Neuroradiol 1993; 14(4):822–826.

107. Miller JA, Cross DT, Moran CJ, Dacey RG Jr., McFarland JG, Diringer MN. Severe thrombocytopenia following intraarterial papaverine administration for treatment of vasospasm. J Neurosurg 1995; 83(3):435–437.

108. Mathis JM, DeNardo AJ, Thibault L, Jensen ME, Savory J, Dion JE. In vitro evaluation of papaverine hydrochloride incompatibilities: a simulation of intraarterial infusion for cerebral vasospasm. AJNR Am J Neuroradiol 1994; 15(9):1665–1670.

109. Clyde BL, Firlik AD, Kaufmann AM, Spearman MP, Yonas H. Paradoxical aggravation of vasospasm with papaverine infusion following aneurysmal subarachnoid hemorrhage. Case report. J Neurosurg 1996; 84(4):690–695.

110. Biondi A, Ricciardi GK, Puybasset L, et al. Intra-arterial nimodipine for the treatment of symptomatic cerebral vasospasm after aneurysmal subarachnoid hemorrhage: preliminary results. AJNR Am J Neuroradiol 2004; 25(6):1067–1076.

111. Badjatia N, Topcuoglu MA, Pryor JC, et al. Preliminary experience with intra-arterial nicardipine as a treatment for cerebral vasospasm. AJNR Am J Neuroradiol 2004; 25(5):819–826.

112. Feng L, Fitzsimmons BF, Young WL, et al. Intraarterially administered verapamil as adjunct therapy for cerebral vasospasm: safety and 2-year experience. AJNR Am J Neuroradiol 2002; 23(8):1284–1290.

113. Rosenwasser RH, Armonda RA, Thomas JE, Benitez RP, Gannon PM, Harrop J. Therapeutic modalities for the management of cerebral vasospasm: timing of endovascular options. Neurosurgery 1999; 44(5):975–979.

114. Eskridge JM, McAuliffe W, Song JK, Deliganis AV, Newell DW, Lewis DH, Mayberg MR, Winn HR. Balloon angioplasty for the treatment of vasospasm: results of first 50 cases. Neurosurgery 1998; 42(3):510–516.

115. Bejjani GK, Bank WO, Olan WJ, Sekhar LN. The efficacy and safety of angioplasty for cerebral vasospasm after subarachnoid hemorrhage. Neurosurgery 1998; 42(5):979–986.

116. Azmi-Ghadimi H, Heary RF, Farkas JE, Hunt CD. Use of intraventricular tissue plasminogen activator and Guglielmi detachable coiling for the acute treatment of casted ventricles from cerebral aneurysm hemorrhage: two technical case reports. Neurosurgery 2002; 50(2):421–424.

117. Varelas PN, Rickert KL, Cusick J, et al. Intraventricular hemorrhage after aneurysmal subarachnoid hemorrhage: pilot study of treatment with intraventricular tissue plasminogen activator. Neurosurgery 2005; 56(2):205–213.

118. Schwarz S, Schwab S, Steiner HH, Hacke W. Secondary hemorrhage after intraventricular fibrinolysis: a cautionary note: a report of two cases. Neurosurgery 1998; 42(3):659–662.

119. Wang YC, Lin CW, Shen CC, Lai SC, Kuo JS. Tissue plasminogen activator for the treatment of intraventricular hematoma: the dose-effect relationship. J Neurol Sci 2002; 202(1–2):35–41.

120. Deutsch H, Rodriguez JC, Titton RL. Lower dose intraventricular T-PA fibrinolysis: case report. Surg Neurol 2004; 61(5):460–463.

121. Kivisaari RP, Porras M, Ohman J, Siironen J, Ishii K, Hernesniemi J. Routine cerebral angiography after surgery for saccular aneurysms: is it worth it? Neurosurgery 2004; 55(5):1015–1024.

122. Chiang VL, Gailloud P, Murphy KJ, Rigamonti D, Tamargo RJ. Routine intraoperative angiography during aneurysm surgery. J Neurosurg 2002; 96(6):988–992.

123. Lalouschek W, Schnider P, Aull S, et al. Cocaine abuse with special reference to cerebrovascular complications. Wien Klin Wochenschr 1995; 107(17):516–521.

124. Byrne JV, Sohn MJ, Molyneux AJ, Chir B. Five-year experience in using coil embolization for ruptured intracranial aneurysms: outcomes and incidence of late rebleeding. J Neurosurg 1999; 90(4):656–663.

125. Asgari S, Wanke I, Schoch B, Stolke D. Recurrent hemorrhage after initially complete occlusion of intracranial aneurysms. Neurosurg Rev 2003; 26(4):269–274.

126. Birchall D, Khangure MS, Mcauliffe W, Thomas W. Delayed aneurysm rerupture following total endovascular occlusion. Br J Neurosurg 2001; 15(3):269–272.

127. Moller V, Axmann C, Reith W. Clinical course of a partially thrombosed, symptomatic aneurysm of the basilar artery tip with partial recanalization subsequent to coiling. Radiologe 2006; 46(5):417–420.

128. Raymond J, Guilbert F, Weill A, et al. Long-term angiographic recurrences after selective endovascular treatment of aneurysms with detachable coils. Stroke 2003; 34(6):1398–1403.

129. Slob MJ, Sluzewski M, van Rooij WJ, Roks G, Rinkel GJ. Additional coiling of previously coiled cerebral aneurysms: clinical and angiographic results. AJNR Am J Neuroradiol 2004; 25(8):1373–1376.

130. Juvela S, Poussa K, Porras M. Factors affecting formation and growth of intracranial aneurysms: a long-term follow-up study. Stroke 2001; 32(2):485–491.

131. Obray R, Clatterbuck R, Olvi A, Tamargo R, Murphy KJ, Gailloud P. De novo aneurysm formation 6 and 22 months after initial presentation in two patients. AJNR Am J Neuroradiol 2003; 24(9):1811–1813.

132. Davis GG, Swalwell CI. The incidence of acute cocaine or methamphetamine intoxication in deaths due to ruptured cerebral (berry) aneurysms. J Forensic Sci 1996; 41(4):626–628.

133. McEvoy AW, Kitchen ND, Thomas DG. Intracerebral haemorrhage and drug abuse in young adults. Br J Neurosurg 2000; 14(5):449–454.

134. Levine SR, Brust JC, Futrell N, et al. A comparative study of the cerebrovascular complications of cocaine: alkaloidal versus hydrochloride--a review. Neurology 1991; 41(8):1173–1177.

135. Neiman J, Haapaniemi HM, Hillbom M. Neurological complications of drug abuse: pathophysiological mechanisms. Eur J Neurol 2000; 7(6):595–606.

136. Oyesiku NM, Colohan AR, Barrow DL, Reisner A. Cocaine-induced aneurysmal rupture: an emergent negative factor in the natural history of intracranial aneurysms? Neurosurgery 1993; 32(4):518–525.

137. Nanda A, Vannemreddy PS, Polin RS, Willis BK. Intracranial aneurysms and cocaine abuse: analysis of prognostic indicators. Neurosurgery 2000; 46(5):1063–1067.

138. Fessler RD, Esshaki CM, Stankewitz RC, Johnson RR, Diaz FG. The neurovascular complications of cocaine. Surg Neurol 1997; 47(4):339–345.

139. Tamargo RJ, Rigamonti D, Murphy K, Gailloud P, Conway JE, Clatterbuck RE. Treatment of intracranial aneurysms: surgical clipping or endovascular coiling? Ann Neurol 2001; 49(5):682–684.

of the adequacy of cerebral perfusion during aneurysmal exposure and clipping. The main limitation of intraoperative electrophysiologic ischemia monitoring is the lack of specificity, demonstrated by a relatively high rate of false-positive (40–60%) and false-negative (10–30%) detection (11,12).

Patients with aSAH have a high risk for increased ICP throughout the first days after insult. Some centers advocate continuous intraoperative ICP monitoring, e.g., using intraventricular catheters, which also allows for cerebrospinal fluid (CSF) drainage and helps to guide treatment during periods of increased ICP. However, placement of an intraventricular catheter is associated with significant risk of changing transmural pressure (TMP) in the aneurysm wall and potential rupture. In development are new devices designed to prevent rapid efflux of CSF during ventricular catheter placement. Until these devices are a part of common practice, most centers do their best to avoid ICP catheter placement.

Intraoperative angiography provides a means by which to evaluate the result of aneurysmal clip placement and to ensure complete obliteration of the aneurysm neck and patency of the parent arterial trunk and adjacent arterial branches (13). If indicated, the clip can be replaced and the result visualized prior to emergence from anesthesia, which might help to limit the risk for postoperative ischemic complications. The additional equipment necessary requires special organization of airway and monitoring around the head to allow safe C-arm placement during surgery.

Intraoperative positioning of the patient must accommodate surgical access, which, in turn, is determined by the aneurysm location. Most aneurysms originate from, or are in close proximity to, the Circle of Willis. In an effort to prevent devastating perioperative strokes, especially in patients with evidence for arteriosclerosis, it is paramount to limit their head rotation to maintain cerebral perfusion through the contralateral carotid and vertebral arteries, as well as to maintain jugular drainage. Vertebral-basilar aneurysm procedures typically are performed with the patient in the lateral position and frequently require access to both the middle and the posterior fossa. The imminent risk of irritation of, or possible damage to, the brain stem warrants high vigilance toward sudden intraoperative cardiovascular responses, which should be communicated immediately to the neurosurgeon to modify surgical manipulations. Most such procedures are performed with continuous electrophysiologic monitoring (11,12,14).

Induction of Anesthesia

The main goal during anesthesia induction is to pharmacologically induce loss of consciousness and manage the airway without a sudden and profound increase or decrease in arterial blood pressure, coughing, or straining that might lead to rebleeding of the aneurysm (if blood pressure is too high) (15) or cerebral ischemia (if blood pressure is too low) (16). This challenge results from the fact that the TMP of the aneurysm, as well as CPP, is determined by the difference of the same two variables: MABP−ICP = TMP; MABP−ICP = CPP. Thus, the anesthesiologist is confronted with conflicting objectives regarding blood-pressure management and ICP treatment. However, therapeutic interventions must be tailored to the pathophysiologic condition of each patient. Patients with low SAH grades (I and II) usually have normal ICP and CPP and, therefore, might tolerate a modest decrease of MABP (up to 30% from baseline) for limited periods. Patients with higher clinical grades (III and IV) can be assumed to have higher ICP and lower CPP; therefore, their tolerance for periods of low MABP is very limited.

Loss of consciousness is usually induced with thiopental (3–5 mg/kg), propofol (1.5–2.5 mg/kg), or etomidate (0.1–0.2 mg/kg), all of which reduce cerebral metabolism and TMP. However, extra precautions are warranted in patients with high clinical grades (III and IV), who are exceptionally vulnerable to developing cerebral ischemia following a reduction in MABP during induction, as their autoregulation might be impaired and some degree of vasospasm might already be present. Opiates are administered (e.g., fentanyl, 5–10 mcg/kg or sufentanil, 0.5–1.0 mcg/kg) to ameliorate the sympathetic response to laryngoscopy and endotracheal intubation. To further blunt potential systemic hypertension, IV lidocaine (1.5–2.0 mg/kg) is favored by many clinicians. In addition, administration of β-antagonists, such as esmolol (0.5 mg/kg) or labetalol 10–20 mg/kg), a second dose of the induction agent (e.g., thiopental 1–2 mg/kg), or inhalation of a volatile anesthetic (e.g., isoflurane) during bag-mask ventilation can be provided approximately 1 to 2 min prior to airway instrumentation.

Muscle paralysis for tracheal intubation is achieved by most clinicians using a nondepolarizing agent such as rocuronium or vecuronium. No evidence suggests that patients with aSAH are at higher risk of gastroesophageal reflux and aspiration. If rapid sequence induction with cricoid pressure is indicated, use of either rocuronium or succinylcholine is appropriate. Any increase in ICP that might occur with succinylcholine administration is small and has never been demonstrated to be of clinical significance. Awake fiberoptic intubation with regional anesthesia is indicated for aSAH patients who have evidence of a potentially difficult airway. If a difficult airway is encountered unexpectedly, appropriate action is required according to the ASA-airway algorithm and under close monitoring and appropriate treatment of the patient's arterial blood pressure. If bag-mask ventilation is possible, fiberoptic intubation can be achieved by a second clinician, using an appropriate adapter and under maintenance of continuous ventilation. Alternatively, a laryngeal mask airway can be used for the same purpose. If ventilation is not possible ("cannot intubate, cannot ventilate"), transtracheal-jet ventilation should be applied to maintain oxygenation until access to the airway is achieved by either a fiberscope or immediate surgical airway management (cricothyroidotomy and tracheostomy). After successful endotracheal intubation, the tube must be secured, avoiding placement of anything circumferentially around the neck, as this might compromise cerebral venous drainage.

Maintenance

The treatment strategy should allow the anesthesiologist to secure an adequate depth of anesthesia to sympathetic stimulation during every phase of surgery. The agents chosen should facilitate the anesthesiologist's ability to quickly manipulate blood pressure and intracellular water content of the brain (brain relaxation) at any time during the surgery. The maintenance strategy must also allow the anesthesiologist to be successful with his/her plan for rapid postoperative neurologic evaluation in patients with favorable SAH grades (I–II). It is important to note that, during the different phases of aneurysmal surgery, stimulation can vary significantly. Manipulation at the scalp, skull, and dura requires a deeper level of anesthesia than does aneurysmal dissection, which causes little to no stimulation. However, sudden changes in heart rate and blood pressure might occur when the brain stem or cranial nerves are retracted.

For anesthesia maintenance during aneurysmal surgery, clinicians frequently choose a combination of volatile anesthetics in oxygen-enriched air, short-acting opiates (or regional scalp block), and nondepolarizing muscle relaxants ("balanced anesthesia"). As with induction of anesthesia, although the choice of anesthetics might vary between practitioners, the goal remains uniform, i.e., to achieve an appropriate balance between the levels of anesthesia and surgical stimulation to maintain stable hemodynamics and avoid aneurysmal rerupture or cerebral ischemia.

Volatile anesthetics dilate the cerebral vasculature and increase CBF to various extents (17). The potential risk of a subsequent increase in ICP can be balanced with the effects of mild hyperventilation. Isoflurane is probably the most widely used volatile agent in anesthesia for cerebral aneurysmal clipping (18). Desflurane appears to have additional beneficial effects on oxygenation of dependent brain areas during temporary clipping (19), potentially by improved collateral flow. Sevoflurane is unique, in that at clinically relevant doses, it is less detrimental to cerebral autoregulation than are other inhaled anesthetics (20).

Nitrous oxide is less frequently used in aneurysmal surgery, due to vasodilating and cerebral-stimulating effects (21), although no evidence exists that its use negatively affects outcome. In animal models of cerebral ischemia (as would occur during temporary clipping of parent vessels of the aneurysm), nitrous oxide accentuates brain injury. Therefore, many clinicians consider its use undesirable. However, when nitrous oxide is used in combination with IV anesthetics (e.g., propofol and fentanyl infusion), the vasodilatory potential is attenuated (22), and some clinicians implement it to quickly augment anesthesia in the most stimulating phases of the surgical procedure.

Opiates (e.g., fentanyl, remifentanil, and sufentanil) are frequently provided in combination with volatile anesthetics (mean alveolar concentration, 0.5–1) as part of a "balanced anesthesia". No differences have been observed between the different opiates concerning effects on the surgical field, i.e., "tightness" or necessary pressure for brain retraction (23,24). Hypnotics should always be available in bolus doses to cope with unexpected sudden sympathetic stimulation. A continuous infusion of hypnotic agents, i.e., thiopental (5–6 mg/kg/hr), propofol (150–200 µg/kg/hr), or etomidate (0.2–0.3 mg/kg/hr), represents a second tier of intervention when the brain remains "tight," despite more conventional measures (e.g., dehydration).

One of the first challenges after induction of anesthesia is blood-pressure control during application of the Mayfield clamp or a similar fixation device and the final positioning of the patient for surgery. To prevent hypertension during clamp placement, some anesthesiologists recommend preemptive complete scalp block or infiltration anesthesia at the sites of pins. In addition, a bolus dose of, e.g., thiopental or fentanyl 1 to 2 min prior to the procedure might be required to minimize the sympathetic response. The preventive administration of esmolol or labetalol could be considered as an alternative approach. If preemptive treatment is not successful, clamp-associated increases in blood pressure warrant immediate antiadrenergic treatment. During positioning, the head and neck should be positioned relative to the body to ensure adequate perfusion and venous drainage of the brain to minimize the risk of intraoperative stroke or cerebral edema. Less-than-optimal positioning might result in the endotracheal tube migrating into the right main-stem bronchus, requiring the anesthesiologist to confirm bilateral breath sounds prior to surgical draping.

Besides limiting the TMP of the aneurysm, the anesthesiologist must also maintain adequate CPPs throughout the surgical procedure (25–28), an even greater challenge in patients with evidence for vasospasm, particularly prior to aneurysmal clipping. Intraoperative management of patients with vasospasm follows the same treatment strategy as defined in the nonanesthetized patient (see Chapter 4), except that treatment success cannot be assessed with neurologic examination.

Fluid and electrolytes should be balanced throughout the perioperative period. The anesthesiologist must be aware that these patients are prone to salt wasting and hyponatremia (see Chapter 7). It is critical to have crossmatched blood available to the OR prior to aneurysmal clipping, in the event that resuscitation is needed as a result of accidental aneurysmal rupture. The aim, prior to aneurysmal clamping, is to restore and maintain normovolemia by replacing fluid deficits from an overnight fast with iso-osmolar crystalloid solutions. Profound hypovolemia has been associated with perioperative ischemia and neurologic deficits in patients with subarachnoid hemorrhage, particularly if vasospasm was apparent (29). After successful clipping of the aneurysm, the aim is to reach a hypervolemic state to reduce the risk of vasospasm in the postoperative period (30). The advantages of the use of 5% albumin to raise intravascular volume have not been documented to date. However, some clinicians favor hypertonic saline instead, which, in addition to its volume-expanding effect, could positively influence endothelial edema formation, thereby improving the capillary perfusion of the brain (31–33). The use of hetastarch solution, in contrast, might not be advisable during aneurysmal surgery due to the increased risk of intracranial bleeding (34). Electrolytes should be replaced according to the individual needs of the patient (35,36), and glucose levels above 150 mg/dL should be treated appropriately with insulin (37).

Relaxation of the brain can be achieved by hyperventilation (reduction of the cerebral blood volume), dehydration (reduction of the brain tissue volume), and CSF drainage (reduction of CSF volume). Although hyperventilation to lower $PaCO_2$ reduces ICP and improves the surgeon's ability to open the dura, it can also hypothetically cause cerebral ischemia, particularly in patients with preexisting vasospasm. Periods of low perfusion pressures render the brain, particularly vulnerable to ischemia, and normocarbia is suggested prior to deliberate hypotension, especially when vasospasm is suspected (38). Continuous clinical assessment by the anesthesiologist usually allows the fine-tuning between optimal brain relaxation and an acceptable $PaCO_2$ level. Normoventilation should be reinstituted as soon as possible. As with initiation of hyperventilation, changes toward normoventilation should be made slowly to allow adaptation of the vasculature and to avoid a rebound phenomenon, which is characterized by an abrupt increase in cerebral volume and ICP.

Dehydration of the brain tissue is frequently achieved by the application of the osmotic diuretic mannitol (1098 mOsm/L at 20%). In addition, mannitol might also reduce CSF production (39). The drug has a quick onset of action (about 5–10 min after start of the infusion), and the peak decrease in ICP can be anticipated at 30 to 60 min. Mannitol is dosed at a range between 0.5 and 2.0 g/kg, depending on goals for intensity of effect and desired duration of action. Some clinicians have suggested that mannitol should be administered very carefully prior to dural incision to avoid sudden decrease in ICP (because of increased intravascular volume), which might increase the risk of aneurysmal rebleeding due to a proportional increase of TMP (40,41). To potentiate the effects of mannitol, furosemide can be administered at a dose of 0.25 to 0.5 mg/kg intravenously (42). The use of diuretics, especially at these doses, can trigger severe electrolyte abnormalities, in particular with sodium, potassium, chloride, magnesium, and calcium (43). Some clinicians suggest an additional dose of mannitol prior to temporary occlusion of parent arteries (maximum total intraoperative dose, 2 g/kg) (41). Mannitol has been associated with specific neuroprotective effects, which could be related to oxygen radical scavenging properties of the drug, although no long-term benefit has been proven (44,45).

Drainage of CSF through a ventricular or lumbar subarachnoid catheter allows effective reduction in ICP (46), might facilitate dural incision, and optimizes exposure of the brain. However, significant drainage of CSF poses multiple risks to patients with aSAH. Sudden reduction in ICP due to CSF drainage is associated with a proportional increase in TMP and can trigger rerupture of the aneurysm. Lumbar CSF drainage is considered contraindicated in patients with parenchymal hemorrhages due to the risk of uncal and brain stem herniation.

When sufficient brain relaxation cannot be achieved via conventional techniques, a thorough check should be conducted of potential factors associated with brain edema formation in aneurysmal surgery. Before further action is taken, the following should be excluded: arterial hypoxemia, systemic hypertension, impaired cerebral venous drainage (neck position), occlusion of the CSF draining system, or the use of vasodilating agents (e.g., nitrous oxide and nitroprusside) in combination with volatile anesthetics (21,27,28). Additional brain relaxation might be achieved by initiating a head-up position (by 5–30°), which requires direct interaction with the surgeon to determine the safest time to proceed. A bolus of thiopental (2–3 mg/kg) or propofol (1–2 mg/kg) could also be tested for a specific "brain relaxation" effect in this situation. If effective, either of these drugs can also be administered by continuous infusion to maintain brain relaxation during surgical dissection. Ideally, these drugs should be infused to the point of EEG burst suppression, which could significantly delay the postoperative recovery time.

Emergence

The management of patients after open cerebral aneurysmal clipping should be individualized according to both the initial clinical presentation and the course of the surgical procedure. If the operation was uneventful, patients with favorable clinical grades (Hunt & Hess I–II) may be extubated immediately following completion of surgery. Patients with SAH Grade III might tolerate immediate emergence and tracheal extubation if surgery was uneventful, no evidence of brain swelling or increased ICP is apparent, and chances are high that airway control and gas exchange will be sufficient under spontaneous breathing. Patients with higher grades (IV–V) will have a prolonged recovery independent of the course of the surgical procedure and require postoperative intubation and mechanical ventilation until their neurologic status has improved. Similarly, patients with vertebral-basilar aneurysms and those who experience complicating intraoperative events (e.g., aneurysmal rerupture) might require prolonged intensive care for continuous airway support and mechanical ventilation to allow recovery from cranial nerve dysfunction or perioperative ischemia.

The anesthetic goals during emergence from anesthesia are dependent on whether the patient has residual unclipped aneurysms, which might occur in patients who have multiple aneurysms and in whom the surgeon is unable to completely obstruct the operative aneurysm because of complex anatomy. Compulsive prevention of hypertension, coughing, and straining is critical in patients with residual unclipped aneurysm(s). IV lidocaine might help to minimize coughing at emergence, when manipulation of the head is necessary (to apply surgical dressing or extubate the trachea). The recommended dose is 1.5 mg/kg, which can be repeated if necessary. Arterial hypertension is common after aneurysmal repair, is frequently related to preexisting hypertension or triggered by pain and CO_2 retention, and should be treated causally. β-receptor antagonists (labetalol in 5–10 mg increments or esmolol in 0.1–0.5 mg/kg increments) are suggested to stabilize the patient until desired blood-pressure goals are achieved (47,48).

Frequent neurologic evaluations during the immediate postoperative period are critical for early detection of any clinical deterioration. It is important to distinguish between surgical complications and effects of residual anesthesia, so that appropriate diagnostic procedures and therapeutic interventions are initiated as early as possible.

During the immediate postoperative period, the patient should return to his/her preoperative baseline neurologic status. Recovery from anesthesia is a function of various factors, among which are the type of drugs and doses administered and the patient's metabolic capacity and individual sensitivity. Residual volatile anesthetics are unlikely to affect neurologic function after 30 to 60 min of recovery. Narcotics are unlikely to be responsible for delayed emergence from anesthesia in patients presenting with normal respiration pattern and midsized pupils that are reactive to light. High residual doses of sedatives usually affect the neurologic presentation in a more general fashion. The issue of residual anesthetics delaying emergence can be avoided by using inhaled anesthetics with low tissue solubility (e.g., desflurane) and providing analgesia with a scalp block, rather than using narcotics for postoperative pain management. In addition, metabolic causes, such as hypoxia, hypercarbia, or hyponatremia, could be responsible for an overall poor emergence and neurologic depression. The possibility that subclinical seizures are an underlying reason for delayed recovery after aneurysmal surgery can only be ruled out by EEG, and, if discovered, they require immediate treatment. Surgical complications (e.g., subdural hematoma, intracranial hemorrhage, acute hydrocephalus, and pneumocephalus) frequently are associated with focal neurologic deficits, including unequal pupils and hemiparesis. Whereas residual anesthetic effects might be reversed by specific receptor antagonists, any suspicion of a new structural lesion should engender an immediate neurosurgic consult and diagnostic imaging.

SPECIAL PROBLEMS AND TECHNIQUES

Reducing Risk of Rebleeding During Microscopic Dissection and Aneurysmal Clipping

Two techniques—controlled systemic hypotension and temporary occlusion of the major feeding arteries—have been applied to decrease TMP, during the critical part of aneurysmal surgery, theoretically reducing the risk of intraoperative aneurysmal rupture and improving conditions for the final clip placement. Anesthetic considerations for these two techniques differ significantly.

Controlled systemic hypotension has been the traditional approach for several reasons: (i) the aneurysm wall tension increases almost linearly with the MABP (49), and control of the systemic blood pressure is a high priority until final clipping of the aneurysm; (ii) all necessary drugs and techniques are familiar to the anesthesiologist and accessible during aneurysmal surgery; (iii) controlled hypotension might also reduce surgical bleeding, thereby improving visualization during microscopic dissection. However, the risks of perioperative arterial hypotension are significant and include global cerebral ischemia, as well as focal ischemic damage in areas affected by brain retraction (50). In addition, coronary ischemia, reduced hepatic and renal blood flow, hyperglycemia, and, depending on the agent used, inhibition of hypoxic vasoconstriction, have been described (51). After aSAH, the risk for ischemia is especially high due to cerebral vasospasm and impaired autoregulation (52,53). A safe limit of intraoperative hypotension has never been established. Patients with preexisting arterial hypertension, as well as those at risk for cerebral vasospasm, might require a significantly higher MABP to maintain adequate CPP during surgery. Intraoperative neuromonitoring (e.g., EEG and somatosensory-evoked potentials) might help to detect ischemia in areas at risk during deliberate hypotension, but the reliability of these methods is questionable. In addition, the duration of systemic hypotension could be an important confounding factor for adverse outcome (54,55).

Frequently, isoflurane and sodium nitroprusside are administered to reduce blood pressure during aneurysmal surgery (56). Others report the successful use of nitroglycerin, adenosine, prostaglandin E, and β-receptor blockers (labetalol and esmolol) (57). However, the effectiveness of this method to reduce the risk of perioperative rebleeding has never been precisely determined, and its use has declined over the last years, especially with the availability of improved techniques for temporary occlusion of upstream arteries (58). Today, deliberate hypotension should be limited in degree and duration and applied only during short periods immediately prior to aneurysmal clipping; the risk–benefit ratio must be assessed for each patient (59).

Temporary occlusion of the parent artery immediately reduces blood flow, resulting in reduced TMP and attenuated risk of excessive bleeding if the aneurysmal dome is violated during dissection (60). At the same time, it results in various degrees of transient focal ischemia in dependent brain areas. The risk of such a maneuver to trigger permanent neurologic damage is apparent, and controversy exists regarding duration and technique for safe "temporary clipping." Short periods of artery occlusion (5–7 min) are usually well tolerated, although this is not sufficient for every surgical procedure. Currently, it is believed that 15 to 20 min of temporary artery occlusion might represent the critical threshold for the development of cerebral infarction. Longer durations of up to 120 min have been reported without neurologic sequelae, but others report a significant lower ischemia tolerance (maximum, 10 min), e.g., for brain stem and certain nuclei (61). The effects could be strongly related to the area involved and to certain risk factors, such as age >61, unfavorable clinical grades (H&H III–IV), and the state of collateral circulation (62). In addition, hypothermia, the application of arterial hypertension to improve collateral blood flow, or putative neuroprotective pharmacologic agents might increase the tolerance period for temporary vessel occlusion (63). Alternatively, temporary clipping can be interrupted after approximately 7 min and reinstituted after sufficient and profound reperfusion has been accomplished.

Intraoperative Cerebral Protection

The effort to identify appropriate means by which to provide specific neuroprotection beyond adequate cerebral perfusion and oxygenation during aneurysmal surgery has been the focus of a large body of experimental and clinical research (63). Barbiturates have been intensively studied in regard to their potential for intraoperative protection (64). These gamma-aminobutyric acid (GABA)-agonistic agents reduce the cerebral metabolic rate to 50% at minimal electrical brain activity (EEG burst suppression) and, subsequently, reduce CBF and ICP (reduction in blood volume). Barbiturates, such as thiopental, must be provided prior to temporary occlusion in order to exert their potential neuroprotective effects, and their application might be associated with significant arterial hypotension (65), which, in turn, might compromise cerebral perfusion in areas at risk for ischemia due to impaired autoregulation. The mechanism of neuroprotection is controversial and possibly relates to the barbiturates' ability to decrease cerebral metabolism or attenuate ischemia-induced excitotoxic amino acids' mechanisms. However, despite experimental evidence, clinical studies in humans have been unable to provide evidence for an improved aneurysmal surgery outcome with intraoperative barbiturate therapy. Etomidate has been used for the same purpose and results in better hemodynamic stability, but its neuroprotective potential remains questionable (66). Propofol exhibits similar neuroprotective properties as thiopental and etomidate when applied at doses that result in burst suppression EEG (67). However, some experimental evidence has challenged the concept that the neuroprotective effects of these drugs are only demonstrated by a silent or nearly silent EEG (68).

Volatile anesthetics, such as isoflurane, sevoflurane, and desflurane, are frequently used during aneurysmal surgery. They are thought to exert mild neuroprotective effects via GABA-agonism and opening of K–ATP channels, with the latter potentially resulting in hyperpolarization of brain cells, suggesting that these drugs might be useful for brain preconditioning prior to surgery (18,69). CBF is generally increased by volatile anesthetics, but coupling between CBF and metabolism is maintained with moderate doses. Recently, desflurane (compared to IV agents) has been shown to improve oxygenation of brain areas at risk during temporary clipping, possibly by improving collateral blood flow. However, the neuroprotective potential of anesthetics appears to be limited. It is generally accepted that temporary occlusion for <10 min is well tolerated, independent of the agent used (41). Addition of IV hypnotics (barbiturates or etomidate) to a balanced anesthetic regimen (volatile anesthetics and opiates) might increase the "safe" occlusion time up to 19 min. Occlusion times exceeding 30 min, however, appear to always result in clinically relevant neurologic damage (61).

Hypothermia has long been proposed to convey neuroprotection after various brain insults (70,71), including during open surgical repair of ruptured cerebral aneurysms (72,73). Mild-to-moderate hypothermia is believed to reduce cerebral metabolic demands for both neuronal activity and maintenance of cellular integrity. In addition, hypothermia has been shown to reduce the release of ischemia-induced excitotoxic neurotransmitters. Potential severe complications include myocardial depression and arrhythmias, coagulopathy, and infections, including pneumonia and sepsis. Spurred by evidence from a large volume of related experimental research and positive preliminary clinical data (74), a large, randomized, international, multicentered clinical trial was recently conducted on the effects of moderate hypothermia during aneurysmal surgery in patients after aSAH (International Hypothermia in Aneurysm Surgery Trial) (75). A total of 1001 patients from 30 centers (WFNS Grades I–III), who required open aneurysmal surgery, were assigned to hypothermia (target temperature 33°C, surface cooling) or normothermia (37°C) during the operation. No difference was reported between the treatment groups in regard to incidence and severity of postoperative neurologic recovery and overall outcome (duration of ICU stay, total length of hospitalization, destination at discharge, Glasgow Outcome Score at 90 days, and death). In contrast, avoidance of cerebral hyperthermia (>38°C) is paramount during aneurysmal surgery, because it worsens ischemic and traumatic brain injury in both animals and humans (76–79).

Management of Intraoperative Aneurysmal Rupture

Sudden rerupture of an aneurysm after aSAH occurs quite frequently (2–19%) (80–82) and presents a life-threatening emergency that requires immediate communication and very close cooperation between the surgeon and the anesthesiologist until the situation is resolved. The use of video monitors that transmit the surgical view to the anesthesiologist greatly facilitates management of this crisis. The time of rupture determines immediate treatment options, morbidity, mortality, and outcome prognosis, whether it happens during induction, prior to aneurysmal dissection, or during final clip application. The critical timepoint for rerupture is during induction of anesthesia, which accounts for only 7% of all perioperative aneurysmal ruptures (80,81). Clinical signs include abrupt and dramatic increase in blood pressure, sudden bradycardia, seizures, or signs of cerebral herniation. Surgery is frequently postponed to reestablish control over ICP and cerebral perfusion and to allow for a neurologic reevaluation. The prognosis is generally poor, although some institutions have reported more favorable outcomes with the so-called "rescue clipping" approach after aneurysmal rupture during induction of anesthesia (25).

Approximately half of all intraoperative ruptures (48%) occur during aneurysmal dissection, whereas 45% are associated with final clip placement when the aneurysm is fully exposed (80). As would be expected, bleeding does not influence outcome if it is controlled quickly. The surgeon may provide suction and apply a final clip to the neck of the aneurysm. Alternatively, the feeding arteries can be temporarily clipped to allow final aneurysmal clipping in a more controlled fashion. If an aneurysm reruptures before it is fully dissected, temporary clipping is not an option, and if the bleeding is massive, other means must be considered. The anesthetic goals are twofold: maintain adequate cerebral perfusion and facilitate fast surgical control. One option is to rapidly reduce MABP to 50 mmHg or lower, which might reduce bleeding, improve surgical orientation in the field, allow further dissection, and, ultimately, aneurysmal clipping. However, this maneuver poses the risk of cerebral ischemia and, therefore, could impair neurologic recovery more than would temporarily clipping the feeding arteries, which clearly is the preferred technique (59), because it allows prior administration of putative neuroprotective agents to limit neurologic damage, as explained above.

The situation is very different if blood loss is significant and hemodynamic stability is lost. Rapid fluid resuscitation and transfusion of blood products is indicated to restore adequate cerebral perfusion. Deliberate hypotension and administration of IV hypnotics for neuroprotection could further worsen cerebral perfusion and should be withheld until the intravascular volume is appropriately restored. If temporary clipping is applied to stop bleeding, vasoactive drugs should be used to attain normotension and allow for adequate collateral perfusion, especially in the presence of limited intravascular volume (80).

Anesthetic Considerations for Aneurysmal Embolization in the Radiology Suite

During the last years, endovascular ablation of aneurysms has become a popular alternative to the classic surgical approach. Recent studies show a similar, or even improved, outcome after endovascular aneurysmal therapy (83,84). The definitive roles of microsurgical and endovascular treatments, however, remain to be defined, as only future follow-up studies of the two treatment paradigms will be able to evaluate the long-term risk for rerupture and rebleeding, the necessity for repeat procedures, and the long-term development of neurologic function and subsequent quality of life (85,86). During an endovascular aneurysmal procedure, the goals of anesthetic management are as follows: (i) comprehensive management during the course of the intervention, including safe transport between the radiology suite and the ICU, (ii) providing for patient immobility and tolerance of the procedure, (iii) providing physiologic homeostasis throughout, (iv) manipulating systemic and CBF, (v) controlling anticoagulation, (vi) managing all unexpected procedural complications, and (vii) allowing rapid recovery after the procedure.

The best anesthetic technique is a matter of controversy (87). Some centers use IV sedation, and others request general anesthesia for these procedures; but no scientific evidence suggests that one technique over the other improves outcome. Frequently, patients require general anesthesia, including endotracheal intubation, because advancement of the endovascular instruments requires the patient's head and neck to be in a neutral position, which, in turn, might compromise the airway of a moderately sedated patient. Moreover, the procedure is very sensitive to motion artifacts, and it is not likely that a patient will tolerate a long period of lying supine and remaining motionless throughout. Even small head and neck movements elicited by spontaneous breathing can compromise the therapeutic result. In addition, general anesthesia might improve the tolerance of short, deliberate interruptions of cerebral perfusion, sometimes necessary to allow placement and securing of embolic material. Some teams provide short cardiac pauses by application of escalating doses of adenosine to allow a short (10–20 sec) cessation of cerebral perfusion (88). The introduction of Guglielmi detachable coils (2) for embolization has reduced the need for profound hypotension during neuroradiologic aneurysmal repair.

The anesthesiologist also plays an important role during the management of procedure-related crises. For example, in case of an accidental aneurysmal perforation, the anesthesiologist must provide rapid reversal of anticoagulation to minimize aSAH. Similarly, if embolic material is displaced and threatens to occlude cerebral vessels, the blood pressure might need to be increased immediately to improve collateral blood flow. The respective drugs should be prepared and available at all times.

CONCLUSION

aSAH presents a complex disease process that affects various organ systems, with critical impairment of cerebrovascular, cardiovascular, and pulmonary function, and carries a significant risk for life-long neurologic sequelae and disability. Intraoperative management aims at preventing sudden changes in transmural aneurysmal pressure to prevent rebleeding and at providing adequate CBF during the surgical intervention to prevent cerebral ischemia and secondary brain insults. In parallel, the anesthesiologist provides means to relax the brain, monitor the neurologic function, provide cerebral protection, manipulate the CBF, and provide emergency treatment in the event of an intraoperative aneurysmal rupture. During emergence from surgery, frequent neurologic evaluation is imperative to detect neurologic deterioration as early as possible, allowing immediate therapeutic intervention.

REFERENCES

1. Dott NM. Intracranial aneurysms cerebral arterio-radiography and surgical treatment. Edingb Med J 1933; 40:219–234.
2. Guglielmi G, Vinuela F, Duckwiler G, et al. Endovascular treatment of posterior circulation aneurysms by electrothrombosis using electrically detachable coils. J Neurosurg 1992; 77:515–524.
3. Molyneux A, Kerr R, Stratton I, et al. International Subarachnoid Aneurysm Trial (ISAT) Collaborative Group. International Subarachnoid Aneurysm Trial (ISAT) of neurosurgical clipping versus endovascular coiling in 2143 patients with ruptured intracranial aneurysms: a randomised trial. Lancet 2002; 360:1267–1274.
4. Albuquerque FC, Fiorella DJ, Han PP, Deshmukh VR, Kim LJ, McDougall CG. Endovascular management of intracranial vertebral artery dissecting aneurysms. Neurosurg Focus 2005; 18:E3.
5. Sugiu K, Tokunaga K, Watanabe K, Sasahara W, Ono S, Tamiya T, Date I. Emergent endovascular treatment of ruptured vertebral artery dissecting aneurysms. Neuroradiology 2005; 47:158–164.
6. Hunt WE, Hess RM. Surgical risk as related to time of intervention in the repair of intracranial aneurysms. J Neurosurg 1968; 28:14–20.
7. Anonymous. Report of World Federation of Neurological Surgeons Committee on a Universal Subarachnoid Hemorrhage Grading Scale. J Neurosurg 1988; 68:985–986.
8. Matta BF, Lam AM, Mayberg TS, Shapira Y, Winn HR. A critique of the intraoperative use of jugular venous bulb catheters during neurosurgical procedures. Anesth Analg 1994; 79:745–750.
9. Clavier N, Schurando P, Raggueneau JL, Payen DM. Continuous jugular bulb venous oxygen saturation validation and variations during intracranial aneurysm surgery. J Crit Care 1997, 12:112–119.
10. Moss E, Dearden NM, Berridge JC. Effects of changes in mean arterial pressure on SjO2 during cerebral aneurysm surgery. Br J Anaesth 1995; 75:527–530.
11. Manninen PH, Lam AM, Nantau WE. Monitoring of somatosensory evoked potentials during temporary arterial occlusion in cerebral aneurysm surgery. J Neurosurg Anesthesiol 1990; 2:97–104.
12. Lam AM, Keane JF, Manninen PH. Monitoring of brainstem auditory evoked potentials during basilar artery occlusion in man. Br J Anaesth 1985; 57:924–928.
13. Martin N, Doberstein C, Bentson J, Vinuela F, Dion J, Becker D. Intraoperative angiography in cerebro-vascular surgery. Clin Neurosurg 1991; 37:312–331.
14. Manninen PH, Patterson S, Lam AM, Gelb AW, Nantau WE. Evoked potential monitoring during posterior fossa aneurysm surgery: a comparison of two modalities. Can J Anaesth 1994; 41:92–97.

15. Kassell NF, Torner JC, Jane JA, Haley EC Jr., Adams HP. The International Cooperative Study on the Timing of Aneurysm Surgery. Part 2: Surgical results. J Neurosurg 1990; 73:37–47.
16. Cole DJ, Drummond JC, Shapiro HM, Zornow MH. Influence of hypotension and hypotensive technique on the area of profound reduction in cerebral blood flow during focal cerebral ischaemia in the rat. Br J Anaesth 1990; 64:498–502.
17. Artru AA, Lam AM, Johnson JO, Sperry RJ. Intracranial pressure, middle cerebral artery flow velocity, and plasma inorganic fluoride concentrations in neurosurgical patients receiving sevoflurane or isoflurane. Anesth Analg 1997; 85:587–592.
18. Meyer FB, Muzzi DA. Cerebral protection during aneurysm surgery with isoflurane anesthesia. Technical note. J Neurosurg 1992; 76:541–543.
19. Hoffman WE, Charbel FT, Edelman G. Desflurane increases brain tissue oxygenation and pH. Acta Anaesthesiol Scand 1997; 41:1162–1166.
20. Cho S, Fujigaki T, Uchiyama Y, Fukusaki M, Shibata O, Sumikawa K. Effects of sevoflurane with and without nitrous oxide on human cerebral circulation. Transcranial Doppler study. Anesthesiology 1996; 85:755–760.
21. Lam AM, Mayberg TS, Eng CC, Cooper JO, Bachenberg KL, Mathisen TL. Nitrous oxide-isoflurane anesthesia causes more cerebral vasodilation than an equipotent dose of isoflurane in humans. Anesth Analg 1994; 78:462–468.
22. Van Hemelrijck J, Fitch W, Mattheussen M, Van Aken H, Plets C, Lauwers T. Effect of propofol on cerebral circulation and autoregulation in the baboon. Anesth Analg 1990; 71:49–54.
23. Mutch WA, Ringaert KR, Ewert FJ, White IW, Donen N, Hudson RJ. Continuous opioid infusions for neurosurgical procedures: a double-blind comparison of alfentanil and fentanyl. Can J Anaesth 1991; 38:710–716.
24. From RP, Warner DS, Todd MM, Sokoll MD. Anesthesia for craniotomy: a double-blind comparison of alfentanil, fentanyl, and sufentanil. Anesthesiology 1990; 73:896–904.
25. Tsementzis SA, Hitchcock ER. Outcome from "rescue clipping" of ruptured intracranial aneurysms during induction anaesthesia and endotracheal intubation. J Neurol Neurosurg Psychiatry 1985; 48:160–163.
26. Origitano TC, Wascher TM, Reichman OH, Anderson DE. Sustained increased cerebral blood flow with prophylactic hypertensive hypervolemic hemodilution ("triple-H" therapy) after subarachnoid hemorrhage. Neurosurgery 1990; 27:729–739.
27. Strandgaard S, Jones JV, MacKenzie ET, Harper AM. Upper limit of cerebral blood flow autoregulation in experimental renovascular hypertension in the baboon. Circ Res 1975; 37:164–167.
28. Sundt TM Jr., Kobayashi S, Fode NC, Whisnant JP. Results and complications of surgical management of 809 intracranial aneurysms in 722 cases. Related and unrelated to grade of patient, type of aneurysm, and timing of surgery. J Neurosurg 1982; 56:753–765.
29. Rinkel GJ, Feigin VL, Algra A, van Gijn J. Circulatory volume expansion therapy for aneurysmal subarachnoid haemorrhage. Cochrane Database Syst Rev 2004; 18:CD000483.
30. Sen J, Belli A, Albon H, Morgan L, Petzold A, Kitchen N. Triple-H therapy in the management of aneurysmal subarachnoid haemorrhage. Lancet Neurol 2003; 2:614–621.
31. Zausinger S, Thal SC, Kreimeier U, Messmer K, Schmid-Elsaesser R. Hypertonic fluid resuscitation from subarachnoid hemorrhage in rats. Neurosurgery 2004; 55:679–686.
32. Horn P, Munch E, Vajkoczy P, et al. Hypertonic saline solution for control of elevated intracranial pressure in patients with exhausted response to mannitol and barbiturates. Neurol Res 1999; 21:758–764.
33. Tseng MY, Al-Rawi PG, Pickard JD, Rasulo FA, Kirkpatrick PJ. Effect of hypertonic saline on cerebral blood flow in poor-grade patients with subarachnoid hemorrhage. Stroke 2003; 34:1389–1396.
34. Trumble ER, Muizelaar JP, Myseros JS, Choi SC, Warren BB. Coagulopathy with the use of hetastarch in the treatment of vasospasm. J Neurosurg 1995; 82:44–47.
35. Cole CD, Gottfried ON, Liu JK, Couldwell WT. Hyponatremia in the neurosurgical patient: diagnosis and management. Neurosurg Focus 2004; 16:E9.
36. Claassen J, Vu A, Kreiter KT, et al. Effect of acute physiologic derangements on outcome after subarachnoid hemorrhage. Crit Care Med 2004; 32:832–838.
37. Dorhout Mees SM, van Dijk GW, Algra A, Kempink DR, Rinkel GJ. Glucose levels and outcome after subarachnoid hemorrhage. Neurology 2003; 61:1132–1133.
38. Lang EW, Diehl RR, Mehdorn HM. Cerebral autoregulation testing after aneurysmal subarachnoid hemorrhage: the phase relationship between arterial blood pressure and cerebral blood flow velocity. Crit Care Med 2001; 29:158–163.
39. Polderman KH, van de Kraats G, Dixon JM, Vandertop WP, Girbes AR. Increases in spinal fluid osmolarity induced by mannitol. Crit Care Med 2003; 31:584–590.
40. Heuer GG, Smith MJ, Elliott JP, Winn HR, LeRoux PD. Relationship between intracranial pressure and other clinical variables in patients with aneurysmal subarachnoid hemorrhage. J Neurosurg 2004; 101:408–416.

41. Lam AM. Cerebral aneurysms: anesthetic considerations. In: Cotrell JE, Smith DS, eds. Anesthesia and Neurosurgery. 5th ed. St. Louis: Mosby, 2004:367–396.
42. Samson D, Beyer CW Jr. Furosemide in the intraoperative reduction of intracranial pressure in the patient with subarachnoid hemorrhage. Neurosurgery 1982; 10:167–169.
43. van den Bergh WM, Algra A, Rinkel GJ. Electrocardiographic abnormalities and serum magnesium in patients with subarachnoid hemorrhage. Stroke 2004; 35:644–648.
44. Bereczki D, Liu M, do Prado GF, Fekete I. Mannitol for acute stroke. Cochrane Database Syst Rev 2001; 1:CD001153.
45. Bereczki D, Liu M, Prado GF, Fekete I. Cochrane report: A systematic review of mannitol therapy for acute ischemic stroke and cerebral parenchymal hemorrhage. Stroke 2000; 31:2719–2722.
46. Klimo P Jr., Kestle JR, MacDonald JD, Schmidt RH. Marked reduction of cerebral vasospasm with lumbar drainage of cerebrospinal fluid after subarachnoid hemorrhage. J Neurosurg 2004; 100:215–224.
47. Drummond JC. Anesthesia for intracranial aneurysm surgery. 2004 Annual Meeting Refresher Course Lectures. ASA Annual Meeting 2004, Las Vegas; Lecture 219:1–7.
48. Bendo AA. Intracranial vascular surgery. Anesthesiology Clin N Am 2002; 20:377–388.
49. Ferguson GG. The rational for controlled hypotension. In: Varkey GP, ed. Anesthetic Considerations in the Surgical Repair of Intracranial Aneurysms. Boston: Little Brown, 1982 (cited according to 41).
50. Lownie S, Wu X, Karlik S, Gelb AW. Brain retractor edema during induced hypotension: the effect of the rate of return of blood pressure. Neurosurgery 1990; 27:901–905.
51. Drummond JC. Deliberate hypotension for intracranial aneurysm surgery: changing practices. Can J Anaesth 1991; 38:935–936.
52. Aaslid R. Hemodynamics of cerebrovascular spasm. Acta Neurochir Suppl 1999; 72:47–57.
53. Dernbach PD, Little JR, Jones SC, Ebrahim ZY. Altered cerebral autoregulation and CO2 reactivity after aneurysmal subarachnoid hemorrhage. Neurosurgery 1988; 22:822–826.
54. Hitchcock ER, Tsementzis SA, Dow AA. Short- and long-term prognosis of patients with a subarachnoid haemorrhage in relation to intra-operative period of hypotension. Acta Neurochir (Wien) 1984; 70:235–42.
55. Chang HS, Hongo K, Nakagawa H. Adverse effects of limited hypotensive anesthesia on the outcome of patients with subarachnoid hemorrhage. J Neurosurg 2000; 92:971–975.
56. Abe K. Vasodilators during cerebral aneurysm surgery. Can J Anaesth 1993; 40:775–790.
57. Hamann G, Haass A, Schimrigk K. Beta-blockade in acute aneurysmal subarachnoid haemorrhage. Acta Neurochir (Wien) 1993; 121:119–122.
58. Ogilvy CS, Carter BS, Kaplan S, Rich C, Crowell RM. Temporary vessel occlusion for aneurysm surgery: risk factors for stroke in patients protected by induced hypothermia and hypertension and intravenous mannitol administration. J Neurosurg 1996; 84:785–791.
59. Giannotta SL, Oppenheimer JH, Levy ML, Zelman V. Management of intraoperative rupture of aneurysm without hypotension. Neurosurgery 1991; 28:531–535.
60. Engelhard HH, Andrews CO, Slavin KV, Charbel FT. Current management of intraventricular hemorrhage. Surg Neurol 2003; 60:15–21.
61. Lavine SD, Masri LS, Levy ML, Giannotta SL. Temporary occlusion of the middle cerebral artery in intracranial aneurysm surgery: time limitation and advantage of brain protection. J Neurosurg 1997; 87:817–24.
62. Taylor CL, Steele D, Kopitnik TA Jr., Samson DS, Purdy PD. Outcome after subarachnoid hemorrhage from a very small aneurysm: a case-control series. J Neurosurg 2004; 100:623–625.
63. Kett-White R, Hutchinson PJ, Al-Rawi PG, et al. Cerebral oxygen and microdialysis monitoring during aneurysm surgery: effects of blood pressure, cerebrospinal fluid drainage, and temporary clipping on infarction. J Neurosurg 2002; 96:1013–1019.
63. Frietsch T, Kirsch JR. Strategies of neuroprotection for intracranial aneurysms. Best Pract Res Clin Anaesthesiol 2004; 18:595–630.
64. Spetzler RF, Hadley MN. Protection against cerebral ischemia: the role of barbiturates. Cerebrovasc Brain Metab Rev 1989 Fall; 1:212–229.
65. Todd MM, Drummond JC, Hoi SU. Hemodynamic effects of high dose pentobarbital: studies in elective neurosurgical patients. Neurosurgery 1987; 20:559–563.
66. Cheng MA, Theard MA, Tempelhoff R. Intravenous agents and intraoperative neuroprotection. Beyond barbiturates. Crit Care Clin 1997; 13:185–199.
67. Bayona NA, Gelb AW, Jiang Z, Wilson JX, Urquhart BL, Cechetto DF. Propofol neuroprotection in cerebral ischemia and its effects on low-molecular-weight antioxidants and skilled motor tasks. Anesthesiology 2004; 100:1151–1159.
68. Warner DS, Takaoka S, Wu B, et al. Electroencephalographic burst suppression is not required to elicit maximal neuroprotection from pentobarbital in a rat model of focal cerebral ischemia. Anesthesiology 1996; 84:1475–1484.
69. Zaugg M, Lucchinetti E, Garcia C, Pasch T, Spahn DR, Schaub MC. Anaesthetics and cardiac preconditioning. Part II. Clinical implications. Br J Anaesth 2003; 91:566–576.

70. Olsen TS, Weber UJ, Kammersgaard LP. Therapeutic hypothermia for acute stroke. Lancet Neurol 2003; 2:410–416.
71. Hypothermia after Cardiac Arrest Study Group. Mild therapeutic hypothermia to improve the neurologic outcome after cardiac arrest. N Engl J Med 2002; 346:549–556.
72. Kimme P, Fridrikssen S, Engdahl O, Hillman J, Vegfors M, Sjoberg F. Moderate hypothermia for 359 operations to clip cerebral aneurysms. Br J Anaesth 2004; 93:343–347.
73. Young WL, Lawton MT, Gupta DK, Hashimoto T. Anesthetic management of deep hypothermic circulatory arrest for cerebral aneurysm clipping. Anesthesiology 2002; 96:497–503.
74. Hindman BJ, Todd MM, Gelb AW, et al. Mild hypothermia as a protective therapy during intracranial aneurysm surgery: a randomized prospective pilot trial. Neurosurgery 1999; 44:23–32.
75. Todd MM, Hindman BJ, Clarke WR, Torner JC. Intraoperative Hypothermia for Aneurysm Surgery Trial (IHAST) Investigators. Mild intraoperative hypothermia during surgery for intracranial aneurysm. N Engl J Med 2005; 352:135–145.
76. Thompson HJ, Tkacs NC, Saatman KE, Raghupathi R, McIntosh TK. Hyperthermia following traumatic brain injury: a critical evaluation. Neurobiol Dis 2003; 12:163–173.
77. Reith J, Jorgensen HS, Pedersen PM, Nakayama H, Raaschou HO, Jeppesen LL, Olsen TS. Body temperature in acute stroke: relation to stroke severity, infarct size, mortality, and outcome. Lancet 1996; 347:422–425.
78. Cormio M, Citerio G, Spear S, Fumagalli R, Pesenti A. Control of fever by continuous, low-dose diclofenac sodium infusion in acute cerebral damage patients. Intensive Care Med 2000; 26:552–557.
79. Suehiro E, Povlishock JT. Exacerbation of traumatically induced axonal injury by rapid posthypothermic rewarming and attenuation of axonal change by cyclosporin A. J Neurosurg 2001; 94:493–498.
80. Batjer H, Samson D. Intraoperative aneurysmal rupture: incidence, outcome, and suggestions for surgical management. Neurosurgery 1986; 18:701–707.
81. Houkin K, Kuroda S, Takahashi A, et al. Intra-operative premature rupture of the cerebral aneurysms. Analysis of the causes and management. Acta Neurochir (Wien) 1999; 141:1255–1263.
82. Eng CC, Lam AM, Byrd S, Newell DW. The diagnosis and management of a perianesthetic cerebral aneurysmal rupture aided with transcranial Doppler ultrasonography. Anesthesiology 1993; 78:191–194.
83. Rabinstein AA, Pichelmann MA, Friedman JA, et al. Symptomatic vasospasm and outcomes following aneurysmal subarachnoid hemorrhage: a comparison between surgical repair and endovascular coil occlusion. J Neurosurg 2003; 98:319–325.
84. Hoh BL, Topcuoglu MA, Singhal AB, et al. Effect of clipping, craniotomy, or intravascular coiling on cerebral vasospasm and patient outcome after aneurysmal subarachnoid hemorrhage. Neurosurgery 2004; 55:779–786.
85. Sade B, Mohr G. Critical appraisal of the International Subarachnoid Aneurysm Trial (ISAT). Neurol India 2004; 52:32–35.
86. Bellebaum C, Schafers L, Schoch B, et al. Clipping versus coiling: neuropsychological follow up after aneurysmal subarachnoid haemorrhage (SAH). J Clin Exp Neuropsychol 2004; 26:1081–1092.
87. Hashimoto T, Gupta DK, Young WL. Interventional neuroradiology: anesthetic considerations. Anesthesiol Clin North America 2002; 20:347–359.
88. Hashimoto T, Young WL, Aagaard BD, Joshi S, Ostapkovich ND, Pile-Spellman J. Adenosine-induced ventricular asystole to induce transient profound systemic hypotension in patients undergoing endovascular therapy. Dose-response characteristics. Anesthesiology 2000; 93:998–1001.

7 | Medical Management of Subarachnoid Hemorrhage

Yekaterina K. Axelrod, MD, Fellow
Department of Neurosciences Critical Care, Washington University School of Medicine, St. Louis, Missouri, USA

Michael N. Diringer, MD, Professor[a] and Director[b]
[a]*Departments of Neurology and Neurological Surgery,* [b]*Neurocritical Care Unit, Washington University School of Medicine, St. Louis, Missouri, USA*

PRESENTATION

A sudden dramatic elevation of intracranial pressure (ICP) accounts for the classic presentation of acute aneurysm rupture—the instantaneous onset of a severe headache often described by patients as "the worst headache of my life" (1). Headache frequently presents during physical exertion and is often associated with nausea and vomiting. Syncope (mainly due to increased ICP) is seen in about half of cases and is usually followed by a gradual improvement in the level of consciousness. Focal neurologic signs appear in only 10% to 15% of cases and typically represent mass effect from a giant aneurysm (e.g., an enlarging posterior communicating artery aneurysm pressing upon the third cranial nerve), intraparenchymal hemorrhage, subdural hematoma, or a large localized subarachnoid clot. There may be a report of a seizure, but it is often unclear as to whether these episodes are true epileptic events or abnormal posturing. Up to 20% of patients with subarachnoid hemorrhage (SAH) may develop intraocular hemorrhages (2).

EVALUATION AND INITIAL MANAGEMENT

The initial steps in the assessment of a patient with suspected SAH should always focus on the level of neurologic function and the ability to protect the airway. The Hunt and Hess Scale and the more recently developed World Federation of Neurological Surgeons Scale are the most widely used measures of the patient's clinical condition (Tables 1 and 2).

Diagnostic Evaluation

The best initial diagnostic test is a noncontrasted computed tomography (CT) scan, which is able to detect more than 95% of subarachnoid bleeds on the day of onset (3,4). Blood typically appears as a high-density signal in the perimesencephalic, interpeduncular, and basal cisterns, Sylvian fissure, and sulci of the brain (Fig. 1). CT scans may be falsely negative under certain circumstances: if hemorrhage occurred several days prior (sensitivity drops to 50% in a week) (5), if the amount of extravasated blood is small, or if hematocrit is below 27% (6). The amount of subarachnoid blood is graded by Fisher Scale (Table 3), which is also used to predict the risk of vasospasm. At this stage, the size of the third ventricle and the temporal horns of the lateral ventricles should be evaluated to detect and promptly treat early hydrocephalus.

Lumbar puncture should only be performed in cases of high clinical suspicion of SAH in the context of negative CT. It may be difficult to distinguish a traumatic lumbar puncture from a true SAH. The presence of xanthochromia, best determined by spectrophotometry (4), reflects high levels of either cerebrospinal fluid (CSF) protein (>200dL mg/dL) or bilirubin, the end product of hemoglobin conversion (a complex process that takes up to 12 hr). Determining if cell count declines from the first to last collected tube of CSF does not reliably distinguish between traumatic tap and SAH.

With the current emphasis on early surgical or endovascular treatment of aneurysms, conventional angiography should be performed as soon as possible (Fig. 2). As multiple aneurysms are present in approximately 20% of cases (7,8), selective four-vessel angiography is

Table 1 Hunt and Hess Scale

Grade	Symptoms
I	Asymptomatic or mild headache
II	Moderate to severe headache, nuchal rigidity, with or without cranial nerve deficits
III	Confusion, lethargy, or mild focal symptoms
IV	Stupor and/or hemiparesis
V	Comatose and/or extensor posturing

Table 2 World Federation of Neurological Surgeons

Grade	Glasgow Coma Scale	Motor deficits
I	15	Absent
II	14–13	Absent
III	14–13	Present
IV	12–7	Present or absent
V	6–3	Present or absent

necessary. Magnetic resonance (MR) and CT angiography are not presently sufficiently sensitive to replace conventional angiography, but the techniques are rapidly advancing (9,10). CT and MR angiograms may serve as an additional tool with which to plan surgery (11).

In 15% to 20% of patients, the cause of nontraumatic SAH remains undetermined even after angiography. In a few instances, this may be due to vasospasm or inadequate views incapable of detecting smaller aneurysms. Repeat angiography is therefore often recommended in a few days to two weeks. In patients whose bleeding is confined to the perimesencephalic and ambient cisterns, a source of bleeding might not be evident despite high-quality angiograms. Such hemorrhages are referred to as "perimesencephalic SAH" and have been attributed to venous rather than arterial bleeding (12). However, detecting the typical perimesencephalic pattern of SAH on CT should not prevent one from pursuing angiography, because this pattern may be seen with aneurysmal rupture (13,14), especially in the posterior circulation (15).

Initial Stabilization

Patient's clinical condition must be carefully assessed and stabilized prior to diagnostic testing. If the patient is lethargic or agitated, management of the airway should be addressed first. During angiography, sedation is frequently used, which could lead to airway obstruction in lethargic patients. To facilitate a safe and rapid study for agitated patients, elective endotracheal intubation should be considered.

Generalized sympathetic activation with high catecholamine levels, as well as pain and anxiety, generally cause elevated blood pressure after SAH. Because hypertension is associated with aneurysmal rerupture, it requires prompt treatment; however, headache should be addressed first. Nimodipine, used routinely for prevention of vasospasm, and analgesics may be sufficient for blood pressure control in some patients, whereas others may require the administration of additional antihypertensive medications. The most widely employed agents are combined α-1 and β-blocker labetalol or other general β-blockers, none of which raises ICP.

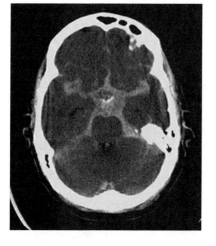

Figure 1 Computed tomography scan of a patient with a subarachnoid hemorrhage.

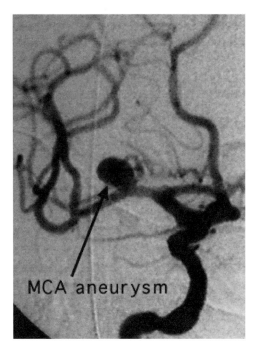

MCA aneurysm

Figure 2 Angiographic image of an aneurysm of the MCA. *Abbreviation*: MCA, middle cerebral artery.

In the presence of a mass lesion or elevated ICP, the use of vasodilators engenders concern, especially venous dilators, such as sodium nitroprusside, which can raise ICP to a significant degree (16). Debate is ongoing regarding the appropriateness of administering agents that are pure arterial dilators, e.g., hydralazine, nicardipine, and angiotensin-converting enzyme inhibitors; yet many centers routinely use them (17). One trial demonstrated an improved outcome after SAH with the use of high doses of β-blockers (18). A notable exception to vigorous management of hypertension is made when patients develop hydrocephalus with potentially higher ICP, in which case, elevated blood pressure helps to maintain adequate cerebral perfusion. Only after the treatment of hydrocephalus should hypertension be addressed.

Cardiac abnormalities are common in the first 24 to 48 hr following SAH, and they are almost always completely reversible. Electrocardiographic alterations, including tall-peaked T-waves ("cerebral T-waves"), QT segment prolongation, and ST segment elevation/depression, are frequent; they have been linked to excessive levels of circulating catecholamines (19). Cardiac enzymes may be elevated in up to one-third of patients and are variably associated with echocardiographic abnormalities. These disturbances may occur in the absence of coronary artery disease. Myocardial lesions (mainly contraction band necrosis) that have been reported in cases of SAH are pathologically distinct from ischemic lesions (20). Arrhythmias are frequently seen; however, life-threatening arrhythmias such as ventricular tachycardia have been only rarely noted (21). Cardiac wall motion abnormalities have also been detected in up to one-third of patients (22). In rare cases, a picture of a "stunned myocardium" develops, with severe pump

Table 3 Fisher Scale (Based on Initial CT Appearance and Quantification of Subarachnoid Blood)

Grade	CT Description
1	No subarachnoid blood on CT
2	Broad diffusion of subarachnoid blood, no clots, and no layers of blood greater than 1 mm
3	Either localized blood clots in the subarachnoid space or layers of blood greater than 1 mm
4	Intraventricular and intracerebral blood present, in the absence of significant subarachnoid blood

Abbreviation: CT, computed tomography.

failure, poor cardiac output, pulmonary edema, and hypotension. The most important predictors of cardiac dysfunction are those that reflect the severity of the hemorrhage.

EARLY CRITICAL CARE MANAGEMENT

Routine Care and Monitoring
The routine monitoring of all patients with acute SAH should include serial neurologic examinations, continuous CARDIAC monitoring, and frequent determinations of blood pressure, electrolytes, body weight, fluid balance, and, in many centers, cerebral blood flow velocity by transcranial Doppler (TCD). Adequate hydration should be maintained with isotonic saline to avoid volume contraction. Monitoring of daily fluid balance, body weight, and hematocrit is important to ascertain stable intravascular volume.

Anticonvulsants
The risks and implications of seizures associated with SAH are not well defined, and the need for and efficacy of routinely administered anticonvulsants following SAH for seizure prophylaxis are yet to be established. A large number of seizure-like episodes are associated with aneurysmal rupture. It is unclear, however, whether these episodes are truly epileptic in origin. In a large prospective study, early seizures were reported to occur in 6% of patients (23). A retrospective review found that the majority of early seizures occurred before medical presentation; in-hospital seizures were rare in patients who were administered prophylactic anticonvulsants (24).

The routine use of prophylactic anticonvulsants during the perioperative period has been evaluated in several studies. Nonrandomized studies of patients who underwent craniotomy indicated a benefit of prophylactic anticonvulsants (25–27); however, the number of patients with SAH in these reports was too small to address the issue. A study of patients who underwent coil embolization of an aneurysm (rather than surgery) reported no periprocedural seizures and a delayed *de novo* seizure rate of 1.7% (28). Risk factors for seizures after SAH include middle cerebral artery aneurysms (29,30), intraparenchymal hematoma (25,29,31), infarcts (32), and a history of hypertension (33). Noteworthily, a recent study found that phenytoin routinely administered to patients following SAH for seizure prophylaxis was associated with worse neurologic and cognitive outcome (34).

Steroids
Dexamethasone is widely used to reduce meningeal irritation and intra- and postoperative edema, but no convincing evidence that documents its efficacy exists. A prospective, randomized, controlled trial of tirilazad mesylate, a nonglucocorticoid 21-aminosteroid, failed to show any benefit (35,36).

Rebleeding
The risk of rebleeding is highest immediately following hemorrhage (4–6% over the first 24 hrs) and declines over the next few days. At two weeks, the cumulative risk approaches 20%. Rebleeding rates are highest in women and in those with poor medical condition and with elevated systolic blood pressure. Almost a half of the patients who rebleed do not survive.

In the past, antifibrinolytic agents, such as epsilon-aminocaproic or tranexamic acid, were routinely administered to prevent rebleeding. It is clear that these agents do reduce the incidence of rebleeding; however, this benefit was offset by an increase in hydrocephalus and more ischemic infarctions from vasospasm (37). A meta-analysis of several trials revealed no overall effect on outcome (38). With the advent of early surgical and endovascular management, the use of these agents has declined dramatically. Still, short-term use of antifibrinolytics has been suggested for patients awaiting surgery or endovascular treatment. The data are mixed as to whether short courses are also associated with more vasospasm.

Anecdotally, rerupture has been associated with systemic hypertension and sudden drops or elevations of ICP, the latter caused by coughing, sneezing, straining, and Valsalva maneuvers. Hence, initial management focuses on avoiding these factors. Measures should be taken to minimize coughing and straining. In intubated patients, verifying the position of the endotracheal tube and administering antitussives and local anesthetics may be necessary if patients cough excessively. Stool softeners are given routinely to prevent straining. Slow CSF drainage during lumbar puncture or ventriculostomy is recommended.

Excessive stimulation of patients has traditionally been avoided to prevent fluctuations in blood pressure. Although adverse effects of such stimulation have never been established, it seems prudent to medicate agitated or combative patients. Ideally, they should be sedated to the point of drowsiness but should remain responsive to stimulation. Care must be taken to prevent oversedation, so that clinical deterioration can be easily recognized. Opiates provide not only sedation but also analgesia for treating headache; long-acting sedative agents, such as barbiturates, should be avoided.

Definitive prevention of rebleeding is accomplished by aneurysm repair. The old notion that surgery is more difficult and results in a worse outcome when performed early (within three days of hemorrhage) has not been supported by careful analysis. Outcome of patients with Hunt and Hess grades II and III is improved with early surgery. Additionally, repair of aneurysms has the further advantage of permitting safe elevation of blood pressure to treat vasospasm.

A multicenter, randomized trial recently compared one-year outcomes in acute SAH patients who were randomized to have their aneurysm repaired either by surgical or endovascular means. Of the almost 10,000 patients screened, only approximately 2000 met the inclusion criteria, which required that the treating physicians agree that the aneurysm could be successfully repaired by either means. At one-year, outcome was somewhat better in patients treated by endovascular coiling, and long-term follow-up is underway to assess rebleeding rates (39).

Hydrocephalus

Acute hydrocephalus (ventricular enlargement within 72 hr) is reported to occur in about 20% to 30% of patients (40–43). The ventricular enlargement is often accompanied by intraventricular blood (44,45), whereas hydrocephalus without intraventricular hemorrhage is associated with the amount and distribution of cisternal blood (46,47). Acute hydrocephalus is more frequent in patients with poor clinical grade and a higher Fischer grade (40–43).

The clinical significance of acute ventriculomegaly after SAH is uncertain, because many patients are apparently asymptomatic and do not deteriorate (48). Yet, in patients with diminished level of consciousness, 40% to 80% show some degree of improvement after ventriculostomy (45,48,49). Based on two small series, the placement of a ventriculostomy may (50) or may not (51) be associated with rebleeding.

Delayed hydrocephalus requiring permanent shunting procedures is reported at rates of 18% to 26% of surviving patients (42,52,53). The need for permanent CSF diversion is associated with older age, early ventriculomegaly, presence of intraventricular hemorrhage, poor clinical condition on presentation, and female gender (54–58). Two single center series suggest that routine fenestration of the lamina terminalis during microsurgical aneurysm repair reduces the incidence of chronic hydrocephalus (59,60). On the other hand, rates are no different in patients who undergo clipping or endovascular treatment of their aneurysms (52,53). Ventriculoatrial, ventriculoperitoneal, or lumboperitoneal shunts may improve clinical status in this group of patients (61,62).

Stunned Myocardium

In rare cases, myocardial contractility may be impaired after SAH, leading to a fall in cardiac output and blood pressure, with subsequent pulmonary edema. Even though this condition has been referred to as "stunned myocardium," an element of neurogenic pulmonary edema may also be seen. The management of this condition is similar to treatment of acute pump failure of other etiologies and includes administration of inotropic agents, diuretics, high concentrations of oxygen, and positive end-expiratory pressure. This state is surprisingly transient and is usually completely reversed in an average of four days.

Pulmonary Complications

Pulmonary complications are frequent in patients with SAH and represent a significant cause of morbidity and mortality. Among the most common are nosocomial and aspiration pneumonia, pulmonary edema (neurogenic and cardiogenic), and pulmonary embolism (21,63). Older patients with worse Hunt and Hess grade and lower Glasgow Coma Scale score on admission are at higher risk for developing pulmonary complications (63).

Patients with pulmonary complications were shown to have a greater incidence of symptomatic vasospasm.

Most cases of pneumonia are seen in patients who require mechanical ventilation. Extubation should be performed as early as clinically possible. Care must be taken to prevent accidental extubation. Nasally placed endotracheal tubes should be avoided to diminish risk of sinusitis. All mechanically ventilated patients should be maintained in semirecumbent position to prevent aspiration. Adequate enteral nutrition is crucial; however, large gastric volumes should be avoided (64).

Neurogenic pulmonary edema may be seen acutely, within hours of the initial ictus, or a few days after the onset of aneurysmal rupture. Clinical features are nonspecific and similar to those of cardiogenic pulmonary edema with respiratory distress, tachycardia, and hypotension. Treatment is generally supportive and includes the administration of both supplemental oxygen, to maintain adequate tissue oxygenation, and diuretics; patients with severe hypoxemia require ventilatory support with high positive end-expiratory pressure. Insertion of a pulmonary artery catheter may be warranted, especially if hemodynamic therapy for vasospasm is required. Neurogenic pulmonary edema is often reversible within 48 to 72 hrs.

LATE COMPLICATIONS

Venous Thromboembolism
Multiple risk factors are associated with venous thromboembolism in this population, including craniotomy, lower limb paralysis, advanced age, and prolonged ICU stay with indwelling venous catheters. Methods of mechanical prophylaxis (graduated compression stockings and pneumatic compression devices) have been proven to be safe and effective. Adjunct of low-molecular-weight heparins is a more efficacious option at the expense of an additional mild risk of intracranial hemorrhagic complications (65–67).

Glucose Management
Hyperglycemia has been associated with poor functional outcome in patients with SAH (68,69). An aggressive approach to achieve normoglycemia should be instituted early. A large randomized study of intensive insulin therapy in surgical critically ill patients demonstrated a significant reduction in morbidity and mortality (70).

Fever
Fever is commonly seen in patients with SAH even without infections; its detrimental effects on neurologic outcome, mortality, and vasospasm have been recognized (71,72). Both novel physical (intravascular catheters) (73) and conventional pharmacologic means of lowering body temperature are useful; however, many patients after SAH remain refractory to any efforts to achieve normothermia. A multicenter study of intraoperative hypothermia to 33°C that did not follow postoperative fever management failed to show benefit in neurologic outcome (74).

Hyponatremia and Intravascular Volume Contraction
Hyponatremia occurs in up to one-third of patients following SAH. Although originally attributed to the syndrome of inappropriate secretion of antidiuretic hormone, the picture is more complex. Disturbances of humoral and neural regulation of sodium, intravascular volume, and water in SAH lead to intravascular volume contraction and hyponatremia, sometimes referred to as cerebral salt wasting. When administered the usual 2 to 3 L of fluids per day, up to half of patients develop intravascular volume contraction. The important clinical consequences include a higher rate of symptoms in patients with angiographic vasospasm and an increase in the number of delayed ischemic deficits that progress to infarction.

Levels of several circulating natriuretic factors are elevated following SAH, yet antidiuretic hormone levels remain elevated during hyponatremia. Administration of large volumes of isotonic fluids can prevent volume contraction and appears to limit the severity of the hyponatremia. Hyponatremia can frequently be managed with restriction of all free water by giving only isotonic or hypertonic intravenous fluids (1.25–3.0% saline), minimizing oral liquids, and using concentrated enteral feedings.

Two randomized, controlled trials have evaluated the ability of the mineralocorticoid fludrocortisone to correct hyponatremia and fluid balance. One (75) found that it helped correct the negative sodium balance but not volume contraction or hyponatremia; the second (76) reported a reduced need for fluids and improved sodium levels with fludrocortisone.

Vasospasm

In the context of SAH, the term "vasospasm" refers to a condition that is much more complex than simply constriction of blood vessels. Additional contributing factors include pathologic changes in arterial walls, with narrowing of the lumen and impairing vascular relaxation, altered vascular reactivity, and hypovolemia. The term "delayed ischemic deficit" (DID) more aptly describes the situation in which these multiple factors conspire to result in cerebral ischemia.

Vasospasm may be defined on the basis of angiographic, TCD, or clinical criteria. Angiographic segmental or diffuse narrowing of vessels occurs in up to 70% of patients. These changes are usually seen 5 to 14 days after the hemorrhage but may occur from as early as day 2 and as late as 3 weeks following the bleed. TCD criteria define vasospasm, using absolute linear blood flow velocity (LBFV), as mild (>120 cm/sec), moderate (>160 cm/sec), or severe (>200 cm/sec). The rate of rise in the LBFV may be a more sensitive indicator of vasospasm. When compared to angiography, TCD has a sensitivity of about 80%, reflecting that it samples only a small segment of the vasculature.

DIDs develop in approximately one-third of SAH patients, primarily in those with large amounts of subarachnoid blood. The syndrome presents as either a gradual decline in level of consciousness or the appearance of new focal neurologic deficits. These findings may fluctuate and can be exacerbated by hypovolemia or hypotension.

The disparity between the incidence of angiographic, TCD, and clinical vasospasm complicates management. All agree that when clinical symptoms develop, they should be treated aggressively; however, there is disagreement about how to respond to elevated TCD velocities or angiographic vasospasm in the absence of symptoms.

The management of vasospasm involves both the routine "prophylactic" measures used for all patients and the more aggressive intervention reserved for situations with signs of active vasospasm. Routine measures include the administration of the centrally acting calcium channel blocker nimodipine, avoidance of intravascular volume contraction, and mechanical means to remove subarachnoid blood at the time of surgery.

Nimodipine has been shown to reduce the incidence of ischemic infarctions and improve outcome in several prospective controlled studies; it is routinely administered to all patients (77). Hypotension is infrequent with the usual doses (60 mg every 4 hr), especially if patients are well hydrated. In those treated with vasopressors for symptomatic vasospasm, dips in blood pressure following nimodipine administration could be more of a problem; therefore, changing the dose to 30 mg every 2 hr might be helpful.

It is routine practice to remove subarachnoid blood at surgery. Subarachnoid administration of recombinant tissue plasminogen activator completely prevented vasospasm in experimental models; however, in a randomized controlled trial of SAH patients, it did not alter neurologic outcome. Preliminary reports suggest a beneficial effect of a variation on this approach, using head shaking combined with cisternal irrigation with urokinase (78). Another recent study found improved outcome with reintroduction of the old practice of draining large volumes of CSF from the lumbar space to help clear subarachnoid blood (79).

Prophylactic Hypervolemia

A number of recent studies have addressed the use of "prophylactic" hypervolemia. In one prospective, randomized trial, routine administration of albumin to keep central venous pressure greater than 7 mmHg did not improve cerebral blood flow or outcome (80). Another report suggested that outcome worsened after the discontinuation of the routine use of albumin (81). Due to concern about hyperchloremic metabolic acidosis developing after administration of large amounts of saline, some clinicians partially replace chloride with acetate.

Other Prophylactic Measures

The implantation of prolonged release implants at the time of surgical repair of the aneurysm might help reduce the incidence of vasospasm. Preliminary work with implants impregnated with papaverine (82) and nicardipine (83) is promising. A small trial with enoxaparin suggested a reduction in DID (84). A more aggressive approach, the prophylactic use of transluminal balloon angioplasty in patients with Fisher Grade 3 SAH, was reported to markedly reduce the rate of vasospasm in this high-risk group of patients (85).

Hemodynamic Augmentation

Currently the mainstay of treatment of symptomatic vasospasm in patients with repaired aneurysms is hemodynamic augmentation (HA). HA consists of some combination of large volumes of fluids, vasopressors, and inotropic agents; however, the optimal combination is unknown. This intervention has never been tested in a randomized, controlled setting and is based on a number of case series that focused on different aspects of HA.

Once the threshold for aggressive treatment has been crossed, any possible hypovolemia should be corrected rapidly. The use of colloids is controversial, with no clear data to support their efficacy. Although it appears that the correction of hypovolemia is important, no data clearly indicate benefits of hypervolemia over euvolemia. Some degree of acute volume expansion may be helpful in improving cardiac output and blood pressure, but this effect in one study plateaued at pulmonary capillary wedge pressure of 14 mmHg (86). If fluid administration produces no immediate response, vasoactive agents should be employed, either inotropic agents (dobutamine) to improve cardiac output or vasopressors (phenylephrine) or combined agents (dopamine and norepinephrine) to augment systemic blood pressure.

At issue is the hemodynamic parameter that is best to augment. One approach is to place a pulmonary artery catheter to determine which parameter is most amenable to augmentation. Use of a Swan-Ganz catheter is also helpful in patients with cardiac disease to help guide therapy and prevent fluid overload or congestive heart failure. Although preliminary reports indicated a high complication rate with this therapy, subsequent studies have found that, with close monitoring, complications were low (87).

The major focus of all of these therapeutic maneuvers is to improve neurologic function. If a hemodynamic goal is reached, but no neurologic improvement is observed, the therapeutic maneuver should be reassessed. It should be emphasized that the use of hypertensive therapy is usually not recommended in patients with unclipped aneurysms. The use of HA appears safe in patients with recently coiled aneurysms (88). Weaning hemodynamic augmentation should be performed gradually, usually over several days, the rate of withdrawal being guided, again, by the neurologic status.

Endovascular Treament of Delayed Ischemic Deficits

Endovascular approaches to treatment of vasospasm are continuously evolving. It is now a routine practice to perform angioplasty on the proximal segments of the vasospastic cerebral vessels. The angiographic changes following angioplasty are impressive and appear to be long lasting (Fig. 3). However, clinical efficacy has been difficult to establish, as this procedure is utilized in conjunction

(A)   **(B)**

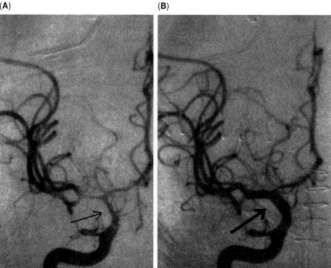

Figure 3   Vasospasm before and after angioplasty. (**A**) Angiogram with vasospasm in the middle cerebral artery territory (*thin arrow*). (**B**) Angiogram after angioplasty with improvement in vasospasm (*thick arrow*).

with HA. In addition to angioplasty, intra-arterial infusion of papaverine results in vasodilation and improvement in global blood flow, but the response is transient and repeated treatments are often necessary. Calcium channel blockers have also been employed with good angiographic results.

The most efficacious point at which to move to endovascular interventions remains unsettled. Most centers initiate hemodynamic augmentation first, and, if no response occurs in a matter of hours, proceed to endovascular interventions. Patients with poor cardiac function, however, might be candidates for prompt endovascular management, because they are at a high risk of complications from hemodynamic augmentation.

CONCLUSION

SAH is a complex multisystemic disorder. Medical complications of SAH may be extremely difficult to treat; morbidity and mortality are high. Frequently, physicians are faced with challenging dilemmas, in which the patient's general medical condition might be put at risk for the benefit of neurologic status. For example, raising blood pressure and maintaining hypervolemia for treatment of vasospasm could be detrimental to patients with severe pump failure. A multidisciplinary team of neurosurgeons, neurointensivists, and neuroradiologists is almost always necessary to achieve success in treating this multifaceted disease.

REFERENCES

1. Kassell NF, Torner JC, Haley EC Jr, et al. The International Cooperative Study on the Timing of Aneurysm Surgery. Part 1: Overall management results. J Neurosurg 1990; 73(1):18–36.
2. Frizzell RT, Kuhn F, Morris R, et al. Screening for ocular hemorrhages in patients with ruptured cerebral aneurysms: a prospective study of 99 patients. Neurosurgery 1997; 41(3):529–533.
3. Adams HP Jr, Kassell NF, Torner JC, et al. CT and clinical correlations in recent aneurysmal subarachnoid hemorrhage: a preliminary report of the Cooperative Aneurysm Study. Neurology 1983; 33:981–988.
4. Morgenstern LB, Luna-Gonzales H, Huber JC Jr, et al. Worst headache and subarachnoid hemorrhage: prospective, modern computed tomography and spinal fluid analysis. Ann Emerg Med 1998; 32(3 Pt 1):297–304.
5. van Gijn J, van Dongen KJ. The time course of aneurysmal haemorrhage on computed tomograms. Neuroradiology 1982; 23(3):153–156.
6. Noguchi K, Seto H, Kamisaki Y, et al. Comparison of fluid-attenuated inversion-recovery MR imaging with CT in a simulated model of acute subarachnoid hemorrhage. Am J Neuroradiol 2000; 21(5):923–927.
7. Kaminogo M, Yonekura M, Shibata S. Incidence and outcome of multiple intracranial aneurysms in a defined population. Stroke 2003; 34(1):16–21.
8. Qureshi AI, Suarez JI, Parekh PD, et al. Risk factors for multiple intracranial aneurysms. Neurosurgery 1998; 43(1):22–26.
9. Hoh BL, Cheung AC, Rabinov JD, et al. Results of a prospective protocol of computed tomographic angiography in place of catheter angiography as the only diagnostic and pretreatment planning study for cerebral aneurysms by a combined neurovascular team. Neurosurgery 2004; 54(6):1329–1340.
10. Villablanca JP, Jahan R, Hooshi P, et al. Detection and characterization of very small cerebral aneurysms by using 2D and 3D helical CT angiography. Am J Neuroradiol 2002; 23(7):1187–1198.
11. Hochmuth A, Spetzger U, Schumacher M. Comparison of three-dimensional rotational angiography with digital subtraction angiography in the assessment of ruptured cerebral aneurysms. Am J Neuroradiol 2002; 23(7):1199–1205.
12. van der Schaaf IC, Velthuis BK, Gouw A, et al. Venous drainage in perimesencephalic hemorrhage. Stroke 2004; 35(7):1614–1618.
13. Van Calenbergh F, Plets C, Goffin J, et al. Nonaneurysmal subarachnoid hemorrhage: prevalence of perimesencephalic hemorrhage in a consecutive series. Surg Neurol 1993; 39(4):320–323.
14. Alen JF, Lagares A, Lobato RD, et al. Comparison between perimesencephalic nonaneurysmal subarachnoid hemorrhage and subarachnoid hemorrhage caused by posterior circulation aneurysms. J Neurosurg 2003; 98(3):529–535.
15. Kallmes DF, Clark HP, Dix JE, et al. Ruptured vertebrobasilar aneurysms: frequency of the nonaneurysmal perimesencephalic pattern of hemorrhage on CT scans. Radiology 1996; 201(3):657–660.
16. Turner JM, Powell D, Gibson RM, et al. Intracranial pressure changes in neurosurgical patients during hypotension induced with sodium nitroprusside or trimetaphan. Br J Anaesth 1977; 49(5):419–425.

17. Tietjen CS, Hurn PD, Ulatowski JA, et al. Treatment modalities for hypertensive patients with intra-cranial pathology: options and risks. Crit Care Med 1996; 24(2):311–322.
18. Neil-Dwyer G, Walter P, Cruickshank JM. Beta-blockade benefits patients following a subarachnoid haemorrhage. Eur J Clin Pharmacol Suppl 1985; 28:25–29.
19. Deibert E, Barzilai B, Braverman AC, et al. Clinical significance of elevated troponin I levels in patients with nontraumatic subarachnoid hemorrhage. J Neurosurg 2003; 98(4):741–746.
20. Doshi R, Neil-Dwyer G. A clinicopathological study of patients following a subarachnoid hemorrhage. J Neurosurg 1980; 52:295–301.
21. Solenski NJ, Haley EC Jr, Kassell NF, et al. Medical complications of aneurysmal subarachnoid hem-orrhage: a report of the multicenter, cooperative aneurysm study. Participants of the Multicenter Cooperative Aneurysm Study. Crit Care Med 1995; 23(6):1007–1017.
22. Miss JC, Kopelnik A, Fisher LA, et al. Cardiac injury after subarachnoid hemorrhage is independent of the type of aneurysm therapy. Neurosurgery 2004; 55:1244–1251.
23. Pinto AN, Canhao P, Ferro JM. Seizures at the onset of subarachnoid haemorrhage. J Neurol 1996; 243:161–164.
24. Rhoney DH, Tipps LB, Murry KR, et al. Anticonvulsant prophylaxis and timing of seizures after aneu-rysmal subarachnoid hemorrhage. Neurology 2000; 55:258–265.
25. Kvam DA, Loftus CM, Copeland B, et al. Seizures during the immediate post operative period. Neurosurgery 1983; 12:14–17.
26. Matthew E, Sherwin AL, Welner SA, et al. Seizures following intracranial surgery: incidence in the first post-operative week. Can J Neurol Sci 1980; 7:285–290.
27. Sethi H, Moore A, Dervin J, et al. Hydrocephalus: comparison of clipping and embolization in aneu-rysm treatment. J Neurosurg 2000; 92:991–994.
28. Byrne JV, Boardman P, Ioannidis I, et al. Seizures after aneurysmal subarachnoid hemorrhage treated with coil embolization. Neurosurgery 2003; 52:545–552.
29. Rose FC, Sarner M. Epilepsy after ruptured intracranial aneurysm. Brit Med J 1965; 1:18–21.
30. Ukkola V, Heikkinen ER. Epilepsy after operative treatment of ruptured cerebral aneurysms. Acta Neurochirurgica 1990; 106:115–118.
31. Cabral RJ, King TT, Scott DF. Epilepsy after two different neurosurgical approaches to treatment of ruptured intracranial aneurysm. J Neurol Neurosurg Psych 1976; 39:1052–1056.
32. Kotila M, Waltimo O. Epilepsy after stroke. Epilepsia 1992; 33:495–498.
33. Ohman J. Hypertension as a risk factor for epilepsy after aneurysmal subarachnoid hemorrhage and surgery. Neurosurg 1990; 27:578–581.
34. Naidech AM, Kreiter KT, Janjua N, et al. Phenytoin exposure is associated with functional and cog-nitive disability after subarachnoid hemorrhage. Stroke 2005; 36(3):583–587.
35. Haley EC Jr, Kassell NF, Apperson-Hansen C, et al. A randomized, double-blind, vehicle-controlled trial of tirilazad mesylate in patients with aneurysmal subarachnoid hemorrhage: a cooperative study in North America. J Neurosurg 1997; 86(3):467–474.
36. Lanzino G, Kassell NF. Double-blind, randomized, vehicle-controlled study of high-dose tirilazad mesylate in women with aneurysmal subarachnoid hemorrhage. Part II. A cooperative study in North America. J Neurosurg 1999; 90(6):1018–1024.
37. Kassell NF, Torner JC, Adams HP Jr. Antifibrinolytic therapy in the acute period following aneu-rysmal subarachnoid hemorrhage. Preliminary observations from the Cooperative Aneurysm Study. J Neurosurg 1984; 61(2):225–230.
38. Roos YB, Rinkel GJ, Vermeulen M, et al: Antifibrinolytic therapy for aneurysmal subarachnoid haemo-rrhage. Cochrane Database Syst Rev 2003; (2): CD001245.
39. Molyneux A, Kerr R, Stratton I, et al. International Subarachnoid Aneurysm Trial (ISAT) Collaborative Group. International Subarachnoid Aneurysm Trial (ISAT) of neurosurgical clipping versus endovas-cular coiling in 2143 patients with ruptured intracranial aneurysms: a randomised trial. Lancet 2002; 360(9342):1267–1274.
40. Lin CL, Kwan AL, Howng SL. Acute hydrocephalus and chronic hydrocephalus with the need of postoperative shunting after aneurysmal subarachnoid hemorrhage. Kaohsiung J Med.Sci 1999; 15:137–145.
41. Mehta V, Holness RO, Connolly K, et al. Acute hydrocephalus following aneurysmal subarachnoid hemorrhage. Can J Neurol.Sci 1996; 23:40–45.
42. Sheehan JP, Polin RS, Sheehan JM, et al. Factors associated with hydrocephalus after aneurysmal subarachnoid hemorrhage. Neurosurgery 1999; 45:1120–1127.
43. Suarez-Rivera O: Acute hydrocephalus after subarachnoid hemorrhage. Surg.Neurol 1998; 49:563–565.
44. Hasan D, Vermeulen M, Wijdicks EF, et al. Effect of fluid intake and antihypertensive treatment on cerebral ischemia after subarachnoid hemorrhage. Stroke 1989; 20:1511–1515.
45. Rajshekhar V, Harbaugh RE. Results of routine ventriculostomy with external ventricular drainage for acute hydrocephalus following subarachnoid haemorrhage. Acta Neurochirurgica 1992; 115:8–14.

46. Hasan D, Tanghe HL. Distribution of cisternal blood in patients with acute hydrocephalus after subarachnoid hemorrhage. Ann.Neurol 1992; 31:374–378.
47. Rinkel GJ, Wijdicks EF, Vermeulen M, et al. Acute hydrocephalus in nonaneurysmal perimesencephalic hemorrhage: evidence of CSF block at the tentorial hiatus. Neurology 1992; 42:1805–1807.
48. Hasan D, Vermeulen M, Wijdicks EF, et al. Management problems in acute hydrocephalus after subarachnoid hemorrhage. Stroke 1989; 20:747–753.
49. Milhorat TH. Acute hydrocephalus after aneurysmal subarachnoid hemorrhage. Neurosurgery 1987; 20:15–20.
50. Pare L, Delfino R, Leblanc R. The relationship of ventricular drainage to aneurysmal rebleeding. J Neurosurg 1992; 76:422–427.
51. McIver JI, Friedman JA, Wijdicks EF, et al. Preoperative ventriculostomy and rebleeding after aneurysmal subarachnoid hemorrhage. J Neurosurg 2002; 97(5):1042–1044.
52. Gruber A, Reinprecht A, Bavinzski G, et al. Chronic shunt-dependent hydrocephalus after early surgical and early endovascular treatment of ruptured intracranial aneurysms. Neurosurgery 1999; 44:503–509.
53. Sethi H, Moore A, Dervin J, et al. Hydrocephalus: comparison of clipping and embolization in aneurysm treatment. J Neurosurg 2000; 92:991–994.
54. Dorai Z, Hynan LS, Kopitnik TA, et al. Factors related to hydrocephalus after aneurysmal subarachnoid hemorrhage. Neurosurgery 2003; 52:763–769.
55. Schmieder K, Koch R, Lucke S, et al. Factors influencing shunt dependency after aneurysmal subarachnoid haemorrhage. Zentralbl Neurochir 1999; 60:133–140.
56. Vale FL, Bradley EL, Fisher WS, III. The relationship of subarachnoid hemorrhage and the need for postoperative shunting. J Neurosurg 1997; 86:462–466.
57. Widenka DC, Wolf S, Schurer L, et al. Factors leading to hydrocephalus after aneurysmal subarachnoid hemorrhage. Neurol NeurochirPol 2000; 34:56–60.
58. Yoshioka H, Inagawa T, Tokuda Y, et al. Chronic hydrocephalus in elderly patients following subarachnoid hemorrhage. Surg Neurol 2000; 53:119–124.
59. Andaluz N, Zuccarello M. Fenestration of the lamina terminalis as a valuable adjunct in aneurysm surgery. Neurosurgery 2004; 55(5):1050–1059.
60. Komotar RJ, Olivi A, Rigamonti D, et al. Microsurgical fenestration of the lamina terminalis reduces the incidence of shunt-dependent hydrocephalus after aneurysmal subarachnoid hemorrhage. Neurosurgery 2002; 51:1403–1413.
61. Black PM. Hydrocephalus and vasospasm after subarachnoid hemorrhage from ruptured intracranial aneurysms. Neurosurgery 1986; 18:12–16.
62. van Gijn J, Hijdra A, Wijdicks EF, et al: Acute hydrocephalus after aneurysmal subarachnoid hemorrhage. J Neurosurg 1985; 63:355–362.
63. Friedman JA, Pichelmann MA, Piepgras DG, et al. Pulmonary complications of aneurysmal subarachnoid hemorrhage. Neurosurgery 2003; 52(5):1025–1031.
64. Dodek P, Keenan S, Cook D, et al. Evidence-based clinical practice guideline for the prevention of ventilator-associated pneumonia. Ann Intern Med 2004; 141(4):305–313.
65. Agnelli G, Piovella F, Buoncristiani P, et al. Enoxaparin plus compression stockings compared with compression stockings alone in the prevention of venous thromboembolism after elective neurosurgery. N Engl J Med 1998; 339(2):80–85.
66. Nurmohamed MT, van Riel AM, Henkens CM, et al. Low molecular weight heparin and compression stockings in the prevention of venous thromboembolism in neurosurgery. Thromb Haemost 1996; 75:233–238.
67. Kleindienst A, Harvey HB, Mater E, et al. Early antithrombotic prophylaxis with low molecular weight heparin in neurosurgery. Acta Neurochir (Wien) 2003; 145(12):1085–1090.
68. Claassen J, Vu A, Kreiter KT, et al. Effect of acute physiologic derangements on outcome after subarachnoid hemorrhage. Crit Care Med 2004; 32(3):832–838.
69. Lanzino G, Kassell NF, Germanson T, et al. Plasma glucose levels and outcome after aneurysmal subarachnoid hemorrhage. J Neurosurg 1993; 79(6):885–891.
70. van den Berghe G, Wouters P, Weekers F, et al. Intensive insulin therapy in the critically ill patients. N Engl J Med 2001, 345:1359–1367.
71. Weir B, Disney L, Grace M, et al. Daily trends in white blood cell count and temperature after subarachnoid hemorrhage from aneurysm. Neurosurgery 1989; 25:161–165.
72. Oliveira-Filho J, Ezzeddine MA, Segal AZ, et al. Fever in subarachnoid hemorrhage: Relationship to vasospasm and outcome. Neurology 2001; 56:1299–1304.
73. Diringer MN; Neurocritical Care Fever Reduction Trial Group. Treatment of fever in the neurologic intensive care unit with a catheter-based heat exchange system. Crit Care Med 2004; 32(2):559–564.
74. Todd MM, Hindman BJ, Clarke WR, et al. Mild intraoperative hypothermia during surgery for intracranial aneurysm. N Engl J Med 2005; 352(2):135–145.

75. Hasan D, Lindsay KW, Wijdicks EF, et al. Effect of fludrocortisone acetate in patients with subarachnoid hemorrhage. Stroke 1989; 20(9):1156–1161.
76. Mori T, Katayama Y, Kawamata T, et al. Improved efficiency of hypervolemic therapy with inhibition of natriuresis by fludrocortisone in patients with aneurysmal subarachnoid hemorrhage. J Neurosurg 1999; 91(6):947–952.
77. Mayberg MR, Batjer HH, Dacey R, et al. Guidelines for the management of aneurysmal subarachnoid hemorrhage. A statement for healthcare professionals from a special writing group of the Stroke Council, American Heart Association. Stroke 1994; 25(11):2315–2328.
78. Kawamoto S, Tsutsumi K, Yoshikawa G, et al. Effectiveness of the head-shaking method combined with cisternal irrigation with urokinase in preventing cerebral vasospasm after subarachnoid hemorrhage. J Neurosurg 2004; 100(2):236–243.
79. Klimo P Jr, Kestle JR, MacDonald JD, et al. Marked reduction of cerebral vasospasm with lumbar drainage of cerebrospinal fluid after subarachnoid hemorrhage. J Neurosurg 2004; 100:215–224.
80. Lennihan L, Mayer SA, Fink ME, et al. Effect of hypervolemic therapy on cerebral blood flow after subarachnoid hemorrhage : a randomized controlled trial. Stroke 2000; 31(2):383–391.
81. Suarez JI, Shannon L, Zaidat OO, et al. Effect of human albumin administration on clinical outcome and hospital cost in patients with subarachnoid hemorrhage. J Neurosurg 2004; 100(4):585–590.
82. Dalbasti T, Karabiyikoglu M, Ozdamar N, et al. Efficacy of controlled-release papaverine pellets in preventing symptomatic cerebral vasospasm. J Neurosurg 2001; 95(1):44–50.
83. Kasuya H, Onda H, Takeshita M, et al. Efficacy and safety of nicardipine prolonged-release implants for preventing vasospasm in humans. Stroke 2002; 33(4):1011–1015.
84. Wurm G, Tomancok B, Nussbaumer K, et al. Reduction of ischemic sequelae following spontaneous subarachnoid hemorrhage: a double-blind, randomized comparison of enoxaparin versus placebo. Clin Neurol Neurosurg 2004; 106(2):97–103.
85. Muizelaar JP, Zwienenberg M, Rudisill NA, et al. The prophylactic use of transluminal balloon angioplasty in patients with Fisher Grade 3 subarachnoid hemorrhage: a pilot study. J Neurosurg 1999; 91:51–58.
86. Levy ML, Day JD, Zelman V, et al. Cardiac performance enhancement and hypervolemic therapy. Neurosurg Clin N Am 1994; 5(4):725–739.
87. Miller JA, Dacey RG Jr, Diringer MN. Safety of hypertensive hypervolemic therapy with phenylephrine in the treatment of delayed ischemic deficits after subarachnoid hemorrhage. Stroke 1995; 26(12):2260–2266.
88. Aiyagari V, Cross DT III, Deibert E, et al. Safety of hemodynamic augmentation in patients treated with Guglielmi detachable coils after acute aneurysmal subarachnoid hemorrhage. Stroke 2001; 32(9):1994–1997.

8 | Clinical Trials in Subarachnoid Hemorrhage

Nader Pouratian, MD, PhD, Resident
Aaron S. Dumont, MD, Fellow
Department of Neurological Surgery,
University of Virginia School of Medicine, Charlottesville, Virginia, USA

Thomas P. Bleck, MD, FCCM, Ruth Cain Ruggles Chairman[a], Vice Chairman[b], Professor[b]
[a] *Department of Neurology, Evanston Northwestern Healthcare,*
[b] *Departments of Neurology, Neurosurgery, and Internal Medicine,*
Northwestern University Feinberg School of Medicine, Chicago, Illinois, USA

INTRODUCTION

Aneurysmal subarachnoid hemorrhage (aSAH) continues to be associated with an unacceptably high rate of morbidity and mortality. For those patients who survive the initial insult of the subarachnoid hemorrhage (SAH), further neurologic deterioration or death can still occur due to early rebleeding of the ruptured aneurysm and posthemorrhagic vasospasm. Medical and surgical management is aimed at reducing the incidence of early rebleeding and symptomatic vasospasm. Unfortunately, appropriate management remains challenging. Although animal models and anecdotal experience are helpful in beginning to define appropriate treatment regimens, clinical trials of new management strategies and interventions are essential. Such trials are critical because they offer an opportunity to unequivocally evaluate whether a management scheme based on theories or animal models truly impacts and improves patient outcome. Unfortunately, despite a number of Phase 3 clinical trials, proven efficacious treatments remain minimal.

In this chapter, we critically appraise the significant clinical trials that have been published in the management of SAH and specifically evaluate the inherent strengths and limitations of these trials (including their design, outcomes assessment, and interpretation). Through such a review, we can begin to appreciate why inconsistent conclusions are being drawn regarding the appropriate management of SAH patients and how clinical trials can be used to advance the provision of care for such patients.

PREVENTION OF REBLEEDING

Early SAH management is largely aimed at preventing early rebleeding, including controlling blood pressure, ensuring adequate hemostasis, and minimizing stimulation. Many management measures are theoretical and have not been challenged in a clinical trial due to ethical considerations of withholding the standard of care. However, several large-scale clinical trials have evaluated significant questions in the management of early rebleeding.

Timing of Intervention

Aneurysms are at highest risk for re-rupture in the first 24 hours following the initial hemorrhage. Consequently, the natural instinct has been to exclude aneurysms from the systemic circulation as early as possible to prevent rebleeding and allow aggressive treatment of vasospasm. However, early surgery is complicated by theoretical concerns of increased surgical morbidity and mortality due to the edematous and inflamed state of the brain and the presence of diffuse, thick blood in the operative field. Clinical trials, therefore, have sought to determine whether the timing of surgery affects outcomes (1).

In the only randomized, prospective trial of the timing of aneurysmal surgery (2), 216 patients with anterior circulation aneurysms and Hunt and Hess Grades I to III were assigned to either early (zero to three days), intermediate (four to seven days), or late (more than seven days) surgery. The researchers reported significantly better clinical outcomes (functional and mortality) in the early-surgery group than in the intermediate- and late-surgery groups. Even though mortality was 5.6% in the early-surgery group, it was 12.9% in the late-surgery group. Likewise, those who underwent early surgery had a higher rate of functional independence at three months than did other patients. Unfortunately, the number of patients studied was small and did not include all SAH patients. Therefore, some view these results with reservation.

The International Cooperative Study on the Timing of Aneurysm Surgery is the largest clinical trial to date addressing this issue. It was an international prospective, observational clinical trial that observed 3521 patients who had either early or late surgery (0–3 or 11–14 days, respectively) (3). Despite theories of the benefit of early surgery to prevent rebleeding, the results indicated no significant differences in functional outcomes or death between early and late surgery; the risks of early surgery were equivalent to the risks of rebleeding and vasospasm that are associated with late surgery. However, a subanalysis of the North American patients in this trial (772 patients) suggested an improved rate of good clinical outcomes in the early-surgery group and nearly twice the mortality in the late-surgery group (4). The lack of randomization in these trials calls into question the possibility of selection bias in the observed outcomes. Nevertheless, for a combination of reasons, early surgery or endovascular coiling has been adopted as the preferred contemporary management plan to prevent *early* rebleeding. The true benefit of early surgery might never be clarified, as further randomized clinical trials to study the timing of aneurysmal surgery are unlikely for ethical considerations (1).

Modality of Intervention

Since the introduction of endovascular therapy for ruptured aneurysms, a controversial debate has ensued regarding the optimal approach for excluding aneurysms from the systemic circulation to prevent rebleeding. Numerous trials have been conducted to characterize the risks of both endovascular and surgical treatment of aneurysms, but only one randomized trial has been conducted and reported—that of the International Subarachnoid Aneurysm Trial (ISAT) (5).

The ISAT trial was an international, randomized trial that compared the safety and efficacy of endovascular and surgical management for ruptured cerebral aneurysms (5). A total of 2143 patients were enrolled, randomly assigned to surgery or endovascular management (with groups well matched for presentation and distribution of aneurysms), and followed for one year, ascertaining for functional outcomes (as assessed by the modified Rankin scale) and secondary endpoints (as described below). The trial was stopped early due to an increased rate of death and dependence in the surgically treated patients (30.6% vs. 23.7%). Although the rate of death and dependence was higher in the surgical cohort, endovascular management involved other complications, including a lower rate of successful initial treatment (92.5% vs. 97.8% in the surgical group), an increased rate of requiring a second procedure (12.6% vs. 3.2% in the surgical group), and a higher rate of bleeding after definitive intervention (68 cases in the endovascular group vs. 43 in the surgical group). The reported rebleeding after endovascular treatment necessitates a closer examination of the rate of SAH after endovascular occlusion to gain a better understanding of the effectiveness of each intervention.

The ISAT trial has been extensively criticized for its design, including subjective enrollment criteria (of both patients and treating physicians), patients undergoing surgery before being enrolled in the trial, and the fact that it was largely conducted outside of the United States (its applicability to the North American population, therefore, questioned) (6). For example, the rate of rebleeding in the first year following surgery appears much higher than reported by North American centers with high caseloads. A review of the critiques of the ISAT trial provides great insight into the limitations of clinical trials and their implications. Most have concluded from this study that endovascular management offers an effective treatment modality for ruptured aneurysms but that such patients need to be selected carefully and advised appropriately. Further trials and long-term outcomes of the ISAT are expected.

Antifibrinolytic Therapy

Antifibrinolytics, such as tranexamic acid, are a theoretically beneficial adjunct drugs that could help prevent the lysis of clot, thereby preventing a ruptured aneurysm from rebleeding. However, by disrupting the hemostatic balance, these drugs might also promote clot formation and complicate vasospasm management. Therefore, clinical trials have been conducted to clarify the role of these medications in the management of aSAH.

The earliest such study of tranexamic acid was conducted (in a double-blinded, placebo-controlled manner) in 51 patients who sustained SAH with tranexamic acid to prevent early rebleeding (7). Based on a three-month endpoint and analysis of outcomes, the authors concluded that tranexamic acid administration was associated with no significant change in outcomes. Since then, most trials of antifibrinolytic therapy (both randomized and observational), with enrollment ranging from approximately 60 to more than 600, have found that, although the antifibrinolytic might reduce early rebleeds, it is also associated with an increased rate of symptomatic vasospasm and relatively no difference in overall outcomes and mortality (8–12). Because of the increased rate of delayed ischemic neurologic deficits (DINDs), most centers opt for early surgical intervention rather than administering antifibrinolytics.

Recently, factor VIIa has received attention as a possible means of preventing early rebleeding. It is a hemostatic therapy that promotes local hemostasis at sites of vascular injury, even in individuals in whom the coagulation cascade is otherwise normal. Randomized trials to assess the value of this therapy in patients with SAH have yet to be reported; however, a dose-escalation study has been published, with report of an ischemic complication halting the study (13).

PREVENTION AND TREATMENT OF VASOSPASM

Beyond rebleeding, vasospasm is one of the most feared consequences of aSAH because of its high rate of morbidity and mortality (14). Vasospasm occurs due to a complex cascade of parallel, yet interacting, biochemical pathways, likely including (i) endothelium-derived factors (including nitric oxide and oxygen free radicals), (ii) vascular smooth muscle–derived factors (e.g., calcium-channel activation and protein kinase C (PKC) activation), (iii) pro-inflammatory mediators (e.g., cysteines, histamine, and bradykinin), and (iv) stress-induced gene activation (e.g., heat shock proteins and heme oxygenase-1) (15). Ultimately, these pathways result in vascular constriction, vascular smooth muscle proliferation, reduced perfusion, and neuronal injury. Consequently, developing pharmacologic agents or interventions that target the underlying biochemical pathways that mediate vasospasm has become a major focus of aSAH research.

Triple-H Therapy
Triple-H therapy is used in the treatment of hypertension, hypervolemia, and hemodilution, with the goal of maintaining cerebral perfusion even in the face of vasospasm. It has been proven to be ethically inappropriate to withhold triple-H therapy in the face of active vasospasm, making it impossible to conduct a clinical trial of its efficacy once vasospasm has been diagnosed. Nevertheless, a handful of studies have investigated the utility of triple-H therapy as a means of preventing symptomatic vasospasm. At least two prospective, randomized trials of triple-H therapy versus normovolemic therapy have suggested that triple-H therapy offers no prophylactic benefit (16,17). The power and validity of these studies, however, is significantly limited by the small number of patients enrolled in each (32 and 82) and incomplete reporting of endpoints. In a recent systematic review of prospective, comparative trials of triple-H prophylaxis (18), four trials were identified (only two of which were randomized). Across studies, they reported triple-H prophylaxis was associated with a reduced risk of symptomatic vasospasm [relative risk (RR), 0.45; 95% confidence interval (CI), 0.32–0.65] and mortality (RR, 0.68; 95% CI 0.53–0.87), but no difference in DINDs (RR, 0.54; 95% CI, 0.20–1.49). Interestingly, the difference in mortality maintained statistical significance only when the two randomized trials were analyzed (RR, 0.4; 95% CI, 0.14–0.66), even though neither study found a statistical difference between groups when analyzed individually. This highlights the limitations of study power when limited samples sizes are used. It was noted that meaningful comparisons between studies are difficult due to nonstandard definitions and reporting. In light of the possible benefits and lack of significant risks (if the aneurysm has been secured), most institutions will prophylactically employ some components of triple-H therapy.

Intra-arterial Therapy
Intra-arterial therapy, including papaverine, verapamil, and angioplasty, has become a regular part of the arsenal of therapeutics to counteract vasospasm. In the first reported use of intra-arterial papaverine in 1992, 34 of 37 targeted vascular territories were successfully dilated and 8 out of 10 patients showed neurologic improvement (19). The prospectively collected database of the North American Trial of Tirilazad for Aneurysmal SAH was used to compare 31 patients treated with intra-arterial papaverine with matched patients (according to degree of vasospasm

and Glasgow Coma Scale scores) who received only medical management (20). Despite the early report of angiographic improvement, no statistical difference was found in the three-month Glasgow Outcome Scale (GOS) scores between the groups. These trials, although not randomized, demonstrate the importance of selecting appropriate endpoints in evaluating the efficacy of a new treatment modality. Although papaverine indeed dilates spastic cerebral vessels, these studies suggest that the dilation is not sustained and does not alter long-term outcomes. Current interest surrounds the benefits of intra-arterial verapamil (which preliminarily results in both angiographic and clinical improvement), although this has not yet been assessed in a prospective manner (21).

Angioplasty consists of physically dilating constricted vessels with a balloon that has been placed within the lumen of the artery (via femoral cannulation). As a follow-up to a number of reports that angioplasty successfully dilates vessels, researchers investigated whether this intervention affected outcomes (22). Using a prospectively collected database, they compared 38 patients treated with angioplasty with 38 matched controls and found no significant difference in GOS scores at three months of follow-up. Despite its lack of observed clinical effect (which might have been masked by a small sample size), most institutions continue to use angioplasty regularly, as few other alternatives exist. Some have reported an interest in prophylactic balloon angioplasty (for which a pilot study was reported with excellent outcomes), but a formal clinical trial has not yet been reported (23).

Clot Evacuation

The amount of blood in the basal cisterns is one of the most consistent predictors of posthemorrhagic vasospasm (see Chapter 3 for further details). Therefore, one of the earliest hypothesized strategies for prevention of vasospasm was to remove the subarachnoid blood to evacuate the putative spasmogenic substrate. The first report of using intracisternal fibrinolytics [recombinant tissue plasminogen activator (rtPA)] to evacuate subarachnoid blood was an observational study of 15 patients, 14 of whom had complete or partial cisternal clot clearing [by computed tomography (CT) scan]. The patient who did not have a clear clot was the only one to experience symptomatic vasospasm (24). The same authors provided the first multicentered, randomized, blinded, placebo-controlled trial of the role of intracisternal fibrinolytics (25). Studying 100 patients, they reported, contrary to earlier reports, that the *overall* incidence of angiographic vasospasm was similar between the two groups (74.4% in placebo vs. 64.6% in treated). When only those patients with thick clots were considered, the authors reported a 56% RR reduction in the incidence of severe vasospasm in the treated group ($p<0.05$). Other clinically important trends in the rtPA-treated group (that did not reach statistical significance) include reduced delayed neurologic worsening, a lower 14-day mortality rate, and improved three-month outcome rate. The major limitation of this study, as the authors themselves suggest, is that they largely focused on radiographic endpoints rather than clinical endpoints.

A prospective, randomized trial of coil embolization followed by intrathecal urokinase infusion in 110 patients reported symptomatic vasospasm in 9.4% of treated and 28.1% of untreated subjects ($p=0.012$) and improved outcomes in the treated groups (90.6%), compared to the untreated group (75.4%; $p=0.036$), but no significant difference in mortality between the groups (3.8% vs. 5.3%, respectively). The authors therefore reported a benefit of fibrinolysis, resulting in a lower rate of permanent neurologic deficits, despite no difference in mortality (26). This latest study highlights the need for further investigation of the role of fibrinolytics in SAH to prevent vasospasm and its sequelae.

Antiplatelet Therapy

The use of antiplatelet therapy to prevent DINDs and to improve outcomes after SAH has been motivated by the theoretical advantage of limiting platelet aggregation in an already constricted vessel and the report that some antiplatelet agents might inhibit vasoconstriction mediated through oxyhemoglobin (one of the implicated pathways in vasospasm) (27). In an observational study, it was reported that the RR of cerebral infarct after SAH (as determined by CT scanning) was 0.18 (95% CI 0.04–0.84) in those patients who had been on aspirin before the SAH, compared to those with no history of aspirin use, suggesting a benefit to antiplatelet therapy in the face of SAH (28). Five studies to date have investigated the benefit of anitplatelet therapy in a randomized, controlled design (29–33), and they unanimously report no difference in long-term outcomes in patients treated with antiplatelet agents, as opposed to placebo. Only three trials reported DINDs rates, and only one (31) demonstrated a significant difference between treatment groups. A meta-analysis suggests that the RR of DINDs in patients treated with antiplatelet therapy across trials (RR, 0.65; 95% CI 0.47–0.89) is still significantly less than those not given antiplatelet therapy (34). Unfortunately, for the most part, study samples were prohibitively small (sometimes as small as 11 patients). Accordingly, a more thorough randomized trial is needed to assess the validity and usefulness of antiplatelet therapy in altering outcomes after SAH.

Anticoagulant Therapy

Trials have also been conducted to evaluate the efficacy of enoxaparin, a low-molecular-weight heparin, in the prevention of DINDs. The first trial was a double-blinded, randomized trial of 170 patients who were treated with either placebo or enoxaparin for 10 days after aneurysm occlusion. The authors found no difference in neurologic outcomes between the two groups at three months (35). A subsequent double-blinded, randomized trial was conducted in 120 consecutive patients who received a lower dose of enoxaparin for a longer period of time (three weeks); the patients were followed for one year instead of only three months (36). In the later study, enoxaparin administration was associated with a reduced rate of DINDs (8.8% vs. 66.7%; $p < 0.001$) and improved clinical outcomes at one-year follow-up. Unfortunately, the two groups were not precisely matched, with the placebo group having a significantly worse Hunt and Hess admission score, making it difficult to interpret the significance of these improved outcomes (as this was not controlled for in their statistical analysis). Nonetheless, with longer follow-up, lower-dose enoxaparin appears to possess some efficacy.

Blocking Vascular Smooth Muscle Activation

The literature suggests that after 24 to 48 hours, vasospasm is largely mediated by vascular and smooth muscle activation, triggered by the release of endothelin and subsequent initiation of a VEGF-mediated cascade, the activation of rho kinase II pathways, and the presence of reactive oxygen species.

Endothelin/VEGF Cascade

It is hypothesized that oxyhemoglobin released from lysed erythrocytes in the subarachnoid space causes vessel contraction, which is potentiated by endothelin-1 (ET-1). The downstream effects of ET-1 are likely mediated by the release of vascular endothelial growth factor (VEGF), one of the most potent mediators of cerebral angiogenesis (37). Studies have implicated this pathway in vitro by measuring cerebrovascular smooth muscle contraction in the presence of varying amounts of ET-1 and inhibitors of the endothelin receptor (38–41). Studies have also shown that plasma ET-1 concentrations correlate with the incidence of DINDs after SAH (42). Based on these studies, a double-blinded Phase 2 trial of an endothelin receptor antagonist (TAK-044), consisting of 420 randomized patients, has been reported (43). Endpoints included DINDS within 10 days and three months of first dose of medication, evidence of new cerebral infarct (on CT or postmortem), GOS at three months, and adverse events. The authors reported a lower incidence of DINDs at three months in the treatment group (29.5% vs. 36.6%, RR, 0.8; 95% CI 0.61–1.06), with no other significantly different endpoints. The authors intend to conduct a full Phase 3 trial, with appropriate power (43). Data from a Phase 2a trial, soon to be published, demonstrate that a selective ET-A receptor antagonist (clazosentan) reduces the frequency and severity of vasospasm and is well tolerated. A major clinical trial involving North American centers is about to be launched to further examine this agent.

Reactive Oxygen Species

Owing to the release of oxyhemoglobin by hemolyzed erythrocytes in the subarachnoid space, many hypothesize that the concentration of reactive oxygen species increases in the subarachnoid environment, thereby contributing to vasospasm (44). A multicentered, placebo-controlled, double-blinded clinical trial of 162 patients was conducted to verify the beneficial effects of free radical scavenging on DINDs and the overall outcomes (45). The authors reported a reduction in the incidence of DINDs in the treated group compared to placebo (35.5% vs. 54.2%, $p < 0.05$), a significantly improved GOS at one month ($p<0.05$), a marginal improvement in outcomes at three months, and a significantly reduced cumulative incidence of death ($p<0.05$) (45).

NEUROPROTECTION

Calcium-Channel Antagonists

Several prospective, randomized, placebo-controlled, double-blinded, randomized trials have investigated the efficacy of calcium-channel antagonists to reduce mortality and DINDs (46–49). Early studies consistently demonstrated a significant improvement in morbidity in patients treated with nimodipine (relative to placebo). Despite differences in morbidity, the placebo and nimodipine-treated groups consistently showed no difference in angiographic vasospasm, suggesting a neuroprotective effect rather than a vasodilating mechanism (46,47). Despite some studies reporting clinical efficacy, the Cooperative Aneurysm Study reported that, although patients treated with high-dose intravenous calcium antagonists had a reduction in symptomatic vasospasm, the two groups had similar outcomes at three months (48,49). Despite these negative findings, the authors conclude that calcium-channel antagonists still reduce the risk of symptomatic cerebral vasospasm in a significant proportion of patients and, therefore, still have a role in treating and preventing vasospasm. The inconsistency across studies probably arises from a lack of power to detect a small but statistically and clinically significant difference between the two treatment groups. Although some have questioned the quality of the evidence for the role of nimodipine in preventing and protecting against the sequelae of vasospasm, many argue that the risks (largely that of hypotension) are minimal in light of its potential benefit (50).

Tirilazad

Tirilazad is a potent inhibitor of oxygen free radical-induced, iron-catalyzed lipid peroxidation in microvascular and nervous tissue. It has been shown to be neuroprotective in animal models of ischemic stroke (51). The clinical trial was undertaken based on the laboratory-based mechanistic studies. Based on the theoretical benefits that this drug could confer, several clinical trials were also conducted with tirilazad in patients with SAH.

The first Phase 3 clinical trial investigating the efficacy of tirilazad serves as a model for a well-designed, randomized, double-blinded, placebo-controlled clinical trial, with adequate enrollment (1023 patients) to ensure adequate power (52). The group receiving 6 mg/kg/day demonstrated a reduced mortality ($p=0.01$), an improved three-month GOS ($p=0.01$), and a trend toward decreased symptomatic vasospasm ($p=0.048$). Interestingly, the benefits were predominately in men. Because of the decreased efficacy of tirilazad in women in the original clinical trial and the apparent dose–response relationship from the original study, follow-up trials were conducted, both internationally (819 patients) and within North America (832 patients) (53,54). As before, the international study revealed a statistically significant mortality advantage among patients who were Hunt and Hess Grade IV or V at the time of admission and were treated with tirilazad, compared to placebo-treated patients (24.6% vs. 43.4%, respectively, $p=0.016$) (53). Interestingly, the outcomes advantage was not seen in the North American trial; although a significant reduction in symptomatic vasospasm was observed, three-month mortality was not different in this accompanying study. The authors attribute this difference to the possibility that placebo-treated patients were more aggressively managed in the North American trial (54).

Fasudil

Fasudil was originally designed as an intracellular calcium antagonist, with the intent of achieving vasodilation. Despite extensive investigations, the precise mechanism of action of fasudil remains unclear. A possible more clinically significant role for fasudil in vasospasm might be its role in Rho kinase II inhibition, thereby preventing the activation of pathways that promote vascular smooth muscle cell contraction and proliferation. Rho Kinase is thought to play a critical role in ET-1–mediated vasoconstriction and proliferation.

The first clinical trial using fasudil was reported from Japan in 1992; 267 patients with Hunt and Hess grades I to IV were randomized to either receive fasudil or placebo (55). The groups were matched clinically and demographically. Fasudil reportedly reduced angiographic vasospasm by 23% (61% vs. 38%, p=0.0023), ischemic CT lesions by 22% (38% vs. 16%, p=0.0013), and symptomatic vasospasm by 15% (50% vs. 35%, p=0.0247). More importantly, the authors report that treated patients had improved rate of good GOS scores (26% vs. 12%, p=0.0152) (55). This study promoted the widespread use of fasudil in Japan to reduce the rate of vasospasm and its pathophysiologic consequences.

Magnesium

Hypomagnesemia is frequent after SAH and has been noted to be associated with the severity of vasospasm following aSAH. Moreover, hypomagnesemia between postbleed days 2 and 12 is predictive of DINDs (56). Magnesium might increase cerebral blood flow, reduce the contraction of cerebral arteries caused by various stimuli, and act as a nonspecific neuroprotectant (57). A prospective, randomized, single-blinded clinical trial of high-dose magnesium therapy following aSAH in 40 patients reported a trend (not statistically significant) in which a higher percentage of patients treated with magnesium attained GOS scores of 4 or 5 (compared to controls). As the authors suggest, a larger study is needed to evaluate this trend, as the power of this study is limited by an n of 40 (58).

WHY HAVE PREVIOUS CLINICAL TRIALS IN ANEURYSMAL SUBARACHNOID HEMORRHAGE FAILED?

Much of the difficulty in addressing the management of SAH and the pathophysiologic consequences of vasospasm arises from the multifactorial nature of the disease process. It is not surprising that clinical trials that target only a single part of this complex cascade fail or report only partial success, at best. One would expect greater success from clinical trials that plan to target either multiple parts of this complex cascade simultaneously or a final common pathway, such that compensatory mechanisms do not out-compete the proposed therapeutic interventions. Similarly, the management of SAH and vasospasm is complicated by ostensibly competing interests. Although initially the goal of therapy is to prevent rebleeding (e.g., antifibrinolytics), the goal of later-phase therapy is to ensure perfusion. Unfortunately, the interventions introduced during the early phase might result in poorer perfusion later in the disease course (as discussed in section "Antifibrinolytic Therapy").

However, the failure of so many trials is not limited to the complexity of vasospasm but can also be attributed to several shortcomings in study design. Most importantly, the majority of studies have been underpowered. To account for inherent heterogeneity of samples, it is critical to use large sample sizes (on the order of that used by the Cooperative Aneurysm Study) in order to detect clinically significant changes associated with a specific therapeutic regimen. Multivariate analysis is therefore critical for informed analysis and interpretation of studies.

Finally, as discussed in the previous section, for clinical trials to be useful, it is critical that appropriate endpoints (and intermediate, or surrogate, endpoints) be measured so that the true efficacy of a particular therapeutic regimen can be evaluated. As illustrated well in the case of investigations of nimodipine and fasudil, depending on the outcomes assessed, the conclusions of a study can be markedly different: both seemingly alter outcomes without evidence of angiographic resolution of vasospasm. Recently, interest has increased in the use of neuropsychologic assessment in clinical studies, as these tests can offer a more sensitive and specific means of assessing patients and identifying small, but clinically significant, differences in functional outcomes (59).

CONCLUSION AND FUTURE DIRECTIONS

Despite numerous clinical trials, most studies have shown little, no, or inconsistent benefits of proposed interventions, compared to placebo. The failure of these trials is multifactorial, related to the underlying complexity of the disease, inadequate power, and the lack of appropriate, sensitive, and specific measures of clinical endpoints. Nevertheless, clinical trials must continue, because the morbidity and mortality of early rebleeding and vasospasm remain theoretically preventable. With increased attention to detail, outcomes, and study design, as well as an improved understanding of the biochemical pathways that result in vasospasm, effective interventions will surely be developed and tested successfully in future clinical trials.

REFERENCES

1. de Gans K, Nieuwkamp DJ, Rinkel GJ, et al. Timing of aneurysm surgery in subarachnoid hemorrhage: a systematic review of the literature. Neurosurgery 2002; 50(2):336–340; discussion 340–342.
2. Ohman J, Heiskanen O. Timing of operation for ruptured supratentorial aneurysms: a prospective randomized study. J Neurosurg 1989; 70(1):55–60.
3. Kassell NF, Torner JC, Jane JA, et al. The international cooperative study on the timing of aneurysm surgery. Part 2: Surgical results. J Neurosurg 1990; 73(1):37–47.
4. Haley EC Jr., Kassell NF, Torner JC. The international cooperative study on the timing of aneurysm surgery. The North American experience. Stroke 1992; 23(2):205–214.
5. Molyneux A, Kerr R, Stratton I, et al. International subarachnoid aneurysm trial (ISAT) of neurosurgical clipping versus endovascular coiling in 2143 patients with ruptured intracranial aneurysms: a randomised trial. Lancet 2002; 360(9342):1267–1274.
6. Ausman JI. Isat study: is coiling better than clipping? Surg Neurol 2003; 59(3):162–165; discussion 165–173; author reply 173–175.
7. van Rossum J, Wintzen AR, Endtz LJ, et al. Effect of tranexamic acid on rebleeding after subarachnoid hemorrhage: a double-blind controlled clinical trial. Ann Neurol 1977; 2(3):238–242.
8. Kaste M, Ramsay M. Tranexamic acid in subarachnoid hemorrhage. A double-blind study. Stroke 1979; 10(5):519–522.
9. Fodstad H. Antifibrinolytic treatment in subarachnoid haemorrhage: present state. Acta Neurochir (Wien) 1982; 63(1–4):233–244.
10. Kassell NF, Torner JC, Adams HP, Jr. Antifibrinolytic therapy in the acute period following aneurysmal subarachnoid hemorrhage. Preliminary observations from the cooperative aneurysm study. J Neurosurg 1984; 61(2):225–230.
11. Roos Y. Antifibrinolytic treatment in subarachnoid hemorrhage: a randomized placebo-controlled trial. Star study group. Neurology 2000; 54(1):77–82.
12. Vermeulen M, Lindsay KW, Murray GD, et al. Antifibrinolytic treatment in subarachnoid hemorrhage. N Engl J Med 1984; 311(7):432–437.
13. Pickard JD, Kirkpatrick PJ, Melsen T, et al. Potential role of novoseven in the prevention of rebleeding following aneurysmal subarachnoid haemorrhage. Blood Coagul Fibrinolysis 2000; 11(suppl 1): S117–S120.
14. Kassell NF, Sasaki T, Colohan AR, et al. Cerebral vasospasm following aneurysmal subarachnoid hemorrhage. Stroke 1985; 16(4):562–572.
15. Bhardwaj A. Sah-induced cerebral vasospasm: unraveling molecular mechanisms of a complex disease. Stroke 2003.
16. Egge A, Waterloo K, Sjoholm H, et al. Prophylactic hyperdynamic postoperative fluid therapy after aneurysmal subarachnoid hemorrhage: a clinical, prospective, randomized, controlled study. Neurosurgery 2001; 49(3):593–605; discussion 605–606.
17. Lennihan L, Mayer SA, Fink ME, et al. Effect of hypervolemic therapy on cerebral blood flow after subarachnoid hemorrhage: a randomized controlled trial. Stroke 2000; 31(2):383–391.
18. Treggiari MM, Walder B, Suter PM, et al. Systematic review of the prevention of delayed ischemic neurological deficits with hypertension, hypervolemia, and hemodilution therapy following subarachnoid hemorrhage. J Neurosurg 2003; 98(5):978–984.
19. Kaku Y, Yonekawa Y, Tsukahara T, et al. Superselective intra-arterial infusion of papaverine for the treatment of cerebral vasospasm after subarachnoid hemorrhage. J Neurosurg 1992; 77(6):842–847.
20. Polin RS, Hansen CA, German P, et al. Intra-arterially administered papaverine for the treatment of symptomatic cerebral vasospasm. Neurosurgery 1998; 42(6):1256–1264; discussion 1264–1267.
21. Feng L, Fitzsimmons BF, Young WL, et al. Intraarterially administered verapamil as adjunct therapy for cerebral vasospasm: Safety and 2-year experience. Am J Neuroradiol 2002; 23(8):1284–1290.
22. Polin RS, Coenen VA, Hansen CA, et al. Efficacy of transluminal angioplasty for the management of symptomatic cerebral vasospasm following aneurysmal subarachnoid hemorrhage. J Neurosurg 2000; 92(2):284–290.
23. Muizelaar JP, Zwienenberg M, Rudisill NA, et al. The prophylactic use of transluminal balloon angioplasty in patients with fisher grade 3 subarachnoid hemorrhage: a pilot study. J Neurosurg 1999; 91(1):51–58.
24. Findlay JM, Weir BK, Kassell NF, et al. Intracisternal recombinant tissue plasminogen activator after aneurysmal subarachnoid hemorrhage. J Neurosurg 1991; 75(2):181–188.
25. Findlay JM, Kassell NF, Weir BK, et al. A randomized trial of intraoperative, intracisternal tissue plasminogen activator for the prevention of vasospasm. Neurosurgery 1995; 37(1):168–176; discussion 177–178.
26. Hamada J, Kai Y, Morioka M, et al. Effect of cerebral vasospasm of coil embolization followed by microcatheter intrathecal urokinase infusion into the cisterna magna. A prospective randomized study. Stroke 2003; 34:2549–2554.

27. Kawakami M, Kodama, Toda N. Suppression of the cerebral vasospastic actions of oxyhemoglobin by ascorbic acid. Neurosurgery 1991; 28(1):33–39; discussion 39–40.
28. Juvela, S. Aspirin and delayed cerebral ischemia after aneurysmal subarachnoid hemorrhage. J Neurosurg 1995; 82(6):945–952.
29. Shaw MD, Foy PM, Conway M, et al. Dipyridamole and postoperative ischemic deficits in aneurysmal subarachnoid hemorrhage. J Neurosurg 1985; 63(5):699–703.
30. Mendelow AD, Stockdill G, Steers AJ, et al. Double-blind trial of aspirin in patient receiving tranexamic acid for subarachnoid hemorrhage. Acta Neurochir (Wien); 1982; 62(3–4):195–202.
31. Suzuki S, Sano K, Handa H, et al. Clinical study of oky-046, a thromboxane synthetase inhibitor, in prevention of cerebral vasospasms and delayed cerebral ischaemic symptoms after subarachnoid haemorrhage due to aneurysmal rupture: A randomized double-blind study. Neurol Res 1989; 11(2):79–88.
32. Tokiyoshi K, Ohnishi T, Nii Y. Efficacy and toxicity of thromboxane synthetase inhibitor for cerebral vasospasm after subarachnoid hemorrhage. Surg Neurol 1991; 36(2):112–118.
33. Hop JW, Rinkel GJ, Algra A, et al. Randomized pilot trial of postoperative aspirin in subarachnoid hemorrhage. Neurology 2000; 54(4):872–878.
34. Dorhout Mees SM, Rinkel GJ, Hop JW, et al. Antiplatelet therapy in aneurysmal subarachnoid hemorrhage: A systematic review. Stroke 2003; 34(9):2285–2289.
35. Siironen J, Juvela S, Varis J, et al. No effect of enoxaparin on outcome of aneurysmal subarachnoid hemorrhage: a randomized, double-blind, placebo-controlled clinical trial. J Neurosurg 2003; 99(6):953–959.
36. Wurm G, Tomancok B, Nussbaumer K, et al. Reduction of ischemic sequelae following spontaneous subarachnoid hemorrhage: a double-blind, randomized comparison of enoxaparin versus placebo. Clin Neurol Neurosurg 2004; 106(2):97–103.
37. Josko J. Cerebral angiogenesis and expression of vegf after subarachnoid hemorrhage (SAH) in rats. Brain Res 2003; 981(1–2):58–69.
38. Lan C, Das D, Wloskowicz A, et al. Endothelin-1 modulates hemoglobin-mediated signaling in cerebrovascular smooth muscle via rhoa/rho kinase and protein kinase c. Am J Physiol Heart Circ Physiol 2004; 286(1):H165–H173.
39. Zimmermann M, Jung CS, Vatter H, et al. Effect of endothelin-converting enzyme inhibitors on big endothelin-1 induced contraction in isolated rat basilar artery. Acta Neurochir (Wien) 2002; 144(11):1213–1219.
40. Zimmermann M, Jung CS, Vatter H, et al. [d-val22]big et-1[16-38] inhibits endothelin-converting enzyme activity: a promising concept in the prevention of cerebral vasospasm. Neurosurg Rev 2003; 26(2):125–132.
41. Vatter H, Zimmermann M, Weyrauch E, et al. Cerebrovascular characterization of the novel nonpeptide endothelin-a receptor antagonist lu 208075. Clin Neuropharmacol 2003; 26(2):73–83.
42. Juvela, S. Plasma endothelin and big endothelin concentrations and serum endothelin-converting enzyme activity following aneurysmal subarachnoid hemorrhage. J Neurosurg 2002; 97(6):1287–1293.
43. Shaw MD, Vermeulen M, Murray GD, et al. Efficacy and safety of the endothelin, receptor antagonist tak-044 in treating subarachnoid hemorrhage: A report by the steering committee on behalf of the uk/netherlands/eire tak-044 subarachnoid haemorrhage study group. J Neurosurg 2000; 93(6):992–997.
44. Shishido T, Suzuki R, Qian L, et al. The role of superoxide anions in the pathogenesis of cerebral vasospasm. Stroke 1994; 25(4):864–868.
45. Asano T, Takakura K, Sano K, et al. Effects of a hydroxyl radical scavenger on delayed ischemic neurological deficits following aneurysmal subarachnoid hemorrhage: results of a multicenter, placebo-controlled double-blind trial. J Neurosurg 1996; 84(5):792–803.
46. Philippon J, Grob R, Dagreou F, et al. Prevention of vasospasm in subarachnoid haemorrhage. A controlled study with nimodipine. Acta Neurochir (Wien) 1986; 82(3–4):110–114.
47. Petruk KC, West M, Mohr G, et al. Nimodipine treatment in poor-grade aneurysm patients. Results of a multicenter double-blind placebo-controlled trial. J Neurosurg 1988; 68(4):505–517.
48. Haley EC Jr., Kassell NF, Torner JC. A randomized trial of nicardipine in subarachnoid hemorrhage: angiographic and transcranial doppler ultrasound results. A report of the cooperative aneurysm study. J Neurosurg 1993; 78(4):548–553.
49. Haley EC Jr., Kassell NF, Torner JC. A randomized controlled trial of high-dose intravenous nicardipine in aneurysmal subarachnoid hemorrhage. A report of the cooperative aneurysm study. J Neurosurg 1993; 78(4):537–547.
50. Rinkel GJ, Feigin VL, Algra A, et al. Calcium antagonists for aneurysmal subarachnoid haemorrhage. Cochrane Database Syst Rev 2002; (4):CD000277.
51. Xue D, Slivka A, Buchan AM. Tirilazad reduces cortical infarction after transient but not permanent focal cerebral ischemia in rats. Stroke 1992; 23(6):894–899.

52. Kassell NF, Haley EC Jr., Apperson-Hansen C, et al. Randomized, double-blind, vehicle-controlled trial of tirilazad mesylate in patients with aneurysmal subarachnoid hemorrhage: a cooperative study in Europe, Australia, and New Zealand. J Neurosurg 1996; 84(2):221–228.

53. Lanzino G, Kassell NF. Double-blind, randomized, vehicle-controlled study of high-dose tirilazad mesylate in women with aneurysmal subarachnoid hemorrhage. Part ii. A cooperative study in north america. J Neurosurg 1999; 90(6):1018–1024.

54. Lanzino G, Kassell NF, Dorsch NW, et al. Double-blind, randomized, vehicle-controlled study of high-dose tirilazad mesylate in women with aneurysmal subarachnoid hemorrhage. Part i. A cooperative study in Europe, Australia, New Zealand, and South Africa. J Neurosurg 1999; 90(6):1011–1017.

55. Shibuya M, Suzuki Y, Sugita K, et al. Effect of at877 on cerebral vasospasm after aneurysmal subarachnoid hemorrhage. Results of a prospective placebo-controlled double-blind trial. J Neurosurg 1992; 76(4):571–577.

56. van den Bergh WM, Algra A, van der Sprenkel JW, et al. Hypomagnesemia after aneurysmal subarachnoid hemorrhage. Neurosurgery 2003; 52(2):276–281; discussion 281–282.

57. Macdonald RL, Curry DJ, Aihara Y, et al. Magnesium and experimental vasospasm. J Neurosurg 2004; 100(1):106–110.

58. Veyna RS, Seyfried D, Burke DG, et al. Magnesium sulfate therapy after aneurysmal subarachnoid hemorrhage. J Neurosurg 2002; 96(3):510–514.

59. Morris PG, Wilson JT, Dunn L. Anxiety and depression after spontaneous subarachnoid hemorrhage. Neurosurgery 2004; 54(1):47–52; discussion 52–54.

Prognosis and Outcomes Following Aneurysmal Subarachnoid Hemorrhage

Richard E. Temes, MD, Fellow
J. Michael Schmidt, PhD, Assistant Professor of Neuropsychology (in Neurology)
Neurological Intensive Care Unit, Columbia University College of Physicians and Surgeons, Columbia University Medical Center, New York, New York, USA

Stephan A. Mayer, MD, Associate Clinical Professor[a] and Director[b]
[a]Departments of Neurology and Neurosurgery, [b]Neurological Intensive Care Unit, Columbia University College of Physicians and Surgeons, Columbia University Medical Center, New York, New York, USA

INTRODUCTION

Aneurysmal subarachnoid hemorrhage (aSAH) is an important public health problem, with more than 25,000 cases occurring annually in the United States (1). Despite advances in medical therapy, aSAH remains a deadly disease. Although mortality among hospitalized patients has fallen from 50% to 20% over the past 25 years, patients are still frequently left with significant cognitive and emotional disability (2,3). Despite these improvements in mortality, the burden of aSAH is magnified by the fact that this disease primarily affects individuals in the prime of their lives, between the ages of 30 and 60 years (4).

CLINICAL GRADING SCALES

Until recently, the most relevant measure of outcome after aSAH had been mortality, and it had long been appreciated that the risk of dying from this disease is primarily determined by the severity of the initial bleeding event. Several clinical grading scales have been designed over the years to evaluate the severity of the initial hemorrhage. The World Federation of Neurological Surgeons (WFNS) and the Hunt and Hess grading scales are two of the more common scales in use today (Table 1). The WFNS scale is based on the Glasgow Coma Scale (see Chapter 4), with an additional axis to acknowledge the presence of a focal neurologic deficit (5). Clinical assessment of 1519 patients demonstrated that it is a good predictor of outcomes. Patients with WFNS grade I had good recovery rates of 87% and mortality of 3%, whereas grades IV and V correlated with much poorer results, regardless of the intensity of treatment (6). The patient's Hunt and Hess grade (7) has also been shown to be a good predictor of in-hospital mortality (Table 2). Initially developed as an aid in assessment of surgical risk and timing for surgery in aSAH patients, this scale takes into account the severity of meningeal irritation, level of arousal, presence of a neurologic deficit, and presence of serious comorbid disease. It has the benefit of being easier to utilize than the WFNS scale.

Regardless of the scale used, admission clinical grade predicts mortality. However, aSAH is a complex disease, with many causes of secondary deterioration, including rebleeding, delayed ischemia from vasospasm, hydrocephalus, cerebral edema, and a host of medical complications. For this reason, a patient's worst clinical grade during the course of hospitalization has a closer correlation with outcome than the admission grade (8). In addition to clinical grade, other important predictors of mortality and poor outcome after aSAH include age, aneurysm size, rebleeding, intraventricular hemorrhage, global cerebral edema, and physiologic derangements, such as hypertension or hypotension, hypoxia, hyperglycemia, and fever (9).

DELAYED CEREBRAL ISCHEMIA

Infarction due to vasospasm remains an especially feared complication of aSAH and has received special attention from neurosurgeons over the years because it is a particularly vexing

Table 1 Clinical Grading Scales for Aneurysmal Subarachnoid Hemorrhage

Grade	Hunt and Hess	World Federation of Neurological Surgeons
1	Asymptomatic or minimal headache and slight nuchal rigidity	GCS 15, no motor deficit
2	Moderate to severe headache nuchal rigidity, no neurologic deficit other than cranial nerve palsy	GCS 13–14, no motor deficit
3	Drowsy, confusion, or mild focal deficit	GCS 13–14, with motor deficit
4	Stupor, moderate to severe hemiparesis, possible early decerebrate rigidity and deficit vegetative disturbances	GCS 7–12, with/without motor
5	Deep coma, decerebrate rigidity, moribund appearance	GCS 3–6, with/without motor deficit

Note: Systemic disease, such as hypertension, severe arteriosclerosis, chronic pulmonary disease, and vasospasm on angiography, results in placement in next less favorable category.
Abbreviation: GCS, Glasgow Coma Scale.

complication in good-grade patients who have undergone successful aneurysmal repair. In 1980, the Fisher Scale (10) was developed to predict risk of vasospasm following aSAH (Table 3). The scale assigns a grade based on the amount of blood seen on CT imaging and was initially evaluated in a small population of 50 patients. The main power of the scale is that it identifies patients with thick cisternal clot in the anterior interhemispheric fissure and sylvian stem, in the immediate vicinity of the anterior and middle cerebral arteries. These patients, designated Fisher grade 3, are at especially high risk for developing symptomatic vasospasm. However, the scale has limitations, including the lack of a reliable criterion by which to identify grade 3 patients (Fisher defined it as blood thicker than 1 mm on the actual CT films, without scaling this measurement to the patient) and the fact that thick intracerebral and intraventricular blood is not independently accounted for in the grading system. In light of evidence that intraventricular hemorrhage also increases the risk of symptomatic vasospasm (Table 4), a modification of the original Fisher scale has been proposed in which the highest risk group (grade 4) has the combination of thick cisternal aSAH and bilateral intraventricular hemorrhage (11).

HIERARCHY OF CLINICAL AND FUNCTIONAL OUTCOMES AFTER aSAH

As mortality rates have fallen over the years, stroke research has increasingly focused on patient-centered outcomes that assess functional disability and health-related quality of life (QOL) among survivors (12–14). Outcome assessment after stroke is conceptualized in terms of *global outcome* (the entire spectrum from death to complete recovery), *impairment* (loss of neurologic function), *disability* (loss of independence in activities of daily livings, ADLs), *handicap* (limitation of social or societal role function), and health-related *QOL* (a multidimensional

Table 2 In-Hospital Mortality by Hunt and Hess Grading System

Grade		Hospital mortality (%)		
		1968	1997	2001
1	Mild headache	11	1	4
2	Moderate to severe headache	26	5	5
3	Lethargic, mild focal signs	37	19	17
4	Stupor	71	42	31
5	Coma	100	71	78
	Total	35	18	22

Note: Data from 275 patients reported by Hunt and Hess in 1968, 214 patients from Johns Hopkins in 1997, and 534 patients enrolled in the Columbia Subarachnoid Hemorrhage Outcomes Project in 2001.

Table 3   The Fisher Scale

Grade	Computed tomography scan
1	No blood visualized
2	A diffuse deposition or thin layer, with all vertical layers of blood less than 1 mm in thickness
3	Localized clots and/or vertical layers of blood 1 mm or greater in thickness
4	Diffuse thin or no subarachnoid blood, but with intracerebral or intraventricular clots

Note: The 1-mm criterion for differentiating thick versus thin aneurysmal subarachnoid hemorrhage (aSAH) was based on actual millimeters measured on the printed computed tomography films and, thus, is not generalizable to patients' millimeters. Grade 4 excludes patients with thick aSAH, hence a patient with a large ventricular or intracerebral clot and thick cisternal aSAH would be classified as grade 3.

assessment of the patient's perceived physical, social, and emotional health status and well being) (Table 5). Disability can be further categorized into loss of independence in self-care ADLs, such as walking, toileting, and eating, and loss of higher level instrumental ADLs, such as using the telephone, shopping, and housekeeping.

GLOBAL OUTCOME SCALES

The modified Rankin Scale (mRS) and Glasgow Outcome Scale (GOS) (Table 6) are perhaps the two most common measures of *global outcome* used in aSAH research. The mRS (15) is increasingly being adopted as a primary endpoint in stroke clinical trials and has significant advantages over the GOS for evaluating aSAH patients because it has a smaller ceiling effect than the GOS. The scale describes death and 6 grades of disability and is able to describe the full spectrum of limitations after injury. The highest level includes patients who have no disability or symptoms related to their hemorrhage. Although inter-rater reliability meets criteria for satisfactory clinical assessment, there is room for improvement (15). The mRS has been used extensively in aSAH research. The GOS (16) was originally developed as an outcome scale for traumatic brain injury. Although it is still widely used, the categories tend to be broad, making it difficult to capture subtle improvements. In contrast to the mRS, the highest level of outcome on the GOS includes independent patients who continue to suffer from mild physical disability. However, it is well documented that patients in this best level of outcome may still suffer from devastating cognitive impairment (17).

NEUROLOGIC IMPAIRMENT AFTER aSAH

Assessment of *impairment* is critical for detection of a positive treatment effect in clinical trials, because it is the measure of outcome that most directly reflects neurologic injury. Unfortunately, scales used to evaluate impairment after ischemic stroke, such as the NIHSS,

Table 4   The Modified Fisher Scale

Grade	Criteria	Percentage (n) of patients	Frequency DCI	Infarction
0	No aSAH or IVH	5% (15)	0% (0/15)	0% (0/15)
1	Minimal/thin aSAH, no IVH in both lateral ventricles	30% (83)	12% (10/83)	6% (5/83)
2	Minimal/thin aSAH, *with* IVH in both lateral ventricles	5% (14)	21% (3/14)	14% (2/14)
3	Thick aSAH, no IVH in both lateral ventricles	43% (117)	19% (22/117)	12% (14/117)
4	Thick aSAH, *with* IVH in both lateral ventricles	17% (47)	40% (19/47)	28% (13/47)

Abbreviations: aSAH, aneurysmal subarachnoid hemorrhage; IVH, intraventricular hemorrhage; DCI, delayed cerebral ischemia.
Source: From Ref. 11.

Table 5 World Health Organization Hierarchy of Stroke Outcomes

Level of outcome	Description	Typical scales used in subarachnoid hemorrhage research
Global outcome	Death to full recovery	Modified Rankin Score, Glasgow Outcome Scale
Impairment	Loss of normal neurologic function	National Institutes of Health Stroke Scale, Telephone Interview of Cognitive Status, Folstein Mini–Mental Status Examination
Disability	Loss of independence in basic or instrumental activities of daily living	Barthel Index, Lawton Scale
Handicap	Loss of interpersonal, social, or societal role function	Return to work,[a] change in marital status[a]
Quality of life	Multidimensional and often subjective assessment of physical, emotional, social well-being	Sickness Impact Profile, Short Form-36

[a]Handicap is generally evaluated via questionnaire, rather than a specific scale.

are inadequate for aSAH (18), because they focus primarily on impairment related to focal neurologic deficits, which occur in only 15% of aSAH survivors (19). By contrast, most neurologic impairment after aSAH is related to cognitive dysfunction, which is best detected by detailed neuropsychometric evaluations. For example, the Cooperative Nicardipine Study (20) assessed levels of impairment at 3 months using both the NIHSS and the Mini–Mental State Score (MMS). A ceiling effect developed, with nearly half of patients scoring a perfect 30 on the MMS and over half scoring a perfect 0 on the NIHSS.

Comprehensive neuropsychologic testing (Table 7) can reveal cognitive impairment following aSAH and is invaluable in characterizing the extent of impairment in individual patients. However, several problems are associated with the use of detailed neuropsychometric testing in aSAH clinical trials. First, testing can be long, arduous, and difficult to complete by severely impaired individuals, potentially leading to missing data, which may result in selection bias, as the most severely impaired patients are unable to complete the evaluation. Second, tests used multiple times can yield variable scores that can be difficult to interpret. Ideally, the extent of cognitive impairment in each patient should be expressed as a single score, but no standardized or well-validated method exists for accomplishing this. Third, testing must be performed in person and can therefore increase missing data due to difficulty in ensuring this level of patient follow-up. Finally, and possibly most important of all, test performance is highly influenced by age, race, and educational background (3). An ideal measure of aSAH-induced

Table 6 Measures of Global Outcome

Grade	Modified Rankin Scale	Glasgow Outcome Scale
0	No symptoms at all	
1	No significant disability despite symptoms—able to carry out all usual duties	Dead
2	Slight disability—unable to carry out all previous activities but able to look after own affairs without assistance	Dependent, vegetative—unable to interact meaningfully with environment or obey simple commands
3	Moderate disability—requires some help but able to walk without assistance	Dependent, severe disability—able to follow commands but unable to live independently
4	Moderately severe disability—unable to walk without assistance and unable to attend to own bodily needs without assistance	Independent, moderate disability—able to live independently; unable to return to work or school
5	Severe disability—bedridden, incontinent and requiring constant nursing care	Independent, good recovery—able to return to work or school
6	Dead	

Table 7 Selected Neuropsychometric Tests Used in Subarachnoid Hemorrhage Research

Global mental status	Telephone Interview of Cognitive Status
	Verbal Sustained Attention Test
	Short Blessed Test of Orientation, Memory, and Concentration
	Neurobehavioral Cognitive Status Examination
	Mattis Dementia Rating Scale
Visual memory	Wechsler Memory Scale-III (WMS-III): Visual Reproduction II
	Rey Osterrieth Complex Figure Test (RCFT): Delayed Recall
	Wechsler Adult Intelligence Scale–III: Digit Symbol Recall
Verbal memory	California Verbal Learning Test
Reaction time	California Computerized Assessment Package
Motor function	Grooved Pegboard Test
	Trails Making Test—Part A
Executive function	Modified Wisconsin Card Sorting Test
	Trails Making Test—Part B
	RCFT: Copy
Visual-spatial function	Wechsler Adult Intelligence Scale-III: Block Design
	WMS-III: Visual Reproduction Copy
Language function	Boston Naming Test
	Token Test
	American National Adult Reading Test
	Word Accentuation Test
	Wechsler Test of Adult Reading
	Cambridge Contextual Reading Test
	Spot Word Test

cognitive impairment for clinical trials would generate a single global score, be applicable to both severely injured and highly functional patients, be resistant to demographic bias, have good inter-rater and test-retest reliability, and possess construct validity, so that poor scores are associated with worse neuropsychologic test performance, increased disease severity, and reduced QOL. One study evaluated 3 simple tests of global cognitive status in a cohort of aSAH patients and found that The Telephone Interview of Cognitive Status (21) comes closest to meeting the above criteria (19).

Unlike ischemic cerebral infarction and intracerebral hemorrhage, aSAH oftentimes causes a more subtle form of diffuse brain injury. Although one might guess that the vast majority of patients are affected in a subtle way, in fact, it appears more likely that a subset of 20% to 30% of patients suffers from severe forms of cognitive impairment, with the remainder doing relatively well (19,22). These problems frequently encompass all domains of cognitive functioning, including processing speed, attention and concentration, verbal and visual memory, visual-spatial skills, and executive function (2,3,19,22–26). It has been found that an estimated from 25% to 50% of patients will have significant cognitive impairment at 3 months (3,22). Many studies have identified predictors of cognitive impairment after aSAH. The most consistently identified risk factors include cerebral infarction, global cerebral edema, thick aSAH clot, intraventricular hemorrhage, hydrocephalus, and anterior circulation aneurysmal location (2,3,22–26).

DISABILITY AND HANDICAP AFTER aSAH

As stated previously, disability is conceptualized as a limitation in performing personal functions, also known as ADLs. ADLs can further be divided into basic functions, such as walking, eating, and toileting, and so-called instrumental functions, such as shopping, performing housework, using a telephone, or paying the bills. The Barthel Index (27) is the most widely used scale for evaluating basic ADL performance after aSAH. However, it is poorly suited for this evaluation, because it is heavily weighted toward limitations that result from physical and motor impairment, which are largely unaffected in most patients. The result is a very large ceiling effect, with the majority scoring a top score of 100 on the scale. For instance, in the Columbia University SAH Outcomes Project, 86% of aSAH survivors had a top score of 100 on the Barthel

Index 3 months after hemorrhage (unpublished data). Much more often, patients suffer from disability related to loss of independence in performing higher level instrumental ADLs after aSAH. Scales that are well suited to evaluate instrumental ADLs include the Lawton Scale (28) and the Pfeffer scale (29). Even with these more sensitive scales of disability, substantial ceiling effects exist, with more than 50% of patients scoring a top score.

Handicap is often confused with *disability*, but it refers specifically to loss of interpersonal or societal role function, due to either an impairment or disability. For example, a person may be impaired due to moderate memory loss and dysarthria, which may result in instrumental disability due to loss of independence for traveling outside the house and taking care of personal finances. These problems, in turn, can result in handicap in terms of fulfilling one's role as a husband, father, and wage earner. Handicap is common after aSAH. Even among good-grade patients, only 50% return to the same level of work prior to their hemorrhage (30), and significant strains are often placed on interpersonal relationships, primarily due to behavioral changes, such as irritability, apathy, and impulsivity (31).

QUALITY OF LIFE AFTER aSAH

QOL refers to a multidimensional assessment of the patient's perceived physical, social, and emotional health status and well-being (32). Although QOL may be the single aspect of recovery that is most relevant to the patient, it is important to remember that QOL assessments can be highly subjective. Thus, QOL measurements are less directly related than impairment or disability to the outcome of a specific disease process. For example, 2 individuals with aSAH may suffer from the same degree of moderate residual cognitive impairment. One is a happily married 70-year-old retiree, and his main daily activity is reading the paper, going for a walk, and feeding the pigeons. He can continue to do these things without much difficulty and reports a good QOL after his hemorrhage. The other individual is an intense, high-powered, 42-year-old banking executive who works in a highly competitive work environment. The moderate cognitive impairment has devastating consequences on his ability to maintain his high productivity and compete in the workplace. He reports his QOL as terrible. Although QOL is an essential and highly relevant aspect of outcomes assessment after aSAH, it is better suited as a secondary, rather than a primary, outcome measure, because it can have a weak relationship to the extent of neurologic impairment directly resulting from brain injury.

QOL can be measured with many different scales. The most commonly used scales in aSAH outcomes research are the Sickness Impact Profile (SIP) (32) and the Short-Form 36 (SF-36) (33), which are multi-item questionnaires that take 20 to 40 min to administer. They yield scores related to a broad number of domains of QOL, such as pain, mobility, sleep and rest, eating, social interaction, and work, as well as summary scores related to global physical and psychosocial function.

Regardless of the instrument used, it is clear that QOL is adversely affected by aSAH. For example, it has been reported that, compared to a reference population, SIP and SF-36 scores were adversely affected in 80% of aSAH survivors (34). In a comparison for their suitability for aSAH research, it was found that the SIP has greater sensitivity to QOL problems and better construct validity (correlation with acute disease severity and concurrent mRS scores) (35) than the SF-36. Another advantage to the SIP is that, unlike the SF-36, it is largely an objective rather than subjective instrument, making it reliable when administered by proxy to more severely affected stroke (36) and aSAH patients (37) who cannot complete the testing on their own.

When QOL scales are administered to aSAH patients, it is interesting that the domains most consistently affected generally relate to physical problems (38–40), which is counterintuitive, because aSAH primarily causes cognitive deficits. This can be understood by the consistent complaints of aSAH patients with regard to mental and physical fatigue, decreased energy, and reduced stamina, which in general make it harder to "do things."

CONCLUSIONS AND FUTURE DIRECTIONS

The use of appropriate outcome measures is critical for clinical trial success. The use of an inappropriate, nongeneralizable, or insensitive outcome measure can prevent detection of an important treatment effect. Thus, the identification of optimal outcome measures for aSAH will increase the likelihood of identifying effective therapies in the future. Stroke investigators have identified desirable characteristics of outcome measures for use in clinical trials (12,13). First, clinical outcome measures should be relevant to the patient, focusing on survival, disability, handicap, and QOL. Second, response variables should include items that relate to a single aspect of outcome, as a mixture of different aspects within a single scale can be confusing and difficult to interpret clinically. Third, outcome measures should be valid, reliable, and responsive to change when following patients over time. Fourth, outcome measures should be easily applied to all patients regardless of degree of injury. The use of complex neuropsychologic tests and QOL scales can be especially problematic in this regard. Finally, measures of outcome are best expressed as a single dichotomous, ordinal, or continuous variable.

In the past, most aSAH clinical trials and cohort studies have relied on global outcome scales that suffer from profound ceiling effects and are insensitive to subtle, but disabling, cognitive deficits. Much needs to be done to improve upon and standardize outcome assessment scales for aSAH. The goal should be to develop widely applicable and standardized instruments that correlate appropriately with increased disease severity, meaningful cognitive impairment, instrumental disability, handicap, and QOL.

REFERENCES

1. Mayberg MR, Batjer HH, Dacey R, et al. Guidelines for the management of aneurysmal subarachnoid hemorrhage. A statement for healthcare professionals from a special writing group of the Stroke Council, American Heart Association. Circulation 1994; 90:2592–2605.
2. Ogden JA, Mee EW, Henning M. A prospective study of impairment of cognition and memory and recovery after subarachnoid hemorrhage. Neurosurgery 1993; 33:572–587.
3. Kreiter KT, Copeland DL, Bernardini GL, et al. Predictors of cognitive dysfunction after subarachnoid hemorrhage. Stroke 2002; 33:200–209.
4. Quality of Care and Outcomes Research in CVD and Stroke Working Groups. Measuring and improving quality of care: a report from the American Heart Association/American college of cardiology first scientific forum on assessment of healthcare quality in cardiovascular disease and stroke. Stroke 2000; 31:1002–1012.
5. Drake CG, Hunt WE, Sano K, et al. Report of the World Federation of Neurological Surgeons committee on a universal subarachnoid hemorrhage grading scale. J Neurosurg 1988; 68:985–986.
6. Sano K. Grading and timing of surgery for aneurysmal subarachnoid hemorrhage. Neurol Res 1994; 16:23–26.
7. Hunt WE, Hess RM. Surgical risk as related to time of intervention in the repair of intracranial aneurysms. J Neurosurg 1968; 28:14–20.
8. Chiang VL, Claus EB, Awad IA. Toward more rational prediction of outcome in patients with high-grade subarachnoid hemorrhage. Neurosurgery 2000; 46:28–35.
9. Claassen J, Vu A, Kreiter KT, et al. Impact of acute physiologic derangements on outcome after subarachnoid hemorrhage. Crit Care Med 2004; 32:832–838.
10. Fisher CM, Kistler JP, Davis JM. Relation of cerebral vasospasm to subarachnoid hemorrhage visualized by computerized tomographic scanning. Neurosurgery 1980; 6:1–9.
11. Claassen J, Bernardini GL, Kreiter K, et al. Effect of cisternal and ventricular blood on risk of delayed cerebral ischemia after subarachnoid hemorrhage: the Fisher scale revisited. Stroke 2001; 32:2012–2020.
12. Roberts L, Counsell C. Assessment of clinical outcomes in acute stroke trials. Stroke 1998; 29:986–991.
13. Lyden PD, Lau GT. A critical appraisal of stroke evaluation and rating scales. Stroke 1991; 22:1345–1352.
14. Wolfe CDA, Taub NA, Woodrow EJ, Burney PGJ. Assessment of scales of disability and handicap for stroke patients. Stroke 1991; 22:1242–1244.
15. Van Swieten JC, Koudstaal PJ, Visser MC, Schouten HJ, van Gijn J. Interobserver agreement for the assessment of handicap in stroke patients. Stroke 1988; 19:604–607.
16. Jennett B, Bond M. Assessment of outcome after severe brain injury: a practical scale. Lancet 1975; 480–484.
17. Hutter BO, Gilsbach JM. Which neuropsychological deficits are hidden behind a good outcome (Glasgow = I) after aneurysmal subarachnoid hemorrhage? Neurosurgery 1993; 33:999–1005.
18. Brott T, Adams HP, Olinger CP, et al. Measurements of acute cerebral infarction: a clinical examination scale. Stroke 1989; 20:864–870.
19. Mayer SA, Kreiter KT, Copeland DL, et al. Global and domain-specific cognitive impairment and outcome after subarachnoid hemorrhage. Neurology 2002; 59:1750–1758.
20. Droy JM, Daridon E, Leroy J, Massari P. Acute nicardipine and nifedipine poisoning. Multicenter study. Cooperative study by the french poison control centers and the ARIT. J Toxicol Clin Exp 1990; 10(4):249–256.

21. Brandt J, Spencer M, Folstein M. The telephone interview for cognitive status. Neuropsychiatr Neuropsychol Behav Neurol 1988; 1:111–117.
22. Stabell KE, Magnaes B. Neuropsychological course after surgery for intracranial aneurysms: a prospective study and critical review. Scand J Psychol 1997; 38:127–137.
23. Hutter BO, Kreitschmann-Andermahr I, Mayfrank L, Rohde V, Spetzger U, Gilsbach JM. Functional outcome after aneurysmal subarachnoid hemorrhage. Acta Neurochir Suppl (Wien) 1999; 72:157–174.
24. Hadjivassiliou M, Tooth CL, Romanowski CAJ, et al. Aneurysmal SAH: cognitive outcome and structural damage after clipping or coiling. Neurology 2001; 56:1672–1677.
25. Richardson JTE. Cognitive performance following rupture and repair of intracranial aneurysm. Acta Neurol Scand 1991; 83:110–122.
26. Vilkki J, Holst P, Ohman J, et al. Social outcome related to cognitive performance and computed tomographic findings after surgery for a ruptured intracranial aneurysm. Neurosurgery 1990; 26:579–585.
27. Mahony FT, Barthel DW. Functional evaluation: Barthel Index. Md Med J 1965; 14:61–65.
28. Lawton MP, Brody EM. Assessment of older people: self-maintaining and instrumental activities of daily living. Gerontologist 1969; 9:179–186.
29. Pfeffer RI, Kurosaki TT, Harrah CH, Chance JM, Filos S. Measurement of functional activities in older adults in the community. J Gerontol 1982; 37:323–329.
30. Ropper AH, Zervas NT. Outcome 1 year after SAH from cerebral aneurysm. J Neurosurg 1984; 60: 909–915.
31. Buck D, Jacoby A, Massey A, Ford G. Evaluation of measures used to assess quality of life after stroke. Stroke 2000; 31:2004–2010.
32. Damiano AM. Sickness impact profile. In: User's Manual and Interpretation Guide. Baltimore: The Johns Hopkins University, 1996.
33. Ware JE Jr., Sherbourne CD. The MOS 36-item short-form health survey (SF-36). I. Conceptual framework and item selection. Med Care 1992; 30:473–483.
34. Hop JW, Rinkel GJE, Algra A, van Gijn J. Changes in functional outcome and quality of life in patients and caregivers after aneurysmal subarachnoid hemorrhage. J Neurosurg 2001; 95:957–963.
35. Copeland D, Kreiter K, Peery S, et al. What's the best scale for assessing quality of life after subarachnoid hemorrhage? [abstract]. Ann Neurol 2000; 48:21.
36. Sneeuw KCA, Aaronson NK, de Haan RJ, Limburg M. Assessing quality of life after stroke: the value and limitations of proxy ratings. Stroke 1997; 28:1541–1549.
37. Ostapkovich N, Kreiter K, Peery S, Connolly ES, Mayer SA. Are proxy ratings valid for assessing quality of life after subarachnoid hemorrhage? [abstract]. Ann Neurol 2001; 50:S78–S79.
38. Hackett ML, Anderson CS. Health outcomes 1 year after subarachnoid hemorrhage. Neurology 2000; 55:658–662.
39. Deane M, Pigott T, Dearing P. The value of the Short Form 36 score in the outcome assessment of subarachnoid haemorrhage. Br J Neurosurgery 1996; 10:187–191.
40. Carter BS, Buckley D, Ferraro R, Rordorf G, Ogilvy CS. Factors associated with reintegration to normal living after subarachnoid hemorrhage. Neurosurgery 2000; 46:1326–1334.

10 | Animal Models of Intracerebral Hemorrhage

Kenneth R. Wagner, PhD, Research Associate Professor
Department of Neurology, University of Cincinnati College of Medicine, and
Veterans Affairs Medical Center, Medical Research Service, Cincinnati, Ohio, USA

Thomas G. Brott, MD, Professor
Department of Neurology, Mayo Clinic College of Medicine,
Jacksonville, Florida, USA

INTRODUCTION

Experimental study of intracerebral hemorrhage (ICH) in animal models has increased dramatically in the last several years. A PubMed search on January 1, 2005, for articles with the keywords "intracerebral hemorrhage" or "hematoma" and "animals" generated almost 300 references written since 1968. Two-thirds of these reports appeared in the last 5 years. These citations by researchers worldwide demonstrate a wide range of investigations examining all aspects of the disorder. The importance of experimental animal models for ICH research is that they permit a detailed examination of the pathophysiologic, biochemical, and molecular processes, as well as the mechanisms underlying brain tissue injury. They also enable testing of new pharmacologic and surgical therapies.

A comprehensive review of experimental ICH models was published by Kaufman and Schochet in 1992 (1). In 2002, we published an updated review (2). Since then, several reports that describe new models of ICH in the mouse have appeared (3,4). In addition, recent reports have described interesting new findings using knockout mice, such as the matrix metalloproteinase (MMP)-9-deficient mouse (5). Thiex et al. (6) examined the extent of edema formation in a murine model of collagenase-induced ICH, which included recombinant tissue plasminogen activator (rtPA)-deficient and wild-type mice. Interestingly, a new mouse model has been reported in which mouse embryos genetically null for all α-V-integrins develop ICH due to defective interactions between blood vessels and brain parenchymal cells (7). Several other recent studies have reported on new ICH treatments in animal models that test local (8) and global (9) brain hypothermia and the use of glutamate receptor antagonists (10), a statin (11), a cyclooxygenase-2 inhibitor (12), and metalloporphyrin heme oxygenase inhibitors (13–15). Another group (16) reported that intraventricular transplantation of embryonic stem (ES) cell-derived neural stem cells in rats with ICH generated ES-derived neurons and astrocytes around the hematoma cavities. The transplants were performed 7 days after the ICH, and 28 days later, ES-derived neurons and astrocytes could be detected in all 10 rats that received grafts.

MODELS AND SPECIES: OVERVIEW

The classic method of inducing ICH in experimental animals has been to directly infuse autologous blood into a specific brain region, usually the basal ganglia. This method has been employed in a variety of species, including rat, rabbit, cat, dog, pig, primate (reviews in Refs. 1 and 2), and, most recently, mouse (3,4). We have developed a large animal lobar ICH model in the pig, in which we infuse up to 3.0 mL of arterial blood into the frontal hemispheric white matter (17), and we have used this model to examine ICH pathophysiology and pathochemistry and surgical clot evacuation (17–19) (reviews in Refs. 20 and 21). A second commonly used model employs bacterial collagenase usually injected locally into the basal ganglia (22,23). Collagenase dissolves the extracellular matrix, leading to blood vessel rupture and an intracerebral bleed.

Overall, these models have significantly contributed to our knowledge of ICH-induced injury. Specifically, they have provided information on the roles of mass effect and elevated intracranial pressure (ICP), alterations in blood flow and metabolism, and the impact of specific blood components on brain edema formation and blood-brain barrier (BBB) disruption. Along with providing details of ICH-induced biochemical and molecular events, these models also enable testing of potential therapies, both surgical and pharmacologic.

In this chapter, the classic blood infusion models are described, and the collagenase model is reviewed. Each model section contains a detailed description of the findings that have been obtained with individual species. The brain pathologic responses to ICH that are present in the various animal models are described and compared with observations in human ICH. Lastly, the limitations of animal models and their ability to fully address various aspects of human ICH are discussed.

INTRACEREBRAL BLOOD INFUSION ICH MODELS

Intraparenchymal infusion (or injection) of autologous blood is the classic technique by which to create an intracerebral hematoma. Clearly, this method does not reproduce the bleeding event of spontaneous ICH in humans, i.e., arterial vessel rupture. However, this model does enable the infused blood volume to be controlled and, therefore, generates reasonably reproducible hematoma sizes and mass effects. These models have been very useful for studying the pathophysiologic and biochemical events that result from the presence of blood in the brain tissue. Disadvantages of blood infusion models are the potential for ventricular rupture and for backflow of the infused blood along the needle track (24,25). Such events during blood infusion can lead to intraventricular and/or subarachnoid leakage of blood. This problem was addressed by a double hemorrhage method, in which a small volume of blood is initially infused into the caudate at a slow rate, followed by a 7-min pause to allow the blood to clot along the needle track, and then infusion of the remaining blood to produce a hematoma (24). The clotting of blood around the shaft of the needle prevents the backflow of blood into the subarachnoid space during the subsequent infusion, thereby enhancing the production of reproducible hematoma volumes. This double-infusion approach has been employed by several groups (3,26).

Rats

The most frequently used species for experimental ICH studies has been the rat, and the most commonly injected site has been the basal ganglia. Some of the earliest ICH studies in rat, conducted in the mid-to-late 1980s, examined relationships between mass effect, perihematomal blood flow, and ICP (27–31). In addition, microballoons were employed to examine the relationships between mass volumes, elevations of ICP, and local perfusion (32). Overall, investigators concluded that perihematomal blood flow was markedly reduced in their model. Based on their findings, it was suggested that ischemia was responsible for secondary damage after ICH (reviews in Refs. 33 and 34).

However, not all investigators have concluded that ischemia is responsible for perihematomal tissue injury after ICH. Although initial ischemia of 20% to 30% below baseline has been noted in a rat model, recovery of flow and hyperemia in the hours following ICH were described (35). More recently, Yang et al. measured local cerebral blood flow (CBF) using [14C]-iodoantipyrine (25). They reported that CBF was reduced to 50% of control at 1 hr after ICH, returned to control values by 4 hr, but then decreased to <50% of control in the subacute phase between 24 and 48 hr. They concluded that although some degree of ischemia occurs in the early minutes to a few hours following ICH, the degree of ischemia is neither severe nor the basis for the development of perihematomal edema (25). Furthermore, in human ICH (36,37), Positron Emission Tomography studies demonstrated that, although blood flow might be reduced, this reduction is coupled with a reduction in metabolism in perihematomal tissue; therefore, cerebral ischemia is not present.

Some investigators have reported that hyperemia is present following ICH in rats (30), and we observed hyperemia in our porcine ICH model (20,38). A recent report that increased glucose metabolism in perihematomal rat brain in the early hours after ICH is due to glutamate receptor activation (10) might explain the hyperemia and the marked increases in perihematomal lactate previously reported in a porcine ICH model (18).

Studies in rats over the past decade have established that activation of the coagulation cascade and specific plasma proteins are required for both acute and delayed development of perihematomal edema. The plasma protein thrombin, when infused into brain, produces edema that is comparable to that generated by infusions of whole blood (39). The importance of the coagulation cascade in ICH-induced perihematomal edema formation was demonstrated both in rat and in porcine ICH models (40). Heparinized blood infusions generated very little edema when compared to infusions of unheparinized blood. As demonstrated in models in which packed red cells alone were infused (40), the contribution by erythrocytes to edema formation is delayed. Red cells infused into the basal ganglia in rats did not produce a dramatic increase in edema until 3 days postinfusion (40). In contrast, infusions of lysed autologous erythrocytes into the rat brain produced marked edema 24 hr after infusion. In the rat model, whereas hemoglobin infusions produce severe edema, packed erythrocytes do not. Similarly, in a porcine ICH model, lysed blood causes severe brain edema and death, presumably as a result of high concentrations of released hemoglobin (41).

Complement activation and membrane attack–complex formation also appear to contribute to perihematomal edema formation, as N-acetylheparin, which inhibits complement activation, diminished this edema (42). Importantly, these results in an animal ICH model suggest that the complement system could be targeted for future ICH treatment.

Lastly, studies in a rat cortical ICH model demonstrate the additional toxicity of hemorrhage, as compared to cerebral ischemic insults (43). These investigators showed that extravasated whole blood causes a greater degree of cell death and inflammation than do ischemic lesions of similar size (44).

Cats

Autologous blood infusions have been used to produce experimental ICH in cats. An early experimental ICH study demonstrated an important relationship between the size and location of an intracerebral hematoma, functional deficits, and ICP elevations (45). Other findings demonstrated that increased ICP was the main cause of blood volume/flow reductions shortly after hematoma induction in the basal ganglia (46). The relationship between neurologic deficits and hematoma volume was also observed, and it was found that urokinase-induced resolution of internal capsule hematomas also improved neurologic outcome (47). These findings in cats support those in human ICH, which reported a strong relationship between hematoma size and clinical outcome (48).

Rabbits

Hematoma volumes in rabbits were studied using autologous blood stereotactically injected into the thalamus, and it was found that these animals would tolerate clots with a volume of 3% to 5% of their brain volume, which approximates a 50-cc clot in humans (49). In one of the earliest studies of the efficacy of hematoma removal with thrombolytics the authors demonstrated 86% efficacy in lysing intracranial hematomas with urokinase in a rabbit ICH model, whereas only 3 of the 13 controls showed evidence of hematoma resolution with saline injections into the clot (50). Furthermore, histologically, no increased damage or inflammation was noted between these animals and 22 additional rabbits treated with urokinase or saline 24 hr after clot injection. The authors concluded that urokinase could be employed safely and effectively for the lysis of intracranial hematomas and that a delay in therapy of up to 24 hr does not significantly compromise its efficacy. The efficacy of urokinase in stereotactic human ICH treatment was further demonstrated by Zuccarello et al. (51).

In a very detailed examination of the cellular activation in the perifocal reactive zone in a rabbit ICH model, Koeppen et al. (52) found that experimental hematomas resolved much more slowly after the injection of whole blood than after the injection of red blood cells, suggesting that proteins in the coagulated blood contribute to the injury process.

Imaging studies of ICH in rabbits demonstrated that susceptibility-weighted gradient-echo imaging at 1.5 T is highly sensitive in detecting hyperacute parenchymal, as well as subarachnoid and intraventricular hemorrhages (53). A rabbit lobar ICH model in which arterial pressure was used to infuse autologous blood into the deep frontal white matter, served to investigate the degree of neuronal injury inside and outside the hematoma at 24 hr (54).

Dogs

Canines were among the earliest-used animals for studying experimental ICH. A 1975 study of the tolerance of the dog's brain to blood injection in different sites—the brain parenchyma and the ventricles—found different lethal volumes for each specific ICH site (55). The authors found that 8 mL was lethal in the dog brain parenchyma and concluded that that death was not a random event but was due to the failure of vital functions as a result of elevated ICP. Further detailed studies demonstrated the evolution of brain injury following ICH in a canine parietal lobe hematoma model by high-resolution sonography, CT, and neuropathologic examinations (56). These authors found a correlation between the sequence of changes on CT and sonography images in their ICH model and the findings following ICH in patients. In early MRI studies in canine ICH models, venous and arterial blood infusions and intraventricular locations of blood were compared, and it was concluded that gradient-echo sequences would be highly useful in detecting and delineating hemorrhages in human ICH patients (57).

In histologic and CT studies of internal capsule hematomas conducted in dogs, 3 distinct stages were identified on histology and CT: (i) in the acute stage (≤5 days), homogeneous high density was present at the periphery of the hematoma on CT, while histologically, a necrotic layer of tissue existed at the boundary of the clot; (ii) in the subacute stage (5–14 days), perihematomal density was decreased with ring enhancement after contrast injection and corresponded to the appearance of immature connective tissue with argentophilic fibers; (iii) in the chronic stage (>15 days), contraction of the enhancing ring was noted, corresponding to the development of mature connective tissue with collagen fibers (58).

Using a mongrel dog ICH model, another study (59) determined the effect of massive ICH on regional CBF (rCBF) and metabolism by testing the hypothesis put forward by Mendelow and coworkers from their studies in rats (27–34) regarding intracerebral bleed-induced perihematomal ischemia. Interestingly, these investigators found no evidence for an ischemic penumbra within the first 5 hr after hemorrhage, despite prominent increases in ICP and mean arterial blood pressure (MABP) following hematoma induction, indicative of a Cushing response.

Other investigators found that hypertonic saline, at 3% and 23.4% concentrations, was as effective as mannitol in controlling intracranial hypertension in a dog model (60). In addition, 3% hypertonic saline appeared to have a longer effect than either 23.4% saline or mannitol. No effect on rCBF or cerebral metabolism was observed with any of the agents. In their study of the pharmacologic reduction of MABP, the same group using the same canine model found that reducing MABP with intravenous labetalol within the normal autoregulatory curve of CPP had no adverse effects on ICP and perihematomal or distant rCBF (54). They concluded that MABP reduction is safe within autoregulation limits in the acute period after ICH.

Monkeys

Hematomas were generated in the caudate nucleus of vervet monkeys by allowing femoral arterial blood to enter the structure via a stereotactically implanted needle (61). ICP peaked at 51 ± 8 mmHg at 3 min after the bleed and remained high throughout the 3 hr procedure. rCBF was significantly reduced in all brain regions for 1 hr after the ictus, with the lowest values in the periphery of the hematoma. Some rCBF values were below the ischemic threshold for 90 min after the hemorrhage. Another group (62) reported an early thrombolytic treatment study in Macaque monkeys in abstract form in 1982. They found that urokinase promoted basal ganglia hematoma resorption that correlated with improvement in the clinical exam.

Pigs

Our group has developed and extensively studied the pathophysiology, pathochemistry, and treatment of ICH in a porcine white-matter (lobar ICH) model (17) (reviews in Refs. 20 and 21). The advantages of using the pig for an ICH model include its large gyrated brain and large amount of hemispheric white matter, its relatively low cost, and its noncompanion animal status. The pig's large brain enables the production of hematoma volumes up to approximately 3 cc by slowly (10–15 mins) infusing autologous arterial blood through a plastic catheter into the frontal white matter. We have used this model to investigate ICH pathophysiology and pathochemistry, edema development, the role of blood components, and metabolism (18,20,63) (reviews in Refs. 21 and 64). The large hematoma volumes that can be generated in this model make it useful to investigate studies of neurosurgical clot evacuation (19,65).

This lobar ICH model in the pig is clinically relevant for several reasons: (i) bleeds into the white matter are common in human ICH and occur with almost similar frequency to basal ganglia bleeds (66); (ii) lobar ICH is the most frequent hemorrhage site in the young (67); (iii) white-matter damage is an important contributor to long-term morbidity following ICH

(68,69). Because white matter is more vulnerable to vasogenic edema development than is gray matter (70), this model is especially applicable for studying edema-associated injury.

Studies in the porcine ICH model have demonstrated the important role of clot formation, retraction, and plasma protein accumulation in perihematomal edema development (17,20). The importance of coagulation in animal models is translatable to patients who developed ICH after thrombolytic treatment but failed to develop significant edema despite large intracerebral masses (71). Although whole blood is responsible for the majority of the hematoma's mass effect, infusions of packed red cells alone fail to generate perihematomal edema. As described above, nonclotting blood also produces minimal perihematomal edema in both rat and porcine models. Thus, these results support the conclusion that the early and substantial perihematomal edema that follows ICH does not result from the mass effect and potentially reduced perfusion that are induced by the hematoma. Rather, the findings suggest that this very early edema results primarily from the coagulation cascade and clot retraction. The cellular elements of the hematoma are concentrated at the core as clotting proceeds. The fluid/serum components of the whole blood are extruded to the perimeter (72). Interestingly, it was recently reported (73) that increased rates of water diffusion measured in the perihematomal region by diffusion-weighted MRI in ICH patients suggested that this edema development is plasma derived. These results also are consistent with the experimental and human ICH studies, which show relatively more early edema in the setting of normal coagulation compared with the lesser edema seen in the setting of anticoagulants or thrombolytics (71).

This porcine ICH model has been especially useful for clot evacuation studies. We have demonstrated that early (3.5 hr) clot aspiration after rtPA-induced lysis markedly reduced (by >70%) both clot volume and perihematomal edema and protected the BBB at 24 hr following ICH (19). This reduction in clot volume, achieved with rtPA liquification of the clot, was significantly (>37%) greater than the reduction obtained by mechanical aspiration without rtPA. Lastly, we have used the porcine ICH model to test the Possis AngioJet rheolytic thrombectomy catheter (74). This surgical clot removal study showed that the device was very effective for rapidly removing intracerebral hematomas, producing an average 61% decrease in clot volumes in approximately 30 sec. Other treatments studied in this model include inhibiting heme oxygenase by a metalloporphyrin (13).

BACTERIAL COLLAGENASE MODEL

The bacterial collagenase model employs the local injection of bacterial collagenase into the basal ganglia to induce an intracerebral bleed (22,23,75). This model mimics spontaneous ICH in humans by dissolving the extracellular matrix around capillaries, resulting in active intraparenchymal bleeding. The hemorrhage is simple to produce. The animals develop spontaneous, reproducible hemorrhages, with volumes that correlate with the amount of collagenase injected, and significant blood leakage does not develop along the needle track. A disadvantage is that bacterial collagenase introduces a significant inflammatory reaction (44,76,77) that is more intense than that observed in experimental ICH models that employ blood infusion. The inflammatory response is also more intense than that observed following human ICH (78). The collagenase model also differs from the punctate arterial rupture that produces human ICH, as the collagenase dissolves the extracellular matrix around capillaries to produce hemorrhage.

The collagenase ICH model has been used by several investigators in mouse, rat, and pig. Their reports shed light on the pathochemical events following ICH and describe several new experimental treatments for ICH that have not been examined in the blood infusion model. Recent studies have demonstrated: (i) the role of MMPs in BBB opening and edema development following collagenase-induced ICH and the effectiveness of MMP inhibitors (79,80), (ii) that select MMPs exhibit increased expression after ICH and that minocycline is neuroprotective by suppressing monocytoid cell activation and downregulating MMP-12 expression (81), and (iii) that the tripeptide macrophage/microglial inhibitory factor inhibits microglial activation and results in functional improvement when given before, as well as after, the onset of collagenase-induced ICH (82,83). Various other reports using this model have described detailed studies of the collagenase dose effect (84), imaging features and histopathology (76,85), neurobehavioral results and therapy (86–88), and influence of hyperglycemia (89). Several drug treatments aimed at different molecular mechanisms of injury have also been studied, including free radical scavengers/spin traps (90,91), neurotransmitter receptor agonists (92,93) and antagonists (94), cytokines and inflammation (77,95–98), and neuroprotectives (99).

The collagenase model in rodents has also been extended to pigs (100,101), and the investigators have reported studies of somatosensory-evoked potentials elicited by electrical stimulation of the contralateral snout, as well as changes in DC-coupled potential, which was monitored in the somatosensory region following induction of ICH into the primary sensory cortex.

ISCHEMIA-REPERFUSION HEMORRHAGE MODEL

An interesting and possibly clinically relevant ICH model has been described in rhesus monkeys, in which hematomas were induced during the vasoproliferative stages of a maturing ischemic infarct (102). In this model, elevating MABP at 5 days after permanent middle cerebral artery occlusion caused hemorrhagic infarct conversion. Interestingly, previously middle cerebral artery-occluded animals that were made hypercarbic with 5% CO_2 air at 5 days postischemia had slowly progressive elevation in ICP and MABP and developed intracerebral hematoma involving the putamen, external capsule, and claustrum, occasionally dissecting through to ipsilateral ventricle. Several clinical reports have cited this model, but no further work has been done using it.

BRAIN PATHOLOGIC RESPONSE TO ICH IN ANIMAL MODELS

Overall, the brain pathologic responses to an intracerebral hematoma in experimental animal models are comparable to those seen in human ICH (20,56,58,78,103–105). The three stages of perihematomal tissue injury defined by Spatz in 1939 (104)—initial deformation, edema and necrosis, and clot absorption and scar or cavity formation—have also been regularly described in animal models, albeit at a faster rate. An excellent description of these changes in rat was provided, in which regions of pallor and spongiform change due to edema formation developed adjacent to clots within 2 hr (105). By 6 to 15 hr, disrupted myelinated nerve fibers and degeneration bulbs were present, along with increasing swelling of the corona radiata as edema fluid continued to accumulate. At 24 hr, white-matter edema was more marked and extensive. By 48 hr, hematomas in rat and dog ICH models were surrounded by edema, vacuolation, and acellular plasma accumulations, with astrocytic swelling present adjacent to, and distant from, the hematoma.

In our porcine ICH model, marked, rapidly developing perihematomal edema with a high water content is already present in white matter by 1 hr after ICH (17). This edema produces perihematomal hyperintensity on T2-weighted MRI (20,38) similar to that in ICH patients (106). We observed increases in edema volumes by 50% over the first 24 hr in the porcine ICH model due to delayed BBB opening (17). In the collagenase ICH model, similar hyperintensities on T2-weighted imaging surround hematomas and extend along posterior white-matter fiber tracts (85). Histologically, by 3 days, we observed decreased Luxol fast blue staining in edematous white matter, suggestive of myelin injury, and markedly increased glial fibrillary acidic protein immunoreactivity, indicative of reactive astrocytosis (20). In our porcine model, neovascularization is present at 7 days. By 2 weeks, continued hematoma resolution and glial scar and cyst formation are similar to both rodent and human ICH pathologies. A similar brain pathologic response occurs in porcine white matter, in which only plasma is infused, thereby demonstrating the significance of the blood's plasma protein component in ICH-induced brain injury (20,107).

The time course of inflammation and cell death following infusion of whole blood into the rat striatum has been carefully examined by several groups (44,108). They have also characterized the cellular perihematomal inflammatory response, including the infiltration of immune cells and activation of microglia. Several others have examined DNA fragmentation using terminal deoxynucleotidyl transferase dUTP nick-end labeling staining (107,109–111). In addition, molecular analyses of the proinflammatory transcription factor, nuclear factor-κB, and cytokine responses to ICH have been conducted (26,64,112–114).

An interesting concept of the mechanism of cell death after ICH has been proposed from studies of ICH in rat, i.e., the "black hole" model of hemorrhagic damage by Felberg and coworkers (115). These investigators showed that histologic damage from ICH is very prominent in the immediate perihematomal region. Except for *substantia nigra pars reticulata*, they found no evidence of neuronal loss in distal regions. The term "black hole" refers to this continued destruction of neurons, which occurs over at least 3 days, as the neurons come into proximity to the hematoma.

LIMITATIONS OF ANIMAL MODELS

Several prominent characteristics of human spontaneous ICH are not well mimicked by current animal models. Human ICH is fundamentally linked to advancing age. The incidence of spontaneous ICH is about 25 times higher for those who are age ≥75 years compared to those who are age ≥45 years (116). Thus, ICH models in young animals do not reproduce the pre-existing degenerative changes in small arteries, arterioles, neurovascular units, or surrounding brain tissue. In addition, the human genetic response capability to brain injury is now known to change with advancing age (117). Recently, in an effort to address this problem, the response to ICH was studied in young (3 months) versus aged (18 months) rats, and more severe brain and neurologic deficits were reported in old rats that persisted for 4 weeks after ICH (118). Additionally, older rats had stronger microglial activation and a greater perihematomal induction of the heat-shock proteins HSP-27 and HSP-32. A goal for future research is to determine the degree to which brain tissue responses to ICH in aging animal models mimic those in aging humans.

Human ICH usually occurs in the setting of longstanding comorbidities (e.g., tobacco use, diabetes, hypertension) and commonly in the presence of active drugs (e.g., antiplatelet, anti-coagulant, statin). These conditions cannot be easily reproduced in animal models. For example, even spontaneously hypertensive rats are not likely to reproduce the decades-long effects in humans of elevated arterial pressure. Human ICH also varies by race, in incidence overall, and in incidence by age epoch, suggesting important and yet-to-be-discovered variations in genetic susceptibility. Inferences regarding treatment must also be drawn with caution. Findings have demonstrated significant benefits from mechanical and pharmacologic interventions that have not been reproduced in human trials, whether small and focused (51,119) or large and inclusive (120). Among the several potential explanations for these discrepancies, delay in treating ICH patients is the likeliest. However, toward improving the design of future ICH models, it is important that conductors of future studies in animal models consider the limitations in translating the findings to human ICH treatment.

SUMMARY OF ANIMAL SPECIES AND ICH INDUCTION METHODS

In this review we have described the various animal species that have been employed in ICH research. In addition, we have discussed the several methodologies that have been employed to produce intracerebral hematomas, presenting the pros and cons of the individual species and the ICH induction techniques. In this section, we have summarized these advantages and disadvantages and have suggested the "best" models and methods based on the goals of the study, the experimental plan, the desired hematoma volumes, and the expense.

Rodents have the advantage of being the most commonly used species in ICH research. The literature on neurobehavioral testing is well developed and the reagents for immunocytochemistry and molecular biology have been extensively studied. The recent development of mouse ICH models enables the study of transgenic and knockout animals, which is a clear advantage for uncovering the detailed molecular pathophysiologic events underlying the development of tissue injury following ICH.

Large animals (pigs, dogs, and primates) have certain advantages over rodents in ICH research. These include their large gyrated brains with a significant amount of white matter. Large animals enable the induction of greater hematoma volumes to test the efficacy of surgical evacuation techniques or combined surgery and drug treatments. The well-developed frontal white matter in the pig has been especially useful for pathophysiologic studies of ICH-induced white-matter injury as well as surgical clot evacuation studies. In addition, pigs have the advantage as compared to dogs and cats that they are less expensive to purchase and are considered non-companion animals. Primates are exceedingly expensive to purchase and house and require special facilities and veterinary care.

Regarding the methods for inducing an intracerebral hematoma, as described above, i.e., the two commonly used methods are the classical blood infusion method and the collagenase injection method. Neither method exactly models the human event, i.e., sudden arterial rupture with a rapid intraparenchymal accumulation of blood. Currently, there is no model of intracerebral blood vessel rupture to induce ICH. Although both the direct blood infusion model and the collagenase model have their artificialities, the arterial blood infusion through an indwelling catheter described throughout the review is generally considered to be the method of choice for inducing experimental ICH. The use of the bacterial collagenase enzyme to "dissolve" the extracellular matrix has been considered to be more artificial due to its severe inflammatory response and secondary pathophysiology that occurs in the setting of an already damaged brain parenchyma.

OVERALL SUMMARY AND CONCLUSIONS

As described in this review, experimental animal ICH models reproduce important pathophysiologic events that develop in human ICH, including perihematomal edema, markedly reduced metabolism, and comparable brain tissue pathologic responses. Thus, these animal ICH models are important tools for new understanding of the mechanisms underlying brain injury after an intracerebral bleed. The recent publication from several laboratories describing ICH models in the mouse will enable new investigations into secondary inflammatory responses, intracellular signaling, and molecular events that are expected to provide future therapeutic targets for treating ICH. The continued use of a large noncompanion animal, such as the pig, enables studies of ICH-induced white-matter injury—an important contributor to patient morbidity. The large animal model also permits studies of surgical treatments that could be combined with pharmacologic approaches. A future animal model that would have considerable clinical applicability would be one that mimics the spontaneous enlarging hematoma with continued bleeding that is observed in about 30% of human ICH patients (121).

ACKNOWLEDGMENTS

These studies were supported by funding from the National Institute of Neurological Diseases and Stroke (R01NS-30652) and the Department of Veterans Affairs Medical Research Service.

REFERENCES

1. Kaufman HH, Schochet SS. Pathology, pathophysiology and modeling. In: Kaufman HH, ed. Intracerebral Hematomas: Etiology, Pathophysiology, Clinical Presentation and Treatment. New York: Raven Press, 1992:13–20.
2. Andaluz N, Zuccarello M, Wagner KR. Experimental animal models of intracerebral hemorrhage. Neurosurg Clin N Am 2002; 13:385–393.
3. Belayev L, Saul I, Curbelo K, et al. Experimental intracerebral hemorrhage in the mouse: histological, behavioral, and hemodynamic characterization of a double-injection model. Stroke 2003; 34:2221–2227.
4. Nakamura T, Xi G, Hua Y, et al. Intracerebral hemorrhage in mice: model characterization and application for genetically modified mice. J Cereb Blood Flow Metab 2004; 24:487–494.
5. Tang J, Liu J, Zhou C, et al. MMP-9 deficiency enhances collagenase-induced intracerebral hemorrhage and brain injury in mutant mice. J Cereb Blood Flow Metab 2004; 24:1133–1145.
6. Thiex R, Mayfrank L, Rohde V, et al. The role of endogenous versus exogenous tPA on edema formation in murine ICH. Exp Neurol 2004; 189:25–32.
7. McCarty JH, Lacy-Hulbert A, Charest A, et al. Selective ablation of alpha v integrins in the central nervous system leads to cerebral hemorrhage, seizures, axonal degeneration and premature death. Development 2005; 132:165–176.

8. Wagner KR, Zuccarello M. Focal brain hypothermia for neuroprotection in stroke treatment and aneurysm repair. Neurol Res. 2005; 27:238–245.

9. MacLellan CL, Girgis J, Colbourne F. Delayed onset of prolonged hypothermia improves outcome after intracerebral hemorrhage in rats. J Cereb Blood Flow Metab 2004; 24:432–440.

10. Ardizzone TD, Lu A, Wagner KR, et al. Glutamate receptor blockade attenuates glucose hypermetabolism in perihematomal brain after experimental intracerebral hemorrhage in rat. Stroke 2004; 35:2587–2591.

11. Seyfried D, Han Y, Lu D, et al. Improvement in neurological outcome after administration of atorvastatin following experimental intracerebral hemorrhage in rats. J Neurosurg 2004; 101:104–107.

12. Chu K, Jeong SW, Jung KH, et al. Celecoxib induces functional recovery after intracerebral hemorrhage with reduction of brain edema and perihematomal cell death. J Cereb Blood Flow Metab 2004; 24:926–933.

13. Wagner KR, Hua Y, de Courten-Myers GM, et al. Tin-mesoporphyrin, a potent heme oxygenase inhibitor, for treatment of intracerebral hemorrhage: in vivo and in vitro studies. Cell Mol Biol (Noisy.-le-grand) 2000; 46:597–608.

14. Huang FP, Xi G, Keep RF, et al. Brain edema after experimental intracerebral hemorrhage: role of hemoglobin degradation products. J Neurosurg 2002; 96:287–293.

15. Koeppen AH, Dickson AC, Smith J. Heme oxygenase in experimental intracerebral hemorrhage: the benefit of tin-mesoporphyrin. J Neuropathol Exp Neurol 2004; 63:587–597.

16. Nonaka M, Yoshikawa M, Nishimura F, et al. Intraventricular transplantation of embryonic stem cell-derived neural stem cells in intracerebral hemorrhage rats. Neurol Res 2004; 26:265–272.

17. Wagner KR, Xi G, Hua Y, et al. Lobar intracerebral hemorrhage model in pigs: rapid edema development in perihematomal white matter. Stroke 1996; 27:490–497.

18. Wagner KR, Xi G, Hua Y, et al. Early metabolic alterations in edematous perihematomal brain regions following experimental intracerebral hemorrhage. J Neurosurg 1998; 88:1058–1065.

19. Wagner KR, Xi G, Hua Y, et al. Ultra-early clot aspiration after lysis with tissue plasminogen activator in a porcine model of intracerebral hemorrhage: edema reduction and blood-brain barrier protection. J Neurosurg 1999; 90:491–498.

20. Wagner KR, Broderick JP. Hemorrhagic stroke: pathophysiological mechanisms and neuroprotective treatments. In: Lo EH, Marwah J, eds. Neuroprotection. Scottsdale: Prominent Press, 2001:471–508.

21. Wagner KR, Sharp FR, Ardizzone TD, et al. Heme and iron metabolism: role in cerebral hemorrhage. J Cereb Blood Flow Metab 2003; 23:629–652.

22. Rosenberg GA, Mun-Bryce S, Wesley M, et al. Collagenase-induced intracerebral hemorrhage in rats. Stroke 1990; 21:801–807.

23. Rosenberg GA, Estrada E, Kelley RO, et al. Bacterial collagenase disrupts extracellular matrix and opens blood-brain barrier in rat. Neurosci Lett 1993; 160:117–119.

24. Deinsberger W, Vogel J, Kuschinsky W, et al. Experimental intracerebral hemorrhage: description of a double injection model in rats. Neurol Res 1996; 18:475–477.

25. Yang GY, Betz AL, Chenevert TL, et al. Experimental intracerebral hemorrhage: relationship between brain edema, blood flow, and blood-brain barrier permeability in rats. J Neurosurg 1994; 81:93–102.

26. Hickenbottom SL, Grotta JC, Strong R, et al. Nuclear factor-kappaB and cell death after experimental intracerebral hemorrhage in rats. Stroke 1999; 30:2472–2477.

27. Bullock R, Mendelow AD, Teasdale GM, et al. Intracranial haemorrhage induced at arterial pressure in the rat. Part 1: Description of technique, ICP changes and neuropathological findings. Neurol Res 1984; 6:184–188.

28. Mendelow AD, Bullock R, Teasdale GM, et al. Intracranial haemorrhage induced at arterial pressure in the rat. Part 2: Short term changes in local cerebral blood flow measured by autoradiography. Neurol Res 1984; 6:189–193.

29. Nath FP, Jenkins A, Mendelow AD, et al. Early hemodynamic changes in experimental intracerebral hemorrhage. J Neurosurg 1986; 65:697–703.

30. Nath FP, Kelly PT, Jenkins A, et al. Effects of experimental intracerebral hemorrhage on blood flow, capillary permeability, and histochemistry. J Neurosurg 1987; 66:555–562.

31. Kingman TA, Mendelow AD, Graham DI, et al. Experimental intracerebral mass: description of model, intracranial pressure changes and neuropathology. J Neuropathol Exp Neurol 1988; 47:128–137.

32. Kingman TA, Mendelow AD, Graham DI, et al. Experimental intracerebral mass: time-related effects on local cerebral blood flow. J Neurosurg 1987; 67:732–738.

33. Mendelow AD. Spontaneous intracerebral haemorrhage. J Neurol Neurosurg Psychiatr 1991; 54:193–195.

34. Mendelow AD. Mechanisms of ischemic brain damage with intracerebral hemorrhage. Stroke 1993; 24, I115–I117.

35. Ropper AH, Zervas NT. Cerebral blood flow after experimental basal ganglia hemorrhage. Ann Neurol 1982; 11:266–271.

36. Powers WJ, Zazulia AR, Videen TO, et al. Autoregulation of cerebral blood flow surrounding acute (6 to 22 hours) intracerebral hemorrhage. Neurology 2001; 57:18–24.

37. Zazulia AR, Diringer MN, Videen TO, et al. Hypoperfusion without ischemia surrounding acute intracerebral hemorrhage. J Cereb Blood Flow Metab 2001; 21:804–810.

38. Wagner KR, Hua Y, Xi G, et al. Pathophysiologic mechanisms underlying edema development in experimental intracerebral hemorrhage: magnetic resonance studies. Stroke 1997; 28:264.

39. Lee KR, Kawai N, Kim S, et al. Mechanisms of edema formation after intracerebral hemorrhage: effects of thrombin on cerebral blood flow, blood-brain barrier permeability, and cell survival in a rat model. J Neurosurg 1997; 86:272–278.

40. Xi G, Wagner KR, Keep RF, et al. Role of blood clot formation on early edema development after experimental intracerebral hemorrhage. Stroke 1998; 29:2580–2586.

41. Wagner KR, Xi G, Hua Y, et al. Blood components and acute white matter edema development following intracerebral hemorrhage: Are hemolysates edemogenic? Stroke 2000; 31:345.

42. Hua Y, Xi G, Keep RF, et al. Complement activation in the brain after experimental intracerebral hemorrhage. J Neurosurg 2000; 92:1016–1022.

43. Xue M, Del Bigio MR. Intracortical hemorrhage injury in rats: relationship between blood fractions and brain cell death. Stroke 2000; 31:1721–1727.

44. Xue M, Del Bigio MR. Intracerebral injection of autologous whole blood in rats: time course of inflammation and cell death. Neurosci Lett 2000; 283:230–232.

45. Mohr CP, Lorenz R. The effect of experimentally produced intracerebral hematoma upon ICP. Neurosurgery 1979; 4:468.

46. Kobari M, Gotoh F, Tomita M, et al. Bilateral hemispheric reduction of cerebral blood volume and blood flow immediately after experimental cerebral hemorrhage in cats. Stroke 1988; 19:991–996.

47. Dujovny M, Yokoh ACP. Experimental intracranial hemorrhage: urokinase treatment. Stroke 1987; 18:280.

48. Broderick JP, Brott TG, Duldner JE, et al. Volume of intracerebral hemorrhage. A powerful and easy-to-use predictor of 30-day mortality. Stroke 1993; 24:987–993.

49. Kaufman HH, Pruessner JL, Bernstein DP, et al. A rabbit model of intracerebral hematoma. Acta Neuropathol (Berl) 1985; 65:318–321.

50. Narayan RK, Narayan TM, Katz DA, et al. Lysis of intracranial hematomas with urokinase in a rabbit model. J Neurosurg 1985; 62:580–586.

51. Zuccarello M, Brott T, Derex L, et al. Early surgical treatment for supratentorial intracerebral hemorrhage: a randomized feasibility study. Stroke 1999; 30:1833–1839.

52. Koeppen AH, Dickson AC, McEvoy JA. The cellular reactions to experimental intracerebral hemorrhage. J Neurol Sci 1995; 134(suppl):102–112.

53. Gustafsson O, Rossitti S, Ericsson A, et al. MR imaging of experimentally induced intracranial hemorrhage in rabbits during the first 6 hours. Acta Radiol 1999; 40:360–368.

54. Qureshi AI, Wilson DA, Hanley DF, et al. Pharmacologic reduction of mean arterial pressure does not adversely affect regional cerebral blood flow and intracranial pressure in experimental intracerebral hemorrhage. Crit Care Med 1999; 27:965–971.

55. Steiner L, Lofgren J, Zwetnow NN. Lethal mechanism in repeated subarachnoid hemorrhage in dogs. Acta Neurol Scand 1975; 52:268–293.

56. Enzmann DR, Britt RH, Lyons BE, et al. Natural history of experimental intracerebral hemorrhage: sonography, computed tomography and neuropathology. Am J Neuroradiol 1981; 2:517–526.

57. Weingarten K, Zimmerman RD, Deo-Narine V, et al. MR imaging of acute intracranial hemorrhage: findings on sequential spin-echo and gradient-echo images in a dog model. Am J Neuroradiol 1991; 12:457–467.

58. Takasugi S, Ueda S, Matsumoto K. Chronological changes in spontaneous intracerebral hematoma—an experimental and clinical study. Stroke 1985; 16:651–658.

59. Qureshi AI, Wilson DA, Hanley DF, et al. No evidence for an ischemic penumbra in massive experimental intracerebral hemorrhage. Neurology 1999; 52:266–272.

60. Qureshi AI, Wilson DA, Traystman RJ. Treatment of elevated intracranial pressure in experimental intracerebral hemorrhage: comparison between mannitol and hypertonic saline. Neurosurgery 1999; 44:1055–1063.

61. Bullock R, Brock-Utne J, van Dellen J, et al. Intracerebral hemorrhage in a primate model: effect on regional cerebral blood flow. Surg Neurol 1988; 29:101–107.

62. Segal R, Dujovny M, Nelson D. Local urokinase treatment for spontaneous intracerebral hematoma. Clin Res 1982; 30:412A.

63. Wagner KR, Packard BA, Hall CL, et al. Protein oxidation and heme oxygenase-1 induction in porcine white matter following intracerebral infusions of whole blood or plasma. Dev Neurosci 2002; 24:154–160.

64. Wagner KR, Beiler S, Dean C, et al. NFkB activation and pro-inflammatory cytokine gene upregulation in white matter following porcine intracerebral hemorrhage. In: Krieglstein J, Klumpp S, eds. Pharmacology of Cerebral Ischemia 2004. Stuttgart: Medpharm Scientific Publishers, 2004:185–194.

65. Zuccarello M, Andaluz N, Wagner KR. Minimally invasive therapy for intracerebral hematomas. Neurosurg Clin N Am 2002; 13:349–354.

66. Kase CS, Caplan LR. Intracerebral Hemorrhage. Newton, MA: Butterworth-Heinemann, 1994.

67. Toffol GJ, Biller J, Adams HP Jr. Nontraumatic intracerebral hemorrhage in young adults. Arch Neurol 1987; 44:483–485.

68. Fukui K, Iguchi I, Kito A, et al. Extent of pontine pyramidal tract Wallerian degeneration and outcome after supratentorial hemorrhagic stroke. Stroke 1994; 25:1207–1210.

69. Kazui S, Kuriyama Y, Sawada T, et al. Very early demonstration of secondary pyramidal tract degeneration by computed tomography. Stroke 1994; 25:2287–2289.

70. Kimelberg HK. Current concepts of brain edema. Review of laboratory investigations. J Neurosurg 1995; 83:1051–1059.

71. Gebel JM, Brott TG, Sila CA, et al. Decreased perihematomal edema in thrombolysis-related intracerebral hemorrhage compared with spontaneous intracerebral hemorrhage. Stroke 2000; 31:596–600.

72. Xi G, Keep RF, Hoff JT. Pathophysiology of brain edema formation. Neurosurg Clin N Am 2002; 13:371–383.

73. Butcher KS, Baird T, MacGregor L, et al. Perihematomal edema in primary intracerebral hemorrhage is plasma derived. Stroke 2004; 35:1879–1885.

74. Zuccarello M, Dean C, Packard BA, et al. Minimally invasive removal of intracerebral hematomas: experience with the Possis AngioJet Catheter in a porcine model. Presented at the 51st Annual Meeting of the Congress of Neurological Surgeons, San Diego, CA, 2001.

75. Mun-Bryce S, Kroh FO, White J, et al. Brain lactate and pH dissociation in edema: 1H- and 31P-NMR in collagenase-induced hemorrhage in rats. Am J Physiol 1993; 265:R697–R702.

76. Del Bigio MR, Yan HJ, Buist R, et al. Experimental intracerebral hemorrhage in rats. Magnetic resonance imaging and histopathological correlates. Stroke 1996; 27:2312–2319.

77. Del Bigio MR, Yan HJ, Campbell TM, et al. Effect of fucoidan treatment on collagenase-induced intracerebral hemorrhage in rats. Neurol Res 1999; 21:415–419.

78. Weller RO. Spontaneous intracranial hemorrhage. In: Adams JH, Dunchen LW, eds. Greenfield's Neuropathology. New York: Oxford Univ Press, 1992:269–301.

79. Rosenberg GA, Navratil M. Metalloproteinase inhibition blocks edema in intracerebral hemorrhage in the rat. Neurology 1997; 48:921–926.

80. Rosenberg GA. Matrix metalloproteinases in neuroinflammation. Glia 2002; 39:279–291.

81. Power C, Henry S, Del Bigio MR, et al. Intracerebral hemorrhage induces macrophage activation and matrix metalloproteinases. Ann Neurol 2003; 53:731–742.

82. Wang J, Rogove AD, Tsirka AE, et al. Protective role of tuftsin fragment 1-3 in an animal model of intracerebral hemorrhage. Ann Neurol 2003; 54:655–664.

83. Wang J, Tsirka SE. Tuftsin fragment 1-3 is beneficial when delivered after the induction of intracerebral hemorrhage. Stroke 2005; 36:613–618.

84. Terai K, Suzuki M, Sasamata M, et al. Amount of bleeding and hematoma size in the collagenase-induced intracerebral hemorrhage rat model. Neurochem Res 2003; 28:779–785.

85. Brown MS, Kornfeld M, Mun-Bryce SM, et al. Comparison of magnetic resonance imaging and histology in collagenase-induced hemorrhage in the rat. J Neuroimaging 1995; 5:23–33.

86. Chesney JA, Kondoh T, Conrad JA, et al. Collagenase-induced intrastriatal hemorrhage in rats results in long-term locomotor deficits. Stroke 1995; 26:312–316.

87. DeBow SB, Davies ML, Clarke HL, et al. Constraint-induced movement therapy and rehabilitation exercises lessen motor deficits and volume of brain injury after striatal hemorrhagic stroke in rats. Stroke 2003; 34:1021–1026.

88. Lee HH, Kim H, Lee MH, et al. Treadmill exercise decreases intrastriatal hemorrhage-induced neuronal cell death via suppression on caspase-3 expression in rats. Neurosci Lett 2003; 352:33–36.

89. Song EC, Chu K, Jeong SW, et al. Hyperglycemia exacerbates brain edema and perihematomal cell death after intracerebral hemorrhage. Stroke 2003; 34:2215–2220.

90. Peeling J, Yan HJ, Chen SG, et al. Protective effects of free radical inhibitors in intracerebral hemorrhage in rat. Brain Res 1998; 795:63–70.

91. Peeling J, Del Bigio MR, Corbett D, et al. Efficacy of disodium 4-[(tert-butylimino) methyl] benzene-1,3-disulfonate N-oxide (NXY-059), a free radical trapping agent, in a rat model of hemorrhagic stroke. Neuropharmacology 2001; 40:433–439.

92. Lyden PD, Jackson-Friedman C, Lonzo-Doktor L. Medical therapy for intracerebral hematoma with the gamma-aminobutyric acid-A agonist muscimol. Stroke 1997; 28:387–391.

93. Lyden P, Shin C, Jackson-Friedman C, et al. Effect of ganaxolone in a rodent model of cerebral hematoma. Stroke 2000; 31:169–175.

94. Terai K, Suzuki M, Sasamata M, et al. Effect of AMPA receptor antagonist YM872 on cerebral hematoma size and neurological recovery in the intracerebral hemorrhage rat model. Eur J Pharmacol 2003; 467:95–101.

95. Del Bigio MR, Yan HJ, Xue M. Intracerebral infusion of a second-generation ciliary neurotrophic factor reduces neuronal loss in rat striatum following experimental intracerebral hemorrhage. J Neurol Sci 2001; 192:53–59.

 96. Mayne M, Fotheringham J, Yan HJ, et al. Adenosine A2A receptor activation reduces proinflammatory events and decreases cell death following intracerebral hemorrhage. Ann Neurol 2001; 49:727–735.
 97. Mayne M, Ni W, Yan HJ, et al. Antisense oligodeoxynucleotide inhibition of tumor necrosis factor-alpha expression is neuroprotective after intracerebral hemorrhage. Stroke 2001; 32:240–248.
 98. Rodrigues CM, Sola S, Nan Z, et al. Tauroursodeoxycholic acid reduces apoptosis and protects against neurological injury after acute hemorrhagic stroke in rats. Proc Natl Acad Sci USA 2003; 100:6087–6092.
 99. Clark W, Gunion-Rinker L, Lessov N, et al. Citicoline treatment for experimental intracerebral hemorrhage in mice. Stroke 1998; 29:2136–2140.
100. Mun-Bryce S, Wilkerson AC, Papuashvili N, et al. Recurring episodes of spreading depression are spontaneously elicited by an intracerebral hemorrhage in the swine. Brain Res 2001; 888:248–255.
101. Mun-Bryce S, Roberts LJ, Hunt WC, et al. Acute changes in cortical excitability in the cortex contra-lateral to focal intracerebral hemorrhage in the swine. Brain Res 2004; 1026:218–226.
102. Laurent JP, Molinari GF, Oakley JC. Primate model of cerebral hematoma. J Neuropathol Exp Neurol 1976; 35:560–568.
103. Courville CB. Intracerebral hematoma; its pathology and pathogenesis. AMA Arch Neurol Psychiatr 1957; 77:464–472.
104. Garcia JH, Ho K-L, Caccamo DV. Intracerebral hemorrhage: Pathology of selected topics. In: Kase CS, Caplan LR, eds. Intracerebral Hemorrhage. Boston, MA: Butterworth-Heinemann, 1994:45–72.
105. Jenkins A, Maxwell WL, Graham DI. Experimental intracerebral haematoma in the rat: sequential light microscopical changes. Neuropathol Appl Neurobiol 1989; 15:477–486.
106. Dul K, Drayer BP. CT and MR imaging of intracerebral hemorrhage. In: Kase CS, Caplan LR, eds. Intracerebral Hemorrhage. Boston, MA: Butterworth-Heinemann, 1994:73–98.
107. Wagner KR, Dean C, Beiler S, et al. Plasma infusions into porcine cerebral white matter induce early edema, oxidative stress, pro-inflammatory cytokine gene expression and DNA fragmentation: impli-cations for white matter injury with increased blood-brain barrier permeability. Curr Neurovasc Res. 2005; 2:149–155.
108. Gong C, Hoff JT, Keep RF. Acute inflammatory reaction following experimental intracerebral hemor-rhage in rat. Brain Res 2000; 871:57–65.
109. Matsushita K, Meng W, Wang X, et al. Evidence for apoptosis after intercerebral hemorrhage in rat striatum. J Cereb Blood Flow Metab 2000; 20:396–404.
110. Wagner KR, Bryan DW, Hall CL, et al. White matter injury after intracerebral hemorrhage: infused plasma but not red blood cells induces early DNA fragmentation. J Cereb Blood Flow Metab 1999; 19(suppl 1):S55.
111. Wu J, Hua Y, Keep RF, et al. Oxidative brain injury from extravasated erythrocytes after intracerebral hemorrhage. Brain Res 2002; 953:45–52.
112. Qureshi AI, Suri MF, Ling GS, et al. Absence of early proinflammatory cytokine expression in experi-mental intracerebral hemorrhage. Neurosurgery 2001; 49:416–420.
113. Wagner KR, Knight J, Packard BA, et al. Rapid nuclear factor kappaB activation and cytokine and heme oxygenase-1 gene expression in edematous white matter after porcine intracerebral hemor-rhage. Stroke 2001; 32:327.
114. Wagner KR, Dean C, Beiler S, et al. Rapid activation of pro–inflammatory signaling cascades in peri-hematomal brain regions in a porcine white matter intracerebral hemorrhage model. J Cereb Blood Flow Metab 2003; 23(suppl 1):277.
115. Felberg RA, Grotta JC, Shirzadi AL, et al. Cell death in experimental intracerebral hemorrhage: the "black hole" model of hemorrhagic damage. Ann Neurol 2002; 51:517–524.
116. Broderick JP, Brott T, Tomsick T, et al. The risk of subarachnoid and intracerebral hemorrhages in blacks as compared with whites. N Engl J Med 1992; 326:733–736.
117. Lu T, Pan Y, Kao SY, et al. Gene regulation and DNA damage in the ageing human brain. Nature 2004; 429:883–891.
118. Gong Y, Hua Y, Keep RF, et al. Intracerebral hemorrhage: effects of aging on brain edema and neu-rological deficits. Stroke 2004; 35:2571–2575.
119. Morgenstern LB, Demchuk AM, Kim DH, et al. Rebleeding leads to poor outcome in ultra-early craniotomy for intracerebral hemorrhage. Neurology 2001; 56:1294–1299.
120. Mendelow AD, Gregson BA, Fernandes HM, et al. Early surgery versus initial conservative treatment in patients with spontaneous supratentorial intracerebral haematomas in the International Surgical Trial in Intracerebral Haemorrhage (STICH): a randomised trial. Lancet 2005; 365:387–397.
121. Brott T, Broderick J, Kothari R, et al. Early hemorrhage growth in patients with intracerebral hemor-rhage. Stroke 1997; 28:1–5.

11 | Pathophysiologic Mechanisms of Brain Injury Following Intracerebral Hemorrhage

Gustavo J. Rodríguez, MD, Vascular Neurology Fellow
Jawad F. Kirmani, MD, Assistant Professor
Mustapha A. Ezzeddine, MD, Assistant Professor
Adnan I. Qureshi, MD, Professor of Neurology and Radiology
Department of Neurology and Neurosciences, Zeenat Qureshi Stroke Research Center,
University of Medicine and Dentistry of New Jersey (UMDNJ), Newark, New Jersey, USA

INTRODUCTION

Nontraumatic intracerebral hemorrhage (ICH) accounts for approximately 10% to 15% of all cases of stroke and is associated with high rates of morbidity and mortality (1–5). To date, no proven specific or effective treatment for ICH exists, nor do clear guidelines regarding management of blood pressure and appropriate timing and indications for performing surgery (6). One of the limitations in developing interventional protocols is the fact that we lack knowledge regarding the temporal response of the human brain to ICH because we have no good test to measure it and much of what we know is based on the animal model. A better understanding of the pathophysiology of the perilesion injury is required in order to develop new therapeutic strategies.

We know that, initially, the hemorrhage spreads between planes of white matter, with minimal destruction, leaving nests of intact neural tissue within and surrounding the hematoma (7,8). However, later, the hematoma is known to potentially expand, mainly in the first 24 hr, and cause additional neuronal damage (9,10). In addition to the mass effect observed in the beginning, the presence of a hematoma induces 3 early pathophysiologic changes in the surrounding parenchyma: neuronal and glial cell death, vasogenic edema, and breakdown of the blood–brain barrier (BBB), accounting for more expansion and cell death (11). It is theorized that tissue damage from ICH is related to both the presence of a mass and to mediators that exist in blood, supported by the observations that hematomas of the same size cause different outcomes in different individuals and that no edema was formed in an animal model when a microballoon was inserted in the caudate nucleus, despite increased intracranial pressure and decreased cerebral blood flow (CBF) (12).

In the past (13–15), ischemia from mass effect was thought to be the main process of neuronal injury and edema following ICH. However, it is now accepted that blood and plasma products play a more important role in secondary brain injury after ICH (16–19). Other mediators considered to cause additional brain damage following ICH are excitatory amino acids, matrix metalloproteinases (MMPs), and mediators of inflammation. This chapter reviews current understanding of brain injury mechanisms following ICH in an effort to further the investigation for development of effective therapies for the future.

PATHOLOGY OF HEMATOMA AND MECHANICAL COMPRESSION

Spontaneous ICH commonly occurs in the basal ganglia, thalamus, pons, cerebellum, and cerebral lobes (7). Hematomas are the result of ruptured, small, penetrating arteries that originate from the main intracranial vasculature. The walls of these small arteries present with degeneration of the media and smooth muscle, particularly at bifurcations (20). After hemorrhage, the blood initially spreads between planes of white-matter cleavage and causes minimal destruction, leaving areas of intact neural tissue within and surrounding the hematoma (7,8).

Hematoma formation is not a monophasic event, and it may certainly expand. The cause of hematoma expansion is not yet clear, but it is attributed to progressive bleeding from the primary source, resulting from disruption of surrounding vessels, hypertension, or a coagulation deficit

(21,22). Recently several factors, such as markers of inflammation [e.g., tumor necrosis factor (TNF)-α and interleukin (IL)-6] and of vascular damage, were found to predict hematoma expansion. MMPs and extracellular fibronectin (glycoprotein of extracellular matrices implicated in the adhesion of platelets to fibrin, known as c-Fn) were found to be highly significant predictors of hematoma expansion (23). In general, up to one-third of hematomas expand in the first 24 hr and, more commonly, within the first 3 hr. This expansion causes more neuronal injury and is the main cause of clinical deterioration during the hyperacute phase of ICH (9,10,24,25).

The presence of hematoma initiates edema in the surrounding parenchyma resulting from the release and accumulation of osmotically active serum clotting proteins and proteases causing additional expansion into the brain tissue (26,27). As fluid begins to collect immediately in the region around the hematoma, focal mass effect develops, with subsequent elevation of intracranial pressure; in cases of massive hemorrhage, this may lead to brain herniation (28,29).

Following ICH, lysed red blood cells and blood products from the hematoma initiate different processes that lead to neurotoxicity and more edema (16–19). The adverse effect of an ICH seems to result from a "toxic" effect of blood components to the brain. The pertinent question arises as to whether clot removal is the best therapeutic strategy. Randomized trials have compared best medical treatment with surgical intervention, but this matter is still controversial. It appears that draining hematomas that are deep and do not involve posterior fossa may lead to worse outcomes, whereas, surgical drainage of superficial hemorrhages may improve patient outcome (30–34). Recently, minimally invasive methods have become an investigational procedure of choice. Infusion of recombinant tissue plasminogen activator (rtPA) into hematomas in a pig model at 3 hr after onset of ICH and subsequent aspiration resulted in reduced brain edema volume and BBB disruption (35). In theory, blood products, induced BBB breakdown, and edema formation after ICH are delayed processes, making them more susceptible to therapeutic options; however, thus far in humans, results are contradictory (36,37). Hematomas, if deep or large, may extend into the ventricles (marker of poor prognosis), but it is unclear whether draining of this blood would improve neurologic outcome.

PATHOLOGY OF THE PERIHEMATOMA REGION

The presence of hematoma initiates edema and neuronal damage in the surrounding parenchyma. Perihematoma edema usually persists for up to 5 days (38), although it has been observed for as long as 2 weeks after stroke (39).

Early edema around the hematoma that occurs within 8 hr of onset is interstitial in nature and results from the accumulation of osmotically active serum proteins from the clot and movement of water across an intact BBB into the extracellular space (26). Between 24 and 48 hr after ICH onset, activation of the coagulation cascade and induction of proteolytic enzymes lead to an inflammatory response, resulting in direct cellular toxicity, BBB disruption, and, possibly, depressed metabolic activity, with secondary reduction of CBF (38,40–42).

Cytotoxic edema from cell death and breakdown of the BBB, are most likely the explanation of the late edema formation, which peaks between days 5 and 6 after symptom onset (43). Macroscopically, the parenchyma adjacent to the clot appears edematous, often discolored by hemoglobin degradation products, and histologic sections are characterized by the presence of edema, neuronal damage, macrophages, and neutrophils in the region surrounding the hematoma (7,8).

ROLE OF CEREBRAL BLOOD FLOW CHANGES

The association of cerebral ischemia and edema formation has been well studied. Although, based on experimental animal models, ischemia was initially thought to contribute to edema in ICH (44–48). This theory is currently controversial, and it is becoming more and more evident that ischemia does not play a role in edema formation in ICH.

No good test exists by which to measure the cerebral response at the cellular level in ICH, but emergent technology, such as MRI, single-photon emission computerized tomography

(SPECT), and positron emission tomography (PET), is being used indirectly to help determine the CBF changes during ICH.

On MRI studies, an initial increase in diffusion that affects both hemispheres diffusely appears to occur as early as 6 hr after hemorrhage onset. These changes reflect a rise in water content that may be attributed to the increased hydrostatic pressure that maintains cerebral perfusion. Vasogenic edema also occurs secondary to a diffuse cerebral inflammatory reaction. This global reaction may represent an adaptive process to a new steady state (49). A prospective study, in which perfusion-weighted MRI and diffusion-weighted MRI was used to asses perihematomal blood flow and edema in ICH, showed a reduction in blood flow in the perihematoma region, but this was self-limited, and normalization occurred between days 3 and 5 after onset. No MRI markers of ischemia were associated with high-signal in diffusion-weighted images or apparent diffusion coefficient (ADC), suggesting that early perihematoma edema is plasma derived (50).

SPECT was also used to study the flow in the perihematoma region and showed decreased CBF that peaked at 24 hr and normalized as edema formed during the first 3 days after ICH; the extent of edema correlated with the size of the initial deficit (51), suggesting that hypoperfusion was present and was highest in the early hours following ICH (52,53). PET studies also reported perihematomal CBF reductions, mainly diffuse and in the ipsilateral hemisphere, without evidence of ischemia (54–56). Although evidence of hypoperfusion has been shown in the perihematoma area or in the ipsilateral hemisphere, it seems to be self-limited and without ischemia (50,52,57,58). The mechanism for transient hypoperfusion may be related to a hydrostatic mechanism with normalization of perfusion as elevated tissue pressure normalizes (49), or it may be due to a transient reduction in metabolic rate of oxygen, suggesting that flow changes may represent hypoactive tissue rather than ischemia (59).

Upon resolution of hypoperfusion, vasodilation induced by inflammatory mediators from the blood clot could follow (60), which, although desired to reduce primary injury, could be implicated in the pathogenesis of secondary damage in ICH (Fig. 1) (52,61).Three phases of CBF and metabolism changes can be identified (Fig. 2) (60). First, a hibernation phase, an acute period of concomitant hypoperfusion and hypometabolism, predominantly involving the perihematoma region, is identified within 48 hr of hemorrhage onset. Reductions in CBF and cerebral oxygen consumption in both affected and contralateral cerebral hemispheres have been shown by PET scanning. Second, a reperfusion phase is observed between 48 hr and 14 days, with a heterogeneous pattern of CBF consisting of areas of relatively normal flow, persistent hypoperfusion, and hyperperfusion. Third, a normalization phase is observed after 14 days, with normal CBF reestablished in all regions except those with nonviable tissue. Despite low CBF, the low metabolism in the acute hibernation phase probably prevents development of ischemia in the perihematoma region.

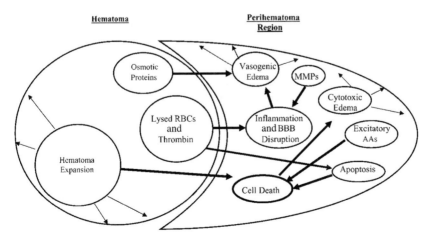

Figure 1   Pathophysiology of neuronal injury in the perihematoma region. *Abbreviations*: BBB, blood–brain barrier; RBCs, red blood cells; AAs, amino acids; MMPs, matrix metalloproteinases.

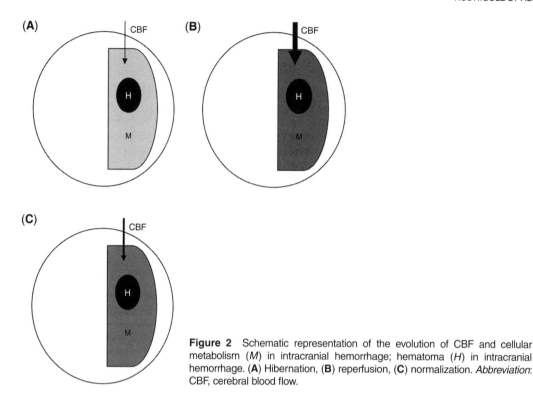

Figure 2 Schematic representation of the evolution of CBF and cellular metabolism (*M*) in intracranial hemorrhage; hematoma (*H*) in intracranial hemorrhage. (**A**) Hibernation, (**B**) reperfusion, (**C**) normalization. *Abbreviation*: CBF, cerebral blood flow.

ROLE OF THROMBIN AND BLOOD PRODUCTS

Blood and blood products seem to consistently produce severe histologic injury, as compared to other inert substances, when injected into brain (17,18). The infusion of packed red blood cells into the cerebral parenchyma produced brain edema in 3 days. Likewise, when lysed blood was injected into brain, edema developed in 24 hr, which is consistent with the hypothesis that some factor within the red blood cell is responsible for causing the edema produced with whole blood injection (16). In addition, injection of intact or lysed red blood cells increases BBB permeability, contributing to edema formation (62).

When thrombin has been reported to cross the damaged BBB it has been associated with the development of inflammation, and perihematoma edema (19,63–65). Thrombin also causes less intense disruption of the BBB, as compared to lysed red blood cells (66). Experimentally depleting cells involved in inflammation, such as leukocytes and platelets, has been shown to ameliorate the extent of ICH-induced brain injury in animal models (67).

Thrombin has also been implicated in apoptosis. In an animal model, when thrombin was injected in brain, the peak to apoptosis preceded the peak that was induced by the injection of autologous blood (68). Apoptosis involves single cells and results in programmed cell death, with subsequent phagocytosis by adjacent normal cells (69,70). Apoptosis has been implicated in ICH in experimental models, persisting for up to 72 hr after the onset of the hemorrhage (71,72), and it has recently been found to be a common feature in ICH in humans, occurring as early as 24 hr after ICH onset. No relationship was found between severity of apoptosis, age, initial Glasgow Coma Scale, hematoma volume, and time between onset and hematoma evacuation. Interestingly, apoptosis was not observed in specimens from cerebellar hematomas, which may reflect differences in cell populations and the spatial distributions of neurons (73).

These observations suggest that apoptotic processes occur in an ongoing delayed manner and are potentially amenable to therapeutic interventions. Further studies are required to define possible mediators of apoptosis (e.g., tumor necrosis factor or caspases) and therapies to inhibit them, as a method to reduce the cellular damage observed with ICH.

ROLE OF INFLAMMATION AND GLUTAMATE

Although expression of cytokines and their contribution to neural injury and inflammatory responses are well characterized in instances of cerebral ischemia and head injury, ICH was not associated with expression of TNF-α, IL-1β, or IL-6, either in the perihematoma region or in other regions of the brain, when blood and cerebrospinal fluid (CSF) were tested 1 hr after the onset of hemorrhage (74). The increase of inflammatory markers only becomes measurable in situations in which the BBB is permeable (75).

Data also supports the probability that the migration of leukocytes and platelets into the perihematoma region, along with the release of vasoactive factors, contributes to secondary injury in ICH. In the animal model, the systemic depletion of platelets and lymphocytes through irradiation can reduce edema formation in the perihematoma region, which suggests a role for circulating leukocytes and platelets in the pathogenesis of edema (75).

The delay in the breakdown of the BBB and development of cerebral edema after ICH strongly suggest the existence of secondary mediators (e.g., glutamate) of both edema and neuronal injury. The neurotoxicity of glutamate and other excitatory amino acids is the result of excessive activation of postsynaptic N-methyl-D-aspartate (NMDA) receptors (76). This activation of NMDA receptors leads to a cellular influx of calcium ions, concurrently activating α-amino-3-hydroxy-5-methyl-4-isoxazolepropionate receptors and facilitating the incorporation of sodium ions into the cells. Intracellular accumulations of calcium and sodium ions give rise to edema and neuronal death (77). In experimental ICH, glutamate and other excitatory amino acids have also been found to accumulate early and transiently in extracellular fluids in the perihematoma region. The role of these amino acids in the pathogenesis of neuronal injury observed in ICH is unclear. Likewise, it is unclear whether this increase in extracellular concentration of amino acids is related to compression of tissue that can be reproduced by intraparenchymal balloon inflation or whether some chemical component is involved that can only be generated by blood and its constituents (78).

ROLE OF MATRIX METALLOPROTEINASES

Breakdown of the BBB has been related to the presence of various MMPs. MMPs are an endogenous family of zinc-dependent enzymes that are responsible for matrix remodeling. The extracellular matrix molecules, including type IV collagen, laminin, and fibronectin, constitute the basement membrane and help maintain the integrity of the BBB. Several types of MMPs have been shown to participate in the degradation of basal lamina and disruption of the BBB in the animal model, and their inhibition has been shown to be helpful in reducing the vasogenic edema in ICH (40,79).

Tissue inhibitor of metalloproteinases (TIMP), especially (TIMP-2), which is found in the brain parenchyma, can be administered in experimental ICH to decrease perihematoma edema by protecting the BBB (80). In humans, a high blood concentration of MMP-9 detected within the first 24 hr of ICH (81) was associated with early edema and edema progression in the subsequent days, whereas high MMP-3 concentration correlated with mortality and residual scar volume (82). MMP-9 concentration was also found to serve as a biologic marker for predicting ICH complications after thrombolytic therapy in human ischemic stroke (83) and hematoma expansion (23), which would suggest that MMPs are predisposing factors for hemorrhage. Interestingly, activation of MMPs was observed in heart transplant recipients when donors died following spontaneous ICH. These heart transplant recipients demonstrated upregulation of MMP-2 and MMP-9, which was associated with cardiac remodeling and subsequent development of coronary vasculopathy (84).

CONCLUSIONS AND FUTURE DIRECTIONS

ICH affects approximately 65,000 individuals in the United States and has higher rates of morbidity and mortality than do ischemic strokes of similar volume. Despite the advances in critical care management, treatment is usually supportive and the prognosis of these patients continues to be poor (85,86), perhaps due to the lack of a consensus for the appropriate management of ICH.

Development of new treatments is required to prevent deterioration of neurologic function after ICH. Potential therapies include prevention of hematoma expansion and limitation of secondary neuronal injury. Although a recent study suggests that the administration of recombinant activated factor VII reduces the growth of hemorrhage, reducing mortality and improving functional outcome, additional data is required to determine safety in patients at risk for thromboembolic disease (87).

The toxic effect of blood and blood products is well known; it induces BBB breakdown and edema formation after ICH. The effect of hematoma evacuation has been studied, and randomized trials have been conducted, but they failed to show clear benefit. A defined indication and more accurate timing for surgical intervention are needed.

At the cellular level, the development of therapies that reduce cerebral edema and neuronal damage may require a better understanding of the pathophysiologic sequence and mediators that produce secondary injuries. Possible therapeutic options for the future include the development of new neuroprotective agents or therapies that would inhibit inflammation, apoptosis, MMPs, or excitatory amino acids.

REFERENCES

1. Broderick JP, Brott TG, Duldner JE, Tomsick T, Huster G. Volume of intracerebral hemorrhage: a powerful and easy-to-use predictor of 30-day mortality. Stroke 1993; 24:987–993.
2. Dennis MS, Burn JP, Sandercock PA, Bamford JM, Wade DT, Warlow CP. Long-term survival after first-ever stroke: the Oxfordshire community stroke project. Stroke 1993; 24:796–800.
3. Qureshi AI, Safdar K, Weil J, et al. Predictors of early deterioration and mortality in black Americans with spontaneous intracerebral hemorrhage. Stroke 1995; 26:1764–1767.
4. Qureshi AI, Tuhrim S, Broderick JP, Batjer HH, Hondo H, Hanley DF. Spontaneous intracerebral hemorrhage. N Engl J Med 2001; 344:1450–1460.
5. Mohr JP, Caplan LR, Melski JW, et al. The Harvard cooperative stroke registry: a prospective registry. Neurology 1978; 28:754–762.
6. Broderick JP, Adams HP, Barsan W, et al. Guidelines for the management of spontaneous intracerebral hemorrhage: a statement for healthcare professionals from a special writing group of the Stroke Council, American Heart Association. Stroke 1999; 30:905–915.
7. Mutlu N, Berry RG, Alpers BJ. Massive cerebral hemorrhage: clinical and pathological correlations. Arch Neurol 1963; 8:644–661.
8. Morris JH. The nervous system. In: Cotran RS, Kumar V, Robbin SL, eds. Pathologic Basis of Disease. 3rd ed. Philadelphia: W.B. Saunders Co., 1999:1385–1450.
9. Brott T, Broderick J, Kothari R, et al. Early hemorrhage growth in patients with intracerebral hemorrhage. Stroke 1997; 28:1–5.
10. Kazui S, Naritomi H, Yamamoto H, Sawada T, Yamaguchi T. Enlargement of spontaneous intracerebral hemorrhage: incidence and time course. Stroke 1996; 27:1783–1787.
11. Qureshi AI, Ling GS, Khan J, et al. Quantitative analysis of injured, necrotic, and apoptotic cells in a new experimental model of intracerebral hemorrhage. Crit Care Med 2001; 29:152–157.
12. Sinar EJ, Mendelow AD, Graham DI, Teasdale GM. Experimental intracerebral hemorrhage: effects of a temporary mass lesion. J Neurosurg 1987; 66:568–576.
13. Qureshi AI, Wilson DA, Hanley DF, Traystman RJ. Pharmacologic reduction of mean arterial pressure does not adversely affect regional cerebral blood flow and intracranial pressure in experimental intracerebral hemorrhage. Crit Care Med 1999; 27:965–971.
14. Qureshi AI, Wilson DA, Hanley DF, Traystman RJ. No evidence for an ischemic penumbra in massive experimental intracerebral hemorrhage. Neurology 1999; 52:266–272.
15. Zazulia AR, Diringer MN, Videen TO, et al. Hypoperfusion without ischemia surrounding acute intracerebral hemorrhage. J Cereb Blood Flow Metab 2001; 21:804–810.
16. Xi G, Keep RF, Hoff JT. Erythrocytes and delayed brain edema formation following intracerebral hemorrhage in rats. J Neurosurg 1998; 89:991–996.
17. Suzuki J, Ebina T. Sequential changes in tissue surrounding ICH. In: Pia HW, Longmaid C, Zierski J, eds. Spontaneous Intracerebral Hematomas. Berlin: Springer-Verlag, 1980:121–128.
18. Jenkins A, Mendelow AD, Graham DI, Nath F, Teasdale GM. Experimental intracranial hematoma: the role of blood constituents in early ischemia. Br J Neurosurg 1990; 4:45–51.
19. Lee KR, Betz AL, Keep RF, Chenevert TL, Kim S, Hoff JT. Intracerebral infusion of thrombin as a cause of brain edema. J Neurosurg 1995; 83:1045–1050.
20. Cole FM, Yates PO. Pseudo-aneurysms in relationship to massive cerebral hemorrhage. J Neurol Neurosurg Psychiatry 1967; 30:61–66.

21. Olson JD. Mechanisms of homeostasis: effect on intracerebral hemorrhage. Stroke 1993; (24 suppl): I109–I114.
22. Kazui S, Minematsu K, Yamamoto H, Sawada T, Yamaguchi T. Predisposing factors to enlargement of spontaneous intracerebral hematoma. Stroke 1997; 28:2370–2375.
23. Silva Y, Leira R, Tejada J, Lainez JM, Castillo J, Dávalos A. Molecular signatures of vascular injury are associated with early growth of intracerebral hemorrhage. Stroke 2005; 36(1):86–91.
24. Fujii Y, Tanaka R, Takeuchi S, Koike T, Minakawa T, Sasaki O. Hematoma enlargement in spontaneous intracerebral hemorrhage. J Neurosurg 1994; 80:51–57.
25. Fehr MA, Anderson DC. Incidence of progression or rebleeding in hypertensive intracerebral hemorrhage. J Stroke Cerebrovasc Dis 1991; 1:111–116.
26. Wagner KR, Xi G, Hua Y, et al. Lobar intracerebral hemorrhage model in pigs: rapid edema development in perihematomal white matter. Stroke 1996; 27:490–497.
27. Wagner KR, Xi G, Hau Y, Kleinholz M, de Courten-Myers GM, Myers RE. Early metabolic alterations in edematous perihematomal brain regions following experimental intracerebral hemorrhage. J Neurosurg 1998; 88:1058–1065.
28. Janny P, Papo I, Chazal J, Colnet G, Barretto LC. Intracranial hypertension and prognosis of spontaneous intracerebral haematomas: a correlative study of 60 patients. Acta Neurochir (Wien) 1982; 61:181–186.
29. Papo I, Janny P, Caruselli G, Colnet G, Luongo A. Intracranial pressure time course in primary intracerebral hemorrhage. Neurosurgery 1979; 4:504–511.
30. Batjer HH, Reisch JS, Allen BC, Plaizier LJ, Su CJ. Failure of surgery to improve outcome in hypertensive putaminal hemorrhage: a prospective randomized trial. Arch Neurol 1990; 47:1103–1106.
31. Juvela S, Heiskanen O, Poranen A, et al. The treatment of spontaneous intracerebral hemorrhage: a prospective randomized trial of surgical and conservative treatment. J Neurosurg 1989; 70:755–758.
32. Auer LM, Deinsberger W, Niederkorn K, et al. Endoscopic surgery versus medical treatment for spontaneous intracerebral hematoma: a randomized study. J Neurosurg 1989; 70:530–535.
33. Morgenstern LB, Frankowski RF, Shedden P, Pasterur WJCG. Surgical treatment for intracerebral hemorrhage (STICH): a single-center, randomized clinical trial. Neurology 1998; 51:1359–1363.
34. Mendelow AD, Gregson BA, Fernandes, et al. STICH investigators. Early surgery versus initial conservative treatment in patients with spontaneous supratentorial intracerebral haematomas in the International Surgical Trial in Intracerebral Haemorrhage (STICH): a randomised trial. Lancet 2005; 365(9457):387–397.
35. Wagner KR, Xi G, Hua Y, et al. Ultra-early clot aspiration after lysis with tissue plasminogen activator in a porcine model of intracerebral hemorrhage: edema reduction and blood-brain barrier protection. J Neurosurg 1999; 90:491–498.
36. Teernstra O, Evers S, Lodder J, Leffers P, Franke C, Blaauw G. Stereotactic treatment of intracerebral hematoma by means of plasminogen activator: a multicentre randomized controlled trial (SICHPA). Stroke 2003; 34:968–974.
37. Hosseini H, Leguerinel C, Hariz M, et al. Stereotactic aspiration of deep intracerebral hematomas under computed tomographic control: a multicentric prospective randomised trial. 12th European Stroke Conference, Valencia, Spain, 2003:57.
38. Yang GY, Betz AL, Chenevert TL, Brunberg JA, Hoff JT. Experimental intracerebral hemorrhage: relationship between brain edema, blood flow, and blood-brain barrier permeability in rats. J Neurosurg 1994; 81:93–102.
39. Zazulia AR, Diringer MN, Derdeyn CP, Powers WJ. Progression of mass effect after intracerebral hemorrhage. Stroke 1999; 30:1167–1173.
40. Rosenberg GA, Navratil M. Metalloproteinase inhibition blocks edema in intracerebral hemorrhage in the rat. Neurology 1997; 48:921–926.
41. Nath FP, Kelly PT, Jenkins A, Mendelow AD, Graham DI, Teasdale GM. Effects of experimental intracerebral hemorrhage on blood flow, capillary permeability, and histochemistry. J Neurosurg 1987; 66:555–562.
42. Lee KR, Colon GP, Betz AL, Keep RF, Kim S, Hoff JT. Edema from intracerebral hemorrhage: the role of thrombin. J Neurosurg 1996; 84:91–96.
43. Sansing LH, Kaznatcheeva EA, Perkins CJ, Komaroff E, Gutman FB, Newman GC. Edema after intracerebral hemorrhage: correlations with coagulation parameters and treatment. J Neurosurg 2003; 98:985–992.
44. Kobari M, Gotoh F, Tomita M, et al. Bilateral hemispheric reduction of cerebral blood volume and blood flow immediately after experimental cerebral hemorrhage in cats. Stroke 1988; 19:991–996.
45. Bullock R, Brock-Utne J, van Dellen J, Blake G. Intracerebral hemorrhage in a primate model: effect on regional blood flow. Surg Neurol 1988; 29:101–107.
46. Nehls DG, Mendelow AD, Graham DI, Sinar EJ, Teasdale GM. Experimental intracerebral hemorrhage: progression of hemodynamic changes after production of a spontaneous mass lesion. Neurosurgery 1988; 23:439–444.
47. Nehls DG, Mendelow AD, Graham DI, Teasdale GM. Experimental intracerebral hemorrhage: early removal of a spontaneous mass lesion improves late outcome. Neurosurgery 1990; 27:674–682.

48. Yang GY, Betz AL, Chenevert TL, Brunberg JA, Hoff JT. Experimental intracerebral hemorrhage: relationship between brain on 18F-fluoromisonidazole PET after intracerebral hemorrhage. Neurology 1999; 53:2179.
49. Kamal AK, Dyke JP, et al. Temporal evolution of diffusion after spontaneous supratentorial intracranial hemorrhage. Am J Neuroradiol 2003; 24:895–901.
50. Butcher KS, Baird T, MacGregor L, Desmond P, Tress B, Davis S. Perihematomal edema in primary intracerebral hemorrhage is plasma derived. Stroke 2004; 35(8):1879–1885.
51. Mayer SA, Lignelli A, Fink ME, et al. Perilesional blood flow and edema formation in acute intracerebral hemorrhage: a SPECT study. Stroke 1998; 29:1791–1798.
52. Sills C, Villar-Cordova C, Pasteur W, et al. Demonstration of hypoperfusion surrounding intracerebral hematoma in humans. J Stroke Cerebrovasc Dis 1996; 6:17–24.
53. Kidwell CS, Saver JL, Mattiello J, et al. Diffusion-perfusion MR evaluation of perihematomal injury in hyperacute intracerebral hemorrhage. Neurology 2001; 57(9):1611–1617.
54. Uemura K, Shishido F, Higano S, et al. Positron emission tomography in patients with a primary intracerebral hematoma. Acta Radiol Suppl 1986; 369:426–428.
55. Videen TO, Dunford-Shore JE, Diringer MN, Powers WJ. Correction for partial volume effects in regional blood flow measurements adjacent to hematomas in humans with intracerebral hemorrhage: implementation and validation. J Comput Assist Tomogr 1999; 23:248–256.
56. Hirano T, Read SJ, Abbott DF, et al. No evidence of hypoxic tissue on 18F-fluoromisonidazole pet after intracerebral hemorrhage. Neurology 1999; 53:2179–2182.
57. Rosand J, Eskey C, Chang Y, Gonzalez RG, Greenberg SM, Koroshetz WJ. Dynamic single-section CT demonstrates reduced cerebral blood flow in acute intracerebral hemorrhage. Cerebrovasc Dis 2002; 14:214–220.
58. Carhuapoma JR, Wang PY, Beauchamp NJ, Keyl PM, Hanley DF, Barker PB. Diffusion-weighted MRI, and proton MR: spectroscopic imaging in the study of secondary neuronal injury after intracerebral hemorrhage. Stroke 2000; 31:726–732.
59. Zazulia AR, Diringer MN, Videen TO, et al. Hypoperfusion without ischemia surrounding acute intracerebral hemorrhage. J Cereb Blood Flow Metab 2001; 21:804–810.
60. Qureshi AI, Hanel RA, Kirmani JF, Yahia AM, Hopkins LN. Cerebral blood flow changes associated with intracerebral hemorrhage. Neurosurg Clin N Am 2002; 13:355–370.
61. Schellinger PD, Fiebach JB, Hoffmann K, et al. Stroke MRI in intracerebral hemorrhage: is there a perihemorrhagic penumbra? Stroke 2003; 34:1674–1679.
62. Xi G, Hua Y, Bhasin RR, Ennis SR, Keep RF, Hoff JT. Mechanisms of edema formation after intracerebral hemorrhage. Effects of extravasated red blood cells on blood flow and blood-brain barrier integrity. Stroke 2001; 32:2932–2938.
63. Lee KR, Betz AL, Kim S, Keep RF, Hoff JT. The role of the coagulation cascade in brain edema formation after intracerebral hemorrhage. Acta Neurochir 1996; 138:396–400; discussion 400–401.
64. Xi G, Wagner KR, Keep RF, et al. Role of blood clot formation on early edema development following experimental intracerebral hemorrhage. Stroke 1998; 29:2580–2586.
65. Lee KR, Kawai N, Kim S, Sagher O, Hoff JT. Mechanisms of edema formation after intracerebral hemorrhage: effects of thrombin on cerebral blood flow, blood-brain barrier permeability, and cell survival in a rat model. J Neurosurg 1997; 86:272–278.
66. Lipton SA, Rosenberg PA. Excitatory amino acids as a final common pathway for neurologic disorders. N Engl J Med 1994; 330:613–622.
67. Kane PJ, Modha P, Strachan RD, et al. The effect of immunosupression on the development of cerebral oedema in an experimental model of intracerebral haemorrhage: whole body and regional irradiation. J Neurol Neurosurg Psychiatry 1992; 55:781–786.
68. Gong C, Boulis N, Qian J, Turner DE, Hoff JT, Keep RF. Intracerebral hemorrhage-induced neuronal death. Neurosurgery 2001; 48:875–882.
69. Beilharz EJ, Williams CE, Dragunow M, Sirimanne ES, Gluckman PD. Mechanisms of delayed cell death following hypoxic-ischemic injury in the immature rat: evidence for apoptosis during selective neuronal loss. Brain Res Mol Brain Res 1995; 29:1–14.
70. Leist M, Nicotera P. Apoptosis, excitotoxicity, and neuropathology. Exp Cell Res 1998; 239:183–201.
71. Matsushita K, Meng W, Wang X, et al. Evidence for apoptosis after intercerebral hemorrhage in rat striatum. J Cereb Blood Flow Metab 2000; 20:396–404.
72. Nakashima K, Yamashita K, Uesugi S, Ito H. Temporal and spatial profile of apoptotic cell death in transient intracerebral mass lesion of the rat. J Neurotrauma 1999; 16:143–151.
73. Qureshi AI, Suri MF, Ostrow PT, et al. Apoptosis as a form of cell death in intracerebral hemorrhage. Neurosurgery 2003; 52:1041–1048.
74. Qureshi AI, Suri MF, Ling GS, Khan J, Guterman LR, Hopkins LN. Absence of early proinflammatory cytokine expression in experimental intracerebral hemorrhage. Neurosurgery 2001; 49:416–421.
75. Castillo J, Davalos A, Alvarez-Sabin J, et al. Molecular signatures of brain injury after intracerebral hemorrhage. Neurology 2002; 58:624–629.

76. Baker AJ, Moulton RJ, MacMillan VH, Shedden PM. Excitatory amino acids in cerebrospinal fluid following traumatic brain injury in humans. J Neurosurg 1993; 79:369–372.
77. Lees KR. Cerestat and other NMDA antagonists in ischemic stroke. Neurology 1997; 49:S66–S69.
78. Mathiasen T, Andersson B, Loftenius A, von Holst H. Increased interleukin-6 levels in cerebrospinal fluid following subarachnoid hemorrhage. J Neurosurg 1993; 78:562–567.
79. Mun-Bryce S, Rosenberg GA. Matrix metalloproteinases in cerebrovascular disease. J Cereb Blood Flow Metab 1998; 18:1163–1172.
80. Rosenberg GA, Kornfeld M, Estrada E, Kelley RO, Liotta LA, Stetler-Stevenson WG. TIMP-2 reduces proteolytic opening of blood-brain barrier by type IV collagenase. Brain Res 1992; 576:203–207.
81. Abilleira S, Montaner J, Molina CA, Monasterio J, Castillo J, Alvarez-Sabin J. Matrix metalloproteinase concentration after spontaneous intracerebral hemorrhage. J Neurosurg 2003; 99:65–70.
82. Alvarez-Sabín J, Delgado P, Abilleira S, et al. Temporal profile of matrix metalloproteinases and their inhibitors after spontaneous intracerebral hemorrhage. Stroke 2004; 35:1316–1322.
83. Montaner J, Molina CA, Monasterio J, et al. Matrix metalloproteinase-9 pretreatment level predicts intracranial hemorrhagic complications after thrombolysis in human stroke. Circulation 2003; 107:598–603.
84. Yamani MH, Starling RC, Cook DJ, et al. Donor spontaneous intracerebral hemorrhage is associated with systemic activation of matrix metalloproteinase-2 and matrix metalloproteinase-9 and subsequent development of coronary vasculopathy in the heart transplant recipient. Circulation 2003; 108:1724–1728.
85. Sacco RL, Mayer SA. Epidemiology of intracerebral hemorrhage. In: Feldmann E, ed. Intracerebral Hemorrhage. Mount Kisco: Futura, 1994:3–23.
86. Folkes PA, Wolf TR, Price, Mohr JP, Hier DB. The stroke data bank: design, methods and baseline characteristics. Stroke 1988; 19:547–554.
87. Mayer SA, Brun NC, Begtrup K, et al. Recombinant activated factor VII for acute intracerebral hemorrhage. N Engl J Med 2005; 352:777–785.
88. Qureshi AI, Ali Z,Suri MF, Shuaib A,Baker G, Todd K, Guterman LR, Hopekins LN.Extracellular glutamate and other amino acids in experimental intracerebral hemorrhage: an in vivo microdialysis study. Crit Care Med 2003; (31):1482–1489.

12 | Surgical Management of Intracerebral Hemorrhage

Gavin W. Britz, MD, MPH, Assistant Professor
Department of Neurological Surgery, Harborview Medical Center,
University of Washington, Seattle, Washington, USA

Arthur M. Lam, MD, FRCPC, Professor, Anesthesiologist-in-Chief
Departments of Anesthesiology and Neurological Surgery, Harborview
Medical Center, University of Washington, Seattle, Washington, USA

INTRODUCTION

Stroke is an important health issue in the United States. More than 700,000 strokes occur per year in the United States, making it the third leading cause of death (1,2). Spontaneous supratentorial intracerebral hemorrhage (ICH) accounts for 20% of all stroke-related sudden neurologic deficits (3) and carries a particularly poor prognosis, with more than one-third of patients dying within 1 month after onset of symptoms and only 20% regaining functional independence (4). The appropriate roles of medical and surgical ICH treatment remain controversial. Medical treatment is largely supportive and often necessitates intensive care. Emerging data has shown that lowering of blood pressure might prevent additional hemorrhage (5) and that recombinant activated factor VII is a promising new therapy that can limit hematoma enlargement and, consequently, reduce morbidity and mortality (5,6). Cerebral edema following an ICH might be another target for medical therapy in this dynamic process. Although, overall, the surgical evacuation of an ICH has not been shown to improve patient outcome, certain patient group subsets might benefit from this procedure. This chapter will discuss surgical management and related factors.

ETIOLOGIC FACTORS FOR INTRACEREBRAL HEMORRHAGE

An ICH, classified as either primary or secondary, can be caused by a variety of factors (Table 1). Primary ICH refers to spontaneous hemorrhage from systemic hypertension. Hypertensive ICH usually occurs in middle-aged to older patients, and the hemorrhage might be attributed to small aneurysmal dilatations on the small, perforating cerebral arteries. These aneurysms are usually multiple, tend to occur in arteries <25 μm in diameter, and might attain a diameter of up to 2 mm. These microaneurysms are usually seen in hypertensive patients and are occasionally seen in normotensive patients and in those over 65 years of age. Secondary ICH can occur due to a variety of underlying structural abnormalities, including a ruptured cerebral aneurysm, arteriovenous malformation, other vascular malformation, cerebral amyloid angiopathy, tumors, trauma, and vasculitis. ICH can also occur secondary to coagulopathy that results from thrombocytopenia and anticoagulant therapy. Thrombolytic therapy for ischemic stroke is associated with a significant risk for ICH. Finally, sympathomimetic agents, such as cocaine and amphetamines, can cause an acute intense increase in blood pressure, resulting in ICH.

PATHOPHYSIOLOGY

In 80% of patients, the hypertensive ICH is located in the region of the basal ganglia; in the remainder of cases, the hemorrhage occurs in the hindbrain, in either the pons or cerebellum. As the hemorrhage is arterial, it enlarges rapidly, causes considerable destruction of the brain, and can result in herniation and death within the first 24–48 hr after initial hemorrhage. The hematoma can also rupture into the ventricles, resulting in acute hydrocephalus, which further aggravates the raised intracranial pressure (ICP). After the initial hemorrhage, natural history studies have demonstrated that continued expansion of the hematoma is common (7,8).

Table 1 Etiologic Factors for Intracerebral Hemorrhage

Primary	Acute and chronic hypertension
Secondary	Structural
	Cerebral aneurysm
	Arteriovenous malformation
	Other vascular malformations
	Cerebral amyloid angiopathy
	Tumors
	Functional-coagulopathy
	Thromobolytic therapy
	Coumadin therapy
	Aspirin-antiplatelet therapy
	Sympathomimetic drugs
	Cocaine
	Amphetamines

An increase in volume of >33% is detectable on repeated computed tomography (CT) in 38% of patients initially scanned within 3 hr after onset, and increase is evident within 1 hr in two-thirds of cases (9). This early hematoma growth occurs in the absence of coagulopathy and appears to result from continued bleeding or rebleeding at multiple sites within the first few hours after onset.

Therefore, the progress of an ICH is a dynamic process, and the consequent-associated neuronal injury is related to both the primary and the secondary injury. The primary injury is related to the direct tissue damage from the expanding hematoma, and causes for secondary injury include inflammation, edema formation, and intraventricular extension of the hemorrhage and accompanying hydrocephalus (Table 2).

DIAGNOSIS OF INTRACEREBRAL HEMORRHAGE

Patients with ICH often have a decreased level of consciousness, with progressive decline in neurologic status as the ICH expands. In addition to obtaining a thorough medical history and neurologic examination, the most useful diagnostic test is a CT scan. Except in patients with very low hematocrit or with a very acute hemorrhage, ICH typically presents as an enhanced lesion in the scan. CT and magnetic resonance angiography might be helpful in excluding secondary causes of ICH. Contrast angiography, however, is required for the definitive diagnosis of secondary causes, such as aneurysm or arteriovenous malformation.

SURGICAL VS. MEDICAL MANAGEMENT

The role of surgical management of a patient with an ICH has not been defined. In general, prognosis is poor when ICH is located in the posterior fossa, when the patient is old (age>65), and when the admission Glasgow Coma Scale score is low. In addition to these factors, however, it is known that the volume of an ICH has consistently been shown to be a powerful predictor of poor outcome, regardless of clot location, patient age, and neurologic condition (10–12). Larger

Table 2 Pathophysiologic Mechanisms of Brain Injury in Intracerebral Hemorrhage

Primary injury	Local effect
	Direct destruction of parenchyma
Secondary injury	Mass effect
	Expansion of hematoma
	Edema formation from release of vasoactive substances
	Elevation of intracranial pressure
	Decrease in cerebral perfusion pressure
	Hydrocephalus
	Herniation

hematomas result in more profound and longer-lasting alterations in adjacent brain parenchyma, attributable in part to mass effect and focal edema. The rationale for surgical evacuation of an ICH is that the reduction of the clot volume could improve neurologic recovery and clinical outcome. Despite this rationale, the results after surgical evacuation have been poorer than medical therapy in the majority of patients.

The only patients who have been demonstrated to be aided by surgery are those with very large supratentorial ICH and those who have deteriorated neurologically from an infratentorial hemorrhage. In those patients with large ICH, extreme ICPs (either supratentorially or infratentorially) result in herniation and inevitable death if not surgically evacuated (Fig. 1A and 1C). The decision to treat or not to treat in those situations is dependent on other variables, such as age of the patient, associated comorbidities, patient's neurologic status, and the wishes of the patient/ family. In situations in which the patient is found to be brain dead or has minimal function from a large, dominant-hemisphere hemorrhage or a posterior-fossa hemorrhage that includes the brain stem, surgical evacuation is unlikely to make any difference, and the family should be informed of the futility of surgery. This is particularly true in older patients. However, with younger and healthier patients who are deemed viable, surgical evacuation is the only option.

In most patients in whom the ICH consists of small- or intermediate-sized hemorrhages, whether to treat surgically or medically is less clearly defined (Fig. 1). Continued interest exists in the surgical treatment of these hemorrhages, as they are structural lesions that exert both local and diffuse mass effect. The development of increased ICP and the associated reduction

(A)   (B)

(C)   (D)

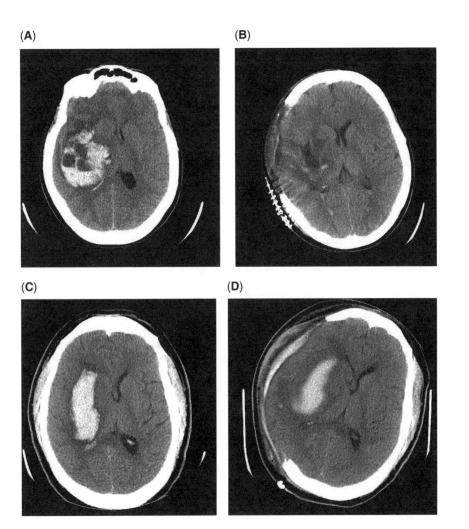

Figure 1 Two examples of intracerebral hemorrhage before (**A** and **C**) and after evacuation (**B** and **D**) and decompressive craniectomy. Note the improvement of adjacent structures following the surgical procedure.

in cerebral perfusion pressure have been shown to result in a poor outcome in patients with ICH. Moreover, as mentioned earlier, the volume of the hematoma has been found to be a critical determinant of mortality and functional outcome after an ICH. Furthermore, hematoma growth is also an important cause of neurologic deterioration. However, the recent clinical trial with recombinant activated factor VII also demonstrated the efficacy of this therapy to limit expansion of hematoma and improve outcome (6). Another potential reason that surgical treatment would benefit the patient is that evacuation of the hematoma might improve the recovery of the ischemic penumbra adjacent to the hematoma and, therefore, result in the improvement of patient outcome. A large amount of controversy relates to this penumbra of functionally impaired (but potentially viable) tissue around the hematoma (3). Such an ischemic penumbra is associated with brain edema related to the presence of thrombin (9,13), and simulated experimental removal of the mass lesion has been shown to improve perfusion in the surrounding brain tissue (14,15). However, clinical studies have yielded conflicting results regarding the importance of such a penumbra (16,17). If a penumbra exists in patients with spontaneous ICH, clot evacuation could theoretically restore function to the surrounding brain tissue and improve outcome; however, clinical imaging studies have failed to provide conclusive evidence to substantiate this theory (3).

CLINICAL TRIALS

Although many surgeons historically believed that surgical evacuation is indicated in those patients with large- and moderate-sized ICH, as stated earlier, the benefits of surgical evacuation have not been proven with a randomized, controlled trial. In 1961, in the first prospective, randomized, controlled trial that compared surgical treatment with medical management, the authors (18) reported that operative treatment was associated with a worse outcome than conservative treatment for patients with spontaneous supratentorial ICH. In 1989, opposite results were reported in a trial of endoscopic removal of hemorrhage in 100 patients (19). However, a different 1989 study reported results that supported the results of the 1961 study (20). Further trials have since been completed, and none has reported any firm conclusions regarding the role of operative treatment in the management of patients with an ICH (21).

Recently, a large International Surgical Trial in Intracerebral Hemorrhage (STICH) was conducted to assess whether a policy of early surgical evacuation of the hematoma in patients with spontaneous supratentorial ICH would improve outcome, in terms of death and disability, compared with a policy of initial conservative treatment (3). This study included 1033 patients from 83 centers in 27 countries, who were randomized to early surgery (503) or initial conservative treatment (530). At 6 months, 51 patients were lost to follow-up, and 17 were alive with unknown status. Of 468 patients randomized to early surgery, 122 (26%) had a favorable outcome, compared with 118 (24%) of 496 patients randomized to initial conservative treatment. These results demonstrated that patients with spontaneous supratentorial ICH in neurosurgical units show no overall benefit from early surgery when compared with initial conservative treatment (3). Results from one subset of patients, however, did favor surgery in patients with hematomas that were <1 cm from the cortical surface. These patients were more likely to have a favorable outcome from early surgery than those who received medical management. The clearest and most disappointing result was the uniformly poor outcome in patients presenting with ICH in coma.

INDICATIONS FOR SURGICAL THERAPY

Based on the current literature and the authors' experience, surgical treatment for ICH might be indicated under the following conditions:

1. ICH located <1 cm from the cortical surface
2. ICH in the posterior fossa
3. Large ICH in patients admitted in good neurologic condition with subsequent deterioration from expansion of the hematoma
4. Patients with elevated ICP refractory to conventional treatment and at risk of herniation

ANESTHETIC CONSIDERATIONS

The anesthetic management of patients with ICH can be complex, depending on the patient's neurologic status, the size of the ICH, and its systemic manifestations, as well as the preexisting comorbidities.

Decrease in level of consciousness might indicate elevated ICP, which can lead to nausea and vomiting, resulting in pneumonitis. The high ICP might invoke Cushing's reflex, with increased systemic blood pressure and bradycardia, possibly accompanied by systemic hypovolemia. Induction of general anesthesia in these patients can result in catastrophic systemic hypotension.

Most patients presenting for surgical evacuation of ICH have decreased neurologic status and high ICP, necessitating endotracheal intubation and mechanical ventilation before being taken to the operating room. In those who are not intubated, induction of anesthesia and intubation of trachea can be accomplished with thiopental, propofol or etomidate, and succinylcholine or rocuronium, using a rapid-sequence technique. Direct arterial blood pressure monitoring should be instituted in addition to routine monitoring. Central venous pressure monitoring might be indicated in patients who are hypovolemic and in those with cardiac disease. Anesthesia can be maintained with propofol infusion for maximal cerebral vasoconstriction or low-dose inhaled anesthetics under mild hyperventilation. The choice might be dependent on the operating conditions. Fluid and electrolytes, as well as serum glucose, must be monitored intraoperatively, because the use of mannitol and hypertonic saline might result in electrolyte disturbances.

SURGICAL TECHNIQUES

In ICH patients for whom surgical evacuation is indicated, the goal of the operation is to remove the hematoma. This is theoretically beneficial, because it reduces the clot volume (14,22), lowers the ICP (23), and reduces the chance of edema formation—all believed to improve perfusion in the affected hemisphere (3,14,22).

The Traditional Approach

The traditional surgical treatment of an ICH consists of a formal craniotomy over the hemorrhage site by making a large opening in the skull. A corticectomy is then performed over the hemorrhage site by coagulating and opening the brain tissue to obtain access to the hematoma, which is then evacuated with suction and irrigation. Although superficial ICH can be removed with minimal destruction of normal brain tissue, the usual deep-seated, basal ganglia hemorrhages require removal of the overlying normal brain to obtain access to the deep hematomas. The larger the brain opening or corticectomy, the more the normal brain tissue is disturbed. Although this traditional approach disturbs more normal brain, it has the distinct advantage of being effective in removing the ICH.

Minimally Invasive Approach

Newer, minimally invasive techniques for management of ICH have been developed and are now receiving a great deal of interest. These techniques theoretically can obtain the benefits of surgical clot removal, without incurring damage to the normal surrounding and overlying brain. A further advantage is that this procedure can often be performed under local anesthesia, or at least with a shorter anesthetic time, with the associated benefits of decreasing the perioperative risk (22). Minimally invasive surgical ICH evacuation is performed through either stereotaxic aspiration or endoscopic surgery. Stereotaxic aspiration consists of creating a small (1–2 cm) opening in the skull and, using a small (5 mm) needle or catheter, accessing and aspirating the hematoma. Early results of stereotactic surgery aimed at simple clot aspiration failed to accomplish satisfactory volume reduction of an ICH (24,25). Other refinements of the technique have led to the adjunct use of fibrinolytic agents as a means of enhancing clot lysis and catheter drainage. Since the introduction of direct instillation of urokinase after stereotaxic aspiration to liquefy the hematoma, several reports have favorably described its usefulness in ICH volume reduction (26). Consequently, agreement is uniform concerning the use of local, directly applied thrombolytics, such as urokinase and plasminongen activator, to liquefy the ICH, which is then aspirated using stereotaxic surgery (26–28). The endoscopic evacuation of an ICH is one of the newer, less-invasive techniques; it requires the performance of a small (1–2 cm) craniotomy and the passage of an endoscope through a small opening in the overlying brain tissue, thereby minimizing damage to this normal brain tissue. Endoscopic evacuation is then performed with suction, ultrasound, and irrigation, with or without concomitant thrombolytics (29). Although these minimally invasive techniques have the advantage of limiting brain injury, efficacy of minimally invasive surgical evacuation is still less than in open procedures. However, continued research will enhance the results of these newer techniques. Indeed, researchers commenting on the recent STICH trial suggest that, with improvement in endoscopic design and surgical technique, it might be possible to evacuate deep clots without causing brain destruction, making the deep lesions as accessible as those superficial clots that are <1 cm beneath the cortex (30).

CONCLUSIONS

Despite improvements in anesthesia, surgery, intensive care, and medical therapy, the outcome in patients with spontaneous ICH remains poor. Surgical evacuation is clearly indicated in viable patients who are herniating from large, supratentorial hemorrhages and in patients who deteriorate neurologically from an infratentorial hemorrhage. However, in the majority of patients who have small- and moderate-sized hemorrhages, the benefit of surgery has not been demonstrated, except with clots that are within 1 cm from the surface. Advances in newer and less-invasive surgical techniques might change that paradigm and result in improved outcome in patients with spontaneous ICH. Newer surgical techniques and improved medical treatments should remain a health-care priority, as the incidence of spontaneous ICH is likely to increase with the aging population.

REFERENCES

1. Warlow CP. Epidemiology of stroke. Lancet 1998; 352 (suppl 3):SIII1–SIII4.
2. Broderick JP. Practical considerations in the early treatment of ischemic stroke. Am Fam Physician 1998; 57(1):73–80.
3. Mendelow AD, Gregson BA, Fernandes HM, et al. STICH Investigators. Early surgery versus initial conservative treatment in patients with spontaneous supratentorial intracerebral haematomas in the International Surgical Trial in Intracerebral Haemorrhage (STICH): a randomised trial. Lancet 2005; 365(9457):387–397.
4. Dennis MS. Outcome after brain haemorrhage. Cerebrovasc Dis 2003; 16(suppl 1):9–13.
5. Grotta JC. Management of Primary Hypertensive Hemorrhage of the Brain Curr Treat Options. Neurol 2004; 6(6):435–442.
6. Mayer SA, Brun NC, Broderick J, et al. Europe/AustralAsia NovoSeven ICH Trial Investigators. Safety and feasibility of recombinant factor VIIa for acute intracerebral hemorrhage. Stroke 2005; 36(1):74–79.
7. Brott T, Broderick J, Kothari R, et al. Early hemorrhage growth in patients with intracerebral hemorrhage. Stroke 1997; 28(1):1–5.
8. Becker KJ, Baxter AB, Bybee HM, Tirschwell DL, Abouelsaad T, Cohen WA. Extravasation of radiographic contrast is an independent predictor of death in primary intracerebral hemorrhage. Stroke 1999; 30(10):2025–2032.
9. Xi G, Wagner KR, Keep RF, et al. Role of blood clot formation on early edema development after experimental intracerebral hemorrhage. Stroke 1998; 29(12):2580–2586.
10. Hankey GJ, Hon C. Surgery for primary intracerebral hemorrhage: is it safe and effective? A systematic review of case series and randomized trials. Stroke 1997; 28(11):2126–2132.
11. Broderick JP, Brott TG, Duldner JE, Tomsick T, Huster G. Volume of intracerebral hemorrhage. A powerful and easy-to-use predictor of 30-day mortality. Stroke 1993; 24(7):987–993.
12. Kothari RU, Brott T, Broderick JP, et al. The ABCs of measuring intracerebral hemorrhage volumes. Stroke 1996; 27(8):1304–1305.
13. Xi G, Keep RF, Hoff JT. Erythrocytes and delayed brain edema formation following intracerebral hemorrhage in rats. J Neurosurg 1998; 89(6):991–996.
14. Nehls DG, Mendelow DA, Graham DI, Teasdale GM. Experimental intracerebral hemorrhage: early removal of a spontaneous mass lesion improves late outcome. Neurosurgery 1990; 27(5):674–682; discussion 682.

15. Kingman TA, Mendelow AD, Graham DI, Teasdale GM. Experimental intracerebral mass: time-related effects on local cerebral blood flow. J Neurosurg 1987; 67(5):732–738.
16. Siddique MS, Fernandes HM, Wooldridge TD, Fenwick JD, Slomka P, Mendelow AD. Reversible ischemia around intracerebral hemorrhage: a single-photon emission computerized tomography study. J Neurosurg 2002; 96(4):736–741.
17. Heiss WD. Ischemic penumbra: evidence from functional imaging in man. J Cereb Blood Flow Metab 2000; 20(9):1276–1293.
18. Mckissock W, Richardson A, Taylor J. Primary intracerebral hæmorrhage: a controlled trial of surgical and conservative treatment in 180 unselected cases. Lancet 1961; 278:221–226.
19. Auer LM, Deinsberger W, Niederkorn K, et al. Endoscopic surgery versus medical treatment for spontaneous intracerebral hematoma: a randomized study. J Neurosurg 1989; 70(4):530–535.
20. Juvela S, Heiskanen O, Poranen A, et al. The treatment of spontaneous intracerebral hemorrhage. A prospective randomized trial of surgical and conservative treatment. J Neurosurg 1989; 70(5):755–758.
21. Fernandes HM, Gregson B, Siddique S, Mendelow AD. Surgery in intracerebral hemorrhage. The uncertainty continues. Stroke 2000; 31(10):2511–2516.
22. Teernstra OP, Evers SM, Lodder J, Leffers P, Franke CL, Blaauw G. Multicenter randomized controlled trial (SICHPA). Stereotactic treatment of intracerebral hematoma by means of a plasminogen activator: a multicenter randomized controlled trial (SICHPA). Stroke 2003; 34(4):968–974.
23. Chambers IR, Banister K, Mendelow AD. Intracranial pressure within a developing intracerebral haemorrhage. Br J Neurosurg 2001; 15(2):140–141.
24. Backlund EO, von Holst H. Controlled subtotal evacuation of intracerebral haematomas by stereotactic technique. Surg Neurol 1978; 9(2):99–101.
25. Kandel EI, Peresedov VV. Stereotaxic evacuation of spontaneous intracerebral hematomas. J Neurosurg 1985; 62(2):206–213.
26. Mohadjer M, Braus DF, Myers A, Scheremet R, Krauss JK. CT-stereotactic fibrinolysis of spontaneous intracerebral hematomas. Neurosurg Rev 1992; 15(2):105–110.
27. Montes JM, Wong JH, Fayad PB, Awad IA. Stereotactic computed tomographic-guided aspiration and thrombolysis of intracerebral hematoma: protocol and preliminary experience. Stroke 2000; 31(4):834–840.
28. Niizuma H, Otsuki T, Johkura H, Nakazato N, Suzuki J. CT-guided stereotactic aspiration of intracerebral hematoma—result of a hematoma-lysis method using urokinase. Appl Neurophysiol 1985; 48(1–6):427–430.
29. Nakano T, Ohkuma H, Ebina K, Suzuki S. Neuroendoscopic surgery for intracerebral haemorrhage—comparison with traditional therapies. Min Invasive Neurosurg 2003; 46(5):278–283.
30. Nakano T, Ohkuma H. Surgery versus conservative treatment for intracerebral haemorrhage—is there an end to the long controversy? Lancet 2005; 365(9457):361–362.

13 | Medical Management of Intracerebral Hemorrhage

Neeraj S. Naval, MD, Instructor
J. Ricardo Carhuapoma, MD, Assistant Professor
Division of Neurosciences Critical Care, Departments of Neurology, Neurological Surgery, and Anesthesiology/Critical Care Medicine, Johns Hopkins University School of Medicine, Baltimore, Maryland, USA

INTRODUCTION

Intracerebral hemorrhage (ICH) is associated with the highest mortality of all cerebrovascular events, with morbidity and mortality as high as 40%. Furthermore, the majority of ICH survivors never regain functional independence (1). The guidelines for the management of spontaneous ICH, released by a Special Writing Group of the American Heart Association (AHA) in 1999, have set the framework for the care of ICH patients and for future clinical research in this area of cerebrovascular neurology (2). This chapter is largely based on the fundamental principles developed by this AHA group, as well as on the report from the National Institutes of Neurological Disorders and Stroke (NINDS) Workshop, which studied the priorities for clinical research in this field (3).

The management of patients with ICH can be broadly divided into the following categories:

1. *Emergent management*
   Airway
   Breathing
   Circulation
2. *Prevention of hematoma growth*
   Blood pressure management
   Correction of coagulopathies
   Hemostasis manipulation (clot lysis, recombinant Factor VIIa)
3. *Treatment of secondary complications*
   Increased intracranial pressure (ICP)
   Herniation syndromes
   Cerebral edema
   Seizures
4. *Treatment of precipitating factor*
   Aneurysms, arteriovenous malformations, hypertension
5. *Other*
   Management of fever
   Deep venous thrombosis (DVT), gastrointestinal (GI) prophylaxis
   Rehabilitation.

DIAGNOSIS

Computerized Tomography and Magnetic Resonance Imaging

Distinguishing between ICH and ischemic stroke becomes a daunting task if only clinical criteria are used, though the presence of headache, nausea, and vomiting significantly elevated blood pressure, and an early reduction in the patient's level of consciousness favor the diagnosis of ICH. Brain computerized tomography (CT) is essential for making the diagnosis of ICH and for guiding patient-risk allocation and management based on the location of the bleed. An ICH > 30 cc is usually an indicator of poor prognosis, with mortality rates increasing significantly if ICH volume is more than 60 cc; in particular, if the initial Glasgow Coma Scale (GCS) is ≤8 (4). Calculation of hematoma volume is based on the "ABC" method, in which A is the length of the clot, B is the diameter perpendicular to A (width), and C is its thickness (based on the number of slices on CT multiplied by the thickness of each slice) (5). Hematoma location is also critical from a treatment perspective. For example, patients with a cerebellar hemorrhage >3 cm in diameter have better outcomes with early surgical evacuation (2).

Although magnetic resonance imaging (MRI) sequences continue to be studied as a radiologic tool to diagnose ICH, the most clinically relevant role of MRI remains enabling estimation of the age of the hemorrhage and assessment of possible etiologies (aneurysm, arterio-venous malformation (AVM), and tumor). Brain CT remains the initial diagnostic study of choice in patients with suspected ICH (6).

Cerebral Angiography

In certain clinical circumstances (young age, absence of hypertension, primary intraventricular hemorrhage (IVH), and unusual anatomic hemorrhage locations), the use of conventional cerebral angiography to evaluate patients with ICH is justified (7). MRI should be incorporated as the initial diagnostic modality in the assessment of ICH patients with a known history of neoplastic disease. Given the risks of conventional angiography, less-invasive alternatives have evolved, such as CT angiography (CTA). CTA is highly reliable (sensitivity 96%) in detecting aneurysms >3 mm in diameter (8), and the diagnostic accuracy of this technique is similar for anterior and posterior circulation aneurysms.

EARLY MANAGEMENT

The first steps in managing patients with ICH, as in patients with other forms of acute brain injury, are the careful assessment and provision of airway patency, respiratory support (if needed), and hemodynamic stability.

Patients with ICH might require endotracheal intubation for several reasons:

1. Airway protection due to reduced level of consciousness
2. Presence of mechanical brainstem injury (herniation syndromes) and elevated ICP that require hyperventilation
3. Other forms of oxygenatory or ventilatory failure, such as aspiration pneumonia, cardiogenic/neurogenic pulmonary edema, or acute lung injury/adult respiratory distress syndrome.

Once the patency of the patient's airway has been secured, arterial blood gases must be obtained to assess adequate gas exchange and to ensure that adequate ventilation is being provided, either by the patient's spontaneous respiration or by assisted ventilation. Normalization of P_aCO_2 and P_aO_2 is critical in patients with reduced cranial compliance due to the risk of hypercarbia and hypoxia triggering increased ICP.

Blood Pressure Management

The accurate assessment of the hemodynamic state in ICH patients is of primary importance during their early management. The vast majority of acute stroke patients present with elevated blood pressure as clinical manifestation of a long-standing premorbid condition, as a physiologic response to the acute neurologic insult, or as a combination of both. In the unusual situation in which hypotension occurs, etiologic causes, such as hypovolemia, neuro/cardiogenic cardiac dysfunction, or significant bleeding at a remote site, must be investigated and treated aggressively, once demonstrated. Vascular access must be adequate for all diagnostic and therapeutic interventions. Central venous access should be considered for patients who require administration of vasoactive drugs or who have inadequate peripheral vein caliber to accommodate the large-bore catheters that are necessary for resuscitation. Insertion of an arterial catheter should be considered in patients in whom measurement of beat-to-beat blood pressure or frequent measurement of arterial blood gases is necessary. Adequate management of the elevated blood pressure that follows the ictus in patients with ICH remains a controversial subject, mainly due to the paucity of clear evidence supporting well-defined targets of care. Hematoma growth (Fig. 1) has been found to occur in 38% of patients in the first 20 hr after the bleed and has been attributed to the acute and poorly controlled hypertension that is

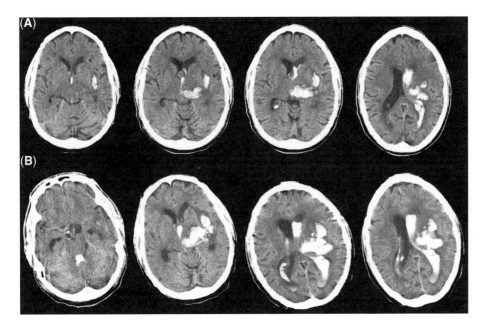

Figure 1 Admission brain CT of a patient with spontaneous ICH showing a left basal ganglia hemorrhage with intraventricular extension (**A**). Eight hours following admission, the patient developed worsening level of consciousness. Follow-up brain CT demonstrated significant hematoma enlargement as well as worsening intraventricular hemorrhage (**B**).

common in these patients (9). Thus, the intuitive response to this clinically meaningful threat has been the attempt to aggressively treat hypertension in this group of patients, though it is now unclear if a true correlation exists between these two events. Furthermore, overaggressive treatment of blood pressure could decrease blood supply to viable perihematoma tissue (perihematoma ischemia) and, in a more global setting, critically reduce cerebral perfusion pressure (global ischemia), especially if the ICP is already elevated. This biologically plausible mechanism of secondary brain injury found a clinical correlate when worse clinical outcome was documented in ICH patients who underwent early rapid and aggressive blood pressure lowering following the ictus (10). Another study using positron-emission tomography, found stable perihematomal cerebral blood flow and oxygen extraction ratio during a 15% to 20% reduction in mean arterial blood pressure of hypertensive patients with small- to moderate-sized hemorrhages. These results suggest that perihematoma ischemia, if present, is far from a universal occurrence in these patients during moderate blood pressure lowering (11,12).

Based on limited clinical evidence that is available in the literature, a Writing Group of the Stroke Council for the AHA recommended maintaining mean arterial blood pressure below 130 mmHg in ICH patients with a history of hypertension (2). Recommended drugs include sodium nitroprusside (0.5–10 µg/kg/min) in the treatment of systolic blood pressure greater than 230 mmHg or diastolic blood pressure greater than 140 mmHg (Table 1). Nevertheless, treating practitioners should be aware of the potential of this agent to further raise ICP. For systolic blood pressure between 180 and 230 mmHg, recommended drugs include intravenous labetalol, hydralazine, esmolol, and enalapril. The choice of agents to treat acute hypertension following ICH is derived from preexisting guidelines for the treatment of hypertension following acute ischemic stroke (13). The availability of intravenous nicardipine and its relative ease of use make it another suitable alternative in the treatment of elevated blood pressure in these patients.

Current research in the field aimed at assessing outcomes in ICH patients who are randomized following the ictus to different target blood pressure goals is being driven by both the lack of prospective studies that address clinically meaningful blood pressure targets and the results of recent clinical investigations that suggest that aggressive pharmacologic treatment of acute hypertension in patients with ICH could lead to a low rate of neurologic deterioration due to hematoma expansion (14).

Table 1 Blood Pressure Management in Intracerebral Hemorrhage

Elevated blood pressure (suggested medications)	
Labetalol	5–100 mg/hr by intermittent bolus doses of 10–40 mg or continuous drip (2–8 mg/min)
Esmolol	500 µg/kg as a load; maintenance use, 50–200 µg kg^{-1} min^{-1}
Nitroprusside	0.5–10 µg kg min
Hydralazine	10–20 mg every 4–6 hr
Enalapril	0.625–1.2 mg every 6 hr as needed
Labetalol	5–100 mg/hr by intermittent bolus doses of 10–40 mg or continuous drip (2–8 mg/min)

The following algorithm adapted from guidelines for antihypertensive therapy in patients with acute stroke may be used in the first few hours of ICH (level of evidence V, grade C recommendation):

1. If systolic blood pressure (BP) is >230 mmHg or diastolic BP >140 mmHg on 2 readings 5 min apart, institute nitroprusside.

2. If systolic BP is 180 to 230 mmHg, diastolic BP 105 to 140 mmHg, or mean arterial BP ≥130 mmHg on 2 readings 20 min apart, institute intravenous labetalol, esmolol, enalapril, or other smaller doses of easily titratable intravenous medications, such as diltiazem, lisinopril, or verapamil.

3. If systolic BP is <180 mmHg and diastolic BP <105 mmHg, defer antihypertensive therapy, choice of medication depends on other medical contraindications (e.g., avoid labetalol in patients with asthma).

4. If ICP monitoring is available, cerebral perfusion pressure should be kept at >70 mmHg.

Low blood pressure:
Volume replenishment is the first line of approach. Isotonic saline or colloids can be used and monitored with central venous pressure or pulmonary artery wedge pressure. If hypotension persists after correction of volume deficit, continuous infusions of pressors should be considered, particularly for low systolic blood pressure, such as <90 mmHg.

Phenylephrine	2–10 µg kg^{-1} min^{-1}
Dopamine	2–20 µg kg^{-1} min^{-1}
Norepinephrine	Titrate from 0.05–0.2 µg kg^{-1} min^{-1}

Source: From Ref. 95.

COAGULOPATHIES

The presence of an associated coagulopathy in the setting of ICH complicates the management of these patients, not only by facilitating hematoma enlargement but also by preventing or delaying emergent invasive procedures, such as the placement of intraventricular catheters (IVC) for ICP monitoring and treatment of obstructive hydrocephalus. Coagulopathies could also delay any emergent surgical treatment in these patients. The most common cause of coagulopathy in the setting of ICH remains the use of systemic anticoagulation. It becomes critical that the coagulopathy be reversed emergently by using fresh frozen plasma and vitamin K to normalize prolongation of the International Normalized Ratio (INR) to < 1.4, with plasma producing a faster, albeit shorter, lasting effect.

ACTIVATED RECOMBINANT FACTOR VIIA

Preliminary studies suggest that activated recombinant factor VII (rFVIIa) is capable of promoting hemostasis at sites of vascular injury, thus minimizing hematoma growth after ICH. The overall frequency of ICH growth in a study of 48 patients (defined as larger than 33%, or more than 12.5 cc from the original hematoma volume) was 20% at 24 hours. following the administration of rFVIIa (15). These results compare favorably with the 38% hematoma enlargement reported previously (9). Subsequently a large, multicentered trial of similar design comparing 40-, 80-, and 160-µg/kg rFVIIa and placebo was undertaken in nearly 400 patients to determine the ability of this treatment to effectively limit ICH growth (16). This study demonstrated a statistically significant decrease in hematoma growth in the group treated with rFVIIa compared with the placebo group. A significant reduction in mortality (18–29%) and poor outcomes was also reported. Notably, serious thromboembolic adverse events (myocardial or cerebral infarction) occurred in 7% of rFVIIa-treated patients, as compared with 2% of those given placebo. Thus, the recommended dose of this drug in the acute treatment of ICH remains unclear at this time.

INTRAVENTRICULAR THROMBOLYSIS

Intraventricular hemorrhage occurs in 40% patients with ICH and 15% with Subarachnoid hemorrhage (SAH), adding to the already elevated morbidityand mortality of these diseases (17). Based on a preliminary report that intraventricular urokinase might significantly improve 30-day survival in IVH patients (18), a double-blinded, placebo-controlled, multicentered study using intraventricular thrombolysis to treat IVH was undertaken (19). The results of an ongoing study assessing the effect of intraventricular thrombolysis on neurologic outcome of ICH patients are eagerly awaited before this intervention can be incorporated into management of patients with IVH.

SURGICAL TREATMENT AND ICH THROMBOLYSIS

Hematoma evacuation remains the treatment of choice when the hematoma is >3 cm in diameter, located in the cerebellum, and causes hydrocephalus or brainstem compression (20). In any other clinical scenario, surgical hematoma evacuation is a therapeutic option but lacks definitive proof of efficacy at this time. Although the AHA attempts to address the indications for surgical hematoma evacuation, the strength of the recommendations provided in the Guidelines for the Management of Supratentorial ICH (2) is insufficient to generalize them to all ICH patients. Biologically, the removal of a "neurotoxin," such as thrombin, that is capable of generating inflammatory brain edema and other forms of secondary neuronal injury (e.g., apoptosis) seems a plausible goal. These mechanisms of neurotoxicity ("hemotoxicity") have been reproduced in several experimental paradigms with similar results (21–27). The clinical application of these concepts has been the driving force behind several attempts of early removal of intraparenchymal clots in ICH patients with open craniotomy. The recently released results of the International Surgical Trial in ICH, which showed no overall benefit from early surgery when compared with initial conservative treatment in a study of 1033 patients (28), reflect what has been the almost uniform finding of smaller studies that started as early as the 1960s, when Mckissock carried out the first clinical trial in the best treatment of ICH (29).

In recent years, growing interest has been developed in testing minimally invasive surgical techniques to remove intracerebral hematomas (30,31). Various procedures have included simple aspiration using mechanical devices, such as the Archimedes screw, endoscopic evacuation of the clot, and, most recently, the application of fibrinolytic agents into the hematoma (Fig. 2) following the stereotactic placement of a soft catheter (32–40). Several small case series in the United States have suggested the safety and efficacy of fibrinolytic agents, such as urokinase, streptokinase, and recombinant tissue plasminogen activator, being used adjunctively to enhance hematoma drainage. Although other authors have reported preliminary experience using adjunctive thrombolytic therapy for patients with ICH (33,41–43), ICH aspiration and thrombolysis in the United States remains a treatment modality largely restricted to centers

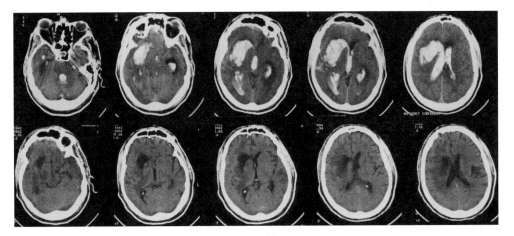

Figure 2 Admission brain CT of a patient with massive spontaneous ICH involving right basal ganglia as well as the ventricular system (*top*). Following the stereotactic placement of an intraclot catheter and the administration of 2 mg of rtPA via this catheter every 12 hours, the follow-up brain CT 5 days later (*bottom*) shows near complete resolution of the parenchymal as well as the intraventricular hemorrhage in this patient.

that are specialized in the advanced treatment of stroke patients. Ongoing prospective research to test this form of therapy for ICH will provide us with contemporary information regarding the actual role of this aggressive and high-risk form of therapy.

INCREASED INTRACRANIAL PRESSURE AND CEREBRAL EDEMA

Intracranial hypertension is operationally defined as sustained ICP >20 mmHg. A patient with suspected elevated ICP and a deteriorating level of consciousness requires invasive ICP monitoring (44). IVCs are considered the gold standard ICP monitor. This form of external ventricular drainage is also useful in treatment of elevated ICP because IVCs allow cerebro-spinal fluid drainage. Recommendations to use antibiotic prophylaxis and to periodically exchange IVCs are largely the result of routine practice, which is institution related rather than data driven. Optimal head position can be adjusted according to ICP values. Evidence in the literature is insufficient to support the prophylactic use of mannitol or hypernatremia; hyponatremia should, however, be avoided to prevent the development or worsening of cerebral edema. In the presence of elevated ICP or herniation syndromes, osmotherapy, using either mannitol with a serum osmolality goal of 310 to 315 mOsm/Lt or hypertonic saline with a serum sodium target of 145 to 155 mEq/Lt, is recommended (45). Controlled hyperventilation with a P_aCO_2 goal of 27 to 30 mmHg lowers ICP faster than osmotherapy, because it causes cere-bral vasoconstriction and an almost immediate reduction in cerebral blood volume, although peak ICP reduction might take up to 30 minutes. The ICP reducing effects of hyperventilation cease when the cerebrospinal fluid pH reaches equilibrium. In practice, however, this might take several hours. Gradual normalization of serum PCO_2 over 24 to 48 hour is recommended, so as to avoid rebound intracranial hypertension.

Corticosteroid use in the management of perihematoma brain edema has failed to dem-onstrate a positive impact on the outcome of ICH patients (46,47). The limitations of these studies, however, are multiple. Current knowledge of outcome predictors following ICH (48) (initial GCS, admission pulse pressure, hematoma volume, presence of IVH, and hydrocepha-lus) were not considered and, therefore, not controlled for in any of these studies, as most of them were performed in the early 1980s, and some even before CT scan technology was available. Contemporary studies on the use of corticosteroids or other immunosuppressant therapy with potential to prevent or treat perihematoma brain edema will certainly improve our knowledge in this area.

Neuromuscular paralysis in combination with adequate sedation can reduce elevated ICP by preventing increases in intrathoracic and venous pressure, commonly associated with coughing, straining, and endotracheal suctioning. If needed, patients with critically elevated ICP should be pretreated with an intravenous bolus of a muscle relaxant or endotracheal lido-caine before airway suctioning is performed. Barbiturate coma remains a treatment option in individual patients when all other forms of ICP control have failed, although few studies have assessed the outcomes of this subgroup of ICH patients with ICP that is refractory to all other forms of therapy (49). Common complications of barbiturate coma include hypotension, pre-disposition to infections, cardiac depression, paralytic ileus, and coagulopathy. Less-studied forms of treatment for elevated ICP include systemic hypothermia and, in certain cases, decom-pressive craniectomy (50,51). Possible indications for emergency decompressive craniotomy are reviewed in Chapter 31.

SEIZURES

The indications for seizure prophylaxis and their management in the setting of ICH are controversial. The reported incidence of seizures and status epilepticus in ICH varies. A large prospective study noted a 10% incidence of seizures in all patients with ICH (52). An expect-edly higher incidence was reported in patients with lobar or extensive ICH (53,54), and another study documented seizure activity in 14% of patients with lobar ICH and in only 4% in patients with deep ICH (55). Additional information favoring the use of seizure prophylaxis derives from a report by investigators who noted an incidence of seizures in 21% of patients with subcortical hemorrhages, as well as seizure association with increased midline shift (56). In its guidelines, the AHA Stroke Council recommended uniform seizure prophylaxis in the acute period after ICH and SAH (2). These guidelines also suggest the dose of phenytoin to be titrated to serum levels of 14 to 23 µg/mL; the discontinuation of prophylaxis after one month is also recommended (57).

Patients who develop seizures after 2 weeks from ictus appear to be at a higher risk of developing epilepsy, and treatment is continued for more than a month (58). The follow-up of these patients might require assessment every 6 months for their need of anticonvulsants (59).

Although concerns about use of anticonvulsant medication in the absence of clear seizure activity are valid (60), the incidence of unrecognized nonconvulsive seizures in obtunded ICH patients supports the use of short-term prophylaxis in these high-risk patients (61,62). An electroencephalogram (EEG) is imperative in patients who are obtunded or have a fluctuating mental status. Preferably, continuous 24-hour EEG monitoring should be obtained.

TREATMENT OF PRECIPITATING FACTORS

Primary and secondary prevention of spontaneous ICH require optimal blood pressure control. The Systolic Hypertension in the Elderly Program study reported that treatment of isolated systolic hypertension in the elderly profoundly decreased the risk of ICH (63). In younger nonhypertensive patients, further investigations, such as cerebral angiography, are warranted due to the high prevalence of aneurysms and AVMs. Older patients are at higher risk for brain tumors, both primary and metastatic, and a brain MRI is recommended in such cases. Amyloid angiopathy is a common etiologic factor in older patients, with multiple lobar hemorrhages, who do not have significant history of hypertension (64). Based on preliminary animal testing (65), the efficacy of the antiamyloidotic agent Cerebril is currently being tested in the setting of lobar hemorrhage related to amyloid angiopathy (Phase II Pilot Study of the Safety, Tolerability, and Pharmacokinetics of Cerebril™ in Patients with Lobar Hemorrhage Related to Cerebral Amyloid Angiopathy). The use of systemic anticoagulation has been associated with an increased risk of ICH and early hematoma expansion. In a 2004 study, an INR < 2 was associated with lower risk for ICH when compared with an INR range between two and three (66). A different study by Rosand and coworkers showed that 68.0% of all warfarin-related hemorrhages occurred at an INR 3 (66). Thus, careful selection and follow-up in patients who require anticoagulation are equally important in minimizing the morbidity associated with this treatment. If necessary, the discontinuation of warfarin therapy for one to two weeks following ICH has a comparatively low probability of embolic events in patients at high embolic risk, such as patients with artificial heart valves.

OTHER GENERAL MEDICAL ASPECTS

Normothermia
Although hyperthermia triggers and enhances several mechanisms of secondary brain damage, the clinical impact of aggressive fever control in these patients remains poorly demonstrated. When critically ill ICH patients are receiving continuous normothermia measures, frequent fluid cultures must be drawn and every instance of breakthrough fever or unexplained leukocytosis should be thoroughly investigated and empirically treated. The initial selection of empiric antibiotic therapy should be properly tailored, once culture results become available, based on infection location and the organism type and its antibiotic susceptibility.

Deep Vein Thrombosis/Pulmonary Embolism Prophylaxis
Patients who are at high risk for DVT and pulmonary embolism (PE) should receive prophylaxis (e.g., thrombo embolic deferrent stockings/sequential compression devices and subcutaneous heparin). If DVT or PE is diagnosed, inferior vena cava filter placement should be considered as an alternative to anticoagulation, especially early after ictus.

Gastrointestinal Prophylaxis
All ICH patients, particularly those with coagulopathy, on mechanical ventilation, and receiving corticosteroids, are at high risk for upper GI bleeding and must be treated with either antacids or proton pump inhibitors to reduce the risk of such a preventable complication.

Long-Term Care

Early surgical establishment of a postpyloric feeding tube and tracheostomy are reasonable options in patients with neurologic deficits that preclude them from safely swallowing and quickly weaning from the ventilator, respectively. Discharge disposition can vary from short-term rehabilitation to long-term ventilator facility placement; therefore, early during the patient's stay in the ICU or hospital, it should be discussed with the physical therapy team, as well as with the treating respiratory therapist and the social work professionals.

CONCLUSION

To generate clinically useful data for the proper medical care of patients with ICH, the NINDS workshop has recently defined three areas of clinical research as imperative (3): the careful evaluation of blood pressure goals in acute ICH, determination of the best approach to reversing antithrombotic-induced coagulopathy, and assessment of therapies to limit cerebral edema. Studies that address these clinical questions are currently being conducted.

Some other areas of clinical research interest, as suggested in the NINDS workshop report, are as follows:

- Identification of appropriate glycemic targets in hemorrhagic stroke
- Assessment of the clinical impact on outcomes that prophylactic, antiepileptic drug administration has in this patient population
- Safety of standard forms of DVT prophylaxis
- Further research in the field of management of hemostatic agents that are specifically directed toward coagulopathy-associated ICH
- Determination of whether normalization of body temperature or induction of hypothermia translates to improved functional outcome. Identification of the best strategy by which to lower core body temperature in these patients should then follow.

It is hoped that future research in these areas will provide the clinician with sufficient data to make clinically directed decisions in patients with ICH. Until then, those who treat patients with this form of stroke will rely on the limited clinical research available and, more importantly, common sense.

REFERENCES

1. Dennis MS. Outcome after brain haemorrhage. Cerebrovasc Dis 2003; 16 (Suppl 1):9–13.
2. Broderick JP, Adams HP Jr., Barsan W, et al. Guidelines for the management of spontaneous intracerebral hemorrhage: A statement for healthcare professionals from a special writing group of the stroke council, american heart association. Stroke 1999; 30:905–915.
3. Priorities for clinical research in intracerebral hemorrhage: Report from a national institute of neurological disorders and stroke workshop. Stroke 2005; 36:e23–e41.
4. Broderick JP, Brott TG, Duldner JE, Tomsick T, Huster G. Volume of intracerebral hemorrhage. A powerful and easy-to-use predictor of 30-day mortality. Stroke 1993; 24:987–993.
5. Broderick JP, Brott TG, Grotta JC. Intracerebral hemorrhage volume measurement. Stroke 1994; 25:1081.
6. Kidwell CS, Chalela JA, Saver JL, et al. Comparison of mri and ct for detection of acute intracerebral hemorrhage. Jama 2004; 292:1823–1830.
7. Zhu XL, Chan MS, Poon WS. Spontaneous intracranial hemorrhage: Which patients need diagnostic cerebral angiography? A prospective study of 206 cases and review of the literature. Stroke 1997; 28:1406–1409.
8. White PM, Wardlaw JM, Easton V. Can noninvasive imaging accurately depict intracranial aneurysms? A systematic review. Radiology 2000; 217:361–370.
9. Brott T, Broderick J, Kothari R, et al. Early hemorrhage growth in patients with intracerebral hemorrhage. Stroke 1997; 28:1–5.
10. Qureshi AI, Bliwise DL, Bliwise NG, Akbar MS, Uzen G, Frankel MR. Rate of 24-hour blood pressure decline and mortality after spontaneous intracerebral hemorrhage: A retrospective analysis with a random effects regression model. Crit Care Med 1999; 27:480–485.

11. Zazulia AR, Diringer MN, Videen TO, et al. Hypoperfusion without ischemia surrounding acute intracerebral hemorrhage. J Cereb Blood Flow Metab. 2001; 21:804–810.

12. Powers WJ, Zazulia AR, Videen TO, et al. Autoregulation of cerebral blood flow surrounding acute (6 to 22 hours) intracerebral hemorrhage. Neurology 2001; 57:18–24.

13. Brott T, Reed RL. Intensive care for acute stroke in the community hospital setting. The first 24 hours. Stroke 1989; 20:694–697.

14. Qureshi AI, Mohammad YM, Yahia AM, et al. A prospective multicenter study to evaluate the feasibility and safety of aggressive antihypertensive treatment in patients with acute intracerebral hemorrhage. J Intensive Care Med 2005; 20:34–42.

15. Mayer SA, Brun NC, Broderick J, et al. Safety and feasibility of recombinant factor viia for acute intracerebral hemorrhage. Stroke 2005; 36:74–79.

16. Mayer SA, Brun NC, Begtrup K, et al. Recombinant activated factor vii for acute intracerebral hemorrhage. N Engl J Med 2005; 352:777–785.

17. Naff NJ. Intraventricular hemorrhage in adults. Curr Treat Options Neurol 1999; 1:173–178.

18. Carhuapoma JR. Thrombolytic therapy after intraventricular hemorrhage: Do we know enough? J Neurol Sci 2002; 202:1–3.

19. Naff NJ, Hanley DF, Keyl PM, et al. Intraventricular thrombolysis speeds blood clot resolution: Results of a pilot, prospective, randomized, double-blind, controlled trial. Neurosurgery 2004; 54:577–583; discussion 583–574.

20. Chen HJ, Lee TC, Wei CP. Treatment of cerebellar infarction by decompressive suboccipital craniectomy. Stroke 1992; 23:957–961.

21. Figueroa BE, Keep RF, Betz AL, Hoff JT. Plasminogen activators potentiate thrombin-induced brain injury. Stroke 1998; 29:1202–1207; discussion 1208.

22. Gong C, Boulis N, Qian J, Turner DE, Hoff JT, Keep RF. Intracerebral hemorrhage-induced neuronal death. Neurosurgery 2001; 48:875–882; discussion 882–873.

23. Hua Y, Xi G, Keep RF, Wu J, Jiang Y, Hoff JT. Plasminogen activator inhibitor-1 induction after experimental intracerebral hemorrhage. J Cereb Blood Flow Metab 2002; 22:55–61.

24. Lee KR, Betz AL, Keep RF, Chenevert TL, Kim S, Hoff JT. Intracerebral infusion of thrombin as a cause of brain edema. J Neurosurg 1995; 83:1045–1050.

25. Lee KR, Betz AL, Kim S, Keep RF, Hoff JT. The role of the coagulation cascade in brain edema formation after intracerebral hemorrhage. Acta Neurochir (Wien) 1996; 138:396–400; discussion 400–391.

26. Lee KR, Colon GP, Betz AL, Keep RF, Kim S, Hoff JT. Edema from intracerebral hemorrhage: The role of thrombin. J Neurosurg 1996; 84:91–96.

27. Lee KR, Drury I, Vitarbo E, Hoff JT. Seizures induced by intracerebral injection of thrombin: A model of intracerebral hemorrhage. J Neurosurg 1997; 87:73–78.

28. Mendelow AD, Gregson BA, Fernandes HM, et al. Early surgery versus initial conservative treatment in patients with spontaneous supratentorial intracerebral haematomas in the international surgical trial in intracerebral haemorrhage (stich): A randomised trial. Lancet 2005; 365:387–397.

29. Fernandes HM, Gregson B, Siddique S, Mendelow AD. Surgery in intracerebral hemorrhage. The uncertainty continues. Stroke 2000; 31:2511–2516.

30. Zuccarello M, Andaluz N, Wagner KR. Minimally invasive therapy for intracerebral hematomas. Neurosurg Clin N Am 2002; 13:349–354.

31. Zuccarello M, Andrioli GG, Trincia G, Pardatscher K. Spontaneous intracerebral haematomas. Aspects of treatment. Zentralbl Neurochir 1983; 44:209–213.

32. Lippitz BE, Mayfrank L, Spetzger U, Warnke JP, Bertalanffy H, Gilsbach JM. Lysis of basal ganglia haematoma with recombinant tissue plasminogen activator (rtpa) after stereotactic aspiration: Initial results. Acta Neurochir (Wien) 1994; 127:157–160.

33. Matsumoto K, Hondo H. Ct-guided stereotaxic evacuation of hypertensive intracerebral hematomas. J Neurosurg 1984; 61:440–448.

34. Miller DW, Barnett GH, Kormos DW, Steiner CP. Stereotactically guided thrombolysis of deep cerebral hemorrhage: Preliminary results. Cleve Clin J Med 1993; 60:321–324.

35. Mohadjer M, Braus DF, Myers A, Scheremet R, Krauss JK. Ct-stereotactic fibrinolysis of spontaneous intracerebral hematomas. Neurosurg Rev 1992; 15:105–110.

36. Montes JM, Wong JH, Fayad PB, Awad IA. Stereotactic computed tomographic-guided aspiration and thrombolysis of intracerebral hematoma: Protocol and preliminary experience. Stroke 2000; 31:834–840.

37. Niizuma H, Otsuki T, Johkura H, Nakazato N, Suzuki J. Ct-guided stereotactic aspiration of intracerebral hematoma--result of a hematoma-lysis method using urokinase. Appl Neurophysiol 1985; 48:427–430.

38. Rohde V, Rohde I, Reinges MH, Mayfrank L, Gilsbach JM. Frameless stereotactically guided catheter placement and fibrinolytic therapy for spontaneous intracerebral hematomas: Technical aspects and initial clinical results. Minim Invasive Neurosurg 2000; 43:9–17.

39. Schaller C, Rohde V, Meyer B, Hassler W. Stereotactic puncture and lysis of spontaneous intracerebral hemorrhage using recombinant tissue-plasminogen activator. Neurosurgery 1995; 36:328–333; discussion 333–325.

40. Tzaan WC, Lee ST, Lui TN. Combined use of stereotactic aspiration and intracerebral streptokinase infusion in the surgical treatment of hypertensive intracerebral hemorrhage. J Formos Med Assoc 1997; 96:962–967.

41. Hondo H, Uno M, Sasaki K, et al. Computed tomography controlled aspiration surgery for hypertensive intracerebral hemorrhage. Experience of more than 400 cases. Stereotact Funct Neurosurg 1990; (54–55):432–437.

42. Hondo H, Matsumoto K, Tomida K, Shichijo F. Ct-controlled stereotactic aspiration in hypertensive brain hemorrhage. Six-month postoperative outcome. Appl Neurophysiol 1987; 50:233–236.

43. Hondo H, Matsumoto K. ct guided stereotactic evacuation of hypertensive and traumatic intracerebral hematomas--experiences with 35 cases. No Shinkei Geka 1983; 11:35–48.

44. Diringer MN. Intracerebral hemorrhage: Pathophysiology and management. Crit Care Med 1993; 21:1591–1603.

45. Bhardwaj A, Ulatowski JA. Cerebral edema: Hypertonic saline solutions. Curr Treat Options Neurol 1999; 1:179–188.

46. Poungvarin N. Steroids have no role in stroke therapy. Stroke 2004; 35:229–230.

47. Poungvarin N, Bhoopat W, Viriyavejakul A, et al. Effects of dexamethasone in primary supratentorial intracerebral hemorrhage. N Engl J Med 1987; 316:1229–1233.

48. Tuhrim S, Horowitz DR, Sacher M, Godbold JH. Volume of ventricular blood is an important determinant of outcome in supratentorial intracerebral hemorrhage. Crit Care Med 1999; 27:617–621.

49. Dereeper E, Berre J, Vandesteene A, Lefranc F, Vincent JL. Barbiturate coma for intracranial hypertension: Clinical observations. J Crit Care 2002; 17:58–62.

50. D'Ambrosio AL, Sughrue ME, Yorgason JG, et al. Decompressive hemicraniectomy for poor-grade aneurysmal subarachnoid hemorrhage patients with associated intracerebral hemorrhage: Clinical outcome and quality of life assessment. Neurosurgery 2005; 56:12–19; dicussion 19–20.

51. McDonald C, Carter BS. Medical management of increased intracranial pressure after spontaneous intracerebral hemorrhage. Neurosurg Clin N Am 2002; 13:335–338.

52. Bladin CF, Alexandrov AV, Bellavance A, et al. Seizures after stroke: A prospective multicenter study. Arch Neurol 2000; 57:1617–1622.

53. Kilpatrick CJ, Davis SM, Hopper JL, Rossiter SC. Early seizures after acute stroke. Risk of late seizures. Arch Neurol 1992; 49:509–511.

54. Kilpatrick CJ, Davis SM, Tress BM, Rossiter SC, Hopper JL, Vandendriesen ML. Epileptic seizures in acute stroke. Arch Neurol 1990; 47:157–160.

55. Labovitz DL, Hauser WA, Sacco RL. Prevalence and predictors of early seizure and status epilepticus after first stroke. Neurology 2001; 57:200–206.

56. Vespa PM, O'Phelan K, Shah M, et al. Acute seizures after intracerebral hemorrhage: A factor in progressive midline shift and outcome. Neurology 2003; 60:1441–1446.

57. Qureshi AI, Tuhrim S, Broderick JP, Batjer HH, Hondo H, Hanley DF. Spontaneous intracerebral hemorrhage. N Engl J Med 2001; 344:1450–1460.

58. Cervoni L, Artico M, Salvati M, Bristot R, Franco C, Delfini R. Epileptic seizures in intracerebral hemorrhage: A clinical and prognostic study of 55 cases. Neurosurg Rev 1994; 17:185–188.

59. Silverman IE, Restrepo L, Mathews GC. Poststroke seizures. Arch Neurol 2002; 59:195–201.

60. Naidech AM, Kreiter KT, Janjua N, et al. Phenytoin exposure is associated with functional and cognitive disability after subarachnoid hemorrhage. Stroke. 2005; 36:583–587

61. Vespa P. Continuous eeg monitoring for the detection of seizures in traumatic brain injury, infarction, and intracerebral hemorrhage: "to detect and protect". J Clin Neurophysiol 2005; 2299–106.

62. Vespa PM, Nuwer MR, Nenov V, et al. Increased incidence and impact of nonconvulsive and convulsive seizures after traumatic brain injury as detected by continuous electroencephalographic monitoring. J Neurosurg 1999; 91:750–760.

63. Perry HM Jr., Davis BR, Price TR, et al. Effect of treating isolated systolic hypertension on the risk of developing various types and subtypes of stroke: The systolic hypertension in the elderly program (shep). Jama 2000; 284:465–471.

64. Mandybur TI. Cerebral amyloid angiopathy: The vascular pathology and complications. J Neuropathol Exp Neurol 1986; 45:79–90.

65. Gervais F, Chalifour R, Garceau D, et al. Glycosaminoglycan mimetics: A therapeutic approach to cerebral amyloid angiopathy. Amyloid 2001; 8 (Suppl 1):28–35.

66. Fang MC, Chang Y, Hylek EM, et al. Advanced age, anticoagulation intensity, and risk for intracranial hemorrhage among patients taking warfarin for atrial fibrillation. Ann Intern Med 2004; 141:745–752.

14 | Clinical Trials in Intracerebral Hemorrhage

Alejandro A. Rabinstein, MD, Associate Professor of Neurology[a], Consultant[b]

[a]*Mayo Clinic College of Medicine,*
[b]*Neurological–Neurosurgical Intensive Care Unit, Saint Mary's Hospital, Rochester, Minnesota, USA*

Eelco F. M. Wijdicks, MD, Professor of Neurology and Chair

Division of Critical Care Neurology, Mayo Clinic College of Medicine, and
Neurological–Neurosurgical Intensive Care Unit, Saint Mary's Hospital, Rochester, Minnesota, USA

INTRODUCTION

Traditionally, the treatment of intracerebral hemorrhage (ICH) has been largely empirical. However, this situation is rapidly changing due to the accumulation of data from rigorously conducted, randomized clinical trials that address old treatment quandaries and assess novel and promising therapeutic modalities. Evidence provided by these trials is likely to generate new standards of care for the management of patients with ICH.

Neurologists and neurosurgeons often share uncertainties when faced with patients with large intracerebral hematomas. Questions about appropriateness and timing of surgical intervention to evacuate the hematoma have been pervasive. Several randomized, controlled trials have addressed these questions, and their results offer valuable information to guide our decisions.

Medical treatment of patients with ICH remains mostly supportive, but ultraearly hemostatic therapy and the use of fibrinolytic drugs to accelerate the dissolution of intraventricular clots are strategies with great potential to improve the outcome of these patients. Confirmation of favorable preliminary results from safety trials that tested these treatment modalities may transform the role of clinicians in the management of ICH after many years of therapeutic nihilism.

SURGICAL EVACUATION

The first randomized trial assessing the value of surgical evacuation in patients with ICH was conducted by McKissock et al. in 1961 (1), before CT technology became available, an important limitation that implies that misdiagnosis at the time of enrollmentlikely resulted in the inclusion of patients without ICH. Actually, the authors recognized several misdiagnosed cases after randomization, reaching a known diagnostic error of 5%. The investigators randomized 180 patients to surgical evacuation (if the hematoma could be localized and was surgically accessible) or to conservative management. The results showed that patients in the surgical group had a 28% increased mortality rate and worse overall functional outcome. The odds ratio (OR) for death or dependency was 2.0, with a 95% confidence interval (CI) of 1.04 to 3.86.

Another study randomized 52 patients with ICH to surgery or medical treatment within 48 hr of symptom onset (2). Upon enrollment, patients were unconscious (but responsive to pain) or had severe hemiparesis or aphasia. Randomization was not well balanced because patients allocated to surgical treatment had larger hematomas and significantly lower Glasgow Coma Scale (GCS) at entry. Both mortality and functional dependence were slightly higher among surgically treated patients. A small number of patients enrolled precluded subgroup analysis. The authors logically concluded that spontaneous ICH should be treated conservatively.

Enrollment in a third trial was interrupted after only 21 patients had been randomized (3). The therapeutic arms were best medical treatment (including routine use of steroids and mannitol), best medical treatment plus ventriculostomy for intracranial pressure monitoring, and surgical evacuation (with attempts to standardize the procedure using a predefined microsurgical technique). The trial was prematurely terminated because of the extremely poor outcome observed in both treatment groups. No differences among the groups were noticed, but the very small number of patients studied impeded any meaningful comparison.

In the only randomized trial that solely used endoscopic aspiration for clot evacuation, favorable results were reported with surgery (4). The investigators randomized 100 patients with symptomatic hematomas >10 cc within 48 hr of symptom onset to partial endoscopic evacuation through a burr hole or medical treatment (including antifibrinolytic agents for 3 days). At 6 months, mortality was significantly lower, and functional outcome was improved in the surgically treated patients. Subgroup analysis showed that the benefit afforded by surgery was restricted to patients younger than 60 years old who presented with lobar hematomas and were not stuporous at entry. The results of this trial have been questioned because outcome assessment was not blinded. However, this study remains the strongest evidence in favor of surgical treatment for spontaneous ICH.

The concept of early surgery has been tested in a few small, randomized studies. One randomized 20 patients (over a 2-year period) with ICH volume >10 cc, focal neurologic deficit, and GCS >4 at the time of enrollment to either surgical evacuation (craniotomy or stereotactic aspiration as decided by the case surgeon) or medical treatment (5). All patients were enrolled within 24 hr of symptom onset and underwent surgery within 3 hr of randomization. Median time from onset of symptoms to surgery was 8 hr and 35 min. Patients' neurologic status at the time of randomization was better than in previous trials; median GCS was 13 (range, 11–14) in the surgical arm and 11 (range, 6–13) in the medical arm ($p=0.06$). At 3 months, a nonsignificant but well-defined trend toward better outcome in the surgically treated patients was apparent on 3 different functional scales. Mortality was only minimally lower in the surgical group, but surgery afforded a significant reduction in residual neurologic deficits, as assessed by the National Institutes of Health stroke scale.

Although intuitively appealing, early surgery to prevent the consequences from hematoma expansion has been formally evaluated with disappointing results. First, a single-center, pilot trial compared craniotomy within 12 hr of symptom onset versus best medical treatment (6). Inclusion criteria required hematoma volume ≥10 cc and presence of impairment of consciousness or severe hemiparesis. A total of 34 patients were randomized, and at 6 months, a trend toward lower mortality and better functional outcome was observed in the surgical group, although it is unclear if outcome assessment was blinded. Albeit modest, the benefits observed with early surgery in this pilot study reasonably led the investigators to postulate that shortening the time window to surgery could maximize the benefit of the intervention. Thus, a subsequent trial enrolled patients for craniotomy and clot evacuation within 4 hr of symptom onset to compare them with the patients who had been randomized to the surgical and medical treatment arms within a 12-hr time window in the previous study (7). Median initial hematoma volume was 40 cc (range, 23–84 cc), and median GCS was 12 (range, 6–15). The trial was prematurely terminated after only 11 patients had undergone surgery within 4 hr because of increased rate of rebleeding (40% compared with 12% among patients who underwent surgery between 4 and 12 hr) and mortality (36% vs. 18% in patients who went to surgery between 4 and 12 hr, including 3 of 4 patients who rebled). The investigators concluded that ultraearly craniotomy for hematoma evacuation cannot be recommended because it is complicated by rebleeding, most likely related to problems with homeostasis.

Several meta-analyses have attempted to systematically review the data of these prospective randomized studies (8–13). The results should be interpreted with caution because of the marked heterogeneity of the original trials, which varied considerably in terms of diagnostic and inclusion criteria, surgical technique, outcome measures, and size of the population studied.

Older meta-analyses (8–10), including the first 4 randomized trials (1–4), concluded that craniotomy showed a tendency to be detrimental. Pooled data from these trials ($n=349$ patients) shows a nonsignificant increase in the odds of death and dependency at 6 months for surgical patients (OR: 1.23; 95% CI: 0.77–1.98). A subsequent meta-analysis (13) included the two more recent trials (5,6) as well as another previously overlooked Chinese study (14). When all trials ($n=530$ patients) were considered, the trend was still toward greater chance of death and dependency among patients undergoing surgery (OR: 1.20; 95% CI: 0.83–1.74). However, when the 2 trials with the most notable methodologic weaknesses were excluded, the results changed sensibly. The oldest study (1) was excluded because of the high diagnostic error rate as a result of the unavailability of CT at the time of the study and the uncertainty about the number of patients allocated to surgery who actually underwent craniotomy. The Chinese study (14) was removed due to concerns about poorly balanced randomization, inclusion of cerebellar hematomas, and possible incorporation into the surgical group of patients who only underwent ventricular drainage. After these exclusions, the resulting meta-analysis ($n = 224$) actually indicated a trend toward a reduction in the odds of death and dependency after surgery (OR: 0.63; 95% CI: 0.35–1.14).

These meta-analyses do not include the most recent trials. A randomized, multicenter trial compared stereotactic blood clot drainage after liquefaction with urokinase (instilled through a catheter into the hematoma every 6 hr for 2 days) with conservative treatment (15). Seventy patients were enrolled within 72 hr of ICH onset. No differences in mortality or severe disability between the treatment groups were observed. However, a significant ICH volume reduction was achieved by neurosurgical intervention (10–20%; $p < 0.05$).

By far, the largest randomized trial evaluating surgical evacuation in the management of ICH, the International Surgical Trial in Intracerebral Hemorrhage was an international (27 countries), multicenter (83 centers) study that enrolled 1033 patients to receive early surgery or initial conservative treatment. Eligible patients had confirmed spontaneous supratentorial ICH that had arisen within the previous 72 hr, with a minimum hematoma diameter of 2 cm and GCS > 4. Patients randomized to the surgical arm underwent hematoma evacuation within the following 24 hr. The trial protocol did not include a standardized surgical technique; thus, the responsible surgeon chose the method used for evacuation in each case. Best medical treatment was similarly left to the discretion of the participating clinicians. Later surgical evacuation was allowed in patients initially treated conservatively, if it was deemed necessary due to neurologic deterioration. Outcome measures were death and functional disability at 6 months, as measured by several validated functional scales and using information obtained through structured postal questionnaires. The investigators adopted a pragmatic prognosis-based outcome to evaluate functional end results; patient outcomes were categorized as good or poor upon randomization, and this classification was considered to establish different outcome expectations. Analysis of results was based on intention-to-treat.

In total, 503 patients were randomized to early surgery and 530 to conservative treatment. Groups were well balanced for meaningful baseline variables. Median age was 62 years, and more than half of all patients were randomized within 20 hr of hematoma onset. Twenty percent of patients were comatose (GCS 5–8) upon enrollment. Hematomas were fairly equally distributed between lobar and ganglionic locations in both treatment groups. Median hematoma volume was 38 mL and comparable in both groups. Ninety-four percent of patients randomized to early surgery actually underwent evacuation. Median time between ictus and surgery was 30 hr, and between randomization and surgery, 5 hr. Meanwhile, 26% of patients randomized to initial conservative treatment eventually went to surgery due to neurologic deterioration after a median interval from ictus of 60 hr. Craniotomy was the procedure chosen for evacuation in 77% of surgical patients.

After excluding patients lost to follow-up or with insufficient follow-up information, the final population analyzed consisted of 468 patients randomized to the surgical arm and 497 patients randomized to the conservative arm. Favorable functional outcome using the extended GCS occurred in 26% of patients who were randomized to early surgery and 24% of those randomized to initial conservative treatment (OR: 0.89; CI: 0.66–1.19; $p = 0.41$). Therefore, early surgery resulted in a nonsignificant absolute benefit of 2.3% and a relative benefit of 10%. Similar results were observed with other functional scales. Mortality rates at 6 months did not differ much between treatment groups (36% vs. 37% for early surgery and initial conservative approach, respectively).

On subgroup analysis, the only remarkable finding was the greater likelihood of favorable outcome with early surgery among patients with superficial hematomas (i.e., located 1 cm or less from the cortical surface). For these patients, early surgery afforded an absolute benefit of 8% over initial medical treatment ($p = 0.02$). Conversely, patients with deep hematomas tended to fare better with conservative treatment. Craniotomy appeared to offer an advantage over other surgical techniques, but the difference was not significant, and the number of patients treated with methods other than conventional craniotomy might have been too small to draw reliable conclusions. In the subpopulation of comatose patients, early surgery was actually associated with a trend toward increased risk of death or disability.

In conclusion, surgical evacuation cannot be advocated as standard treatment of choice for most patients with acute primary ICH. The role of surgery should probably be restricted to patients deteriorating because of mass effect. Nonetheless, future studies may define a particular niche for specific surgical interventions targeted to well-defined subpopulations of patients.

The most important features of the randomized trials on surgical versus medical treatment of ICH are summarized in Table 1.

Table 1 Summary of Published Randomized Trials Comparing Surgical and Medical Treatment for Patients with ICH

Trial	Population	Surgical technique	Results	OR (95% CI) of death/ dependency
McKissock et al. 1961 (1)	n=180 Clinical presentation/LP/ angio consistent with ICH No defined time limit	Craniotomy	No significant difference Death—S: 65%; M: 51% Poor outcome—S: 80%; M: 66%	2.0 (1.0, 3.9)
Juvela et al. 1989 (2)	n=52 Unconscious and/or severe hemiparesis/ dysphasia S within 48 hr	Craniotomy	No significant difference Death—S: 46%; M: 38% Poor outcome—S: 98%; M: 66%	4.39 (0.8, 23.6)
Auer et al. 1989 (4)	n=100 ICH > 10 cc; altered consciousness Ictus within < 48 hr	Endoscopic aspiration	S significantly better Death—S: 42%; M: 70% Poor outcome—S: 58%; M: 74%	0.46 (0.2, 1.0)
Batjer et al. 1990 (3)	n=21 Putaminal ICH >3 cm Altered consciousness or hemiparesis Ictus within < 24 hr	Craniotomy	No significant difference Death—S: 50%; M: 85% Poor outcome—S: 75%; M: 85%	0.55 (0.1, 4.9)
Morgenstern et al. 1998 (6)	n=31 ICH >9 cc, lobar or extending out of thalamus, GCS 5–15 Ictus within 12 hr	Craniotomy	No significant difference Death—S: 24%; M: 18% Poor outcome—S: 69%; M: 50%	0.46 (0.1, 1.9)
Zuccarello et al. 1990 (5)	n=20 ICH > 10 cc; GCS > 4, (+) neuro deficit Ictus within 12 hr	Craniotomy/ stereotactic aspiration	No significant difference Death—S: 22%; M: 27% Poor outcome—S: 44%; M: 64%	0.48 (0.1, 2.7)
Teernstra et al. 2003 (15)	n=70 ICH > 10 cc; GEM 2–10 Ictus within 72 hr	Urokinase installation and stereotactic drainage	No significant difference Death—S: 56%; M: 59% Poor outcome—S: 75%; M: 76%	0.52 (1.2, 2.3)
STICH 2005 (16)	n=1033 ICH >2 cm; GCS>4 Ictus within 72 hr Surgery within 24 hr of enrollment	At the surgeon's discretion (78% craniotomy)	No significant difference Death—S: 36% M: 37% Poor outcome—S: 74%; M: 76%	0.89 (0.7, 1.2)

Abbreviations: CI, confidence interval; ICH, intracerebral hemorrhage; LP, lumbar puncture; M, medical; OR, odds ratio; S, surgery; GCS, Glasgow Coma Scale; GEM, Glasgow Eye Motor Scale; STICH, Surgical Trial in Intracerebral Hemorrhage; Ictus, symptom onset.

MEDICAL TREATMENT

Early Hemostatic Therapy

The use of hemostatic agents designed to arrest ongoing hemorrhage in the hyperacute setting constitutes one of the most promising interventions to improve the outcome of patients with ICH (17). In that, hematoma expansion is most common in the first few hours after bleeding onset, the effectiveness of this treatment depends on its very early administration. Hemostatic agents may theoretically increase the risk of thrombotic complications. Therefore, the results of a recently conducted Phase 2 trial, which proved the feasibility and safety of this therapeutic strategy, are of great importance (18,19). The information yielded from the trial has already become available for the use of activated recombinant factor VII (rFVIIa), which is a genetically altered agent resembling a natural clotting factor.

This randomized, double-blinded, placebo-controlled, dose-escalation trial tested the use of 6 different doses of rFVIIa versus placebo in 47 patients with ICH within 3 hr of ictus onset (18). Mean age of participants was 61 ± 15 years, median GCS was 14, and mean ICH volume was 21 ± 24 mL (range, 1–151 mL). ICH was ganglionic in 72% of cases, and intraventricular extension was present in 45%. Treatment was initiated after a median interval of 181 min (range, 120–265 min) from hematoma onset. ICH growth was documented in 17% at 1 hr and 19% at 24 hr. No differences were observed in hematoma growth or functional outcome among the treatment groups, but the study was not powered to assess efficacy. Twelve serious adverse events occurred, including 5 deaths; all fatalities were primarily caused by the ICH itself. No relationship was detected between the frequency, type, or severity of side effects and rFVIIa dose. Six adverse events were considered possibly related to treatment, but only two were potentially severe (popliteal deep venous thrombosis in the acute phase in one case and T-wave inversion at 24 hr without elevation of creatinine kinase isoenzyme MB (CK-MB) level in the other). No cases of consumption coagulopathy, systemic embolism, or excessive cerebral edema causing neurologic deterioration were reported. The authors reasonably concluded that this small Phase 2 trial did not raise major safety concerns and that a larger trial was justified to confirm the safety and evaluate the effectiveness of rFVIIa in the treatment of acute ICH.

Another Phase 2B (19), dose-ranging, proof-of-concept trial randomized 399 patients with primary ICH (confirmed by CT scan) within 3 hr after onset of symptoms to receive rFVIIa 40 μg/kg body weight (BW; 108 patients), 80 μg/kg BW (92 patients), 160 μg/kg BW (103 patients), or placebo (96 patients) (18). Patients were excluded if they had a GCS>6, history of coagulopathy or recent use of oral anticoagulants, or any history of thrombotic or vaso-occlusive disease. Treatment was started within 1 hr of obtaining the CT scan and administered in a double-blinded fashion. The primary outcome measure was the percentage change in the hematoma volume at 24 hr. Clinical outcomes were assessed at 90 days using various validated scales. Analysis followed the intention-to-treat principle. Baseline characteristics were similar in all groups, although the degree of acute blood pressure elevation was not reported. Location of the hematoma was deep in more than 80% of cases, and median GCS was 14. Mean hematoma volume at baseline was 27 mL (range, 0.4–153 mL). Mean time from symptom onset to initiation of treatment was 167 ± 32 min.

Increase in hematoma volume was lower in the rFVIIa arms than in the placebo group ($p = 0.01$ for the difference between placebo and the combined rFVIIa groups), and the difference was more pronounced with the higher doses of rFVIIa. Mean percentage increase from baseline was 29% with placebo, versus 16%, 14%, and 11% with the 3 escalating doses, respectively. This reflected absolute volume differences of 3.3, 4.5, and 5.8 mL in the 3 treatment doses. Benefit was greater when therapy was initiated within 3 hr of symptom onset. Total lesion volume [ICH + intraventricular hemorrhage (IVH) + edema] was also significantly reduced in the treatment groups; the estimated mean total volume reduction at 72 hr was 11 mL for the combined treatment groups. Mortality at 3 months was 29% in the placebo group versus 18% in the treatment groups combined ($p = 0.02$; relative risk reduction 38%; Fig. 1). Functional outcome was also significantly better in patients who received rFVIIa; a 16% absolute reduction in the number of patients with modified Rankin score of 4 to 6 at 90 days was associated with the use of rFVIIa. In terms of functional outcome, the best dose was 80 μg/kg BW. Severe arterial thromboembolic events were significantly more frequent among patients treated with rFVIIa (5% vs. 0% with placebo; $p = 0.01$), including 2 cases of ischemic stroke that were fatal and 5 more that were disabling. Rates of venous thromboembolic events did not differ between

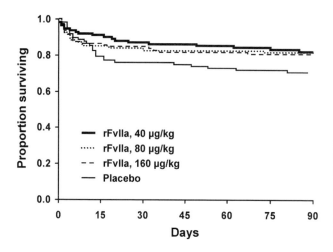

Figure 1 Survival at 90 days according to study group. Mortality was reduced by approximately 35% in each rFVIIa group, as compared to placebo group (p=0.10 by the log-rank test, comparing all 4 groups; p=0.02 by the chi-square test for the comparison of the three rFVIIa groups combined with placebo). *Source*: From Ref. 19.

groups. Only 2% of the serious thromboembolic events were considered possibly or probably related to the drug.

In summary, this trial showed that early infusion of rFVIIa can ameliorate ICH growth, with a resulting favorable impact on functional outcome. However, it did not dispel concerns that the treatment might increase the risk of serious arterial vascular events. The investigators concluded that further research is still needed to identify the best candidates for the safe use of this hemostatic treatment, as well as the ideal dose and optimal time window for its administration. The cost of the drug is high—up to $12 per patient—but may be offset by reduced hospital stay and rehabilitation time.

Intraventricular Thrombolysis

IVH is a poor prognostic factor in patients with ICH (20,21), and a large volume of IVH is predictive of mortality and unfavorable functional outcome (22). Although external ventricular drainage is effective in treating obstructive hydrocephalus, it has never been proven to accelerate resolution of the intraventricular clot. Furthermore, obstruction of the ventriculostomy catheter by the clot is a relatively frequent problem. Therefore, the use of thrombolytic drugs to hasten the removal of intraventricular blood is based on a solid rationale. The safety and efficacy of this strategy has been successfully tested in case series and cohort studies (23,24).

These initial favorable results were confirmed in a Phase 2, multicenter, prospective, controlled trial, in which 12 patients with IVH requiring ventriculostomy were randomized to receive intraventricular injections of urokinase (25,000 IU) or saline solution. Injections were administered every 12 hr starting at between 12 and 24 hr after bleeding onset. They were continued until the ventriculostomy catheter was removed following prespecified criteria (i.e., clamping of catheter for 24 hr without elevation of intracranial pressure above 15 mmHg). IVH volumes were measured on daily CT scans by examiners blinded to treatment assignment. Unfortunately, enrollment had to be stopped when the manufacturer withdrew urokinase from the market. Patients in the urokinase group received a mean of 7.7 injections (range, 4–11 doses). Clot resolution was significantly faster in patients treated with urokinase (p=0.02). After adjustment for baseline differences in gender distribution—which was necessary because faster IVH resolution was also associated with females—a reduction of 3.8 days in the intraventricular clot half-life was observed (i.e., time required for a 50% decrement in the initial volume of the clot). Mean duration of external ventricular drainage tended to be reduced in patients treated with urokinase (170 hr vs. 208 hr in the placebo group). No significant differences in adverse events between groups were observed, and no cases of expansion of ICH or IVH were reported.

A larger (n=48) Phase 2 trial using recombinant tissue plasminogen activator (rtPA) has also offered encouraging results (25). Infusion of rtPA strongly accelerated IVH resolution, and treated patients showed improved levels of consciousness more rapidly and tended to have better functional outcomes. Although symptomatic hemorrhages were more common in the rtPA group, this difference was not significant. In addition, nonhemorrhagic complications occurred more frequently in the placebo group. The results of this study justify the conduction of a Phase 3 trial to establish the role of intraventricular thrombolysis in daily practice.

Treatment of Edema

Edema is responsible for complications from mass effect and may further worsen cerebral blood flow in areas already affected by hypoperfusion. Both cytotoxic and vasogenic edema occur after ICH, and their amelioration was the target of controlled trials that tested the efficacy of glycerol and corticosteroids.

Dexamethasone was tested in two randomized, controlled trials. Tellez and Bauer enrolled 40 patients with a clinical diagnosis of nontraumatic ICH and impaired consciousness to receive dexamethasone (19 patients) or placebo (21 patients) (26). Treatment was started within 48 hr of the ictus, and patients on the active treatment group received a total of 120 mg of dexamethasone over 10 days. Diagnosis was based on history, physical examination, and the finding of more than 200 erythrocytes/mL of cerebrospinal fluid. The mortality was very high in both groups (89% with dexamethasone and 76% with placebo) and uniform among patients presenting with deep stupor or coma, who were treated with corticosteroids. Overall functional outcome upon discharge from the hospital was similarly poor in both groups. Two patients treated with steroids developed episodes of gastrointestinal hemorrhage, versus none in the control group. Limitations of this study included its low population size, lack of confirmation of ICH by brain imaging, and partial blinding (only the last 23 patients were double blinded).

A larger and more scientifically rigorous trial evaluating the effects of dexamethasone in primary supratentorial ICH was subsequently conducted in Thailand (27). This double-blinded, controlled trial randomized patients within 48 hr of the ictus. Diagnosis of ICH was confirmed by CT scan. Patients in the dexamethasone group were scheduled to receive a total of 150 mg of the drug over 9 days. Ninety-three patients were enrolled before the trial was prematurely terminated due to an excess of adverse events among patients treated with the corticosteroid. Groups were well balanced at baseline in terms of age, comorbid conditions, ICH location, and severity of initial clinical presentation. The only notable difference was a larger mean hematoma volume among patients assigned to receive dexamethasone than among those in the control group (72 vs. 59 mL). Neither mortality nor functional recovery after 21 days was different between groups. However, the rate of complications and possible adverse effects was significantly greater in the dexamethasone group, mainly due to the increased frequency of persistent hyperglycemia and infections.

The use of glycerol was assessed in one double-blinded, randomized, placebo-controlled trial that enrolled 120 patients with ICH onset within the previous 24 hr (28). Active treatment consisted of 500 mL of 10% glycerol in a physiologic saline solution administered intravenously over 4 hr for 6 consecutive days. Groups were adequately balanced in terms of clinical severity at presentation (most patients had GCS = 12–15), concomitant illnesses, and hematoma volume (mean = 28–32 mL). Functional outcome at 6 months was not affected by treatment assignment. No subgroup of patients was shown to benefit from receiving glycerol. Hemolysis was the only side effect noticed to be more common in the glycerol-treated patients, but the resulting anemia most often was not clinically meaningful.

Therefore, these trials indicate that the routine use of corticosteroids or glycerol has no role in cases of ICH. Other osmotic agents, including mannitol and hypertonic saline (the two most commonly used in United States), have not been formally tested in randomized, controlled trials. In light of the absence of data supporting their efficacy and the lack of benefit observed with glycerol, the use of these agents should be reserved for cases with documented or highly suspected intracranial hypertension or signs of impending herniation (29).

Acute Reduction of Blood Pressure

No randomized, controlled trials sought to identify the ideal target for acute blood pressure reduction after spontaneous ICH. Current guidelines for the management of this condition recommend keeping the mean arterial pressure below 130 mmHg in patients with history of hypertension but recognize the lack of solid scientific grounds for this advice by rating the level of evidence as V (i.e., data from anecdotal case series) (29).

The rationale for this rather conservative approach lies in the hypothesis that an area of penumbra typically surrounds intraparenchymal hematomas. Reduced cerebral perfusion in the perihematoma region has been demonstrated by various techniques (30–32). However, the existence of an area of true penumbra has been questioned by data obtained from experimental models (33,34) and human studies using positron-emission technology (35,36). It is possible that the hypoperfusion observed around the hematoma does not produce tissue ischemia, but might be the result of regional metabolic depression after the hemorrhage. Meanwhile, hematoma enlargement has been repeatedly noticed to be associated with more elevated blood pressures (37,38). Aggressive early blood-pressure reduction has been successfully tested in a small preliminary study (39). A randomized, controlled trial to evaluate the effects of this approach in a large population of patients with acute primary ICH appears to be the next logical and necessary step.

FUTURE TRIALS

The trials discussed in this chapter indicate that emergent, targeted medical interventions have the potential to greatly improve the outcome of some patients with ICH. However, more research is needed before any of these novel therapies will be ready for introduction in daily clinical practice. A recent National Institute of Neurological Disorders and Stroke ICH workshop identified priorities for clinical research (Table 2) (16). It is hoped that additional trials that test optimized protocols of early hemostasis with rFVIIa, and intraventricular thrombolysis with rtPA, will offer robust data to support their approval for clinical application. Infusion of rFVIIa should also be evaluated for the treatment of ICH induced by excessive anticoagulation. Techniques of minimally invasive surgery in combination with local infusion of a thrombolytic drug deserve further exploration. New studies that test the role of surgery exclusively on patients with superficial hematomas are justified. Prompt administration of neuroprotectants to limit neuronal death is an option that must continue to be studied regardless of the disappointing results so far observed in patients with ischemic infarction. The value of aggressive reduction of blood pressure as soon as ICH is diagnosed should also be formally investigated. It is only reasonable to expect that these clinical trials will hold the key to providing a better outlook for future patients with ICH.

Table 2 Priorities for Clinical Research in ICH

Medical priorities
  Blood-pressure management
  Treatment of hyperglycemia
  Normalization of body temperature
  Prophylactic use of antiepileptic agents
  Safety of prophylactic anticoagulants
  Reversal of antithrombotic- and fibrinolytic-induced ICH
  Evaluation of hemostatic agents in coagulopathy-associated ICH
Surgical priorities
  Mechanical clot removal devices
  Surgical targeting
  Perioperative imaging
  Local delivery of protective restorative agents
  Regional hypothermia
  Intracavitary microdialysis for markers of ongoing injury
  Polymer-based sustained release technology
  Delayed restorative surgical procedures
  Delayed implantation of bionic interfaces

Abbreviation: ICH, intracerebral hemorrhage.
Source: From Ref. 16.

REFERENCES

1. McKissock W, Richardson A, Taylor J. Primary intracerebral hemorrhage: a controlled trial of surgical and conservative treatment in 180 unselected cases. Lancet 1961; 2:221–226.
2. Juvela S, Heiskanen O, Poranen A, et al. The treatment of spontaneous intracerebral hemorrhage. A prospective randomized trial of surgical and conservative treatment. J Neurosurg 1989; 70(5):755–758.
3. Batjer HH, Reisch JS, Allen BC, et al. Failure of surgery to improve outcome in hypertensive putaminal hemorrhage. A prospective randomized trial. Arch Neurol 1990; 47(10):1103–1106.
4. Auer LM, Deinsberger W, Niederkorn K, et al. Endoscopic surgery versus medical treatment for spontaneous intracerebral hematoma: a randomized study. J Neurosurg 1989; 70(4):530–535.
5. Zuccarello M, Brott T, Derex L, et al. Early surgical treatment for supratentorial intracerebral hemorrhage: a randomized feasibility study. Stroke 1999; 30(9):1833–1839.
6. Morgenstern LB, Frankowski RF, Shedden P, et al. Surgical treatment for intracerebral hemorrhage (STICH): a single-center, randomized clinical trial. Neurology 1998; 51(5):1359–1363.
7. Morgenstern LB, Demchuk AM, Kim DH, et al. Rebleeding leads to poor outcome in ultra-early craniotomy for intracerebral hemorrhage. Neurology 2001; 56(10):1294–1299.
8. Hankey GJ, Hon C. Surgery for primary intracerebral hemorrhage: is it safe and effective? A systematic review of case series and randomized trials. Stroke 1997; 28(11):2126–2132.
9. Prasad K, Browman G, Srivastava A, et al. Surgery in primary supratentorial intracerebral hematoma: a meta-analysis of randomized trials. Acta Neurol Scand 1997; 95(2):103–110.
10. Prasad K, Shrivastava A. Surgery for primary supratentorial intracerebral hemorrhage Cochrane Database Syst Rev 2000; (2):CD000200 (Cochrane review).
11. Saver JL. Surgical therapy. In: Feldmann E, ed. Intracerebral Hemorrhage. Armonk, NY: Futura Publishing, 1994:303–332.
12. Saver JL. Surgery for primary intracerebral hemorrhage: Meta-analysis of CT-era studies. Stroke 1998; 29(7):1477–1478.
13. Fernandes HM, Gregson B, Siddique S, et al. Surgery in intracerebral hemorrhage. The uncertainty continues. Stroke 2000; 31(10):2511–2516.
14. Chen X, Yang H, Czherig Z. A prospective randomized trial of surgical and conservative treatment of hypertensive intracranial hemorrhage (Chinese). Acta Acad Med Shanghai 1992; 19:237–240.
15. Teernstra OP, Evers SM, Lodder J, et al. Stereotactic treatment of intracerebral hematoma by means of a plasminogen activator: a multicenter randomized controlled trial (SICHPA). Stroke 2003; 34(4):968–974.
16. Ohwaki K, Yano E, Nagashima H, et al. Blood pressure management in acute intracerebral hemorrhage: relationship between elevated blood pressure and hematoma enlargement. Stroke 2004; 35(6):1364–1367.
17. Priorities for Clinical Research in Intracerebral Hemorrhage: Report From a National Institute of Neurological Disorders and Stroke Workshop. Stroke 2005; 36(3):e23–e41.
18. Mayer SA, Brun NC, Broderick J, et al. Safety and feasibility of recombinant factor VIIa for acute intracerebral hemorrhage. Stroke 2005; 36(1):74–79.
19. Mayer SA, Brun NC, Begtrup K, et al. Recombinant activated factor VII for acute intracerebral hemorrhage. N Engl J Med 2005; 352(8):777–785.
20. Hallevy C, Ifergane G, Kordysh E, et al. Spontaneous supratentorial intracerebral hemorrhage. Criteria for short-term functional outcome prediction. J Neurol 2002; 249(12):1704–1709.
21. Hemphill JC III, Bonovich DC, Besmertis L, et al. The ICH score: a simple, reliable grading scale for intracerebral hemorrhage. Stroke 2001; 32(4):891–897.
22. Tuhrim S, Horowitz DR, Sacher M. Volume of ventricular blood is an important determinant of outcome in supratentorial intracerebral hemorrhage. Crit Care Med 1999; 27(3):617–621.
23. Coplin WM, Vinas FC, Agris JM, et al. A cohort study of the safety and feasibility of intraventricular urokinase for nonaneurysmal spontaneous intraventricular hemorrhage. Stroke 1998; 29(8):1573–1579.
24. Naff NJ, Carhuapoma JR, Williams MA, et al. Treatment of intraventricular hemorrhage with urokinase: effects on 30-day survival. Stroke 2000; 31(4):841–847.
25. Naff NJ, Hanley DF, Keyl PM, et al. Intraventricular thrombolysis speeds blood clot resolution: results of a pilot, prospective, randomized, double–blind, controlled trial. Neurosurgery 2004; 54(3):577–583; discussion 583–584.
26. Tellez H, Bauer RB. Dexamethasone as treatment in cerebrovascular disease. 1. A controlled study in intracerebral hemorrhage. Stroke 1973; 4(4):541–546.
27. Poungvarin N, Bhoopat W, Viriyavejakul A, et al. Effects of dexamethasone in primary supratentorial intracerebral hemorrhage. N Engl J Med 1987; 316(20):1229–1233.
28. Yu YL, Kumana CR, Lauder IJ, et al. Treatment of acute cerebral hemorrhage with intravenous glycerol. A double-blind, placebo-controlled, randomized trial. Stroke 1992; 23(7):967–971.

29. Broderick JP, Adams HP Jr., Barsan W, et al. Guidelines for the management of spontaneous intracerebral hemorrhage: a statement for healthcare professionals from a special writing group of the Stroke Council, American Heart Association. Stroke 1999; 30(4):905–915.

30. Mayer SA, Lignelli A, Fink ME, et al. Perilesional blood flow and edema formation in acute intracerebral hemorrhage: a SPECT study. Stroke 1998; 29(9):1791–1798.

31. Kidwell CS, Saver JL, Mattiello J, et al. Diffusion-perfusion MR evaluation of perihematomal injury in hyperacute intracerebral hemorrhage. Neurology 2001; 57(9):1611–1617.

32. Rosand J, Eskey C, Chang Y, et al. Dynamic single-section CT demonstrates reduced cerebral blood flow in acute intracerebral hemorrhage. Cerebrovasc Dis 2002; 14(3–4):214–220.

33. Qureshi AI, Wilson DA, Hanley DF, Traystman RJ. Pharmacologic reduction of mean arterial pressure does not adversely affect regional cerebral blood flow and intracranial pressure in experimental intracerebral hemorrhage. Crit Care Med 1999; 27(5):965–971.

34. Qureshi AI, Wilson DA, Hanley DF, Traystman RJ. No evidence for an ischemic penumbra in massive experimental intracerebral hemorrhage. Neurology 1999; 52(2):266–272.

35. Zazulia AR, Diringer MN, Videen TO, et al. Hypoperfusion without ischemia surrounding acute intracerebral hemorrhage. J Cereb Blood Flow Metab 2001; 21(7):804–810.

36. Powers WJ, Zazulia AR, Videen TO, et al. Autoregulation of cerebral blood flow surrounding acute (6 to 22 hours) intracerebral hemorrhage. Neurology 2001; 57(1):18–24.

37. Leira R, Davalos A, Silva Y, et al. Early neurologic deterioration in intracerebral hemorrhage: predictors and associated factors. Neurology 2004; 63(3):461–467.

38. Ohwak K, Yano E, Nagashima H, et al. Blood pressure management in acute intracerebral hemorrhage: relationship between elevated blood pressure and hematoma enlargement. Stroke 2004; 35(6):1364–1367.

39. Qureshi AI, Mohammad YM, Yahia AM, et al. A prospective multicenter study to evaluate the feasibility and safety of aggressive antihypertensive treatment in patients with acute intracerebral hemorrhage. J Intensive Care Med 2005; 20(1):34–42.

15 | Prognosis and Outcomes Following Intracerebral Hemorrhage

Stanley Tuhrim, MD, Director[a], Professor[b]

[a] Division of Cerebrovascular Diseases, [b] Department of Neurology,
Mount Sinai School of Medicine, New York, New York, USA

INTRODUCTION

Intracerebral hemorrhage (ICH) is the most lethal form of stroke, with mortality estimates ranging from 23% to 58% in various modern series (1–3). The study of the characteristics, behaviors, and outcomes of ICH has progressed through 3 phases. Early reports concerning outcome were largely descriptive and focused on specific lesion locations. These reports often identified specific clinical findings of prognostic significance. Subsequently, the advent of more sophisticated statistical analysis allowed for the development of multivariate models that provided powerful predictive instruments for large classes of ICH patients. These models have proven useful for estimating the effects of certain characteristics in heterogeneous patient groups (e.g., supratentorial hemorrhages), but they often lack specific clinical detail. Most recently, the prognostic significance of individual factors has been confirmed by clinical trial and observational data from larger data sets. This chapter describes the prognostic information gleaned from these 3 phases.

PROGNOSIS BY SPECIFIC LESION SITE

Putaminal Hemorrhage

ICH occurs primarily in the deep portions of the cerebral hemispheres, most commonly in the putamen (~40%), with a broad spectrum of clinical presentations and a wide range of outcomes. In an early CT-based study of 24 cases of putaminal hemorrhage, pupillary abnormalities, disturbances in extraocular movement, and bilateral Babinski signs were associated with larger hematomas and a poor chance of survival, whereas preserved higher cortical function and partial sparing of motor function were associated with good outcome. Four patients with absent extraocular movements had massive hemorrhages and fatal outcomes. Age, gender, and admission blood pressure were unrelated to outcome (4). Predictive CT scan findings included large hemorrhage size and presence of intraventricular blood. Kanaya, on the basis of extensive experience with medically and surgically treated patients, developed a detailed classification schema based on the involvement of adjacent structures. He indicated that lesions that involve only the anterior limb of the internal capsule (Grades I and II) fare much better than those involving the posterior limb (Grades III and IV) or thalamus (Grade V) (5).

Caudate Hemorrhage

Although the caudate is supplied by deep penetrating branches of larger, superficial arteries, similar to branch vessels supplying putamen and thalamus, hemorrhage originating in the caudate accounts for only 5% to 7% of all ICH. Patients with caudate hemorrhage can be divided into two groups on the basis of initial presentation. One group mimics subarachnoid hemorrhage [due to the invariable presence of intraventricular hemorrhage (IVH), with meningismus, vomiting, headache, and changes in level of consciousness and behavior]. These patients usually recover completely. In addition to the manifestations described above, a second group has hemiparesis and conjugate gaze paresis, indicating compression of the internal capsule. These patients frequently take longer to recover, but mortality remains low (6). The consistently good outcome in these patients, despite IVH, stands in sharp contrast to putaminal hemorrhage, in which such extension is strongly associated with a fatal outcome.

Thalamic Hemorrhage

Thalamic hemorrhage represents 10% to 15% of ICH. Overall survival in thalamic hemorrhage appears comparable to putaminal hemorrhage. In early descriptive studies, hematoma size emerged as the most important predictor of mortality. In the earliest report of the CT scan era, 18 hypertensive thalamic hemorrhages were noted; all of those with a maximum diameter >3.3 cm were fatal, whereas the overall mortality rate was 50% (7). Other reports of a small series suggested 2.5, 3.0, and 3.3 cm as the crucial lesion diameter (8–10). In the largest series to date, Weisberg noted that no patients with maximum-diameter hematoma of <2.5 cm died, whereas those with hematomas >3 cm had ventricular extension, became comatose, and died. Although a precise hematoma size that results in mortality has not been defined, it is apparent that hematoma size correlates with prognosis and that patients with thalamic lesions >3 cm in diameter rarely survive. Ventricular extension occurs in most thalamic hemorrhages and is associated with a variable prognosis, but hydrocephalus, presumably secondary to IVH, is associated with a high mortality rate (10).

Level of consciousness is consistently related to survival. For example, Piepgras and Rieger reported that 6 of 7 patients admitted in coma died, but 5 of 6 with an initially clear sensorium survived (11). Posterior thalamic lesions rarely result in significant permanent deficit. Complete recovery is typical with a described syndrome of posterior thalamic hemorrhage that consists of ipsilateral ptosis and miosis, contralateral sensory neglect and hemiparesis, defective pursuit toward the lesion, and hypometric saccades away from the lesion (12). Similarly, the aphasia associated with left thalamic hemorrhage usually resolves completely (10).

Lobar Hemorrhage

Lobar hemorrhage may carry a lower mortality risk than ICH in other locations. Reported mortality rates range from 9% to 32%. A history of hypertension is present in only approximately one-third of lobar hemorrhage patients (13–16). Patients without a history of hypertension have a substantially better prognosis. In a series of 50 patients, all normotensive patients survived, most with little or no residual disability. Among those with hypertension, 50% worsened in the hospital, 28% died, and 77% of survivors had significant neurologic disability (16). Hypertension was strongly associated with hematoma size. Consciousness level, hemorrhage size, intraventricular extension, and degree of midline shift have been identified as important prognostic variables (13–16).

Pontine Hemorrhage

Pontine hemorrhage accounts for only 5% of ICH (17). Previously, this lesion was universally believed to be almost fatal. Bilateral paramedian pontine hemorrhage with ventricular extension is usually fatal, and those who survive are neurologically devastated. However, modern imaging has demonstrated small hemorrhages limited to the pontine tegmentum or encompassing a small portion of the basis pontis, and patients with these abnormalities typically have signs and symptoms that mimic lacunar syndromes (18). These more lateral lesions are frequently associated with vascular malformations (19). The prognosis in these small hemorrhages is excellent, with full recovery reported (20–22).

Cerebellar Hemorrhage

Cerebellar hemorrhages, accounting for ~10% of ICH, usually occur in the cerebellar hemispheres. Patients who remain conscious fare far better than those who become stuporous or comatose, regardless of whether they undergo evacuation of the hematoma. When patients are operated upon while still arousable, the reported mortality rate is <30%, but evacuation of a cerebellar hematoma after the onset of coma is associated with at least a 72% mortality rate (23,24). Other clinical findings at presentation do not reliably predict outcome. Hemorrhage diameter >3 cm, obstructive hydrocephalus, and IVH are associated with a decreased level of consciousness and a high mortality rate (24). Overall, the survival rate for cerebellar hemorrhage is higher than for other ICH locations. For example, in the National Institute of Neurological Disorder and Stroke Data Bank series, more than 80% of cerebellar hemorrhage patients survived at least 30 days. Frequently, those patients who survive make an excellent recovery (24,25).

GENERAL PROGNOSTIC FEATURES

The information in the preceding section regarding specific hemorrhage locations is based on observations of small groups of patients. Another approach assesses outcome in larger, more heterogeneous groups (e.g., patients with supratentorial hemorrhage). The potential advantage of the second approach is the ability to apply powerful statistical techniques; however, the ability to collect information such as is collectible with small subgroups might be lost.

Several early studies (26–33) performed only univariate analysis of factors associated with outcome. Age, lesion location, electrocardiographic abnormalities, and hypertensive history were inconsistently associated with prognoses, but shift of midline structures on CT scan was associated with fatal outcome in the two studies that evaluated this finding. Ropper noted an association between level of consciousness and degree of horizontal displacement of the pineal body in acute hemispheral mass lesions, mainly ICHs (34). Level of consciousness is the clinical sign most consistently associated with ICH prognosis. The consistent importance of hemorrhage size, level of consciousness or Glasgow Coma Scale (GCS), and IVH extension mirror the prominent role that these factors play in descriptions of specific hemorrhage types.

Studies that employed multivariate analysis (35–43) produced fairly consistent results, despite minor variations in patient selection, variables assessed, and statistical methods. The variables identified as independent predictors of outcome in these studies are listed in Table 1.

Hemorrhage size, intraventricular extension of blood, and GCS or level of consciousness emerge as consistent, independent predictors of survival. Midline shift, oxygen saturation, and electrocardiographic abnormalities have been identified in some models, but too infrequently to be included in the table. Serum glucose and age are frequently examined, but with contradictory results.

LONG-TERM PROGNOSIS

Long-term outcome has been studied less frequently than early mortality for several reasons: (i) there are relatively fewer survivors overall (though short-term prognosis has improved partly because of the ability to identify relatively mildly affected individuals, with modern imaging techniques); (ii) obtaining information at appropriate intervals postdischarge is more difficult than determining early mortality; and (iii) it is more difficult to measure recovery or functional capacity than the clear endpoint of mortality. Many early long-term stroke outcome studies did not separate ICH from infarction; the results of several of the larger studies that did are summarized below. One study reported on 63 of 100 consecutive patients with spontaneous ICH, who survived the first month. Of these, 34 remained paretic (11 plegic), although only 5 of those were not ambulatory. Thirty-five returned to work, and only 6 remained institutionalized. Functional status was largely independent of hemorrhage location but was related to original hematoma size and GCS (29).

Of the 69 survivors from among 104 nonoperated ICH patients followed for 1 year in another study, 51 made a good to excellent recovery (28). The 18 patients with persistent, severe neurologic deficits who had significantly larger hemorrhages were older (mean age 65 vs. 58), and were twice as likely to have had IVH.

Another group followed 42 survivors from a series of 70 ICH patients for an average of 29 months. Another 7 died during the follow-up period; none died of vascular disease, and 5 patients suffered seizures. Only 5 of the 35 surviving patients returned to work, 19 walked without assistance, and 13 ambulated with assistance. The authors noted that functional status of most patients did not change during the follow-up period. The GCS was used to assess functional status following ICH in a cohort of 166 ICH patients, of whom 95 survived 6 months, and 78% of them functioned independently at 6 months. Limb weakness, language disorders, hemorrhage size, and ventricular hemorrhage were related to outcome. Initial survival was unrelated to age, but age was an important determinant of functional recovery (36).

Tuhrim et al. used factors predictive of 30-day survival (GCS, hemorrhage size, pulse pressure, and ventricular extension) to devise a model for predicting long-term outcome. The model correctly classified 95% of patients as having a good (defined as alive, Barthel's index >60) or poor (defined as dead or Barthel's index<60) outcome at 1 year. This study made no attempt to determine if age or premorbid level of function related to long-term outcome (35). Another group did include premorbid Rankin scale in a multivariate analysis of predictors of 6-month outcome and found that it, along with age and GCS, was helpful as a predictor (42).

Given the caveat that the data are more limited, the same factors that determine early mortality appear to be predictive of poor long-term functional outcome. Age may play a greater

Table 1 Predictors of Intracerebral Hemorrhage Outcome

Refs.	Age	Intracerebral hemorrhage (ICH) size	Intraventricular hemorrhage (IVH) +/−	IVH vol	Glasgow Coma Scale (GCS) Loc	Location	Hydro	Blood pressure[a]	Glu	Fourth vent
Dixon et al. (37)	−	+	+	N	+	+	N	−	N	N
Portenoy et al. (38)	N	+	+	N	+	−	N	−	N	N
Senant et al. (39)	+	+	+	N	+	−	N	N	−	N
Daverat et al. (36)	+	+	+	N	+	−	N	+	N	N
Tuhrim et al. (35)	N	+	N	N	+	N	N	−	−	N
Broderick et al. (44)	−	+	N	+	N	−	−	−	N	N
Lisk et al. (45)	+	+	+	+	+	−	−	−	N	N
Shapiro et al. (46)	−	+	+	N	+	N	N	N	N	N
Mase et al. (47)	−	+	+	N	+	−	N	−	N	N
Qureshi et al. (3)	−	+	+	N	+	−	N	−	N	N
Fogelholm et al. (48)	−	−	−	−	−	N	−	+	+	N
Diringer et al. (49)	−	−	−	−	−	−	+	−	N	N
Fujii et al. (50)	+	+[b]	−	−	−	+	N	N	−	N
Razzaq and Hussain (51)	−	+	+	N	+	−	+	+	N	N
Tuhrim et al. (52)	N	+	−	−	+	N	+	+	N	N
Phan et al. (53)	−	+	+	N	+	−	+	−	−	N
Hemphill et al. (41)	+	+	+	N	+	+	N	−	−	N
Hallevy et al. (54)	+	+	+	N	+	−	N	−	N	N
Cheung and Zou (43)	−	−	+	+	+	−	−	+	−	N
Fang[c] et al. (55)	+	−	+	N	+	+	N	−	+	N

[a]Systolic, diastolic, mean arterial blood pressure, or pulse pressure.
[b]ICH growth.
[c]GCS, ICH, IVH, location, and age as composite ICH score.

role in determining functional outcome than in predicting initial survival. Several authors suggest that for a given initial stroke severity, long-term functional recovery is better for ICH survivors than for those who suffer infarctions, but this has not been rigorously studied. However, in recent controlled comparison, outcomes were actually slightly poorer in patients with primary ICH than in ischemic stroke patients matched for prestroke disability, early neurologic impairment, and age (2).

SPECIFIC PROGNOSTIC FEATURES

Hydrocephalus

Hydrocephalus is present in as many as half of ICH patients at some time during the course of their illness; however, it has received relatively little attention as a prognostic factor.

In a descriptive study of 100 patients with thalamic hemorrhage, hydrocephalus was noted as an important predictor of mortality, but a multivariate analysis was not performed (56). Similarly, another descriptive study noted 67% mortality in patients with contralateral ventricular dilatation, compared with 30% overall mortality among 200 consecutive ICH patients (57). In a separate study of the significance of ventricular blood in supratentorial hemorrhage, hydrocephalus correlated with mortality, but external ventricular drainage did not appear to alter outcome (58). A more definitive, multivariate study analyzed 81 ICH patients treated in a neurointensive care setting, creating a detailed method of assessing the degree of hydrocephalus (49). Forty patients with at least some degree of hydrocephalus fared much worse (50% mortality) than those without (2% mortality). Only male gender, GCS, pineal shift, and hydrocephalus were independent predictors of mortality in this patient population. ICH location did not affect outcome or modify the effect of hydrocephalus on outcome. This latter finding is at odds with the findings of a later study that used the same method to quantify hydrocephalus in 100 consecutive ICH patients and then divided them into those with medial (thalamic and caudate) or lateral (putaminal) hemorrhages (53). Hydrocephalus, thus calculated, was present in 86% of those who died and was an independent predictor of mortality in the whole group. However, when the medial and lateral groups were considered separately, hydrocephalus was an independent predictor of outcome only in the lateral group. The authors noted that hydrocephalus in the medical group might be caused by a small dorsomedial thalamic hemorrhage with intraventricular extension, while in the lateral group, hydrocephalus was associated with larger intraparenchymal hemorrhage volume. This implies that hydrocephalus might be confounded with hemorrhage size in that population. In summary, hydrocephalus appears to be a poor prognostic sign in ICH. In the two studies that performed multivariate analyses, hydrocephalus, rather than hemorrhage size, appeared in the final model, although hemorrhage size, as in many other studies, was associated with outcome when considered alone.

Anticoagulant-Related Hemorrhage

Chronic anticoagulation, often for the purpose of preventing ischemic stroke, is a risk factor for ICH. It also appears to be associated with an increased likelihood of a poor outcome in patients who suffer an ICH. Two early reports focused on prognosis in anticoagulant-related hemorrhage. One reported that 20 of 40 patients did not survive, but 18 of 20 survivors recovered completely. Five patients suffered concomitant subdural hematomas, but no patients had multiple ICHs (59). The second report found that 28 of a series of 200 patients with ICH had been taking warfarin at the time of the hemorrhage (57). The mortality of the entire group was 30%, but 57% of those with anticoagulant-related hemorrhages died. The anticoagulant-related hemorrhages were also larger on average (57). A 2004 study attempted to quantify the independent effect, on ICH prognosis, of anticoagulation with warfarin by assessing 435 consecutive ICH patients over age 55, of whom 102 were taking warfarin at the time of hemorrhage (60). The use of warfarin more than doubled the 3-month mortality rate. Higher admission international normalized ratio (INRs) were associated with greater mortality. Hemorrhage size was not measured in this study. Several studies, including the second that is cited above (57), have suggested that patients with anticoagulant-related hemorrhages have larger hemorrhages; thus, warfarin use might simply be acting as a proxy for hemorrhage size. However, in a Taiwanese study that excluded anticoagulated patients, prothrombin times were significantly higher among nonsurvivors after adjusting for initial hemorrhage size (55), suggesting that noniatrogenic coagulopathies might play a more important role in ICH than is currently appreciated. Anticoagulant-related ICH may also have a greater likelihood of expansion (see below). Regardless of the etiology, anticoagulant-related hemorrhages tend to be larger, with a poorer prognosis. Hemorrhage size, IVH, and level of consciousness or GCS continue to predict outcome accurately in these patients, as they do for most patients with ICH.

Hematoma Expansion

Recently recognized to occur in ~one-third of all ICH patients who were scanned repeatedly within 24 hr of onset, hematoma expansion is associated with poor outcome and might account in part for the poorer prognosis in anticoagulant-related hemorrhage. In another recent study of 70 supratentorial ICH patients who were rescanned within 7 days of onset, warfarin use was associated with an increase in hematoma volume of at least 33% from baseline size of the hemorrhage (61). Hematoma expansion was detected later in the hospital course, and expansion was associated with a greater risk of mortality than is typical for spontaneous, idiopathic hemorrhages.

Warfarin use is a major determinant of hematoma expansion, but other factors have also been identified. In a multivariate analysis of 327 ICH patients admitted within 24 hr of onset, Fujii et al. (50) identified time from onset, amount of alcohol consumed, irregular shape of hematoma, decreased level of consciousness, and lower fibrinogen level as risk factors for hematoma expansion. Hematoma expansion was associated with increased mortality. Patients taking anticoagulants or antiplalelet agents were excluded from analysis. The phenomenon of hematoma expansion after initial presentation is better understood due to the advent of rapid evaluation of stroke patients who are studied with intravenous thrombolysis for acute ischemic stroke. The earlier a patient gets to the hospital and undergoes an initial CT scan, the more likely hematoma expansion is to be found (62).

In a study at hospitals participating in acute thrombolysis trials, of 142 patients who presented but were excluded because their CT scans diagnosed ICH within 3 hr of symptom onset, at least 38% had hematoma expansion of at least 33% of the baseline size within 24 hr. This might represent an underestimate, as one-third of the patients did not undergo a follow-up CT scan at 20 hr postbaseline because they were moribund, had undergone surgery, or had died. No significant predictors of hemorrhage growth were identified in this study (63). A recent dose-finding trial that evaluated activated factor VII in preventing hematoma expansion noted that 32% of the placebo group had substantial expansion within 24 hr (and also noted significantly less growth in the group treated with activated factor VII) (64).

Various measures of blood pressure have been associated with poorer prognosis in ICH. In a recent meta-analysis, high systolic blood pressure has been associated with hematoma expansion, as well as worse outcome. One study estimated that patients with high systolic blood pressure had twice the rate of hematoma expansion (65).

In summary, frequently, hematoma expansion occurs within 24 hr of presentation and is associated with a worse outcome. Patients with anticoagulant-related hemorrhage or other evidence of a coagulopathy and those with elevated blood pressure are more likely to suffer hematoma growth and, therefore, have a poorer prognosis. Prevention of hematoma growth may be feasible and could improve outcome.

Blood Pressure

Elevated blood pressure occurs in ~90% of ICH patients early after onset but frequently declines spontaneously (66). A 1997 study demonstrated that the prognostic significance of initial blood pressure readings related to the site of hemorrhage. The mean initial blood pressures in 383 patients with fatal outcomes were compared to those in 1318 patients who survived, and higher blood pressures were found in the fatal putaminal and thalamic hemorrhages but not in the fatal subcortical, cerebellar, or pontine hemorrhages, relative to those who survived (67). Another study not only confirmed that elevated initial mean arterial blood pressure (MABP >145 mmHg) was associated with a worse outcome but also that lowering blood pressure (to MABP <125 mmHg) 2 to 6 hr following admission was associated with a better outcome (68). An effect of blood pressure on hematoma enlargement is one possible explanation for the association of poorer outcome with lowering initially high blood pressure. This was perhaps first suggested by Chen et al., who noted persistent hypertension in 6 out of 8 ICH patients prior to hematoma enlargement, 4 of whom died. In each instance, clinical deterioration was linked to hematoma enlargement (69). Another series linked early hematoma expansion and neurologic deterioration to elevated blood pressure (systolic blood pressure ≥195 mmHg) in 8 patients scanned within 2½ hr of onset (70). A more recent study demonstrated that early neurologic deterioration was associated with enlargement of hemorrhage, IVH, and systolic blood pressure (71). Early neurologic deterioration was itself associated with an 8-fold increase in the probability of a poor functional outcome. This is the most convincing evidence to date that elevated blood pressure could be linked to poor functional outcome by increasing the risk of hematoma expansion.

As Table 1 indicates, in multivariate models predicting outcome in ICH, blood pressure measured in a variety of ways at various times following symptom onset, is inconsistently associated with outcome. However, it is likely that elevated pressure early in the patient's course is associated with a poorer outcome and might be a causative factor. Whether lowering of blood pressure (and to what degree) is beneficial remains to be demonstrated in a controlled trial.

Intraventricular Hemorrhage

Expansion of ICH to the ventricles is associated with poor outcome. This phenomenon was initially observed in descriptive studies, which noted that IVH was associated with larger intraparenchymal hemorrhage size and, therefore, could not determine the relative importance of these factors in affecting outcome (72,73). Subsequent multivariate analyses confirmed the independent contribution of the volume of IVH to poor outcome (35,58,65). As with hydrocephalus, the value of ventriculostomy alone in improving prognosis is unclear, but the use of intraventricular recombinant tissue plasminogen activator results in more rapid clearance of blood and may improve outcome (74).

CONCLUSION

Despite no single proven effective therapy, the prognosis of ICH has appeared to improve in the past 20 years, in part because of the ability to identify smaller hemorrhages by modern imaging but perhaps also because of modern neurointensive care (75). It has even been suggested that the accuracy of some of the models discussed above might reflect a "self-fulfilling prophecy" in which care is not provided to those deemed unlikely to survive, when, in fact, aggressive treatment could result in "reasonable" neurologic outcomes (76). Although this thesis remains difficult to either be verified or disproved, the congruence of many predictors of short-term mortality and long-term disability suggests that even the most sophisticated aggressive care still has a limited impact on outcome, however it is measured. Smaller observational studies have given way to larger, more sophisticated analyses, which have identified factors that can serve as targets for specific interventions, such as hematoma expansion, IVH, hydrocephalus, and elevated blood pressure.

REFERENCES

1. Juvela S. Risk factors for impaired outcome after spontaneous intracerebral hemorrhage. Arch Neurol 1995; 52(12):1193–1200.
2. Barber M, Roditi G, Stott DJ, et al. Poor outcome in primary intracerebral haemorrhage: results of a matched comparison. Postgrad Med J 2004; 80(940):89–92.
3. Qureshi AI, Safdar K, Weil J, et al. Predictors of early deterioration and mortality in black Americans with spontaneous intracerebral hemorrhage. Stroke 1995; 26(10):1764–1767.
4. Hier DB, Davis KR, Richardson EP Jr., et al. Hypertensive putaminal hemorrhage. Ann Neurol 1977; 1(2):152–159.
5. Kanaya H, Kuroda K. Development in neurosurgical approaches to hypertensive intracerebral hemorrhage in Japan. In: Kaufman HH (ed): Intracerebral Hematomas: Etiology, Pathophysiology, Clinical Presentation and Treatment. New York: Raven, 1992: 197–210.
6. Stein RW, Kase CS, Hier DB, et al. Caudate hemorrhage. Neurology 1984; 34(12):1549–1554.
7. Walshe TM, Davis KR, Fisher CM. Thalamic hemorrhage: a computed tomographic-clinical correlation. Neurology 1977; 27(3):217–222.

8. Barraquer-Bordas L, Escartin A, Ruscalleda J, et al. Thalamic hemorrhage. A study of 23 patients with diagnosis by computed tomography. Stroke 1981; 12(4):524–527.

9. Kwak R, Kadoya S, Suzuki T. Factors affecting the prognosis in thalamic hemorrhage. Stroke 1983; 14(4):493–500.

10. Weisberg LA. Thalamic hemorrhage: clinical-CT correlations. Neurology 1986; 36(10):1382–1386.

11. Piepgras U, Riegerand P. Thalamic bleeding: diagnosis, course and prognosis. Neuroradiology 1981; 22(2):85–91.

12. Hirose G, Kosoegawa H, Saeki M, et al. The syndrome of posterior thalamic hemorrhage. Neurology 1985; 35(7):998–1002.

13. Ropper AH, Davis KR. Lobar cerebral hemorrhages: acute clinical syndromes in 26 cases. Ann Neurol 1980; 8(2):141–147.

14. Kase CS, Williams JP, Wyatt DA, et al. Lobar intracerebral hematomas: clinical and CT analysis of 22 cases. Neurology 1982; 32(10):1146–1150.

15. Tanaka Y, Furuse M, Iwasa H, et al. Lobar intracerebral hemorrhage: etiology and a long-term follow-up study of 32 patients. Stroke 1986; 17(1):51–57.

16. Weisberg LA. Subcortical lobar intracerebral haemorrhage: clinical-computed tomographic correlations. J Neurol Neurosurg Psychiatry 1985; 48(11):1078–1084.

17. Silverstein A. Primary pontile hemorrhage. A review of 50 cases. Confin Neurol 1967; 29(1):33–46.

18. Tuhrim S, Yang WC, Rubinowitz H, et al. Primary pontine hemorrhage and the dysarthria-clumsy hand syndrome. Neurology 1982; 32(9):1027–1028.

19. Kilpatrick TJ, Davis SM, Tress BM. Lateral tegmental haemorrhage due to vascular malformations. Cerebrovasc Res 1991; 108.

20. Burns J, Lisak R, Schut L, et al. Recovery following brainstem hemorrhage. Ann Neurol 1980; 7(2):183–184.

21. Payne HA, Maravilla KR, Levinstone A, et al. Recovery from primary pontine hemorrhage. Ann Neurol 1978; 4(6):557–558.

22. Weisberg LA. Primary pontine haemorrhage: clinical and computed tomographic correlations. J Neurol Neurosurg Psychiatry 1986; 49(4):346–352.

23. Ott KH, Kase CS, Ojemann RG, et al. Cerebellar hemorrhage: diagnosis and treatment. A review of 56 cases. Arch Neurol 1974; 31(3):160–167.

24. Little JR, Tubman DE, Ethier R. Cerebellar hemorrhage in adults. Diagnosis by computerized tomography. J Neurosurg 1978; 48(4):575–579.

25. Fisher CM, Picard ED, Polak A. Acute hypertensive cerebellar hemorrhage: diagnosis and treatment. Arch Neurol 1974; 160.

26. Furlan AJ, Whisnant JP, Elveback LR. The decreasing incidence of primary intracerebral hemorrhage: a population study. Ann Neurol 1979; 5(4):367–373.

27. Drury I, Whisnant JP, Garraway WM. Primary intracerebral hemorrhage: impact of CT on incidence. Neurology 1984; 34(5):653–657.

28. Fieschi C, Carolei A, Fiorelli M, et al. Changing prognosis of primary intracerebral hemorrhage: results of a clinical and computed tomographic follow-up study of 104 patients. Stroke 1988; 19(2):192–195.

29. Garde A, Bohmer G, Selden B, et al. Hundred cases of spontaneous intracerebral haematoma. Diagnosis, treatment, and prognosis. Eur Neurol 1983; 22(3):161–172.

30. Steiner I, Gomori JM, Melamed E. The prognostic value of the CT scan in conservatively treated patients with intracerebral hematoma. Stroke 1984; 15(2):279–282.

31. Nath FP, Nicholls D, Fraser RJ. Prognosis in intracerebral haemorrhage. Acta Neurochir (Wien) 1983; 67(1–2):29–35.

32. Mayr U, Bauer P, Fischer J. Non-traumatic intracerebral haemorrhage. Prognostic implications of neurological and computer-tomographical findings in 100 consecutive patients. Neurochirurgia (Stuttg) 1983; 26(2):36–41.

33. Helweg-Larsen S, Sommer W, Strange P, et al. Prognosis for patients treated conservatively for spontaneous intracerebral hematomas. Stroke 1984; 15(6):1045–1048.

34. Ropper AH. Lateral displacement of the brain and level of consciousness in patients with an acute hemispheral mass. N Engl J Med 1986; 314(15):953–958.

35. Tuhrim S, Dambrosia JM, Price TR, et al. Intracerebral hemorrhage: external validation and extension of a model for prediction of 30-day survival. Ann Neurol 1991; 29(6):658–663.

36. Daverat P, Castel JP, Dartigues JF, et al. Death and functional outcome after spontaneous intracerebral hemorrhage. A prospective study of 166 cases using multivariate analysis. Stroke 1991; 22(1):1–6.

37. Dixon AA, Holness RO, Howes WJ, et al. Spontaneous intracerebral haemorrhage: an analysis of factors affecting prognosis. Can J Neurol Sci 1985; 12(3):267–271.

38. Portenoy RK, Lipton RB, Berger AR, et al. Intracerebral haemorrhage: a model for the prediction of outcome. J Neurol Neurosurg Psychiatry 1987; 50(8):976–979.

39. Senant J, Samson M, Proust B, et al. A multi-factorial approach in the vital prognosis of spontaneous intracerebral hematoma. Rev Neurol (Paris) 1988; 144(4):279–283.

40. Tuhrim S, Dambrosia JM, Price TR, et al. Prediction of intracerebral hemorrhage survival. Ann Neurol 1988; 24(2):258–263.
41. Hemphill JC III, Bonovich DC, Besmertis L, et al. The ICH score: a simple, reliable grading scale for intracerebral hemorrhage. Stroke 2001; 32(4):891–897.
42. Garibi J, Bilbao G, Pomposo I, et al. Prognostic factors in a series of 185 consecutive spontaneous supratentorial intracerebral haematomas. Br J Neurosurg 2002; 16(4):355–361.
43. Cheung RT, Zou LY. Use of the original, modified, or new intracerebral hemorrhage score to predict mortality and morbidity after intracerebral hemorrhage. Stroke 2003; 34(7):1717–1722.
44. Broderick JP, Brott TG, Duldner JE, et al. Volume of intracerebral hemorrhage. A powerful and easy-to-use predictor of 30-day mortality. Stroke 1993; 24(7):987–993.
45. Lisk DR, Pasteur W, Rhoades H, et al. Early presentation of hemispheric intracerebral hemorrhage: prediction of outcome and guidelines for treatment allocation. Neurology 1994; 44(1):133–139.
46. Shapiro SA, Campbell RL, Scully T. Hemorrhagic dilation of the fourth ventricle: an ominous predictor. J Neurosurg 1994; 80(5):805–809.
47. Mase G, Zorzon M, Biasutti E, et al. Immediate prognosis of primary intracerebral hemorrhage using an easy model for the prediction of survival. Acta Neurol Scand 1995; 91(4):306–309.
48. Fogelholm R, Avikainen S, Murros K. Prognostic value and determinants of first-day mean arterial pressure in spontaneous supratentorial intracerebral hemorrhage. Stroke 1997; 28(7):1396–1400.
49. Diringer MN, Edwards DF, Zazulia AR. Hydrocephalus: a previously unrecognized predictor of poor outcome from supratentorial intracerebral hemorrhage. Stroke 1998; 29(7):1352–1357.
50. Fujii Y, Takeuchi S, Sasaki O, et al. Multivariate analysis of predictors of hematoma enlargement in spontaneous intracerebral hemorrhage. Stroke 1998; 29(6):1160–1166.
51. Razzaq AA, Hussain R. Determinants of 30-day mortality of spontaneous intracerebral hemorrhage in Pakistan. Surg Neurol 1998; 50(4):336–342; discussion 342–343.
52. Tuhrim S, Horowitz DR, Sacher M, et al. Volume of ventricular blood is an important determinant of outcome in supratentorial intracerebral hemorrhage. Crit Care Med 1999; 27(3):617–621.
53. Phan TG, Koh M, Vierkant RA, et al. Hydrocephalus is a determinant of early mortality in putaminal hemorrhage. Stroke 2000; 31(9):2157–2162.
54. Hallevy C, Ifergane G, Kordysh E, et al. Spontaneous supratentorial intracerebral hemorrhage. Criteria for short-term functional outcome prediction. J Neurol 2002; 249(12):1704–1709.
55. Fang HY, Lin CY, Ko WJ. Hematology and coagulation parameters predict outcome in Taiwanese patients with spontaneous intracerebral hemorrhage. Eur J Neurol 2005; 12(3):226–232.
56. Kumral E, Kocaer T, Ertubey NO, et al. Thalamic hemorrhage. A prospective study of 100 patients. Stroke 1995; 26(6):964–970.
57. Radberg JA, Olsson JE, Radberg CT. Prognostic parameters in spontaneous intracerebral hematomas with special reference to anticoagulant treatment. Stroke 1991; 22(5):571–576.
58. Young WB, Lee KP, Pessin MS, et al. Prognostic significance of ventricular blood in supratentorial hemorrhage: a volumetric study. Neurology 1990; 40(4):616–619.
59. Forsting M, Mattle HP, Huber P. Anticoagulation-related intracerebral hemorrhage. Cerebrovasc Dis 1991:97.
60. Rosand J, Eckman MH, Knudsen KA, et al. The effect of warfarin and intensity of anticoagulation on outcome of intracerebral hemorrhage. Arch Intern Med 2004; 164(8):880–884.
61. Flibotte JJ, Hagan N, O'Donnell J, et al. Warfarin, hematoma expansion, and outcome of intracerebral hemorrhage. Neurology 2004; 63(6):1059–1064.
62. Kazui S, Naritomi H, Yamamoto H, et al. Enlargement of spontaneous intracerebral hemorrhage. Incidence and time course. Stroke 1996; 27(10):1783–1787.
63. Brott T, Broderick J, Kothari R, et al. Early hemorrhage growth in patients with intracerebral hemorrhage. Stroke 1997; 28(1):1–5.
64. Mayer SA, Brun NC, Begtrup K, et al. Recombinant activated factor VII for acute intracerebral hemorrhage. N Engl J Med 2005; 352(8):777–785.
65. Willmot M, Leonardi-Bee J, Bath PM. High blood pressure in acute stroke and subsequent outcome: a systematic review. Hypertension 2004; 43(1):18–24.
66. Wallace JD, Levy LL. Blood pressure after stroke. JAMA 1981; 246(19):2177–2180.
67. Terayama Y, Tanahashi N, Fukuuchi Y, et al. Prognostic value of admission blood pressure in patients with intracerebral hemorrhage. Keio Cooperative Stroke Study. Stroke 1997; 28(6):1185–1188.
68. Dandapani BK, Suzuki S, Kelley RE, et al. Relation between blood pressure and outcome in intracerebral hemorrhage. Stroke 1995; 26(1):21–24.
69. Chen ST, Chen SD, Hsu CY, et al. Progression of hypertensive intracerebral hemorrhage. Neurology 1989; 39(11):1509–1514.
70. Broderick JP, Brott TG, Tomsick T, et al. Ultra-early evaluation of intracerebral hemorrhage. J Neurosurg 1990; 72(2):195–199.
71. Leira R, Davalos A, Silva Y, et al. Early neurologic deterioration in intracerebral hemorrhage: predictors and associated factors. Neurology 2004; 63(3):461–467.

72. Hayashi M, Handa Y, Kobayashi H, et al. Prognosis of intraventricular hemorrhage due to hypertensive hemorrhagic cerebrovascular disease. Zentralbl Neurochir 1988; 49(2):101–108.

73. Weisberg LA, Elliott D, Shamsnia M. Intraventricular hemorrhage in adults: clinical-computed tomographic correlations. Comput Med Imaging Graph 1991; 15(1):43–51.

74. Naff NJ, Hanley DF, Keyl PM, et al. Intraventricular thrombolysis speeds blood clot resolution: results of a pilot, prospective, randomized, double-blind, controlled trial. Neurosurgery 2004; 54(3):577–583; discussion 583–584.

75. Diringer MN, Edwards DF. Admission to a neurologic/neurosurgical intensive care unit is associated with reduced mortality rate after intracerebral hemorrhage. Crit Care Med 2001; 29(3):635–640.

76. Becker KJ, Baxter AB, Cohen WA, et al. Withdrawal of support in intracerebral hemorrhage may lead to self-fulfilling prophecies. Neurology 2001; 56(6):766–772.

16 | Animal Models of Ischemic Stroke

Turgut Tatlisumak, MD, Associate Professor and Vice Chairman
Department of Neurology, University of Helsinki, Helsinki University Central Hospital, Helsinki, Finland

Fuhai Li, MD, Resident
Department of Neurology, Duke University School of Medicine, Duke University Medical Center, Durham, North Carolina, USA

Marc Fisher, MD, Professor
Department of Neurology, University of Massachusetts Medical School, Worcester, Massachusetts, USA

INTRODUCTION

Ischemic stroke is a major public health issue that requires urgent efforts toward development of novel remedies, and focal brain ischemia animal models significantly aid in these efforts. They have been developed with significant effort to closely mimic the changes that occur during and after human stroke. Models help us to learn about the pathogenesis of stroke and to define the biochemical changes in tissue during ischemia, toward potential discovery of mechanisms involved in the evolution of ischemic injury. These discoveries could lead to the development of novel molecules designed to reduce the undesirable consequences of ischemia, and these same animal models can be utilized to test whether the novel molecules have beneficial anti-ischemic effects *in vivo*. When combined with various imaging techniques, such as MRI or positron emission tomography, these models provide versatile information on the evolution of ischemic damage, pathophysiologic aspects, and the size of the lesion. In that human ischemic stroke is often caused by occlusion of the middle cerebral artery (MCA) or one of its branches (1), most focal cerebral ischemia models were developed to induce ischemia within the MCA territory. Ideally, an ischemic stroke animal model satisfies the following criteria (2): (i) the ischemic processes and pathophysiologic changes should be relevant to human ischemic stroke, (ii) the ischemic lesion should be reproducible, (iii) the technique used to induce ischemia should be relatively easy to perform and minimally invasive, (iv) physiologic variables can be monitored and maintained within normal ranges, (v) brain samples should be readily available for outcome measurements, such as histopathologic, biochemical, and molecular biologic evaluation and (vi) the cost and effort should be reasonable.

Focal brain ischemia models can be divided into transient (temporary, ischemia-reperfusion) ischemia and permanent ischemia models. The ability to use one animal model for both types of ischemia is important, because in human stroke, most patients experience recanalization (either spontaneous or treatment induced) at various time points following stroke onset (3).

ANIMAL SELECTION

Although higher species, such as cats, rabbits, dogs, pigs, and nonhuman primates, can be used in focal ischemia models, small animals, such as rats, mice, and gerbils, are more commonly used. The rat is the most commonly used animal in stroke studies owing to numerous reasons, including (i) their resemblance to humans in cerebrovascular anatomy and physiology, (ii) their moderate size, which allows researchers to easily monitor the physiologic parameters and collect the brain specimens, (iii) the low cost of animals, in terms of transportation, storage, and feeding, (iv) the relative homogeneity within strains from inbreeding, (v) their small brain size, which is well suited to fixation procedures and microscopic and macroscopic examination, (vi) the ease of conducting reproducible studies, and (vii) the greater acceptability of their use (compared to subhuman primates and pet animals) from ecologic and ethical perspectives (4–6). Mice have been of increasing interest because of the availability of transgenic technology, which offers new insights into the molecular mechanisms involved in ischemic stroke. The gerbil might not be a good candidate for testing potential neuroprotective agents, as many neuroprotective agents effective in the gerbil failed to protect against ischemic damage in other species (7). Brain infarcts are more uniform in lower animal species, and reproducibility is significantly better when the MCA is occluded proximally, preferably at or near its orifice. Models of MCA occlusion (MCAO) in primates were developed in the 1930s (8). However, because of the relatively higher cost, difficulty in experimental procedures, and ethical concerns, higher species of animals are used more limitedly. Nevertheless, it might be reasonable and necessary to consider testing neuroprotective agents in larger animal stroke models to determine if the compound is broadly effective before beginning clinical trials (7).

The spontaneously hypertensive rat (SHR) and its variant stroke-prone SHR develop larger infarcts with lesser variability following MCAO (9,10). Many SHRs develop large infarcts upon occlusion of the common carotid arteries bilaterally, whereas other rats do not develop macroscopic infarctions (11). The susceptibility of SHRs to developing larger infarcts probably stems from a lack of collateral blood flow. Reduction of infarct volume by experimental agents in SHRs is regarded as a more stringent test than in other rat strains but is more difficult to achieve. Stroke-prone SHRs frequently develop spontaneous infarcts and might be of use in chronic primary prevention studies.

Most researchers use solely male animals for brain ischemia studies, a practice well justified, as this approach avoids experimental variability caused by female hormones. The relationship between biologic sex and ischemic stroke outcome has been greatly explored mainly in rodents. The overwhelming majority of published studies reported that female rodents sustain smaller infarctions than males following focal brain ischemia (12–14), although one study showed no difference between genders (15). The menstrual cycle might be critical, as female rats in proestrus (high endogenous estradiol levels) developed significantly smaller infarcts than those in the metestrus phase (low endogenous estradiol levels), indicating that estrogen itself might have neuroprotective properties (16). Furthermore, gender differences could be abolished following ovariectomy (12) or after menopause (17). Estrogen administration to female, intact male, and castrated male rats reduced infarct sizes in almost all studies (12,14,18). All of this evidence suggests that replicating studies in both sexes might add to our knowledge, but it is not yet known at what stage of the menstrual cycle female animals should undergo ischemia procedures.

APPROACHES FOR INDUCING FOCAL CEREBRAL ISCHEMIA

Focal cerebral ischemia can be induced by many techniques, including intraluminal suture insertion, thromboembolus injection, direct surgical occlusion of the MCA or carotid artery, embolization of microspheres, photochemical thrombosis, and application of endothelin. The primary focus of this discussion will be on MCAO models because of their increasing popularity in developing neuroprotective, thrombolytic, and restorative drugs. Other models will only be briefly mentioned.

Carotid Artery Occlusion

Unilateral carotid artery occlusion in most animals does not lead to ischemic changes unless combined with severe hypotension (19) or asphyxia (20). The same procedure, however, leads to even fatal strokes in gerbils, as the gerbil lacks a functioning Circle of Willis (21,22) and, therefore, gerbil cerebrovascular anatomy is different from human anatomy. Furthermore, the gerbil focal brain ischemia models present several other disadvantages: (i) not all animals develop an infarction (22), (ii) many animals with an infarction develop seizures (23), (iii) the body temperature decreases too easily, and (iv) blood sampling is technically extremely difficult because of the small size (50–80 g) of adult gerbils.

The unilateral carotid artery occlusion model can also be applied in monkeys and dogs, in which the anterior communicating and posterior communicating arteries are ligated first and the common carotid artery (CCA) is subsequently ligated to produce focal cerebral ischemia (24,25). Finally, SHRs develop large infarctions upon bilateral CCA occlusion (11). CCA occlusion models pose no advantages over MCAO models and are seldom used.

Middle Cerebral Artery Occlusion Models

Intraluminal Suture (Monofilament) Middle Cerebral Artery Occlusion Model
The intraluminal suture (monofilament) MCAO model is the most commonly used in focal brain ischemia studies, probably because it is relatively easy to perform and less invasive than other

models. Because a craniectomy is not required, damage from brain retraction, vessel manipulation, temperature loss, and desiccation of exposed brain are all avoided. In this model, the MCA is occluded by inserting a monofilament suture into the internal carotid artery (ICA) to block blood flow to the MCA (Fig. 1). Either permanent or transient MCAO can be simply achieved by maintaining or withdrawing the monofilament suture. This suture MCAO model was originally described in rats in 1986 and later modified (26). Usually, a 3-0 or 4-0 monofilament suture is used as the occluder. The monofilament can be coated with silicone (26,27) or poly-L-lysine (28), or it can be used without coating (29,30). The suture occluder can be inserted through the CCA, the ICA, or the external carotid artery. The length of suture inserted from the bifurcation of the CCA is approximately 17 to 22 mm (31–33), depending on body weight, size of the suture tip, rat strain, and location of the bifurcation.

The typical infarct areas induced by this suture model include both the lateral caudoputamen and frontoparietal cortex (Fig. 2). It is established that a substantial ischemic penumbra exists in this model early after ischemia (34) and that the infarct size induced by prolonged ischemia (>90 min) is relatively reproducible, thus making this model appropriate for testing neuroprotective agents. However, it must be remembered that many factors can affect infarct size. First, one study showed that a slight difference in aspects of the monofilament (i.e., diameter, tensile strength, and extensibility) can cause a significant difference in infarct volume (35). Second, the ischemia induced by a silicone-coated suture is likely more substantial and less variable (28,29); consequently, the infarct volume is more reproducible and larger than that induced by an uncoated suture (29,30). Third, a longer insertion distance of the monofilament suture might give rise to larger infarction because the deeper insertion of the suture can also obstruct blood flow in some branches of the anterior cerebral artery (32). Lastly, inadvertent premature reperfusion might also cause variability of infarct volume (36). It is therefore important that consistent and standardized surgical procedures and techniques be used to generate reproducible lesions.

The suture MCAO method was also successfully applied to mice because transgenic or knockout mice provide unique avenues for basic research into the molecular mechanisms that

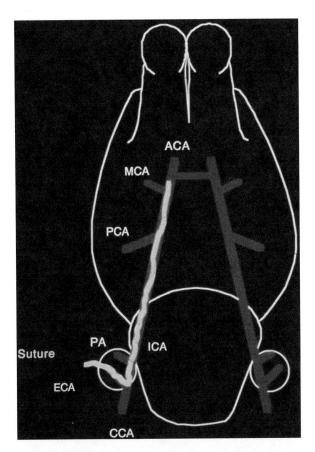

Figure 1 A schematic representation of the suture-occlusion model, demonstrating occlusion of the entire middle cerebral artery. *Abbreviations*: ACA, anterior carotid artery; MCA, middle cerebral artery; PA, plasminogen activator; ICA, internal carotid artery; CCA, common carotid artery.

contribute to ischemic cell damage and development of novel therapeutic interventions (37–39). Usually, a 5-0 monofilament nylon suture or 8-0 suture coated with silicone is used to occlude blood flow to the MCA territory. The insertion depth from the bifurcation of the CCA is approximately 9 to 11 mm (38,39). The lesion is reproducible and its distribution is similar to that of the rat. Recently, the suture occlusion model could successfully be applied to neonatal rats that weigh 14 to 19 g (40) and to adult rabbits (41).

Another important role for this MCAO method is that it can be modified to induce ischemia in an MRI unit by remotely advancing the suture occluder, the so-called "in-bore suture MCAO model" (33,42–44). Combined with new MRI techniques, this in-bore occlusion method enables researchers to monitor *in vivo* ischemic changes at a very early time point after the onset of ischemia and to acquire both pre- and postischemic data for later pixel-by-pixel comparison. The in-bore MCAO method was improved recently and achieved a high success rate (33).

Similar to the intraluminal suture occlusion model, some investigators used a silicone plastic catheter as a plug to occlude the MCA in dogs via the left ICA (45). In this study, MCAO and reperfusion upon withdrawal of the catheter could be demonstrated by angiography in all 19 mongrel dogs. Unfortunately, infarct sizes and locations varied largely (45). Various catheter models with inflating balloon tips have been used to occlude the MCA in several species.

Some disadvantages and complications are associated with the intraluminal suture MCAO model. Subarachnoid hemorrhage might occur because of inadvertent arterial rupture caused by the suture, a complication that is likely to have higher incidence with uncoated sutures than with silicone-coated sutures (28,36). In addition, spontaneous hyperthermia occurs when the ischemic duration lasts >2 hr, most likely due to ischemic damage of the hypothalamus, which is caused by blockage of small branches to the hypothalamus by suture insertion (46,47). Finally, the inner surface of vessels might be mechanically injured by the suture, which can complicate reperfusion.

Application of laser-Doppler flowmetry or electroencephalography during and after induction of ischemia in this model substantially reduced the incidence of complications, such as subarachnoid hemorrhage, incomplete MCAO, or premature reperfusion (36). Ipsilateral cortical laser-Doppler flowmetry signal immediately and abruptly decreases to approximately 20% of baseline following MCAO and substantially recovers following premature or induced reperfusion. Similarly, MCAO causes severe suppression of the ipsilateral hemispheric electroencephalographic signal, with a delay of 5 to 10 sec and recovers after reperfusion. Both methods could substantially increase successful MCAO rates and reduce the complications sometimes associated with this model (36).

Thromboembolic Model
Focal ischemia induced by thromboemboli is of great interest because of its resemblance to human ischemic stroke (approximately 80% of which are caused by thromboembolism) (48) and because of its role in evaluating thrombolytic therapy. Thrombolytic therapy, with recombinant tissue plasminogen activator (rtPA) administered intravenously within 3 hr after onset of ischemic stroke, improves neurologic outcome in humans (49) and is a standard therapy in carefully selected

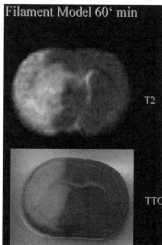

Figure 2 Demonstration of infarction on T2-weighted MRI and with TTC staining from a rat subjected to the suture-occlusion model. *Abbreviation*: TTC, 2,3,5-triphenyltetrazolium chloride.

patients. Thromboembolic animal models are therefore playing an increasingly important role. Single-clot embolization models were developed for several species, including rabbit (50), dog (51,52), rat (53,54), mouse (55,56), guinea pig (57), and monkey (58,59).

Thromboembolic ischemia can be produced by a photochemical approach or by injection of autologous or heterologous thrombi. The photochemical method produces an arterial lesion in the CCA that results in formation of a platelet-rich thrombus, which can then dislodge and embolize to distal vessels (60,61). The photochemically induced thromboemboli are platelet-rich and, therefore, might not be amenable to thrombolytic therapy with rtPA.

The most commonly used thromboembolic model is blood-clot injection (Fig. 3) in the rat. In the early versions of this model, a suspension of microembolic clot was injected, causing diffuse and inhomogeneous infarction in the MCA territory because of peripheral branch microembolization. Scattered, multifocal lesions were also observed in the territories of the anterior cerebral artery and posterior cerebral artery and even in the contralateral hemisphere (53,54). In addition, early spontaneous recanalization frequently occurred, which made evaluation of thrombolytic therapy difficult. The early autolysis of blood clots might be due to a more fragile red thrombus formed *in vitro* by whole blood. To overcome these problems, a more resistant white thrombus was produced by using a mobile, high-pressure, closed compartment system (PE-10 polyethylene tube, 0.28 mm in inner diameter) (62). Using white thrombi, a substantial reduction of cerebral blood flow (CBF) was demonstrated in the affected region, with no spontaneous recanalization at 2 hr after embolization, a condition necessary for studying thrombolytic treatment (62). However, infarct size was variable and ischemia caused by multiple small clots did not mimic typical clinical ischemic stroke. An ideal thromboembolic model should employ a blood clot that appropriately lodges in the proximal segment of the MCA, with the distal branches remaining open. Smaller clots embolize distally into the cerebral vessels, whereas larger clots lodge in vessels too proximal from the origin of MCA. Therefore, the size (length and diameter) and characteristics (i.e., more rigid fibrin-rich clot) of blood clots are crucial in this model. Recently (63), a rat clot model was developed in which 12 medium-sized (1.5 × 0.35 mm), fibrin-rich autologous clots formed in a PE-50 catheter (0.58 mm in inner diameter) were injected to produce reliable occlusion of the proximal MCA. Consistent reduction of CBF and histologic damage in the MCA territory were observed. Visual inspection demonstrated no early spontaneous clot lysis in the ipsilateral vessels and no clots in the contralateral vessels at 3 hr

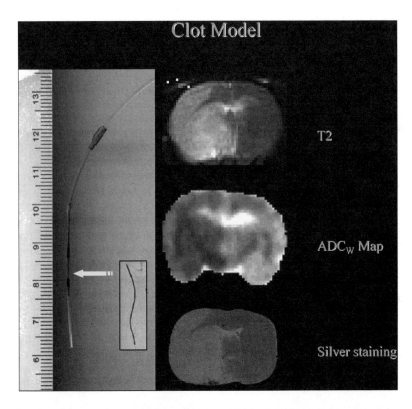

Figure 3 A clot in polyethylene tubing (*left*). An infarct on MRI and with silver staining (*right*). *Abbreviation*: ADC, apparent diffusion coefficient.

after injection. It was demonstrated that thrombolytic therapy with rtPA (63) or prourokinase (64) can recanalize the occluded MCA. By inserting a modified tube into the ICA 2 to 3 mm proximal to the MCA origin, a single, fibrin-rich clot (25×0.1 mm) could also be selectively introduced into the proximal part of the MCA (65), or a thrombosis could be induced at the origin of the MCA (66), thus causing typical MCAO. Using this single-clot model, a significant reduction of CBF in the MCA territory was demonstrated, and the blood clot in the MCA trunk was found at 24 hr after embolization (66). This single clot was also applied to occlude the proximal MCA in mouse (55), but one disadvantage is the relatively high incidence of subarachnoid and intraparenchymal hemorrhage. The very same model was successfully transferred to monkeys and led to the development of reproducible infarctions without hemorrhagic complications (59).

In conclusion, these single-clot or medium-sized, multiple-clot models induce predictable and reproducible infarcts in both extent and size in the MCA territory, similar to those caused by the intraluminal suture model. Embolization of the proximal MCA trunk by a single, fibrin-rich clot is similar to human embolic ischemia, because the majority of human ischemic strokes are caused by a single embolus in the MCA territory (1). Therefore, the single-clot model is promising for studying the pathogenesis of ischemic stroke and thrombolytic therapy.

Direct Surgical Middle Cerebral Artery Occlusion Model

Direct surgical MCAO is invasive, as it requires a craniectomy. In this model, ischemia can be induced by directly ligating, coagulating, clipping, or snaring the MCA trunk or its branches. The MCAO in the rat can be permanent or transient (67–69), can be performed under anesthesia or in awake animals and has been performed in nonhuman primates (70,71), dogs (25,72), rabbits (73,74), cats (75,76), rats (77), and mice (78). The rat is the most common species on which surgical MCAO has been performed.

Many models of focal brain ischemia have utilized temporary or permanent occlusion of the MCA in various animal species, with various routes described, including the subfrontal route (8), the retro-orbital route (79), and the transorbital route (71,80). With all of these large-animal models, the fundamental problem was the extreme variability of infarct size among animals. Among the first studies with reproducible infarct sizes was the description of a cat model with left MCAO via a transorbital approach, combined with bilateral ligation of internal carotid arteries (81). The transorbital method requires removal of the eyeball but is otherwise considered to be atraumatic, because it is not necessary to retract the brain for exposure of the vessel. The postorbital approach to the MCA in cats was developed later and revealed reproducible infarct sizes (82). The advantage of this model is that it does not necessitate enucleation of the eye, but it is technically much more complicated.

Direct ligation of the distal MCA at the rhinal fissure in the rat (77) was first described in 1975. The typical ischemic injury induced by such a method is in the frontoparietal cortex, but the extent of lesion is quite variable, ranging from 1 to 5 mm in diameter. Surgical occlusions more proximally in the MCA trunk were performed through a subtemporal craniectomy (83,84). Occluding the main trunk of the MCA proximal to the lenticulostriatal branches that supply the lateral caudoputamen results in an infarction always involving both the frontal cortex and the lateral part of the caudoputamen. A more distal occlusion of the MCA (sparing the lenticulostriate branches) restricts the infarction to the cortex (68). Tandem occlusion of the MCA and the ipsilateral CCA improves the reproducibility of infarction (85). Similarly, simultaneous occlusions of the MCA and the ipsilateral CCA, combined with transient occlusion of the contralateral CCA, leads to good reproducibility of infarcts (86). Use of microclips, hooks, or ligature snares instead of electrocoagulation allows for later reperfusion (67,87,88). The infarction areas induced by a proximal MCAO appear to be larger and less variable, compared with those induced by distal MCAO. As focal occlusion of the MCA might not always produce infarction, even when the occlusion is performed at the proximal MCA trunk, researchers have refined this model and demonstrated that both the site and extent of MCAO affect the neuropathologic outcome and are critical factors in producing reproducible infarction (89). Occlusion of a very short segment (1–2 mm) of the MCA resulted in greater variability of infarction, and the rate of infarction was low when focal MCAO was performed at the origin of the MCA. This might relate to the persistence of abundant collateral circulation. Furthermore, because MCA branching is variable (90), such a focal occlusion at one point might not really involve both the lenticulostriatal and cortical branches. Interestingly, in the young (36 days) rat, MCAO beyond the point of origin of the lenticulostriate branches did not cause neuronal injury, probably because of better collateral supply (5).

A long, segmental occlusion of the MCA (3–6 mm) beginning proximal to the olfactory tract, however, induces uniform infarction in both extent and location in all rats. This extensive occlusion involves the lenticulostriate and small cortical branches and, therefore, produces reproducible infarction. However, the ischemic penumbra in this model might be small (91) and less amenable to testing neuroprotective compounds. This model is appropriate for investigating cerebrovascular function after focal ischemia (92). Because of higher long-term survival of rats due to the relatively small lesion, this model is a good option for screening stroke restorative drugs (7). Interestingly, in one study, MCAO alone led to infarction in only 50% of mongrel dogs, whereas 75% developed infarcts upon tandem occlusion of the MCA and the ipsilateral carotid artery (93).

Some disadvantages are associated with direct surgical MCAO models. First, performing this model is more difficult and requires more experience and technical skill due to varying MCA anatomic patterns (84). Second, direct exposure of brain to air after craniectomy might change intracranial pressure and blood–brain barrier permeability (5). Third, a small amount of subarachnoid hemorrhage around the MCA trunk can occur (84). Although these models had been extensively used, they have now been largely replaced by the intraluminal suture MCAO model.

Nonclot Embolus Models

Many materials, such as plastic microspheres, silicone cylinders, viscous silicone, collagen, and air, can be injected to induce ischemic injury as emboli via the CCA or the ICA (94–96). The magnitude and severity of ischemic damage induced by these embolic models depends on the number and size of the embolic particles injected (97). The injection of sodium arachidonate into the ICA of rats induced widespread intravascular cerebral thrombosis (98). Previously, diffuse distribution and inhomogeneous infarction were the neuropathologic hallmarks of these models, making histologic evaluation difficult. However, these models have recently been refined, and injection of 6 ceramic spheres, 0.3 to 0.4 mm in diameter, into the CCA via the external carotid artery leads to reproducible infarcts (99). The advantage of this model is the lack of potential hyperthermia, but the disadvantage is that it does not allow reperfusion. Single silver or golden ball injections into the ICA, which leads to MCAO, have already been used for decades in larger animals (100).

Various amounts of microfibrillar collagen, which was frequently used in neurosurgery as a topical hemostatic agent, were injected directly into the left CCA and resulted in cerebral infarcts of various sizes, shapes, locations (within the MCA territory), and number in 9 out of 10 mongrel dogs (101). A catheter with an inflatable balloon tip that was inserted into the MCA of baboons and was kept in place for 3 hr led to formation of an *in situ* thrombosis (102). Similarly, artificial embolic materials have successfully been used for inducing MCA-territory ischemia in several species, including monkeys (103).

Photochemically Induced Thrombosis Model

In this model, the ischemic injury is induced by vascular injection of a photoactive dye, such as rose bengal (104) or photofrin (105), in combination with irradiation with a light beam at a specific wavelength. It has been shown that a reaction between the circulating dye and the light engenders free radicals, leading to platelet aggregation and thrombosis (104). The location and extent of photochemically induced lesions can be well controlled by selectively illuminating the brain tissue and by using different intensities of light and different doses of dye. A typical lesion in this model is a sharply circumscribed infarct that involves only the cortex. However, this model results in a small penumbral region. In addition, breakdown of the blood–brain barrier and vasogenic edema occur very early in this model (106,107). It is debatable whether the lesion induced by this model is secondary to an ischemic event. Although this model was used to test neuroprotective agents (108), its usefulness is limited, because it is believed that the pathophysiologic processes induced in this model are likely to be less relevant to those in human ischemic stroke.

Endothelin-Induced Middle Cerebral Artery Occlusion Model

Endothelin-1 is a 21-amino acid peptide with a potent vasoconstrictor effect (109). Application of endothelin-1 to the exposed MCA induces a significant decrease in CBF. Furthermore, microinjection of endothelin-1 into areas near the MCA through a cannula also decreases CBF in the

MCA territory. The distribution of ischemic infarct induced by this method is similar to that following permanent surgical ligation of the MCA (110). Interestingly, CBF around the ischemic core significantly increases in this model. The advantage of this model is that ischemia can be induced in conscious rats, which excludes the confounding effects of general anesthesia. However, the ischemic damage is variable due to different responses of vessels to endothelin-1 (109), and the duration of ischemia is not controllable, as endothelin-1–mediated vasoconstriction gradually disappears (111). Furthermore, this model requires craniectomy. These limitations inhibit the use of this model in drug development, although it was used to test drug efficacy (110). A modification of this model was developed for the rat by utilizing endothelin-3 instead of endothelin-1 (112), but this model probably suffers from the same limitations. It was recently reported that application of endothelin-1 topically onto the M2 segment of the MCA in marmosets led to marked hemiparesis and both cortical and subcortical infarcts (113).

Cerebral Venous Thrombosis Models

Cerebral venous thrombosis (CVT) is a relatively rare cause of stroke. The most common site for CVT is the superior sagittal sinus (SSS). It is characterized by an *in situ* thrombotic occlusion of one or more sinus, elevated brain parenchymal pressure caused by venous congestion (stasis), elevated cerebral blood volume and decreased regional CBF, blood–brain barrier disruption, and increased net capillary filtration that leads to progressive brain edema. CVT is frequently associated with venous infarctions with or without hemorrhagic transformation, intracerebral hemorrhage, and even subarachnoid hemorrhage. The severity of parenchymal damage is dependent on the degree of involvement of the venous drainage (114).

In the first reported CVT model in 1836, both jugular veins of a rabbit were tied, and the animal died 7 days after the operation (115). Early models concentrated on injecting the SSS with sclerosing substances, such as lard oil, hot paraffin, sodium morhuate, ethanolamine, cyanoacrylate, etc., or on mechanical obstruction of the SSS by electrocoagulation or muscle and cotton tamponades (116). One group injected thrombin directly into the SSS of the dog to induce *in situ* thrombosis (117). In the rabbit, mechanical direct compression of the SSS led to local thrombus formation, which could subsequently be successfully treated with intravenous rtPA infusion (118). SSS could be successfully occluded by the retrograde insertion of a catheter-balloon system in the pig (119). In a rat model, mechanical obstruction of the SSS at 2 separate and distinct sites was combined with an injection of cephalin-caolin suspension into the SSS (116). Ligation of the SSS at a posterior part appears to be critically important for development of brain damage, and the findings are probably more severe with additional involvement of cortical veins. Similar models were developed for various species, including the gerbil (120) and the cat (121), with good success.

Posterior Cerebral Circulation Models

Most focal ischemia models have concentrated on MCA territory ischemia. However, a few other models were designed for ischemia within the posterior parts of the brain.

Basilar artery occlusion combined with bilateral carotid artery occlusion in the rat was first developed in 1985 (122) as a global brain ischemia model and was further refined in 1991 (123). In this model, a single-point occlusion of the basilar artery, regardless of the location of the occlusion, did not produce infarction and was well tolerated by the rats (123). Two-point occlusion of the basilar artery led to small and variable-sized infarctions within the brain stem which were also well tolerated (123). Intracranial administration of picomole amounts of endothelin-1 was found to induce severe brain stem ischemia in the conscious rat, and CBF could be reduced by up to 85% in the lower brain stem and cerebellum (124). Catheterization of the left vertebral artery (VA) of the rabbit and delivery of a 0.1-cc clot by this route resulted in a clot lodged at the juncture of the basilar artery tip (125). Thromboembolic models are technically demanding and might not be feasible to develop in small-sized animals but might be more appropriate to develop in larger animals. Even though not in widespread use, basilar artery occlusion models might be helpful in mimicking certain clinical conditions.

MONITORING

Animal models eliminate much of the variability associated with the human condition and thereby provide the experimentalist with the degree of control and predictability for hypothesis testing.

In every brain ischemia experiment, several physiologic parameters must be monitored closely to exclude variability and increase reliability of the results. Among them are the precise control of arterial blood pressure, blood gases (pO_2, pH, pCO_2), serum glucose levels, and body or brain temperature (2). Failure to monitor and, failure to control these variables when necessary, confounds the validity of the results. Monitoring of some of these variables is especially difficult in small animals, such as mice and gerbils.

Temperature
Brain temperature is largely determined by the CBF and the core temperature (126). In animal models, even mild hypothermia is neuroprotective (127,128) and hyperthermia worsens outcome (129). Several factors affect brain temperature, and depression of CBF, anesthesia, brain exposure by means of craniectomy (or loss of insulating tissues, such as hair, skin, subcutaneous fat, and bone) are the most important. Larger brains cool down slower than smaller brains. Monitoring and maintaining the rectal temperature within physiologic ranges by means of a heating blanket or a heating lamp will likely suffice in most conditions. However, experiments with novel drugs might necessitate separate measurements of brain temperature and CBF to verify or to exclude possible hypothermic or vasodilatative effects as the primary source of neuroprotection.

Oxygenation
The arterial tensions of CO_2 and O_2 directly alter the severity of cerebral ischemia. Hypoxia/anoxia itself has been used as an ischemia model (20). Hypoxia also increases CBF via vasodilatation. Therefore, arterial blood gases should be monitored and maintained within the normal range during brain ischemia experiments.

Arterial Blood Pressure and Cerebral Blood Flow
Even though CBF can be maintained within the normal range over a large range of arterial blood pressure values, severe decreases in blood pressure cannot be compensated for and eventually lead to low perfusion pressure, aggravating cerebral ischemic changes. Furthermore, novel pharmacologic agents might themselves induce hypotension, which would be undetected if blood pressures were not monitored. Technology for monitoring CBF is not available everywhere; however, CBF measurements are relevant in most brain ischemia experiments for demonstrating adequate reduction of CBF during ischemia, for recovery of CBF following reperfusion, and to rule out potential effects of novel compounds on CBF. A number of techniques are used, including laser-Doppler flowmetry, positron emission tomography, computed tomography perfusion imaging, and MRI. These methods are noninvasive or minimally invasive and usually easy to perform. Among them, laser-Doppler flowmetry is a relatively inexpensive, minimally invasive, and easy-to-perform technique that delivers relative cortical CBF values and can easily be incorporated in most benchtop experiments. Arterial blood pressure and CBF vary among species, strains, and even within the same strain procured from different vendors, and they are dependent on the measurement technique used. Therefore, these parameters should be evaluated within each experiment, with comparison to a separate control group of animals.

Blood Glucose
The relationship of blood glucose levels and focal cerebral ischemia is complex. Elevated blood glucose levels were reported to increase (130), decrease (131), or has no effect on infarct volumes. However, the overwhelming majority of reports in the literature indicate that hyperglycemia is detrimental in focal ischemia models. In human stroke, hyperglycemia is associated with infarct expansion and worse neurologic outcome (132). Monitoring and, when necessary, controlling blood glucose levels eliminate this confounding factor.

OUTCOME MEASURES

Outcome measures should include both functional response and infarct volume (7). Infarct volume can easily and objectively be measured post mortem with a number of histologic techniques or *in vivo* by imaging. Early lesion development can be monitored with MRI techniques, such as diffusion- and perfusion-weighted MRI (133,134), and compared to final infarct volumes measured histologically at time points after induction of ischemia. Long-term experiments are necessary because some drugs might simply delay the maturation of ischemic injury and deliver encouraging results in acute experiments, but the benefit might be lost at later time points (135,136).

Functional Outcome

Functional recovery is the main interest for stroke patients and is universally used as a primary endpoint in clinical trials. In animal models, a number of relatively easy and quick methods exist for evaluating motor deficits (29,31,89), but more complicated behavioral tests, including paw-placement test, foot-fault test, beam-walking test, cylinder test, reaching tests, and Morris water maze test, are increasingly incorporated into experimental stroke studies (137–141).

In Vitro Histopathologic Evaluation

A number of histopathologic methods are used to evaluate infarct volumes. The most frequently used techniques are 2,3,5-triphenyltetrazolium chloride (TTC) staining and hematoxylin eosin (HE) staining. The infarct volume, used as an outcome measure, is calculated by multiplying the area of the lesion by the slice thickness and can be reported as uncorrected (direct) or corrected (indirect) infarct volumes. The direct infarct volume is obtained by summing the volumes of the lesion regions within the coronally cut brain slices, whereas the indirect infarct volume is obtained by subtracting the volume of the unaffected ipsilateral hemisphere from the volume of the contralateral hemisphere. The difference between these 2 methods is that corrected infarct volume is used to compensate for brain edema (142–144), which is essential to exclude the possibility that pharmacologic intervention might reduce edema but might not actually salvage ischemic brain tissue that is at risk of infarction. In addition to absolute infarct volumes, the percentage of the hemisphere involved with ischemia should also be measured, and it can be reported as a percentage of the ipsilateral or contralateral hemispheres.

TTC staining is easier, quicker, and less expensive for determining infarct volume, as compared with HE staining (89,145). Traditionally, a 2% solution of TTC in saline is used to react with brain slices for 30 min at body temperature. TTC is reduced by mitochondrial enzymes (especially by succinyl dehydrogenase) to a red compound that stains the intact brain regions dark red, whereas infarcted regions with damaged mitochondrial enzymes are not stained (remain white), resulting in good contrast between the infarcted and intact brain areas (146). The low density of mitochondria in white matter structures (especially in the corpus callosum) results in a pale staining. TTC staining is reliable between 6 and 72 hr after ischemia, and a good correlation exists between TTC staining and HE staining in delineating infarct volumes (89,143,147). When used earlier than 6 hr after induction of ischemia, this technique might not accurately reflect the full extent of the ischemic tissue because destruction of the mitochondrial enzymes requires time. However, in our experience, TTC can be reliably used, even as early as 4 hr after MCAO in both transient and permanent ischemia models (Tatlisumak et al., unpublished observation). After 72 hr, the infarct volume determined by TTC staining might be underestimated because various cells infiltrate the periphery of the infarcted region and mitochondrial enzymes in these cells react with TTC leading to obscuration of infarct borders (148). TTC penetrates poorly into brain tissue and stains only the surface of brain slices when applied post mortem, as described above. However, when given premortem intravenously, TTC stains the entire intact brain tissue, but the tissue is spoilt for further histochemic or biochemic analysis.

HE staining is a traditional and well-established staining method for evaluating both early and delayed ischemic changes (149,150). In the early phase, cellular swelling and spongiosis are prominent features, with neurons appearing shrunken. In the delayed phase, the neurons are irreversibly damaged and appear eosinophilic (149,150). Pannecrosis occurs 48 to 72 hr after induction of ischemia (149). HE is an accurate method, but it is time consuming and more costly than TTC staining.

A number of other staining procedures have been successfully applied to focal brain ischemia research, including nitroblue tetrazolium (151), Nissl's staining (cresyl violet), toluidine blue (149), and, recently, silver infarct staining (152). Silver infarct staining delineated the ischemic tissue even at the 2 hr time point after MCAO (Fig. 3) and was found to be superior to other staining procedures at early time points (152).

CONCLUSIONS

Overall, focal ischemia models and experimental stroke drug development work have had a great impact on our understanding of stroke and on development of novel therapies during the last 2 decades, but results from experimental work must be interpreted with caution. Experimental and clinical studies have developed interactively regarding the various demands, design, time window, and outcome measures, and those in the field have attempted to establish uniform standards (7,153,154). The very recent advancement in clinical stroke care and research is the development of diffusion- and perfusion-weighted MRI in experimental models and the recent utilization of this superb technology to clinical practice and trials.

ACKNOWLEDGMENTS

Dr. Tatlisumak was supported in part by the University of Helsinki, the Helsinki University Central Hospital, the Finnish Medical Foundation, the Finnish Foundation for Neurology, and the Sigrid Juselius Foundation.

REFERENCES

1. del Zoppo GJ, Poeck K, Pessin MS, et al. Recombinant tissue plasminogen activator in acute thrombotic and embolic stroke. Ann Neurol 1992; 32:78–86.
2. Hsu CY. Criteria for valid preclinical trials using animal stroke models. Stroke 1993; 24:633–636.
3. Saito I, Segawa H, Shiokawa Y, Taniguchi M, Tsutsumi K. Middle cerebral artery occlusion: correlation of computed tomography and angiography with clinical outcome. Stroke 1987; 18:863–868.
4. Yamori Y, Horie R, Handa H, Sato M, Fukase M. Pathogenetic similarity of strokes in stroke-prone spontaneously hypertensive rats and humans. Stroke 1976; 7:46–53.
5. Coyle P. Middle cerebral artery occlusion in the young rat. Stroke 1982; 13:855–859.
6. Ginsberg MD, Busto R. Rodent models of cerebral ischemia. Stroke 1989; 20:1627–1642.
7. Stroke Therapy Academic Industry Roundtable (STAIR). Recommendations for standards regarding preclinical neuroprotective and restorative drug development. Stroke 1999; 30:2752–2758.
8. Peterson JN, Evans JP. The anatomical end results of cerebral artery occlusion; experimental and clinical correlation. Trans Am Neurol 1937; A63:88.
9. Coyle P. Outcomes to middle cerebral artery occlusion in hypertensive and normotensive rats. Hypertension 1984; 6:169–174.
10. Coyle P, Odenheimer DJ, Sing CF. Cerebral infarction after middle cerebral artery occlusion in progenies of spontaneously stroke-prone and normal rats. Stroke 1984; 15:711–716.
11. Ogata J, Fujishima M, Morotomi Y, Omae T. Cerebral infarction following bilateral carotid artery ligation in normotensive and spontaneously hypertensive rats: a pathological study. Stroke 1976; 7:54–60.
12. Alkayed NJ, Harukuni I, Kimes AS, London ED, Traystman RJ, Hurn PD. Gender-linked brain injury in experimental stroke. Stroke 1998; 29:159–165.
13. Li K, Futrell N, Tovar S, Wang LC, Wang DZ, Schultz LR. Gender influences the magnitude of the inflammatory response within embolic cerebral infarcts in young rats. Stroke 1996; 27:498–503.
14. Zhang YQ, Shi J, Rajakumar G, Day AL, Simpkins JW. Effect of gender and estradiol treatment on focal brain ischemia. Brain Res 1998; 784:321–324.
15. Vergouwen MD, Anderson RE, Meyer FB. Gender differences and the effects of synthetic exogenous and non-synthetic estrogens in focal cerebral ischemia. Brain Res 2000; 878:88–97.
16. Carswell HV, Dominiczak AF, Macrae IM. Estrogen status affects sensitivity to focal cerebral ischemia in stroke-prone spontaneously hypertensive rats. Am J Physiol Heart Circ Physiol 2000; 278:H290–H294.
17. Alkayed NJ, Murphy SJ, Traystman RJ, Hurn PD. Neuroprotective effects of female gonadal steroids in reproductively senescent female rats. Stroke 2000; 31:161–168.
18. Fukuda K, Yao H, Ibayashi S, Nakahara T, Uchimura H, Fujishima M. Ovariectomy exacerbates and estrogen replacement attenuates photothrombotic focal ischemic brain injury in rats. Stroke 2000; 31:155–160.
19. Mendelow AD, Graham DI, McCulloch J, Mohamed AA. The distribution of ischaemic damage and cerebral blood flow after unilateral carotid occlusion and hypotension in the rat. Stroke 1984; 15:704–710.
20. Levine S. Anoxic-ischemic encephalopathy in rats. Am J Pathol 1960; 36:1–17.

21. Levine S, Payan H. Effects of ischemia and other procedures on the brain and retina of the gerbil (Meriones unguiculatus). Exp Neurol 1966; 16:255–262.

22. Levine S, Sohn D. Cerebral ischemia in infant and adult gerbils: relation to incomplete circle of Willis. Arch Pathol 1969; 87:315–317.

23. Kaplan H, Miezejeski C. Development of seizures in the Mongolian gerbil (Meriones unguiculatus). J Comp Physiol Psychol 1972; 81:267–273.

24. West CR, Matsen FA. Effects of experimental ischemia on electrolytes of cortical cerebrospinal fluid and on brain water. J Neurosurg 1972; 36:687–699.

25. Suzuki J, Yoshimoto T, Tanaka S, Sakamoto T. Production of various models of cerebral infarction in the dog by means of occlusion of intracranial trunk arteries. Stroke 1980; 11:337–341.

26. Koizumi J, Yoshida Y, Nakazawa T, Ooneda G. Experimental studies of ischemic brain edema 1. A new experimental model of cerebral embolism in which recirculation can be introduced in the ischemic area. Jpn J Stroke 1986; 8:1–8.

27. Takano K, Tatlisumak T, Bergmann AG, Gibson DG, Fisher M. Reproducibility and reliability of middle cerebral artery occlusion using a silicon-coated suture (Koizumi) in rats. J Neur Sci 1997; 153:8–11.

28. Belayev L, Alonso OF, Busto R, Zhao W, Ginsberg MD. Middle cerebral artery occlusion in the rat by intraluminal suture: neurological and pathological evaluation of an improved model. Stroke 1996; 27:1616–1623.

29. Longa EZ, Weinstein PR, Carlson S, Cummins R. Reversible middle cerebral artery occlusion without craniectomy in rats. Stroke 1989; 20:84–91.

30. Laing RJ, Jakubowski J, Laing RW. Middle cerebral artery occlusion without craniectomy in rats: which method works best? Stroke 1993; 24:294–298.

31. Nagasawa H, Kogure K. Correlation between cerebral blood flow and histological changes in a new rat model of middle cerebral artery occlusion. Stroke 1989; 20:1037–1043.

32. Zarow GJ, Karibe H, States BA, Graham SH, Weinstein PR. Endovascular suture occlusion of the middle cerebral artery in rats: effect of suture insertion distance on cerebral blood flow, infarct distribution and infarct volume. Neurol Res 1997; 19:409–416.

33. Li F, Han S, Tatlisumak T, Carano RAD, Irie K, Sotak CH, Fisher M. A new method to improve in-bore middle cerebral artery occlusion in rats. Demonstration with diffusion- and perfusion-weighted imaging. Stroke 1998; 29:1715–1720.

34. Meng X, Fisher M, Shen Q, Sotak CH, Duong TQ. Characterizing the diffusion/perfusion mismatch in experimental focal cerebral ischemia. Ann Neurol 2004; 55:207–212.

35. Kuge Y, Minematsu K, Yamaguchi T, Miyake Y. Nylon monofilament for intraluminal middle cerebral artery occlusion in rats. Stroke 1995; 26:1655–1658.

36. Schmid-Elsaesser R, Zausinger S, Hungerhuber E, Baethmann A, Reulen H-J. A critical reevaluation of the intraluminal thread model of focal cerebral ischemia: evidence of inadvertent premature reperfusion and subarachnoid hemorrhage in rats by laser-Doppler flowmetry. Stroke 1998; 29:2162–2170.

37. Kinouchi H, Epstein CJ, Mizui T, Carlson E, Chen SF, Chan PH. Attenuation of focal cerebral ischemic injury in transgenic mice overexpressing CuZn superoxide dismutase. Proc Natl Acad Sci USA 1991; 88:11158–11162.

38. Yang G, Chan PH, Chen J, et al. Human copper-zinc superoxide dismutase transgenic mice are highly resistant to reperfusion injury after focal cerebral ischemia. Stroke 1994; 25:165–170.

39. Hata R, Mies G, Wiessner C, et al. A reproducible model of middle cerebral artery occlusion in mice: hemodynamic, biochemical, and magnetic resonance imaging. J Cereb Blood Flow Metab 1998; 18:367–375.

40. Wen TC, Rogido M, Gressens P, Sola A. A reproducible experimental model of focal cerebral ischemia in the neonatal rat. Brain Res Brain Res Protoc 2004; 13:76–83.

41. Kong LQ, Xie JX, Han HB, Liu HD. Improvements in the intraluminal thread technique to induce focal cerebral ischaemia in rabbits. J Neurosci Methods 2004; 137:315–319.

42. Roussel SA, van Bruggen N, King MD, Houseman J, Williams SR, Gadian DG. Monitoring the initial expansion of focal ischemic changes by diffusion-weighted MRI using a remote controlled method of occlusion. NMR Biomed 1994; 7:21–28.

43. Kohno K, Back T, Hoehn-Berlage M, Hossmann K-A. A modified rat model of middle cerebral artery thread occlusion under electrophysiological control for magnetic resonance investigations. Magn Reson Imaging 1995; 13:65–71.

44. Röther J, de Crespigny AJ, D'Arceuil H, Moseley ME. MRI detection of cortical spreading depression immediately after focal ischemia in the rat. J Cereb Blood Flow Metab 1996; 16:214–220.

45. Purdy PD, Devous MD, White CL, Batjer HH, Samson DS, Brewer K, Hodges K. Reversible middle cerebral artery embolization in dogs without intracranial surgery. Stroke 1989; 20:1368–1376.

46. Zhao Q, Memezawa H, Smith ML, Siesjö BK. Hyperthermia complicates middle cerebral artery occlusion induced by an intraluminal filament. Brain Res 1994; 649:253–259.

47. Li F, Omae T, Fisher M. Spontaneous hyperthermia and its mechanism in the intraluminal suture middle cerebral artery occlusion model of rats. Stroke 1999; 30:2464–2471.
48. Albers GW. Antithrombotic agents in cerebral ischemia. Am J Cardiol 1995; 75:348–388.
49. The National Institute of Neurological Disorders and Stroke rt-PA Stroke Study Group. Tissue plasminogen activator for acute ischemic stroke. N Engl J Med 1995; 333:1581–1587.
50. Phillips DA, Davis MA, Fisher M. Selective embolization and clot dissolution with tPA in the internal carotid artery circulation of the rabbit. AJNR Am J Neuroradiol 1988; 9:899–902.
51. Hill NC, Millikan CH, Wakim KG, Sayre GP. Studies in cerebrovascular disease. VII. Experimental production of cerebral infarction by intracarotid injection of homologous blood clot; preliminary report. Mayo Clin Proc 1955; 30:625–633.
52. De Ley G, Weyne J, Demeester G, Stryckmans K, Goethals P, Van de Velde E, Leusen I. Experimental thromboembolic stroke studied by positron emission tomography: immediate versus delayed reperfusion by fibrinolysis. J Cereb Blood Flow Metab 1988; 4:539–545.
53. Kudo M, Aoyama A, Ichimori S, Fukunaga N. An animal model of cerebral infarction. Homologous blood clot emboli in rats. Stroke 1982; 13:505–508.
54. Kaneko D, Nakamura N, Ogawa T. Cerebral infarction in rats using homologous blood emboli: development of a new experimental model. Stroke 1985; 16:76–84.
55. Zhang ZG, Chopp M, Zhang RL, Goussev A. A mouse model of embolic focal cerebral ischemia. J Cereb Blood Flow Metab 1997; 17:1081–1088.
56. Kilic E, Hermann DM, Hossmann KA. A reproducible model of thromboembolic stroke in mice. Neuroreport 1998; 13:2967–2970.
57. Heffez D, Sheremata W. Experimental embolic stroke in the guinea pig (Cuvis cobaya). J Neuropathol Exp Neurol 1980; 39:82–87.
58. Kuge Y, Yokota C, Tagaya M, et al. Serial changes in cerebral blood flow and flow-metabolism uncoupling in primates with acute thromboembolic stroke. J Cereb Blood Flow Metab 2001; 21:202–210.
59. Kito G, Nishimura A, Susumu T, et al. Experimental thromboembolic stroke in cynomolgus monkey. J Neurosci Methods 2001; 105:45–53.
60. Futrell N, Watson BD, Dietrich WD, Prado R, Millikan C, Ginsberg MD. A new model of embolic stroke produced by photochemical injury to the carotid artery in the rat. Ann Neurol 1988; 23:251–257.
61. Futrell N. An improved photochemical model of embolic cerebral infarction in rats. Stroke 1991; 22:225–232.
62. Overgaard K, Sereghy T, Boysen G, Pedersen H, Hoyer S, Diemer NH. A rat model of reproducible cerebral infarction using thrombotic blood clot emboli. J Cereb Blood Flow Metab 1992; 12:484–490.
63. Busch E, Kruger K, Hossmann K-A. Improved model of thromboembolic stroke and rt-PA induced reperfusion in the rat. Brain Res 1997; 778:16–24.
64. Takano K, Carano RAD, Tatlisumak T, et al. Efficacy of intra-arterial and intravenous prourokinase in an embolic stroke model evaluated by diffusion-perfusion magnetic resonance imaging. Neurology 1998; 50:870–875.
65. Zhang RL, Chopp M, Zhang ZG, Jiang Q, Ewing JR. A rat model of focal embolic cerebral ischemia. Brain Res 1997; 766:83–92.
66. Zhang ZG, Zhang RL, Jiang Q, Raman SB, Cantwell L, Chopp M. A new rat model of thrombotic focal cerebral ischemia. J Cereb Blood Flow Metab 1997; 17:123–135.
67. Shigeno T, Teasdale GM, McCulloch J, Graham DI. Recirculation model following MCA occlusion in rats. Cerebral blood flow, cerebrovascular permeability, and brain edema. J Neurosurg 1985; 63:272–277.
68. Shigeno T, McCulloch J, Graham DI, Mendelow AD, Teasdale GM. Pure cortical ischemia versus striatal ischemia. Surg Neurol 1985; 24:47–51.
69. Takizawa S, Hakim AM. Animal models of cerebral ischemia. 2. Rat models. Cerebrovasc Dis 1990; 1(suppl 1):16–21.
70. Waltz AG, Sundt TM. The microvasculature and microcirculation of the cerebral cortex after arterial occlusion. Brain 1967; 90:681–700.
71. Hudgins WR, Garcia JH. Transorbital approach to the middle cerebral artery of the squirrel monkey: a technique for experimental cerebral infarction applicable to ultrastructural studies. Stroke 1970; 1:107–111.
72. Michenfelder JD, Milde JH. Influence of anesthetics on metabolic, functional and pathological responses to regional cerebral ischemia. Stroke 1975; 6:405–410.
73. Meyer FB, Anderson RE, Sundt TM, Yaksh TL. Intracellular brain pH, indicator tissue perfusion, electroencephalography, and histology in severe and moderate cortical ischemia in the rabbit. J Cereb Blood Flow Metab 1986; 6:71–78.
74. Slivka A, Pulsinelli W. Hemorrhagic complications of thrombolytic therapy in experimental stroke. Stroke 1987; 18:1148–1156.
75. MacDonald VD, Sundt TM, Winkelmann RK. Histochemical studies in the zone of ischemia following middle cerebral artery occlusion in cats. J Neurosurg 1972; 37:45–54.

76. Hayakawa T, Waltz AG. Immediate effects of cerebral ischemia: evolution and resolution of neurological deficits after experimental occlusion of one middle cerebral artery in conscious cats. Stroke 1975; 6:321–327.

77. Robinson RG, Shoemaker WJ, Schlumpf M, Valk T, Bloom FE. Effect of experimental infarction in rat brain on catecholamines and behaviour. Nature 1975; 255:332–334.

78. Backhauss C, Karkoutly C, Welsch M, Krieglstein J. A mouse model for focal cerebral ischemia for screening neuroprotective drug effects. J Pharmacol Toxicol Methods 1992; 27:27–32.

79. Sundt TM, Waltz AG. Experimental cerebral infarction: retro-orbital, extradural approach for occluding the middle cerebral artery. Mayo Clin Proc 1966; 41:159–168.

80. O'Brien MD, Waltz AG. Transorbital approach for occluding the middle cerebral artery without craniectomy. Stroke 1973; 4:201–206.

81. Bose B, Osterholm JL, Berry R. A reproducible experimental model of focal cerebral ischemia in the cat. Brain Res 1984; 311:385–391.

82. Berkelbach van der Sprenkel JW, Tulleken CAF. The postorbital approach to the middle cerebral artery in cats. Stroke 1988; 19:503–506.

83. Albanese V, Tommasino C, Sparado A, Tomasello F. A transbasisphenoidal approach for selective occlusion of the middle cerebral artery in rats. Experientia 1980; 36:1302–1304.

84. Tamura A, Graham DI, McCulloch J, Teasdale GM. Focal cerebral ischemia in the rat: 1. Description of technique and early neuropathological consequences following middle cerebral artery occlusion. J Cereb Blood Flow Metab 1981; 1:53–60.

85. Brint S, Jacewicz M, Kiessling M, Tanabe J, Pulsinelli W. Focal brain ischemia in the rat: methods for reproducible neocortical infarction using tandem occlusion of the distal middle cerebral and ipsilateral common carotid arteries. J Cereb Blood Flow Metab 1988; 8:474–485.

86. Chen ST, Hsu CY, Hogan EL, Maricq H, Balentine JD. A model of focal ischemic stroke in the rat: reproducible extensive cortical infarction. Stroke 1986; 17:738–743.

87. Dietrich WD, Nakayama H, Watson BD, Kanemitsu H. Morphological consequences of early reperfusion following thrombotic or mechanical occlusion of the rat middle cerebral artery. Acta Neuropathol 1989; 78:605–614.

88. Kaplan B, Brint S, Tanabe J, Jacewicz M, Wang XJ, Pulsinelli W. Temporal thresholds for neocortical infarction in rats subjected to reversible focal cerebral ischemia. Stroke 1991; 22:1032–1039.

89. Bederson JB, Pitts LH, Tsuji M, Nishimura MC, Davis RL, Bartkowski H. Rat middle cerebral artery occlusion: evaluation of the model and development of a neurologic examination. Stroke 1986; 17:472–476.

90. Fox G, Gallacher D, Shevde S, Loftus J, Swayne G. Anatomic variation of the middle cerebral artery in the Sprague-Dawley rat. Stroke 1993; 24:2087–2093.

91. Tyson GW, Teasdale GM, Graham DI, McCulloch J. Focal cerebral ischemia in the rat: topography of hemodynamic and histopathological changes. Ann Neurol 1984; 15:559–567.

92. Tamura A, Graham DI, McCulloch J, Teasdale GM. Focal cerebral ischaemia in the rat. 2. Regional cerebral blood flow determined by 14C-iodoantipyrine autoradiography following middle cerebral artery occlusion. J Cereb Blood Flow Metab 1981; 1:61–69.

93. Diaz FG, Mastri AR, Ausman JI, Chou SN. Acute cerebral revascularization: part I. Cerebral ischemia experimental animal model. Surg Neurol 1979; 12:353–362.

94. Siegel BA, Meidinger R, Elliott AJ, et al. Experimental cerebral microembolism. Multiple tracer assessment of brain edema. Arch Neurol 1972; 26:73–77.

95. Garcia JH. Experimental ischemic stroke: a review. Stroke 1984; 15:5–14.

96. Takeda T, Shima T, Okada Y, Yamane K, Uozumi T. Pathophysiological studies of cerebral ischemia produced by silicone cylinder embolization in rats. J Cereb Blood Flow Metab 1987; 7(suppl):S66.

97. Fukuchi K, Kusuoka H, Watanabe Y, Nishimura T. Correlation of sequential MR images of microsphere-induced cerebral ischemia with histologic changes in rats. Invest Radiol 1999; 34:698–703.

98. Furlow TW, Bass NH. Stroke in rats produced by carotid injection of sodium arachidonate. Science 1975; 187:658–660.

99. Gerriets T, Li F, Silva MD, Meng X, Brevard M, Sotak CH, Fisher M. The macrosphere model. Evaluation of a new stroke model for permanent middle cerebral artery occlusion in rats. J Neurosci Methods 2003; 122:201–211.

100. Hegedus K, Fekete I, Tury F, Molnar L. Experimental focal cerebral ischaemia in rabbits. J Neurol 1985; 232:223–230.

101. Purdy PD, Devous MD, Batjer HH, White CL, Meyer Y, Samson DS. Microfibrillar collagen model of canine cerebral infarction. Stroke 1989; 20:1361–1367.

102. del Zoppo GJ, Copeland BR, Waltz TA, Zyroff J, Plow EF, Harker LA. The beneficial effect of intracarotid urokinase on acute stroke in a baboon model. Stroke 1986; 17:638–643.

103. Watanabe O, Bremer AM, West CR. Experimental regional cerebral ischemia in the middle cerebral artery territory in primates. Part 1: Angio-anatomy and description of an experimental model with selective embolization of the internal carotid artery bifurcation. Stroke 1977; 8:61–70.

104. Watson BD, Dietrich WD, Busto R, Wachtel MS, Ginsberg MD. Induction of reproducible brain infarction by photochemically initiated thrombosis. Ann Neurol 1985; 17:497–504.

105. Yoshida Y, Dereski MO, Garcia JH, Hetzel FW, Chopp M. Neuronal injury after photoactivation of photofrin II. Am J Pathol 1992; 141:989–997.

106. Dietrich WD, Watson BD, Busto R, Ginsberg MD, Bethea JR. Photochemically induced cerebral infarction. I. Early microvascular alterations. Acta Neuropathol (Berlin) 1987; 72:315–325.

107. Dietrich WD, Busto R, Watson BD, Scheinberg P, Ginsberg MD. Photochemically induced cerebral infarction: II. Edema and blood-brain-barrier disruption. Acta Neuropathol (Berlin) 1987; 72:326–334.

108. de Ryck M. Animal models of cerebral stroke: pharmacological protection of function. Eur Neurol 1990; 3(suppl):21–27.

109. Robinson MJ, Macrae IM, Todd M, Read JL, McCulloch J. Reduction of local cerebral blood flow to pathological levels by endothelin-1 applied to the middle cerebral artery in the rat. Neurosci Lett 1990; 118:269–272.

110. Sharkey J, Ritchie IM, Kelly PAT. Perivascular microapplication of endothelin-1: a new model of focal cerebral ischaemia in the rat. J Cereb Blood Flow Metab 1993; 13:865–871.

111. Sharkey J, Butcher SP, Kelly JS. Endothelin-1 induced middle cerebral artery occlusion: pathological consequences and neuroprotective effects of MK801. J Autonom Nerv Syst 1994; 49:S177–S185.

112. Henshall DC, Butcher SP, Sharkey J. A rat model of endothelin-3 induced middle cerebral artery occlusion with controlled reperfusion. Brain Res 1999; 843:105–111.

113. Virley D, Hadingham SJ, Roberts JC, et al. A new primate model of focal stroke: endothelin-1-induced middle cerebral artery occlusion and reperfusion in the common marmoset. J Cereb Blood Flow Metab 2004; 24:24–41.

114. Röther J, Waggie K, van Bruggen N, de Crespigny AJ, Moseley ME. Experimental cerebral venous thrombosis: evaluation using magnetic resonance imaging. J Cereb Blood Flow Metab 1996; 16:1353–1361.

115. Cooper A. Some experiments and observations on tying the carotid and vertebral arteries, and the pneumo-gastric, phrenic, and sympathetic nerves. Grey's Hosp Rep 1836; 1:457–475.

116. Frerichs KU, Deckert M, Kempski O, Schurer L, Einhäupl K, Baethmann A. Cerebral sinus and venous thrombosis in rats induces long-term deficits in brain function and morphology-evidence for a cytotoxic genesis. J Cereb Blood Flow Metab 1994; 14:289–300.

117. Sarwar M, Virapongse C, Carbo P. Experimental production of superior sagittal sinus thrombosis in the dog. AJNR Am J Neuroradiol 1984; 6:19–22.

118. Alexander LF, Yamamoto Y, Ayoubi S, al-Mefti O, Smith RR. Efficacy of tissue plasminogen activator in the lysis of thrombosis of the cerebral venous sinus. Neurosurgery 1990; 26:559–564.

119. Fries G, Wallenfang T, Hennen J, et al. Occlusion of the pig superior sagittal sinus, bridging and cortical veins: multistep evolution of sinus-vein thrombosis. J Neurosurg 1992; 77:127–133.

120. Miyamoto K, Heimann A, Kempski O. Microcirculatory alterations in a Mongolian gerbil sinus-vein thrombosis model. J Clin Neurosci 2001; 8:S97–S105.

121. Schaller B, Graf R, Wienhard K, Heiss W-D. A new animal model of cerebral venous infarction: ligation of the posterior part of the superior sagittal sinus in the cat. Swiss Med Wkly 2003; 133:412–418.

122. Kameyama M, Suzuki J, Shirane R, Ogawa A. A new model of bilateral hemispheric ischemia in the rat-three vessel occlusion model. Stroke 1985; 16:489–493.

123. Wojak JC, DeCrescito V, Young W. Basilar artery occlusion in rats. Stroke 1991; 22:247–252.

124. Macrae IM, Robinson MJ, McAuley M, Reid J, McCulloch J. Effects of intracisternal endothelin-1 injection on blood flow to the lower brain stem. Eur J Pharmacol 1991; 203:85–91.

125. Pan G, Wright KC. Clot embolic stroke in the vertebrobasilar system of rabbits: transfemoral angiographic technique. Cardiovasc Intervent Radiol 1987; 10:285–290.

126. Hasegawa Y, Latour LL, Sotak CH, Dardzinski BJ, Fisher M. Temperature dependent change of apparent diffusion coefficient of water in normal and ischemic brain of rats. J Cereb Blood Flow Metab 1994; 14:383–390.

127. Rosomoff HL. Hypothermia and cerebral vascular lesions. I. Experimental interruption of the middle cerebral artery during hypothermia. J Neurosurg 1956; 4:244–255.

128. Rosomoff HL. Hypothermia and cerebral vascular lesions. II. Experimental middle cerebral artery interruption followed by induction of hypothermia. AMA Arch Neurol Psychiatry 1957; 5:454–464.

129. Kim Y, Busto R, Dietrich WD, Kraydieh S, Ginsberg MD. Delayed postischemic hyperthermia in awake rats worsens the histopathological outcome of transient focal cerebral ischemia. Stroke 1996; 12:2274–2280.

130. de Courten-Myers G, Myers RE, Schoolfield L. Hyperglycemia enlarges infarct size in cerebrovascular occlusion in cats. Stroke 1988; 19:623–630.

131. Ginsberg MD, Prado R, Dietrich WD, Busto R, Watson BD. Hyperglycemia reduces the extent of cerebral infarction in rats. Stroke 1987; 18:570–574.

132. Baird TA, Parsons MW, Phanh T, et al. Persistent poststroke hyperglycemia is independently associated with infarct expansion and worse clinical outcome. Stroke 2003; 34:2208–2214.

133. Tatlisumak T, Li F. Use of diffusion- and perfusion magnetic resonance imaging in drug development for ischemic stroke. Curr Drug Target CNS Neurol Disord 2003; 2:131–141.

134. Tatlisumak T, Strbian D, Abo Ramadan U, Li F. The role of diffusion- and perfusion magnetic resonance imaging in drug development for ischemic stroke: from laboratory to clinics. Curr Vasc Pharmacol 2004; 4:343–355.

135. Valtysson J, Hillered L, Andine P, Hagberg H, Persson L. Neuropathological endpoints in experimental stroke pharmacotherapy: the importance of both early and late evaluation. Acta Neurochir 1994; 129:58–63.

136. Coimbra C, Drake M, Boris-Moller F, Wieloch T. Long lasting neuroprotective effect of post-ischemic hypothermia and treatment with an anti-inflammatory/antipyretic drug. Evidence for chronic encephalopathic processes following ischemia. Stroke 1996; 27:1578–1585.

137. Feeney DM, Gonzales A, Law WA. Amphetamine restores locomotor function after motor cortex injury in the rat. Proc West Pharmacol Soc 1981; 24:15–17.

138. de Ryck M, Van Reempts J, Duytschaever H, van Deuren B, Clincke G. Neocortical localization of tactile/proprioceptive limb placing reactions in the rat. Brain Res 1992; 573:44–60.

139. Markgraf CG, Green EJ, Hurwitz BE, et al. Sensorimotor and cognitive consequences of middle cerebral artery occlusion in rats. Brain Res 1992; 575:238–246.

140. Jones TA, Schallert T. Use-dependent growth of pyramidal neurons after neocortical damage. J Neurosci 1994; 14:2140–2152.

141. Kawamata T, Dietrich WD, Schallert T, et al. Intracisternal basic fibroblast growth factor enhances functional recovery and up-regulates the expression of a molecular marker of neuronal sprouting following focal cerebral infarction. Proc Natl Acad Sci USA 1997; 94:8179–8184.

142. Swanson RA, Morton MT, Tsao-Wu G, Savalos RA, Davidson C, Sharp FR. A semiautomated method for measuring brain infarct volume. J Cereb Blood Flow Metab 1990; 10:290–293.

143. Lin TN, He YY, Wu G, Khan M, Hsu CY. Effect of brain edema on infarct volume in a focal cerebral ischemia model in rats. Stroke 1993; 24:117–121.

144. Tatlisumak T, Takano K, Carano RA, Miller LP, Foster AC, Fisher M. Delayed treatment with an adenosine kinase inhibitor, GP683, attenuates infarct size in rats with temporary middle cerebral artery occlusion. Stroke 1998; 29:1952–1958.

145. Lundy EF, Solik BS, Frank RS, et al. Morphometric evaluation of brain infarcts in rats and gerbils. J Pharmacol Methods 1986; 16:201–214.

146. Li F, Irie K, Anwer MS, Fisher M. Delayed triphenyltetrazolium chloride staining remains useful for evaluating cerebral infarct volume in a rat stroke model. J Cereb Blood Flow Metab 1997; 17:1132–1135.

147. Isayama K, Pitts LH, Nishimura MC. Evaluation of 2,3,5 triphenyltetrazolium tetrachloride staining to delineate rat brain infarcts. Stroke 1991; 22:1394–1398.

148. Liszczak TM, Hedley-Whyte ET, Adams JF, et al. Limitations of tetrazolium salts in delineating infarcted brain. Acta Neuropathol 1984; 65:150–157.

149. Garcia JH, Yoshida Y, Chen H, et al. Progression from ischemic injury to infarct following middle cerebral artery occlusion in the rat. Am J Pathol 1993; 142:623–635.

150. Garcia JH, Liu KF, Ho KL. Neuronal necrosis after middle cerebral artery occlusion in Wistar rats progresses at different time intervals in the caudoputamen and the cortex. Stroke 1995; 26:636–642.

151. Ridenour TR, Warner DS, Todd MM, McAllister AC. Mild hypothermia reduces infarct size resulting from temporary but not permanent focal ischemia in rats. Stroke 1992; 223:733–738.

152. Vogel J, Mobius C, Kuschinsky W. Early delineation of ischemic tissue in rat brain cryosections by high-contrast staining. Stroke 1999; 30:1134–1141.

153. Stroke Therapy Academic Industry Roundtable-II (STAIR-II). Recommendations for clinical trial evaluation of acute stroke therapies. Stroke 2001; 32:1598–1606.

154. Fisher M. Recommendations for advancing development of acute stroke therapies. Stroke Therapy Academic Industry Roundtable 3. Stroke 2003; 34:1539–1546.

17 | Pathogenesis of Brain Injury Following Ischemic Stroke

Xian Nan Tang, MD, Fellow
Zhen Zheng, MD, PhD, Fellow
Midori A. Yenari, MD, Associate Professor

Department of Neurology, University of California–San Francisco, Veterans Affairs Medical Center, San Francisco, and Department of Anesthesia, Stanford University School of Medicine, Stanford, California, USA

INTRODUCTION

Ischemic stroke results when blood flow to the brain is disrupted due to occlusion of the cerebral vessels or cessation of cerebral blood flow (CBF). Normal CBF is approximately 50 mL/100 g brain tissue/min. Cerebral dysfunction begins to occur with CBF reductions in the range of 16 to 20 mL/100 g/min. Ionic pump failure and loss of ion homeostasis occurs with reductions to 10 to 12 mL/100 g/min, and cell death results when CBF is <10 mL/100 g/min (1). The severity of ischemic injury within the cerebrovascular bed can be classified into 2 broad regions depending on the extent of CBF reduction. The area with the most severe CBF reduction is often referred to as the infarct core because of the rapid necrosis seen within vulnerable neurons. The area around the infarct core is sometimes referred to as the penumbra. "Penumbra" is a term used to describe an intermediate area of marginally perfused tissue that might survive if blood flow is restored. The CBF within the penumbra has been estimated to be approximately 12 to 24 mL/100 g/min (Fig. 1) (2). CBF and severity of ischemic injury are also time dependent; increased occlusion time of the parent vessel results in increased damage. However, cells within the penumbra are potentially salvageable in the presence of appropriate cytoprotective strategies (1,3).

Though reperfusion can restore blood flow, reperfusion itself can result in secondary injury due to the influx of neutrophils and abrupt increases in reactive oxygen species (ROS), leading to further damage, as well as edema and hemorrhage. Furthermore, the resulting energy loss leads to mitochondrial dysfunction, causing inadequate handling of sudden high levels of ROS (4). High levels of ROS can activate a variety of cell-death pathways and can directly damage intracellular proteins and DNA through oxidation. Reperfusion also permits the influx of blood elements, including leukocytes, which can mediate a local inflammatory reaction, with subsequent generation of more ROS. Serum and serum proteins might also enter the brain, leading to edema, and when the blood–brain barrier (BBB) is sufficiently disrupted, hemorrhage often results.

The pathogenesis of ischemic stroke involves many complex mechanisms. This chapter will summarize current, established concepts and pathways involved in ischemic brain injury.

EXCITOTOXICITY, INTRACELLULAR CALCIUM, AND ISCHEMIC BRAIN INJURY

Energy failure due to cessation of blood flow can result in calcium accumulation in brain cells via diffusion along electrochemical gradients, depolarization and opening of voltage-dependent calcium channels (VDCC), internal release from organelles [the endoplasmic reticulum (ER) and mitochondria], and via excessive stimulation of glutamate receptors. Ischemia also results in the accumulation and release of excitatory amino acids (EAAs), such as glutamate and aspartate, which contribute to neuronal cell death via entry of calcium and sodium ions. Ischemia-induced calcium toxicity can then lead to cytoskeletal breakdown, altered gene expression, lipolysis, and generation of ROS and reactive nitrogen species (RNS) (Fig. 2) (5).

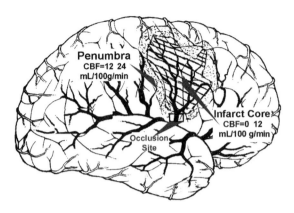

Figure 1 Schematic diagram showing the ischemic penumbra and core. Following occlusion of the middle cerebral artery, CBF decreases to 0 to 12 mL/100 g/min in regions of the most severe injury (core). The peri-infarct area is sometimes termed penumbra, where the CBF is maintained at approximately 12 to 24 mL/100 g/min due to collateral blood flow. It is within this region that brain tissue might be salvageable if blood flow is fully restored or an appropriate cytoprotectant is administered. However, penumbra is a time-dependent concept, as it might shrink if the early blood flow can be restored, or it might be incorporated into the core if ischemia is allowed to persist. *Abbreviation*: CBF, cerebrospinal fluid.

Intracellular Calcium Accumulation

During ischemia, the cytosolic concentration of calcium can increase as much as 1000-fold. Intracellular calcium levels rise via several mechanisms. Calcium influx occurs during cerebral ischemia as a result of the fall in adenosine triphosphate (ATP) levels and membrane depolarization (6), leading to VDCC opening and reversal of the Na^+-Ca^{2+} exchanger (7). Increased release of the EAA glutamate also occurs after ischemia and, by stimulation of glutamate receptors, leads to calcium influx by opening appropriate ion channels. Mitochondria are important sources of intracellular calcium accumulation. Approximately 50% of intracellular calcium is normally stored in the mitochondria and is released under conditions of acidosis and energy depletion. Calcium stored in the ER is released into the cytosol through ischemia-induced activation of phospholipase C (8). Low calcium levels in the ER could impair normal protein folding and processing, leading to ER stress, which in turn, activates the unfolded protein response, involving the activation of 2 kinases that phosphorylate eukaryotic initiation factor 2α, resulting in its inactivation and the shutdown of protein synthesis (9,10).

Excitatory Amino Acids

EAAs, such as glutamate and aspartate, are found in high concentrations in neuronal cells of the central nervous system. EAA receptors are divided into metabotropic and ionotropic receptors. Ionotropic receptors play an important role in neuronal excitotoxicity and include NMDA, AMPA (α-amino-3-hydroxy-5-methyl-4-isoxazole propionic acid), and kainate subtypes. Metabotropic receptors are G-protein–coupled and include a family of receptor subtypes, of which mGlu1 and mGlu2 might play differential roles in ischemic pathogenesis (11). Following energy depletion and anoxic depolarization, massive extracellular glutamate accumulation occurs through presynaptic release and reversal of glutamate transporters in astrocytes (12,13). Once released, glutamate binds to its ionotropic receptors, calcium and sodium enter the cell, and a consequent cascade of damaging events ultimately causes cell death.

The NMDA receptor–channel complex is thought to facilitate calcium entry into the cell after stimulation by glutamate or NMDA. At rest, the NMDA channel is blocked by magnesium, which can be removed by a depolarizing stimulus. In addition to its ligand-binding site, the complex contains glycine, polyamine, and zinc domains, of which a variety of modulators have been studied in the laboratory as potential neuroprotectants (13). Unfortunately, none of the therapeutic strategies aimed at these targets have yielded positive results at the clinical level for treatment of acute stroke (14). Other work in this area suggests that modulation of NMDA subunits during ischemia and related insults might have an important role in their function. NMDA receptors consist of several subunits, including NR1 and NR2. NR1 might facilitate neurotoxicity, as NR1 knockout mice were resistant to glutamate-induced excitotoxicity (15) and rats treated with antisense oligodeoxynucleotides to inhibit the synthesis of NR1 receptors had smaller infarcts following experimental stroke (16). Tyrosine phosphorylation of NR2 has been documented following cerebral ischemia (17,18) and has been implicated in the phenomenon of ischemic tolerance, in which a prior sublethal ischemic insult protects against a subsequent lethal insult (19). NMDA receptors interact with a diversity of intracellular

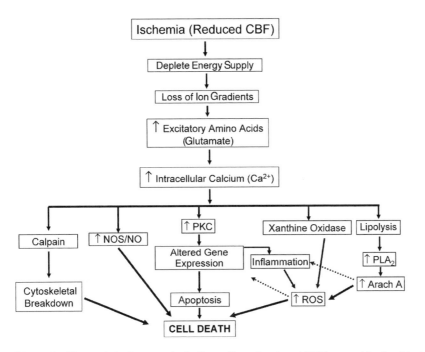

Figure 2 The excitotoxic cascade. In the setting of reduced CBF caused by focal ischemia, energy supplies are depleted, causing membrane depolarization and loss of ionic gradients, which leads to the release of excess excitatory amino acids, such as glutamate. Glutamate activates its ionotropic receptors, permitting entry of large amounts of Ca^{2+}. Excess intracellular Ca^{2+} then activates a series of events that ultimately lead to cell death. Calcium might activate calpain, leading to degradation of several structural proteins. NMDA-receptor stimulation is linked to the activation of NOS, which generates NO. Calcium also triggers various transcription factors that lead to upregulation of many genes. Some of the upregulated genes are involved in apoptosis and inflammation. Inflammatory responses can lead to increases in ROS, which can lead to further transcriptional responses. Calcium can also generate xanthine oxidase, which, in turn, increases intracellular levels of superoxide. Intracellular Ca^{2+} also upregulates lipolysis, which, can trigger inflammation through activation of PLA_2 and the Arach A cascade. *Abbreviations*: CBF, cerebral blood flow; NOS, nitric oxide synthase; ROS, reactive oxygen species; NO, nitric oxide; PLA_2, phospholipase A2; PKC, protein kinase C; Arach A, arachidonic acid.

synaptic and cytoskeletal proteins, and disruption of downstream-signaling pathways also might lead to neuroprotection independent of intracellular calcium changes. NMDA receptor stimulation has been shown to lead to the recruitment of the scaffolding protein postsynaptic density 95 (PSD95), which couples the NMDA receptors to neuronal nitric oxide (NO) synthase (nNOS) (20). nNOS catalyzes the conversion of L-arginine to NO. Prevention of NMDA–PSD95 interactions has led to reduced infarct size and improved neurologic function, without disruption of synaptic transmission or calcium influx. nNOS is now believed to potentiate neuronal cell death in certain settings, as male mice deficient in nNOS have smaller infarcts compared to wild-type mice (21). However, this effect might be gender dependent, as nNOS in female mice might be neuroprotective (22).

AMPA receptors are generally permeable to sodium and impermeable to calcium. However, 8% to 15% of brain neurons express calcium-permeable AMPA receptors due to RNA editing of the GluR2 subunit (23). The presence of the GluR2 subunit appears to render AMPA channels calcium impermeable, and cerebral ischemia appears to downregulate GluR2 expression. Thus, excitotoxicity due to AMPA receptor stimulation might also result from increasing Ca^{2+} influx. Antisense knockdown of GluR2 led to increased calcium influx and increased cell death, even in the absence of ischemia (24). However, the precise role of GluR2 in mediating ischemic injury is not clear. Other studies showed that, although ischemia did reduce GluR2 expression in hippocampal CA1 and CA3 neurons, subsequent neuronal death did not occur (25). Furthermore, mice lacking a functional GluR2 gene did not exhibit increased neurotoxicity, even in the face of increased calcium influx (23). Regardless, AMPA antagonists appear to limit ischemic neuronal damage, especially following global cerebral ischemia (26).

In contrast to the ionotropic receptors, metabotropic receptors are G-coupled proteins with pleitropic effects. The Group 1 mGluRs, including mGluR1 and mGluR5, trigger internal calcium release via phosphoinositol and phospholipase C. mGluR1, in particular, appears to play a damaging role following ischemia, and antagonists are neuroprotective in animal models (11).

Consequences of Excitotoxicity and Calcium Overload

Calcium is known to activate a variety of processes, ultimately leading to ischemic cell death (12). In the setting of ischemia, excess intracellular calcium leads to overactivation of a variety of enzyme systems (lipases, endonucleases, and other proteases) and to formation of ROS or NO, both of which lead to cell death. Calpain, a calcium-activated cysteine protease, can degrade several structural proteins. Pharmacologic inhibitors have been shown to limit injury in several cerebral ischemia models, indicating that calpain might represent an important therapeutic target (27). Calcium also activates phospholipase A_2 (PLA_2) and hydrolyzes glycerophospholipids to release free fatty acids and lysophospholipids. Membrane-bound PLA_2 activity is increased following glutamate exposure. PLA_2 is a key enzyme involved in membrane remodeling, inflammation, and lipid metabolism. The primary substrate for these enzymes is glycerophospholipid, a major constituent of the cell membrane. Following ischemia, PLA_2 not only directly damages cell membranes but also activates arachidonic acid and other cell-death pathways (28). Arachidonic acid metabolism then leads to the generation of ROS and subsequent lipid peroxidation. Additionally, calcium can activate xanthine oxidase, which results in the generation of superoxide.

OXIDATIVE STRESS AND BRAIN ISCHEMIA

The adult human brain constitutes approximately 2% of total body weight but requires approximately 25% of the cardiac output. Because of its high oxygen consumption, the brain is especially vulnerable to oxidative stress. Furthermore, the brain's antioxidant capacity is very low due to low levels of enzymes, such as catalase and glutathione peroxidase, and high levels of iron and unsaturated fatty acids. Following ischemic injury, oxidative stress is a major cause of secondary injury through direct oxidant effects, as well as through activation of a variety of cell-death–signaling pathways (29). Especially in the setting of ischemia followed by reperfusion, pronounced oxidation occurs because large amounts of ROS in oxygenated blood enter the brain through recanalized vessels and through production in activated inflammatory cells. However, even in the absence of reperfusion, the ischemic brain can accumulate ROS. The mitochondrial respiratory chain is one of the main sites of cellular ROS generation, even under physiologic conditions; and, following ischemia, ROS generation further increases due to impaired respiration. ROS can directly react with all macromolecules of the brain cells, causing damage to protein, lipids, and DNA, and can oxidize low-molecular-weight reductants, such as glutathione, ascorbate, and alpha-tocopherol. ROS are also involved in the activation of inflammatory cells and various signaling cascades, thus underscoring their central role in mediating ischemic brain injury (Fig. 3).

Oxidant Systems in the Brain

Many prooxidant and antioxidant enzymes are known to participate in oxidative stress–induced signaling and injury in cerebral ischemia. Prooxidants can be divided into 3 major classes: (i) NOS, which generate NO; (ii) cyclooxygenases (COXs), xanthine dehydrogenase, xanthine oxidase, and NADPH oxidase, which produce superoxide anion; and (iii) myeloperoxidase (MPO) and monoamine oxidase, which generate hypochlorous acid and hydrogen peroxide (H_2O_2), existent in peripheral neutrophils and various brain cells (29). Antioxidants in the brain include the superoxide dismutases (SODs), glutathione peroxidase, and catalase, as well as the low-molecular-weight reductants glutathione, ascorbate (reduced vitamin C), and alpha-tocopherol (reduced vitamin E).

Nitric Oxide Synthase and Nitric Oxide

Three isoforms of NOS generate NO from L-arginine: the neuronal isoform (nNOS) found in neurons, the endothelial isoform (eNOS) found in vessels, and the inducible isoform (iNOS)

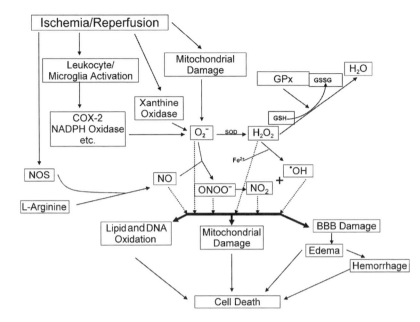

Figure 3 Ischemia-induced oxidative stress. Ischemia, especially followed by reperfusion, leads to increases in reactive oxygen and nitrogen species through a variety of mechanisms. Direct mitochondrial stress can lead to impaired respiratory function and accumulation of ROS. Other sources of ROS include superoxide (O_2^-) generation from inflammatory cell activation of NADPH oxidase and induction of COX-2. Calcium activates xanthine oxidase, whereas NOS converts L-arginine to NO. Superoxide disutase converts O_2^- to hydrogen peroxide (H_2O_2), an oxidant that can react with Fe^{2+} to generate hydroxyl radical ($\cdot$OH). H_2O_2 can be detoxified through glutathione (GSH) in the presence of GPx to form GSSG and H_2O. NO can also react with O_2^- to yield an even more toxic oxidant peroxynitrite (ONOO$^-$). ONOO$^-$ then might further yield 2 other oxidants, NO_2 and $\cdot$OH. All oxidants can then lead to cause oxidation of macromolecules, such as lipids, proteins, and DNA, and cause direct damage to mitochondria. Furthermore, oxidants can lead to BBB damage, causing vasogenic edema and cerebral hemorrhage. *Abbreviations*: COX-2; cyclooxygenase-2; NOS, nitric oxide synthase; NO, nitric oxide; GPx, glutathione peroxidase; GSSG, glutathione disulfide; NO_2; nitric dioxide; BBB, blood–brain barrier.

found in inflammatory cells. In addition to macrophages and microglia, iNOS, under pathologic conditions, can be expressed in other cells, including neurons, astrocytes, and endothelial cells (30). Depending on the isoform and cell type in which NO is produced, NOS plays various roles in ischemic injury (31). nNOS (or NOS1), upregulated in neurons via NMDA receptor–stimulation, mediates early injury, whereas iNOS (or NOS2) is thought to contribute to late injury due to its production in inflammatory cells. eNOS (or NOS3), though expressed at low levels compared to the other isoforms, acts as a vasodilator and is believed to be protective by enhancing CBF. NO can further mediate cell damage by reacting with superoxide anion to form peroxynitrite (ONOO$^-$), which is especially damaging to DNA.

Superoxide-Generating Systems
Superoxide anion is a major oxidant generated in the brain parenchyma after middle cerebral artery occlusion (MCAO) (29). COX-1, COX-2, xanthine dehydrogenase, xanthine oxidase, and NADPH oxidase are all involved in superoxide generation. COX-1 is constitutively expressed, whereas COX-2 is inducible. During prostanoid synthesis, COX-2 generates superoxide ion (32). COX-2 upregulation has been detected following experimental cerebral ischemia (33,34), and COX-2 knockout mice exhibit reduced susceptibility to ischemic brain injury and NMDA-mediated neurotoxicity (35). Furthermore, animals treated with NS-398, an inhibitor of COX-2, also had reduced infarct sizes (36). In contrast, COX-1 might have a beneficial role in ischemia, as COX-1–deficient mice have increased susceptibility, possibly due to downstream effects of prostaglandins on augmenting CBF (37). Superoxide can be generated through xanthine oxidase, which in turn, is generated from xanthine dehydrogenase via a calcium-activated protease. Superoxide is also generated in inflammatory cells, such as peripheral leukocytes and

microglia, via NADPH oxidase as a defense mechanism against microbes. NADPH oxidase is a multicomponent enzyme that consists of 2 membrane-bound subunits (gp91 and p22) and 3 cytosolic subunits (p67, p47, and p40), plus Rac, a small GTPase (38). With appropriate stimuli, the cytosolic subunits translocate to the membrane, where they interact with the membrane-bound subunits to transfer electrons from NADPH to oxygen to form superoxide. NADPH oxidase appears to play a role in mediating ischemic injury, as mice lacking the gp91 subunit have smaller infarcts compared to wildtype (39).

Endogenous Antioxidants

Superoxide Dismutase

The brain has several defensive mechanisms with which to protect itself from oxidative stress. SOD neutralizes superoxide to H_2O_2 (29). Three isoenzymes of SOD are characterized by their subcellular localization and prosthetic metal ions. Cu/Zn-SOD (or SOD1) mainly localizes in cytosol, whereas Mn-SOD (or SOD2) is distributed predominantly in the mitochondria. Extracellular SOD (EC-SOD or SOD3) is found in the extracellular space. The role of SOD1 in focal cerebral ischemia was delineated in studies that used both transgenic SOD1-overexpressing and SOD1-deficient mice. Consistent with a beneficial role, SOD1-transgenic mice exposed to temporary MCAO had smaller infarct sizes than wildtype mice (40). Similarly, SOD1-deficient mice suffered increased neuronal cell death and brain edema after MCAO (41). Similar observations were made in SOD2-knockout mice, which had exacerbated injury (42). EC-SOD is presumed to protect against superoxide produced by membrane-bound NADPH oxidase in inflammatory cells (43). EC-SOD overexpression provides neuroprotection in mice following focal cerebral ischemia (44), whereas EC-SOD–deficient mice have a worsened outcome from experimental stroke (45). Interestingly, SOD does not always protect the brain from ischemia. Neonatal SOD1-transgenic animals had increased injury following hypoxia-ischemia, and this was associated with higher levels of H_2O_2, possibly due to lower levels of downstream antioxidants glutathione peroxidase (GPx) and catalase (46).

Catalase and Glutathione Peroxidase

Whereas SOD dismutates superoxide to H_2O_2 and oxygen O_2, H_2O_2 is another oxidant that can freely cross cell membranes. H_2O_2 is both a product of and a source of free radical reactions. Endogenous H_2O_2 might be converted, either by catalase or GPx, to H_2O, or it might generate the highly reactive free hydroxyl radical ($OH^\bullet$) via the Fenton reaction (47). H_2O_2 is then scavenged by GPx at the expense of reduced glutathione (GSH) to produce H_2O and oxidized glutathione (GSSG). Catalase and GPx are present in the brain (47), with GPx present in the cytosol and catalase localized mainly in peroxisomes (48). Two GPx mimics, ebselen and edaravone, have been shown to be able to reduce infarct volume in experimental focal ischemia (49,50), and viral vector-mediated overexpression of catalase and GPx are associated with improved neuronal survival after experimental stroke (51,52).

Low-Molecular-Weight Reductants

Glutathione, ascorbate, and alpha-tocopherol can reduce H_2O_2 to water and scavenge free radicals; they react preferentially with the chain-propagating radicals to yield a stable radical product of the antioxidants. By donating electrons to free radicals, chain-breaking antioxidants spare other molecules from oxidation. This mechanism is also important in protecting the brain from focal ischemia.

Consequences of Oxidative Damage Following Stroke

Lipid Peroxidation

Phospholipids are major constituents of neuronal membranes, which account for 20% to 25% of the dry weight of the adult brain (53). Phosphatidylcholine and phosphatidylethanolamine comprise >60% of the membrane phospholipids, especially in brain cells. Fatty acids are incorporated into the phosphatidylcholine by combining diacylglycerols, which contain high amounts of such fatty acids as arachidonic and stearic acids. MCAO significantly increases lipid peroxidation in the ischemic hemisphere (54) by hydroxyl radicals and nitrogen dioxide, both of which are generated from ONOO⁻ (55). Lipid peroxidation has many deleterious consequences. Oxidized cell membranes lead to structural compromise, altered permeability, and fluidity, leading to further calcium entry into the cell. Free radicals can cause disruption of membrane-bound receptors and inactivate, and even damage, proteins involved in ion transport (56).

Oxidative DNA Damage

Free radicals can directly damage nucleic acids, causing injury to nuclear DNA, thereby leading to oxidative DNA lesions (ODLs) and DNA strand breaks. Following focal cerebral ischemia, ODLs have been observed mainly in neurons, as well as in astrocytes. They are thought to be caused by hydroxyl radicals and NO (57). Although ODLs are thought to eventually cause neuronal cell death (58), ODLs can be repaired to some degree through nucleotide [nucleotide excision repair (NER)] and base excision repair (BER) (59). Ischemia can trigger NER and BER activity and might represent an important endogenous mechanism in protecting the brain against ischemia-induced oxidative injury (60). If not repaired promptly, ODLs and strand breaks have the potential to trigger various intracellular-signaling pathways and result in brain cell death (58). Not only can such damage interfere with DNA synthesis and gene transcription, but it might also activate poly(ADP-ribose) polymerase-1 (PARP-1) (58,61). Although involved in DNA repair, PARP-1 appears to be detrimental in the setting of brain ischemia (62,63). It is not entirely clear why a repair enzyme might exacerbate ischemic injury, but PARP-1 can deplete ATP and NAD+, leading to further compromises in the cell's energy stores (61,64,65). PARP-1 also appears to mediate caspase-independent apoptosis by facilitating mitochondrial release of apoptosis-inducing factor (AIF) (66,67).

ISCHEMIA-INDUCED GENE EXPRESSION

Cerebral ischemia is generally associated with cessation of gene expression and protein synthesis. However, it is now well recognized that the cell does indeed upregulate new genes and proteins in response to such insults. High-throughput molecular techniques now make it possible to study large numbers of genes that are involved in ischemic pathogenesis. Using such microarray analysis, several groups have documented upregulation of substantial numbers of genes, including the immediate early genes (IEGs) and genes involved in apoptosis, ion channels, inflammation, and others (68–71). Such an approach could lead to the discovery of new pathways and gene families involved in ischemic damage, as well as endogenous mechanisms of protection.

Immediate Early Genes

C-fos, C-jun, and Activator Protein-1

Members of the IEG families, such as c-fos, c-jun, and zinc finger (zif), were among the first genes observed after ischemia onset and are known to be highly upregulated within minutes (72). Mitochondrial membrane depolarization, calcium uptake, and release of factors (e.g., cytochrome c) can ultimately activate activator protein-1 (AP-1) to induce gene expression (73). The induction of IEGs includes several consecutive steps. Ischemia-associated increases in extracellular glutamate and intracellular calcium can lead to the activation of protein kinases (e.g., protein kinase A and protein kinase C), which can phosphorylate DNA binding proteins. DNA binding proteins recognize specific binding domains, which then initiate transcription of the downstream target genes (74). The *c-fos* gene, an IEG that encodes the Fos protein, was found to be upregulated within 30 min after stroke onset (72). Fos protein contains several important structural features, such as a DNA binding region and a leucine zipper. The latter is a region containing leucine residues every 7 amino acids and forms an α-helix with the leucines aligned on one side. Leucine zippers can align with other proteins containing this structure (such as Jun protein families, another IEG) to form dimers. These dimers bind to a specific DNA region known as the AP-1 domain, which regulates the expression of a number of target genes, including the so-called late response genes. Combinations of *c-fos* and *c-jun* family proteins form various dimers that consist of different subunits under certain ischemic circumstances. The composition of the dimer might determine whether the late response gene is turned on or off (75). AP-1, a transcription factor, is formed through dimerization of fos and jun and is thought to be an important component of brain responses to ischemia (76). Whether fos/jun/AP-1 is beneficial or damaging following ischemia is still unclear. Consistent with a beneficial effect, hypothermia, an established neuroprotectant in the laboratory, was associated with early increases in *c-fos* expression and AP-1 DNA binding activity in peri-infarct cortex (77). AP-1 activity is also related to neuronal cell tolerance in ischemia models (78). Furthermore, compounds known to protect the brain were also associated with *c-fos* upregulation (79), and suppression of *c-fos* by an antisense oligonucleotide led to increased tissue damage following cerebral ischemia (80). On the other hand, other studies have shown that transgenic mice that overexpress SOD1 and are protected from experimental stroke have attenuated AP-1 activation, which would be more consistent with a damaging effect (81). The time and regional differences in AP1-binding protein complexes appear to influence final postischemic outcome (82) and might explain why *c-jun* expression has been linked to neuronal apoptosis (83) and to neuronal survival (84).

Activating Transcription Factor

The activating transcription factor (ATF) family includes ATF-1, ATF-2, ATF-3, among which ATF-2 and ATF-3 are reported to be induced by focal cerebral ischemia (85,86). ATF encodes a member of the cAMP response element–binding (CREB) protein family of transcription factors. Members of this family share the same DNA-binding domain (leucine zipper domain) and bind to consensus DNA sequence (TGACGTCA) to form a variety of selective heterodimers with each other via the leucine zipper region (87). ATF-3 is not expressed in the brain under normal conditions but is markedly induced after permanent focal cerebral ischemia. Recent data revealed concurrent expression of ATF-3 and phospho-*c-jun* in neurons (85). ATF-3 represses transcription as a homodimer and activates transcription as a heterodimer with ATF-2 and Jun families (88). Furthermore, ATF-3 has many characteristics of IEGs (89). After MCAO, 98% of ATF-3 immunoreactive neurons simultaneously expressed damage-induced neuronal endopeptidase (DINE) mRNA. In that DINE expression promotes antioxidant activity, these observations suggest that ATF-3 activation upregulates DINE expression and is neuroprotective under ischemic conditions (54).

Additional Immediate Early Genes

Several other IEGs, such as nerve growth factor–induced gene A (NGFI-A, also known as krox24, egr1, and zif268) (74,90) and the orphan nuclear receptor NGFI-B (also known as nur/77) (90,91), have been identified with different structural elements and functions following focal cerebral ischemia. NGFI-B is a member of the steroid receptor superfamily and might have a role coordinating the regulation of the hypothalamic-pituitary-adrenal axis (74). The NGFI-A protein contains a zif that binds to a guanylate-rich DNA consensus sequence. It has been suggested that prolonged NGFI-A expression after an ischemic insult is associated with delayed neuronal degeneration (92).

Heat-Shock Proteins

Following IEG expression, several stress-response genes are upregulated (93–95). Heat-shock proteins (HSPs), among the most studied in the setting of brain ischemia, are a family of chaperone proteins thought to function as the cell's endogenous, self-protecting response to stresses and lethal insults. The inducible HSP70, especially increased following brain ischemia, is a useful marker of stress and correlates to brain regions relatively resistant to injury. In some settings, HSP70 is thought to protect the brain from injury through its chaperone functions by preventing protein malfolding and aggregation (93). However, recent studies suggest that HSP70 might also interfere with cell death pathways, such as apoptosis (96–99), and inhibit expression of damaging proteins, such as the matrix metalloproteinases (MMPs) (100). Whether HSPs can someday be used as a cytoprotective therapy is unclear, but some laboratory data indicate that administration of geldanamycin, a benzoquinone ansamycin that induces HSPs by binding HSP90 and releasing heat-shock factor (HSF) to induce HSP70, ameliorates injury from experimental stroke (101).

APOPTOSIS

Necrosis and apoptosis have both been observed in the brain after stroke, but only recently has it become recognized that apoptosis might also contribute to ischemic damage. Apoptosis, or programmed cell death, is characterized by chromatin condensation and nuclear blebbing. In contrast to necrotic injury, apoptosis involves the activation of specific, energy-dependent cell-death pathways. The best-characterized signaling pathways include the intrinsic (mitochondrial-dependent pathway) and the extrinsic (receptor-mediated pathway) (Fig. 4) (102,103).

Intrinsic Pathway

Following experimental stroke, ischemic injury causes mitochondrial damage that can result in the generation of a permeability transition pore (MPT) (104). The MPT is thought to constitute a large channel in the inner mitochondrial membrane, which is normally closed and can be opened by calcium overload or other factors related to ischemia, such as oxidative stress. Those factors cause translocation of cyclophilin-D from the matrix to the MPT that activates the pore, allowing flux of solutes from the matrix to the intermembrane space (105). Persistent MPT opening allows mitochondrial swelling and disruption of the outer mitochondrial membrane. Release of proapoptotic factors, such as cytochrome c, AIF, endonuclease G, second mitochondria-derived caspase activator (Smac/DIABLO), and high temperature–dependent A2 (HtrA2/Omi, a human serine proteinase), into the cytosol is the ultimate result of MPT opening. Cytochrome c release has been extensively studied as a key factor in mediating ischemia-induced apoptosis (106). Cytochrome c interactswith apoptosis protease–activating factor-1 and dATP/ATP to form the apoptosome, which leads to the activation of procaspase-9, which, in turn, cleaves and activates procaspase-3. This sequence produces further downstream events, including the activation of caspase-activated DNase, that lead to internucleosomal DNA fragmentation.

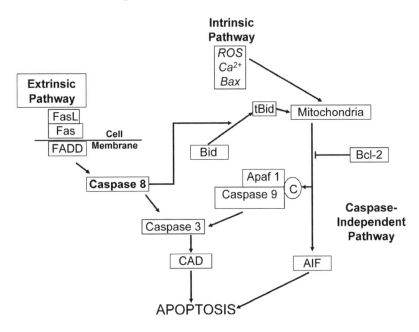

Figure 4 Apoptosis pathways following cerebral ischemia. *Intrinsic pathway*: During brain ischemia and reperfusion, high levels of ROS, calcium ion (Ca²⁺), and proapoptogenic factors, such as Bax, lead to the release of cytochrome c (C). Once released into the cytosol, cytochrome c binds to Apaf-1 and procaspase-9 to form an apoptosome, which, in turn, activates caspase-3, leading to activation of CAD and subsequent cell death. Another pathway is the *caspase-independent pathway*, in which AIF is directly released from the mitochondria and translocates to the nucleus, where it induces apoptosis directly. Bcl-2, a mitochondrial outer membrane protein, is an antiapoptotic protein that can suppress mitochondrial release of cytochrome c and AIF. *Extrinsic pathway*: Several extracellular ligands have now been shown to cause apoptosis through binding their respective receptors. The Fas/FasL system is shown, as this pathway has been the best characterized to date. FasL binds to its respective cell membrane receptor, Fas, which then complexes to an adaptor molecule, FADD, resulting in the recruitment and activation of caspase-8. Caspase-8 then activates caspase-3, leading to cell death. The extrinsic pathway can also interface with the intrinsic pathway because caspase-8 can cleave one of the Bcl-2 family proteins, Bid to tBid. tBid then translocates to mitochondria, where it can trigger cytochrome c (C) and apoptosis-inducing factor release. *Abbreviations*: Apaf-1, apoptotic protease activating factor-1; CAD, caspase-activated DNAse; AIF, apoptosis initiating factor; FasL, Fas ligand; FADD, Fas associate death domain.

AIF, another protein released from the mitochondria, can also produce breakdown of DNA in a caspase-independent fashion (107). Endogenous antiapoptotic proteins of the Bcl-2 family (Bcl-2, Bcl-XL, and others) antagonize mitochondrial release of such apoptogenic factors (108). Interrupting this pathway by blocking cytochrome c release or inhibiting caspase activation appears to reduce injury due to experimental stroke (109,110).

Extrinsic Pathway

The extrinsic, or mitochondrial-independent cell-death, pathway is initiated by the members of death receptor families. Fas/Fas ligand (FasL) is perhaps the most studied pathway with respect to cerebral ischemia. Following experimental stroke, Fas expression has been described, and blocking this pathway by depleting the brain of FasL appears to reduce brain injury (111). This pathway is initiated when the Fas receptor is activated by its corresponding ligand, FasL. Once FasL binds with the Fas receptor, the complex then recruits Fas-associated death domain, a Fas receptor-adaptor protein, from the cytosol and activates caspase-8. Caspase-8 activates caspase-3, leading to DNA damage and cell death in a pathway that is likely identical to the intrinsic pathway. The extrinsic pathway can also interface with the intrinsic pathway, because caspase-8 cleaves Bid, a member of the Bcl-2 family, to form a truncated form (t-Bid), which has the capacity to translocate to the mitochondria and induce cytochrome c release (112).

INFLAMMATION FOLLOWING CEREBRAL ISCHEMIA

Inflammatory cell infiltrates have long been observed in the brain following stroke and have largely been thought to mediate recovery and repair. Inflammation is mostly a nonspecific immunologic reaction and is characterized by peripheral leukocyte influx into the cerebral parenchyma and activation of microglia (1,113). Following stroke, necrotic cells and ROS trigger the innate inflammatory response. Ischemic cells, even ischemic neurons, secrete inflammatory cytokines, which can then lead to adhesion-molecule upregulation in the cerebral vasculature. Various kinds of brain cells also secrete chemokines, which are involved in recruiting peripheral leukocytes and resident microglia to the ischemic lesion. Inflammatory cells can then generate more inflammatory cytokines and potentially cytotoxic substances, leading to more cell damage, as well as disruption of the BBB and extracellular matrix (Fig. 5) (114). Blocking various aspects of the inflammatory cascade has been shown to ameliorate injury from experimental stroke and suggests an important therapeutic target (113), although this has yet to be demonstrated at the clinical level (115).

Adhesion Molecules

Adhesion molecules play a pivotal role in the infiltration of leukocytes into the brain parenchyma after stroke. The interaction between leukocytes and the vascular endothelium is mediated by 3 main groups of cell adhesion molecules: selectins, integrins, and the immunoglobulin superfamily, which includes intercellular adhesion molecule-1 (ICAM-1) (116). When activated, peripheral leukocytes upregulate the CD11/CD18 integrin, which recognizes ICAM-1 on activated vascular endothelia. Selectins mediate rolling of leukocytes on the endothelium of postcapillary venules, which facilitates binding to the cerebral vessel endothelium. Once bound, leukocytes infiltrate and are recruited to necrotic cells by various chemokines (117). Like adhesion molecules, chemokines are also upregulated by NO, ROS, and cytokines produced by ischemic cells. Once activated, the infiltrated leukocytes and resident microglia are able to generate a diversity of potentially toxic substances that lead to such secondary injury as BBB disruption, edema, and hemorrhage. Inflammatory mediators, such as NADPH oxidase and iNOS, can generate more ROS and RNS, respectively. Inflammatory cells also secrete more cytokines and MMPs, proteases thought to cause disruption of the extracellular matrix.

Cytokines

Several cytokines are highly upregulated after stroke. The best-characterized cytokines involved in inflammation after stroke are interleukin (IL)-1, tumor necrosis factor-α (TNF-α), IL-6, IL-10, and transforming growth factor-β (TGF–β). IL-1 appears to play a detrimental role, whereas IL-10 and TGF-β appear to be beneficial. The studies of TNF-α and IL-6 are conflicting.

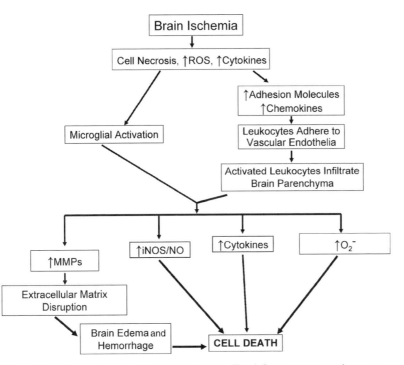

Figure 5 Inflammatory events following stroke. The inflammatory reaction accompanying cerebral ischemia is thought to be triggered by the presence of necrotic cells and ROS. Ischemic brain cells, such as neurons and astrocytes, are also known to secrete inflammatory cytokines, which can rapidly activate microglia. Once activated, microglia generate a variety of inflammatory mediators, such as adhesion molecules and chemokines, which recruit peripheral leukocytes to the brain. Activated leukocytes then infiltrate the ischemic brain parenchyma, which, along with the intrinsic microglia, secrete injurious inflammatory factors, such as MMPs, NO (via iNOS), cytokines, and superoxide (O_2^-, via NADPH oxidase). MMPs lead to disruption of the extracellular matrix, causing brain edema and hemorrhage. *Abbreviations*: ROS, reactive oxygen species; MMP, matrix metalloproteinases; NO, nitric oxide; iNOS, inducible nitric oxide synthase.

IL-1 exists in 2 major isoforms, IL-1α or IL-1β. Their corresponding receptors are IL-1R1 and IL-1R2. IL-1R1 appears to have signaling properties, whereas IL-1R2 does not (118). IL-1 in the ischemic brain appears to potentiate brain injury, as adding exogenous IL-1β exacerbates injury (119). Interestingly, mice lacking both IL-1α and IL-1β exhibited dramatically reduced ischemic infarct volumes compared with wild type (120). However, ischemic damage was not significantly altered in mice lacking either IL-1α or IL-1β, suggesting a requirement for both IL-1α and IL-1β in mediating the effects of IL-1 in acute ischemic stroke brain injury. It has also been suggested that IL-1β acts independently of the IL-1R1 receptor to exacerbate brain injury, as IL-1β exacerbated infarct volume in IL-1R1 knockout mice that was not attenuated by IL-1R antagonist (121). Regardless, IL-1 might prove to be a useful therapeutic target, as an endogenous inhibitor exists, IL-1RA, which, if administered into striatum (122) or delivered via gene therapy to ependymal cells (123), will reduce infarct size.

TNF-α appears to have dual functions in the ischemic brain (124). Inhibition of TNF-α reduces ischemic brain injury (125), whereas administration of recombinant TNF-α protein after stroke onset worsened the ischemic brain damage (126). However, TNF-α might also be beneficial under certain circumstances. It appears to be involved in the phenomenon of ischemic tolerance (127), and mice deficient in TNF receptors have larger infarcts (128,129).

IL-6 is largely thought of as a proinflammatory cytokine, but whether it plays a significant role in ischemic stroke is far from clear. IL-6–deficient mice have similar sized infarcts compared to wild type (130), but other studies suggest either a beneficial (131) or detrimental role (132). IL-10 is an anti-inflammatory cytokine that acts by inhibiting IL-1 and TNF-α, suppressing cytokine receptor expression, and inhibiting receptor activation. It is synthesized in the central nervous system and is upregulated following experimental stroke (133). Both exogenous administration (134,135) and gene transfer of IL-10 (136) in cerebral ischemia models appear to have a protective effect.

TGF-β possesses trophic properties and might be involved in recovery and repair. It is present in the brain after ischemia, and its overexpression is associated with improved neurologic outcome and decreased brain cell injury (137).

Transcriptional Regulation of Inflammation

Nuclear factor-κB (NF-κB) is a major transcription factor involved in the regulation of inflammation induced by focal cerebral ischemia (1). NF-κB is normally located in the cytoplasm and combines with its natural inhibitor, known as the IκB family. The IκB family consists of IκB-α, IκB-β, and IκB-γ. Phosphorylation of IκB-α by an upstream IκB kinase (IKK) liberates NF-κB and allows it to translocate to the nucleus. ROS, cytokines, and excess intracellular Ca^{2+} might activate IKK during stroke. In the nucleus, NFκ-B binds to κB sites, which are specific domains within the promoters of downstream genes to activate their transcription. It is known that a variety of genes involved in inflammation contain functional κB sites within their promoters and are induced by NF-κB; for example, genes that express proteins of TNF-α, ICAM-1, COX-2, and IL-6 are activated by focal ischemia. However, the function of NF-κB in stroke is still controversial. Consistent with a damaging role, mild hypothermia, a robust neuroprotectant, was found to attenuate NFκ-B by inhibiting IKK-β and IKK-γ following transient focal cerebral ischemia (138). Furthermore, mice deficient in NFκ-B's p50 subunit were protected from experimental stroke (139). However, another study reported that rats given an NFκ-B inhibitor, diethyldithiocarbamate, experienced enhanced neuron DNA fragmentation and larger infarct volume, compared with controls (140).

MATRIX METALLOPROTEINASES

Recent work has focused intense study on the MMPs and their contribution to BBB disruption, brain edema, and hemorrhage (141,142). MMPs are a family of extracellular-soluble or membrane-bound proteases that are involved in remodeling the extracellular matrix. MMPs are divided into 4 major classes: (i) interstitial collagenases (MMP-1), (ii) stromelysins (MMP-3), (iii) gelatinases (MMP-2, MMP-7, and MMP-9), and (iv) membrane-type MMP (MMP-14). Several endogenous inhibitors, known as tissue inhibitors of metalloproteinases (TIMPs), also exist. MMP-2, -3, -7, and -9 and TIMP-1, -2 and -3 (143) in relation to cerebral ischemia. MMPs are normally found in the cytosol in a proactivated or inactivated state and are cleaved by proteases, such as plasmin (which is cleaved to its active form from plasminogen by tissue plasminogen activator), to their active state (142). Thus, MMPs might be an important therapeutic target. In fact, prior work has shown that MMP inhibition reduces infarct size, brain edema, and hemorrhage following experimental stroke (144,145). MMP-9 appears to play a more significant role in stroke, compared to MMP-2. Mice deficient in MMP-9 were found to have smaller infarcts compared to wild-type controls (146). MMP-2-deficient mice, on the other hand, fared no better than wild type (147).

MMPs have also been implicated in the disruption of the BBB. Brain edema due to swelling and compromise of adjacent health tissue can worsen outcome from stroke and other neurologic disorders. Accumulated data indicate that increased BBB permeability or disruption results from focal ischemia and induces the formation of vasogenic edema through seepage of serum elements into the brain parenchyma. In the setting of reperfusion, vasogenic edema is thought to play a critical role in brain edema formation due to MMP activation. MMPs, by virtue of their ability to disrupt the extracellular matrix, are thought to contribute to this process. MMP-9 has largely been observed in peripheral leukocytes (148) and microglia (143), thus linking the role of MMPs to the inflammatory system. In fact, peripheral inflammatory cell MMP-9 might contribute significantly to ischemic brain injury, as mice transplanted with bone marrow from MMP-9–deficient mice suffered less injury and less BBB disruption than mice transplanted with marrow containing intact MMP-9 (149). At the clinical level, MMPs might also be important in mediating significant cerebral hemorrhage in the setting of thrombolytic use. In fact, mice treated with a thrombolytic plus an MMP inhibitor suffered less hemorrhagic transformation following embolic stroke, compared to those that only received a thrombolytic (150).

CONCLUSIONS AND FUTURE DIRECTIONS

Ischemic stroke triggers a diversity of signaling pathways related to altered gene expression, inflammation, oxidative stress, mitochondrial function, and programmed cell death. The outcome of ischemic stroke depends on how early the blood flow can be restored and how early the related treatments can be provided. Although no one animal model can completely model the human disease, recent work has taken advantage of the many advances in molecular and cellular biology as tools to better understand the pathogenesis of stroke. Over the past 2 decades, only one treatment (thrombolytic therapy with rtPA) has been available in the United States for patients with acute stroke. However, a better understanding of the involved mechanisms should certainly lead to the identification of appropriate treatments.

ACKNOWLEDGMENTS

This work was supported in part by funds from NIH / NINDS: NS40516 (MAY), American Heart Association grants 0540066N (MAY) and 0325089Y (ZZ), and Stanford University Dean's Postdoctoral Fellowship (XT).

REFERENCES

1. Zheng Z, Lee JE, Yenari MA. Stroke: molecular mechanisms and potential targets for treatment. Curr Mol Med 2003; 3(4):361–372.
2. Bisdas S, Donnerstag F, Ahl B, Bohrer I, Weissenborn K, Becker H. Comparison of perfusion computed tomography with diffusion-weighted magnetic resonance imaging in hyperacute ischemic stroke. J Comput Assist Tomogr 2004; 28(6):747–755.
3. Weinstein PR, Hong S, Sharp FR. Molecular identification of the ischemic penumbra. Stroke 2004; 35(11 suppl 1):2666–2670.
4. Schaller B, Graf R. Cerebral ischemia and reperfusion: the pathophysiologic concept as a basis for clinical therapy. J Cereb Blood Flow Metab 2004; 24(4):351–371.
5. Dirnagl U, Iadecola C, Moskowitz MA. Pathobiology of ischaemic stroke: an integrated view. Trends Neurosci 1999; 22(9):391–397.
6. Schurr A, Rigor BM. The mechanism of cerebral hypoxic-ischemic damage. Hippocampus 1992; 2(3):221–228.
7. Stys PK, Waxman SG, Ransom BR. Na(+)-Ca^{2+} exchanger mediates Ca^{2+} influx during anoxia in mammalian central nervous system white matter. Ann Neurol 1991; 30(3):375–380.
8. Lehotsky J, Kaplan P, Babusikova E, Strapkova A, Murin R. Molecular pathways of endoplasmic reticulum dysfunctions: possible cause of cell death in the nervous system. Physiol Res 2003; 52(3):269–274.
9. Paschen W. Shutdown of translation: lethal or protective? Unfolded protein response versus apoptosis. J Cereb Blood Flow Metab 2003; 23(7):773–779.
10. DeGracia DJ, Kumar R, Owen CR, Krause GS, White BC. Molecular pathways of protein synthesis inhibition during brain reperfusion: implications for neuronal survival or death. J Cereb Blood Flow Metab 2002; 22(2):127–141.
11. Pellegrini-Giampietro DE. The distinct role of mGlu1 receptors in post-ischemic neuronal death. Trends Pharmacol Sci 2003; 24(9):461–470.
12. Choi DW. Calcium-mediated neurotoxicity: relationship to specific channel types and role in ischemic damage. Trends Neurosci 1988; 11(10):465–469.
13. Lipton SA, Rosenberg PA. Excitatory amino acids as a final common pathway for neurologic disorders. N Engl J Med 1994; 330(9):613–622.
14. Hoyte L, Barber PA, Buchan AM, Hill MD. The rise and fall of NMDA antagonists for ischemic stroke. Curr Mol Med 2004; 4(2):131–136.
15. Tokita Y, Bessho Y, Masu M, et al. Characterization of excitatory amino acid neurotoxicity in N-methyl-D-aspartate receptor-deficient mouse cortical neuronal cells. Eur J Neurosci 1996; 8(1):69–78.
16. Wahlestedt C, Golanov E, Yamamoto S, et al. Antisense oligodeoxynucleotides to NMDA-R1 receptor channel protect cortical neurons from excitotoxicity and reduce focal ischaemic infarctions. Nature 1993; 363(6426):260–263.

17. Takagi N, Sasakawa K, Besshoh S, Miyake-Takagi K, Takeo S. Transient ischemia enhances tyrosine phosphorylation and binding of the NMDA receptor to the Src homology 2 domain of phosphatidylinositol 3-kinase in the rat hippocampus. J Neurochem 2003; 84(1):67–76.

18. Matsumoto S, Shamloo M, Isshiki A, Wieloch T. Persistent phosphorylation of synaptic proteins following middle cerebral artery occlusion. J Cereb Blood Flow Metab 2002; 22(9):1107–1113.

19. Shamloo M, Wieloch T. Changes in protein tyrosine phosphorylation in the rat brain after cerebral ischemia in a model of ischemic tolerance. J Cereb Blood Flow Metab 1999; 19(2):173–183.

20. Aarts M, Liu Y, Liu L, et al. Treatment of ischemic brain damage by perturbing NMDA receptor-PSD-95 protein interactions. Science 2002; 298(5594):846–850.

21. Huang Z, Huang PL, Panahian N, Dalkara T, Fishman MC, Moskowitz MA. Effects of cerebral ischemia in mice deficient in neuronal nitric oxide synthase. Science 1994; 265(5180):1883–1885.

22. McCullough LD, Zeng Z, Blizzard KK, Debchoudhury I, Hurn PD. Ischemic nitric oxide and poly (ADP-ribose) polymerase-1 in cerebral ischemia: male toxicity, female protection. J Cereb Blood Flow Metab 2005; 25(4):502–512.

23. Arundine M, Tymianski M. Molecular mechanisms of calcium-dependent neurodegeneration in excitotoxicity. Cell Calcium 2003; 34(4–5):325–337.

24. Tanaka H, Grooms SY, Bennett MV, Zukin RS. The AMPAR subunit GluR2: still front and center-stage. Brain Res 2000; 886(1–2):190–207.

25. Sommer C, Kiessling M. Ischemia and ischemic tolerance induction differentially regulate protein expression of GluR1, GluR2, and AMPA receptor binding protein in the gerbil hippocampus: GluR2 (GluR-B) reduction does not predict neuronal death. Stroke 2002; 33(4):1093–1100.

26. Weiser T. AMPA receptor antagonists with additional mechanisms of action: new opportunities for neuroprotective drugs? Curr Pharm Des 2002; 8(10):941–951.

27. Bartus RT, Elliott PJ, Hayward NJ, et al. Calpain as a novel target for treating acute neurodegenerative disorders. Neurol Res 1995; 17(4):249–258.

28. Phillis JW, O'Regan MH. A potentially critical role of phospholipases in central nervous system ischemic, traumatic, and neurodegenerative disorders. Brain Res Brain Res Rev 2004; 44(1):13–47.

29. Chan PH. Reactive oxygen radicals in signaling and damage in the ischemic brain. J Cereb Blood Flow Metab 2001; 21(1):2–14.

30. Nathan C, Xie QW. Nitric oxide synthases: roles, tolls, and controls. Cell 1994; 78(6):915–918.

31. Iadecola C. Bright and dark sides of nitric oxide in ischemic brain injury. Trends Neurosci 1997; 20(3):132–139.

32. O'Banion MK. Cyclooxygenase-2: molecular biology, pharmacology, and neurobiology. Crit Rev Neurobiol 1999; 13(1):45–82.

33. Kinouchi H, Huang H, Arai S, Mizoi K, Yoshimoto T. Induction of cyclooxygenase-2 messenger RNA after transient and permanent middle cerebral artery occlusion in rats: comparison with c-fos messenger RNA by using in situ hybridization. J Neurosurg 1999; 91(6):1005–1012.

34. Planas AM, Soriano MA, Rodriguez-Farre E, Ferrer I. Induction of cyclooxygenase-2 mRNA and protein following transient focal ischemia in the rat brain. Neurosci Lett 1995; 200(3):187–190.

35. Iadecola C, Niwa K, Nogawa S, et al. Reduced susceptibility to ischemic brain injury and N-methyl-D-aspartate-mediated neurotoxicity in cyclooxygenase-2-deficient mice. Proc Natl Acad Sci USA 2001; 98(3):1294–1299.

36. Sugimoto K, Iadecola C. Delayed effect of administration of COX-2 inhibitor in mice with acute cerebral ischemia. Brain Res 2003; 960(1–2):273–276.

37. Iadecola C, Sugimoto K, Niwa K, Kazama K, Ross ME. Increased susceptibility to ischemic brain injury in cyclooxygenase-1-deficient mice. J Cereb Blood Flow Metab 2001; 21(12):1436–1441.

38. Groemping Y, Rittinger K. Activation and assembly of the NADPH oxidase: a structural perspective. Biochem J 2005; 386(Pt 3):401–416.

39. Walder CE, Green SP, Darbonne WC, et al. Ischemic stroke injury is reduced in mice lacking a functional NADPH oxidase. Stroke 1997; 28(11):2252–2258.

40. Kinouchi H, Epstein CJ, Mizui T, Carlson E, Chen SF, Chan PH. Attenuation of focal cerebral ischemic injury in transgenic mice overexpressing CuZn superoxide dismutase. Proc Natl Acad Sci USA 1991; 88(24):11158–11162.

41. Kondo T, Reaume AG, Huang TT, et al. Reduction of CuZn-superoxide dismutase activity exacerbates neuronal cell injury and edema formation after transient focal cerebral ischemia. J Neurosci 1997; 17(11):4180–4189.

42. Murakami K, Kondo T, Kawase M, et al. Mitochondrial susceptibility to oxidative stress exacerbates cerebral infarction that follows permanent focal cerebral ischemia in mutant mice with manganese superoxide dismutase deficiency. J Neurosci 1998; 18(1):205–213.

43. Oury TD, Ho YS, Piantadosi CA, Crapo JD. Extracellular superoxide dismutase, nitric oxide, and central nervous system O_2 toxicity. Proc Natl Acad Sci USA 1992; 89(20):9715–9719.

44. Sheng H, Bart RD, Oury TD, Pearlstein RD, Crapo JD, Warner DS. Mice overexpressing extracellular superoxide dismutase have increased resistance to focal cerebral ischemia. Neuroscience 1999; 88(1):185–191.

45. Sheng H, Brady TC, Pearlstein RD, Crapo JD, Warner DS. Extracellular superoxide dismutase deficiency worsens outcome from focal cerebral ischemia in the mouse. Neurosci Lett 1999; 267(1):13–16.

46. Fullerton HJ, Ditelberg JS, Chen SF, et al. Copper/zinc superoxide dismutase transgenic brain accumulates hydrogen peroxide after perinatal hypoxia ischemia. Ann Neurol 1998; 44(3):357–364.

47. Sharma Y, Bashir S, Irshad M, Gupta SD, Dogra TD. Effects of acute dimethoate administration on antioxidant status of liver and brain of experimental rats. Toxicology 2005; 206(1):49–57.

48. Warner DS, Sheng H, Batinic-Haberle I. Oxidants, antioxidants, and the ischemic brain. J Exp Biol 2004; 207(Pt 18):3221–3231.

49. Imai H, Graham DI, Masayasu H, Macrae IM. Antioxidant ebselen reduces oxidative damage in focal cerebral ischemia. Free Radic Biol Med 2003; 34(1):56–63.

50. Shichinohe H, Kuroda S, Yasuda H, et al. Neuroprotective effects of the free radical scavenger Edaravone (MCI-186) in mice permanent focal brain ischemia. Brain Res 2004; 1029(2):200–206.

51. Gu W, Zhao H, Yenari MA, Sapolsky RM, Steinberg GK. Catalase over-expression protects striatal neurons from transient focal cerebral ischemia. Neuroreport 2004; 15(3):413–416.

52. Hoehn B, Yenari MA, Sapolsky RM, Steinberg GK. Glutathione peroxidase overexpression inhibits cytochrome c release and proapoptotic mediators to protect neurons from experimental stroke. Stroke 2003; 34(10):2489–2494.

53. Phillis JW, O'Regan MH. The role of phospholipases, cyclooxygenases, and lipoxygenases in cerebral ischemic/traumatic injuries. Crit Rev Neurobiol 2003; 15(1):61–90.

54. Ohba N, Kiryu-Seo S, Maeda M, Muraoka M, Ishii M, Kiyama H. Expression of damage-induced neuronal endopeptidase (DINE) mRNA in peri-infarct cortical and thalamic neurons following middle cerebral artery occlusion. J Neurochem 2004; 91(4):956–964.

55. Beckman JS. -OONO: rebounding from nitric oxide. Circ Res 2001; 89(4):295–297.

56. Zolotarjova N, Ho C, Mellgren RL, Askari A, Huang WH. Different sensitivities of native and oxidized forms of Na+/K(+)-ATPase to intracellular proteinases. Biochim Biophys Acta 1994; 1192(1):125–131.

57. Huang D, Shenoy A, Cui J, Huang W, Liu PK. In situ detection of AP sites and DNA strand breaks bearing 3'-phosphate termini in ischemic mouse brain. Faseb J 2000; 14(2):407–417.

58. Besson VC, Margaill I, Plotkine M, Marchand-Verrecchia C. Deleterious activation of poly(ADP-ribose)polymerase-1 in brain after in vivo oxidative stress. Free Radic Res 2003; 37(11):1201–1208.

59. Kisby GE, Lesselroth H, Olivas A, et al. Role of nucleotide- and base-excision repair in genotoxin-induced neuronal cell death. DNA Repair (Amst) 2004; 3(6):617–627.

60. Lan J, Li W, Zhang F, et al. Inducible repair of oxidative DNA lesions in the rat brain after transient focal ischemia and reperfusion. J Cereb Blood Flow Metab 2003; 23(11):1324–1339.

61. Pieper AA, Verma A, Zhang J, Snyder SH. Poly (ADP-ribose) polymerase, nitric oxide and cell death. Trends Pharmacol Sci 1999; 20(4):171–181.

62. Endres M, Wang ZQ, Namura S, Waeber C, Moskowitz MA. Ischemic brain injury is mediated by the activation of poly(ADP-ribose)polymerase. J Cereb Blood Flow Metab 1997; 17(11):1143–1151.

63. Eliasson MJ, Sampei K, Mandir AS, et al. Poly(ADP-ribose) polymerase gene disruption renders mice resistant to cerebral ischemia. Nat Med 1997; 3(10):1089–1095.

64. Ying W, Alano CC, Garnier P, Swanson RA. NAD+ as a metabolic link between DNA damage and cell death. J Neurosci Res 2005; 79(1–2):216–223.

65. Du L, Zhang X, Han YY, et al. Intra-mitochondrial poly(ADP-ribosylation) contributes to NAD+ depletion and cell death induced by oxidative stress. J Biol Chem 2003; 278(20):18426–18433.

66. Hong SJ, Dawson TM, Dawson VL. Nuclear and mitochondrial conversations in cell death: PARP-1 and AIF signaling. Trends Pharmacol Sci 2004; 25(5):259–264.

67. Alano CC, Ying W, Swanson RA. Poly(ADP-ribose) polymerase-1-mediated cell death in astrocytes requires NAD+ depletion and mitochondrial permeability transition. J Biol Chem 2004; 279(18):18895–18902.

68. Soriano MA, Tessier M, Certa U, Gill R. Parallel gene expression monitoring using oligonucleotide probe arrays of multiple transcripts with an animal model of focal ischemia. J Cereb Blood Flow Metab 2000; 20(7):1045–1055.

69. Jin K, Mao XO, Eshoo MW, et al. Microarray analysis of hippocampal gene expression in global cerebral ischemia. Ann Neurol 2001; 50(1):93–103.

70. Schmidt-Kastner R, Zhang B, Belayev L, et al. DNA microarray analysis of cortical gene expression during early recirculation after focal brain ischemia in rat. Brain Res Mol Brain Res 2002; 108(1–2):81–93.

71. Roth A, Gill R, Certa U. Temporal and spatial gene expression patterns after experimental stroke in a rat model and characterization of PC4, a potential regulator of transcription. Mol Cell Neurosci 2003; 22(3):353–364.

72. Lu XC, Williams AJ, Yao C, et al. Microarray analysis of acute and delayed gene expression profile in rats after focal ischemic brain injury and reperfusion. J Neurosci Res 2004; 77(6):843–857.

73. Mattson MP, Culmsee C, Yu ZF. Apoptotic and antiapoptotic mechanisms in stroke. Cell Tissue Res 2000; 301(1):173–187.

74. Akins PT, Liu PK, Hsu CY. Immediate early gene expression in response to cerebral ischemia. Friend or foe? Stroke 1996; 27(9):1682–1687.

75. Sheng M, Greenberg ME. The regulation and function of c-fos and other immediate early genes in the nervous system. Neuron 1990; 4(4):477–485.

76. Tong L, Toliver-Kinsky T, Rassin D, Werrbach-Perez K, Perez-Polo JR., Hyperoxia increases AP-1 DNA binding in rat brain. Neurochem Res 2003; 28(1):111–115.

77. Akaji K, Suga S, Fujino T, et al. Effect of intra-ischemic hypothermia on the expression of c-Fos and c-Jun, and DNA binding activity of AP-1 after focal cerebral ischemia in rat brain. Brain Res 2003; 975(1–2):149–157.

78. Kapinya K, Penzel R, Sommer C, Kiessling M. Temporary changes of the AP-1 transcription factor binding activity in the gerbil hippocampus after transient global ischemia, and ischemic tolerance induction. Brain Res 2000; 872(1–2):282–293.

79. Cho S, Park EM, Kim Y, et al. Early c-Fos induction after cerebral ischemia: a possible neuroprotective role. J Cereb Blood Flow Metab 2001; 21(5):550–556.

80. Zhang Y, Widmayer MA, Zhang B, Cui JK, Baskin DS. Suppression of post-ischemic-induced fos protein expression by an antisense oligonucleotide to c-fos mRNA leads to increased tissue damage. Brain Res 1999; 832(1–2):112–117.

81. Huang CY, Fujimura M, Chang YY, Chan PH. Overexpression of copper-zinc superoxide dismutase attenuates acute activation of activator protein-1 after transient focal cerebral ischemia in mice. Stroke 2001; 32(3):741–747.

82. Zablocka B, Dluzniewska J, Zajac H, Domanska-Janik K. Opposite reaction of ERK and JNK in ischemia vulnerable and resistant regions of hippocampus: involvement of mitochondria. Brain Res Mol Brain Res 2003; 110(2):245–252.

83. Schenkel J. Activation of the c-Jun transcription factor following neurodegeneration in vivo. Neurosci Lett 2004; 361(1–3):36–39.

84. Herdegen T, Skene P, Bahr M. The c-Jun transcription factor–bipotential mediator of neuronal death, survival and regeneration. Trends Neurosci 1997; 20(5):227–231.

85. Ohba N, Maeda M, Nakagomi S, Muraoka M, Kiyama H. Biphasic expression of activating transcription factor-3 in neurons after cerebral infarction. Brain Res Mol Brain Res 2003; 115(2):147–156.

86. He Q, Csiszar K, Li P. Transient forebrain ischemia induced phosphorylation of cAMP-responsive element-binding protein is suppressed by hyperglycemia. Neurobiol Dis 2003; 12(1):25–34.

87. Liang G, Wolfgang CD, Chen BP, Chen TH, Hai T. ATF3 gene. Genomic organization, promoter, and regulation. J Biol Chem 1996; 271(3):1695–1701.

88. Hai T, Curran T. Cross-family dimerization of transcription factors Fos/Jun and ATF/CREB alters DNA binding specificity. Proc Natl Acad Sci USA 1991; 88(9):3720–3724.

89. Hai T, Wolfgang CD, Marsee DK, Allen AE, Sivaprasad U. ATF3 and stress responses. Gene Expr 1999; 7(4–6):321–335.

90. Johansson IM, Wester P, Hakova M, Gu W, Seckl JR, Olsson T. Early and delayed induction of immediate early gene expression in a novel focal cerebral ischemia model in the rat. Eur J Neurosci 2000; 12(10):3615–3625.

91. Lin TN, Chen JJ, Wang SJ, et al. Expression of NGFI-B mRNA in a rat focal cerebral ischemia-reperfusion model. Brain Res Mol Brain Res 1996; 43(1–2):149–156.

92. Honkaniemi J, States BA, Weinstein PR, Espinoza J, Sharp FR. Expression of zinc finger immediate early genes in rat brain after permanent middle cerebral artery occlusion. J Cereb Blood Flow Metab 1997; 17(6):636–646.

93. Yenari MA. Heat shock proteins and neuroprotection. Adv Exp Med Biol 2002; 513:281–289.

94. Sharp FR, Massa SM, Swanson RA. Heat-shock protein protection. Trends Neurosci 1999; 22(3):97–99.

95. Kelly S, Yenari MA. Neuroprotection: heat shock proteins. Curr Med Res Opin 2002; 18(Suppl 2):s55–s60.

96. Kelly S, Zhang ZJ, Zhao H, et al. Gene transfer of HSP72 protects cornu ammonis 1 region of the hippocampus neurons from global ischemia: influence of Bcl-2. Ann Neurol 2002; 52(2):160–167.

97. Matsumori Y, Hong SM, Aoyama K, et al. Hsp70 overexpression sequesters AIF and reduces neonatal hypoxic / ischemic brain injury. J Cereb Blood Flow Metab 2005; 25:899–910.

98. Ran R, Zhou G, Lu A, et al. Hsp70 mutant proteins modulate additional apoptotic pathways and improve cell survival. Cell Stress Chaperones 2004; 9(3):229–242.

99. Ran R, Lu A, Zhang L, et al. Hsp70 promotes TNF-mediated apoptosis by binding IKK gamma and impairing NF-kappa B survival signaling. Genes Dev 2004; 18(12):1466–1481.

100. Lee JE, Kim YJ, Kim JY, Lee WT, Yenari MA, Giffard RG. The 70 kDa heat shock protein suppresses matrix metalloproteinases in astrocytes. Neuroreport 2004; 15(3):499–502.

101. Lu A, Ran R, Parmentier-Batteur S, Nee A, Sharp FR. Geldanamycin induces heat shock proteins in brain and protects against focal cerebral ischemia. J Neurochem 2002; 81(2):355–364.

102. Graham SH, Chen J. Programmed cell death in cerebral ischemia. J Cereb Blood Flow Metab 2001; 21(2):99–109.
103. Sugawara T, Fujimura M, Noshita N, et al. Neuronal Death / Survival Signaling Pathways in Cerebral Ischemia. Neurorx 2004; 1(1):17–25.
104. Siesjo BK, Elmer E, Janelidze S, et al. Role and mechanisms of secondary mitochondrial failure. Acta Neurochir Suppl 1999; 73:7–13.
105. Tanveer A, Virji S, Andreeva L, et al. Involvement of cyclophilin D in the activation of a mitochondrial pore by Ca^{2+} and oxidant stress. Eur J Biochem 1996; 238(1):166–172.
106. Fujimura M, Morita-Fujimura Y, Murakami K, Kawase M, Chan PH. Cytosolic redistribution of cytochrome c after transient focal cerebral ischemia in rats. J Cereb Blood Flow Metab 1998; 18(11):1239–1247.
107. Joza N, Susin SA, Daugas E, et al. Essential role of the mitochondrial apoptosis-inducing factor in programmed cell death. Nature 2001; 410(6828):549–554.
108. Zhao H, Yenari MA, Cheng D, Sapolsky RM, Steinberg GK. Bcl-2 overexpression protects against neuron loss within the ischemic margin following experimental stroke and inhibits cytochrome c translocation and caspase-3 activity. J Neurochem 2003; 85(4):1026–1036.
109. Yu G, Hess DC, Borlongan CV. Combined cyclosporine-A and methylprednisolone treatment exerts partial and transient neuroprotection against ischemic stroke. Brain Res 2004; 1018(1):32–37.
110. Schulz JB, Weller M, Moskowitz MA. Caspases as treatment targets in stroke and neurodegenerative diseases. Ann Neurol 1999; 45(4):421–429.
111. Martin-Villalba A, Hahne M, Kleber S, et al. Therapeutic neutralization of CD95-ligand and TNF attenuates brain damage in stroke. Cell Death Differ 2001; 8(7):679–686.
112. Ferrer I, Planas AM. Signaling of cell death and cell survival following focal cerebral ischemia: life and death struggle in the penumbra. J Neuropathol Exp Neurol 2003; 62(4):329–339.
113. Han HS, Yenari MA. Cellular targets of brain inflammation in stroke. Curr Opin Investig Drugs 2003; 4(5):522–529.
114. Danton GH, Dietrich WD. Inflammatory mechanisms after ischemia and stroke. J Neuropathol Exp Neurol 2003; 62(2):127–136.
115. Becker KJ. Anti-leukocyte antibodies: LeukArrest (Hu23F2G) and Enlimomab (R6.5) in acute stroke. Curr Med Res Opin 2002; 18(suppl 2):s18–s22.
116. Frijns CJ, Kappelle LJ. Inflammatory cell adhesion molecules in ischemic cerebrovascular disease. Stroke 2002; 33(8):2115–2122.
117. Minami M, Satoh M. Chemokines and their receptors in the brain: pathophysiological roles in ischemic brain injury. Life Sci 2003; 74(2–3):321–327.
118. Rothwell N. Interleukin-1 and neuronal injury: mechanisms, modification, and therapeutic potential. Brain Behav Immun 2003; 17(3):152–157.
119. Stroemer RP, Rothwell NJ. Exacerbation of ischemic brain damage by localized striatal injection of interleukin-1beta in the rat. J Cereb Blood Flow Metab 1998; 18(8):833–839.
120. Boutin H, LeFeuvre RA, Horai R, Asano M, Iwakura Y, Rothwell NJ. Role of IL-1alpha and IL-1beta in ischemic brain damage. J Neurosci 2001; 21(15):5528–5534.
121. Patel HC, Boutin H, Allan SM. Interleukin-1 in the brain: mechanisms of action in acute neurodegeneration. Ann N Y Acad Sci 2003; 992:39–47.
122. Stroemer RP, Rothwell NJ. Cortical protection by localized striatal injection of IL-1ra following cerebral ischemia in the rat. J Cereb Blood Flow Metab 1997; 17(6):597–604.
123. Betz AL, Yang GY, Davidson BL. Attenuation of stroke size in rats using an adenoviral vector to induce overexpression of interleukin-1 receptor antagonist in brain. J Cereb Blood Flow Metab 1995; 15(4):547–551.
124. Hallenbeck JM. The many faces of tumor necrosis factor in stroke. Nat Med 2002; 8(12):1363–1368.
125. Yang GY, Gong C, Qin Z, Ye W, Mao Y, Bertz AL. Inhibition of TNFalpha attenuates infarct volume and ICAM-1 expression in ischemic mouse brain. Neuroreports 1998; 9(9):2131–2134.
126. Barone FC, Arvin B, White RF, et al. Tumor necrosis factor-alpha. A mediator of focal ischemic brain injury. Stroke 1997; 28(6):1233–1244.
127. Ginis I, Jaiswal R, Klimanis D, Liu J, Greenspon J, Hallenbeck JM. TNF-alpha-induced tolerance to ischemic injury involves differential control of NF-kappaB transactivation: the role of NF-kappaB association with p300 adaptor. J Cereb Blood Flow Metab 2002; 22(2):142–152.
128. Gary DS, Bruce-Keller AJ, Kindy MS, Mattson MP. Ischemic and excitotoxic brain injury is enhanced in mice lacking the p55 tumor necrosis factor receptor. J Cereb Blood Flow Metab 1998; 18(12): 1283–1287.
129. Bruce AJ, Boling W, Kindy MS, et al. Altered neuronal and microglial responses to excitotoxic and ischemic brain injury in mice lacking TNF receptors. Nat Med 1996; 2(7):788–794.
130. Clark WM, Rinker LG, Lessov NS, et al. Lack of interleukin-6 expression is not protective against focal central nervous system ischemia. Stroke 2000; 31(7):1715–1720.
131. Herrmann O, Tarabin V, Suzuki S, et al. Regulation of body temperature and neuroprotection by endogenous interleukin-6 in cerebral ischemia. J Cereb Blood Flow Metab 2003; 23(4):406–415.

132. Smith CJ, Emsley HC, Gavin CM, et al. Peak plasma interleukin-6 and other peripheral markers of inflammation in the first week of ischaemic stroke correlate with brain infarct volume, stroke severity, and long-term outcome. BMC Neurol 2004; 4(1):2.

133. Strle K, Zhou JH, Shen WH, et al. Interleukin-10 in the brain. Crit Rev Immunol 2001; 21(5): 427–449.

134. Spera PA, Ellison JA, Feuerstein GZ, Barone FC. IL-10 reduces rat brain injury following focal stroke. Neurosci Lett 1998; 251(3):189–192.

135. Dietrich WD, Busto R, Bethea JR. Postischemic hypothermia and IL-10 treatment provide long-lasting neuroprotection of CA1 hippocampus following transient global ischemia in rats. Exp Neurol 1999; 158(2):444–450.

136. Ooboshi H, Ibayashi S, Shichita T, et al. Postischemic gene transfer of interleukin-10 protects against both focal and global brain ischemia. Circulation 2005; 111(7):913–919.

137. Zhu Y, Yang GY, Ahlemeyer B, et al. Transforming growth factor-beta 1 increases bad phosphorylation and protects neurons against damage. J Neurosci 2002; 22(10):3898–3909.

138. Han HS, Karabiyikoglu M, Kelly S, Sobel RA, Yenari MA. Mild hypothermia inhibits nuclear factor-kappaB translocation in experimental stroke. J Cereb Blood Flow Metab 2003; 23(5):589–598.

139. Schneider A, Martin-Villalba A, Weih F, Vogel J, Wirth T, Schwaninger M. NF-kappaB is activated and promotes cell death in focal cerebral ischemia. Nat Med 1999; 5(5):554–559.

140. Hill WD, Hess DC, Carroll JE, et al. The NF-kappaB inhibitor diethyldithiocarbamate (DDTC) increases brain cell death in a transient middle cerebral artery occlusion model of ischemia. Brain Res Bull 2001; 55(3):375–386.

141. Cunningham LA, Wetzel M, Rosenberg GA. Multiple roles for MMPs and TIMPs in cerebral ischemia. Glia 2005; 50(4):329–339.

142. Rosenberg GA. Matrix metalloproteinases in neuroinflammation. Glia 2002; 39(3):279–291.

143. Lee J, Yoon YJ, Cheng D, Sun GH, Moseley ME, Yenari MA. Mild hypothermia reduces matrix metalloproteinases (MMPs) and increases tissue inhibitor of metalloprotainease-2 (TIMP-2) expression in experimental stroke. J Neurosurg 2005; 103(2):289–297.

144. Pfefferkorn T, Rosenberg GA. Closure of the blood-brain barrier by matrix metalloproteinase inhibition reduces rtPA-mediated mortality in cerebral ischemia with delayed reperfusion. Stroke 2003; 34(8):2025–2030.

145. Lapchak PA, Chapman DF, Zivin JA. Metalloproteinase inhibition reduces thrombolytic (tissue plasminogen activator)-induced hemorrhage after thromboembolic stroke. Stroke 2000; 31(12): 3034–3040.

146. Asahi M, Asahi K, Jung JC, del Zoppo GJ, Fini ME, Lo EH. Role for matrix metalloproteinase 9 after focal cerebral ischemia: effects of gene knockout and enzyme inhibition with BB-94. J Cereb Blood Flow Metab 2000; 20(12):1681–1689.

147. Asahi M, Sumii T, Fini ME, Itohara S, Lo EH. Matrix metalloproteinase 2 gene knockout has no effect on acute brain injury after focal ischemia. Neuroreport 2001; 12(13):3003–3007.

148. Maier CM, Hsieh L, Yu F, Bracci P, Chan PH. Matrix metalloproteinase-9 and myeloperoxidase expression: quantitative analysis by antigen immunohistochemistry in a model of transient focal cerebral ischemia. Stroke 2004; 35(5):1169–1174.

149. Gidday JM, Gasche YG, Copin JC, et al. Leukocyte-derived matrix metalloproteinase-9 mediates blood-brain barrier breakdown and is proinflammatory following transient focal cerebral ischemia. Am J Physiol Heart Circ Physiol 2005; 25:899–910.

150. Sumii T, Lo EH. Involvement of matrix metalloproteinase in thrombolysis-associated hemorrhagic transformation after embolic focal ischemia in rats. Stroke 2002; 33(3):831–836.

18 | Neuroimaging in Ischemic Stroke

José G. Merino, MD, MPhil, Staff Clinician
Steven Warach, MD, PhD, Chief
Section on Stroke Diagnostics and Therapeutics, National Institute of Neurological Disorders and Stroke, Bethesda, Maryland, USA

INTRODUCTION

Neuroimaging plays a critical role in the management of patients with ischemic stroke. The success and safety of pharmacologic and mechanical interventions depends on the precise diagnosis of ischemic stroke and the exclusion of other pathologies. Although CT is currently the most widely available—and thus most commonly used—initial imaging modality, increasing evidence shows that multimodal MRI provides additional clinically relevant diagnostic and prognostic information to optimize patient management. It is also an important research tool with which to study stroke pathophysiology and identify new treatments. In this chapter, we discuss the clinical and research roles of MRI.

MRI IN CLINICAL CARE

A clinical multimodal MRI study for acute stroke takes 20 minutes or less, clearly shows ischemic areas (confirming the diagnosis), and rules out intracranial hemorrhage (ICH) and other pathologies. Several stroke centers rely exclusively on MRI to screen patients for treatment with pharmacologic and mechanical interventions (1). At the NIH Stroke Center, the acute protocol includes the following sequences: diffusion-weighted imaging (DWI), gradient echo (GRE), fluid-attenuated inversion recovery (FLAIR), 3-dimensional, time-of-flight intracranial magnetic resonance angiography (MRA), and perfusion-weighted imaging (PWI). Additionally, if the patient is outside the time window for intravenous recombinant tissue plasminogen activator (rtPA) but is a candidate for other interventions, we perform a contrast-enhanced MRA from the aortic arch to the brain (Fig. 1) (2). Our understanding of the clinical role of this technology is evolving, and the results of several clinical trials that use MRI to determine eligibility, or as an outcome measure, will help to determine its optimal use.

DWI visualizes regions of ischemia within minutes of onset. Ischemia-induced membrane dysfunction and cytotoxic edema restrict the diffusion of water and lead to a decrease in the apparent diffusion coefficient (ADC); the lesion appears dark on ADC maps and hyperintense on DWI. Diffusion imaging has a high degree of sensitivity (88–100%) and specificity (95–100%) for acute ischemia, even at very early time points (3–5). Studies performed in the acute stroke setting show that the accuracy of DWI (95–100%) is higher than that of CT (42–75%) or FLAIR (46%) (6–10). Information on the natural history of lesion growth as seen on DWI comes from clinical trials and case series that show enlargement of the diffusion lesions over time (11–15). Numerous studies show that the initial diffusion lesion volume correlates well with final infarct volume and neurologic and functional outcomes in stroke patients, suggesting that diffusion MR can provide important early prognostic information (12,16–19).

The acute ischemic lesion on DWI is dynamic. Data from experimental models show that acute ischemic changes in ADC might (i) increase in volume and progress to infarct, (ii) regress and normalize, (iii) normalize but later deteriorate despite reperfusion, or (iv) give rise to transient waves of reduced ADC, reflective of the depolarizations of cortical spreading depression that predict lesion growth. In some cases, we observed obvious progression or regression of the lesion over a 10-min period. Defining the rate of infarct evolution is important to determining the relationship of treatment delays and tissue and clinical outcome.

PWI identifies tissue that has decreased perfusion and, when used in conjunction with DWI, shows penumbral tissue that is salvageable if blood flow is restored (20–23). Via the

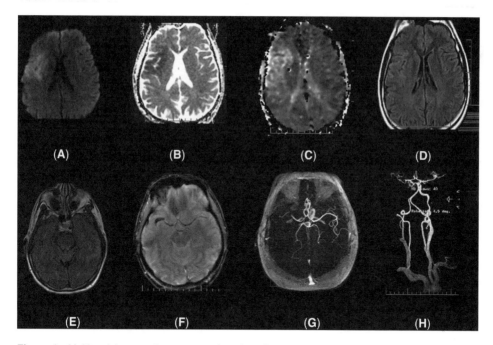

Figure 1 Multimodal magnetic resonance imaging of a 55-year-old man who presented with aphasia, dysarthria, left hemianopsia, and left hemiplegia; the NIHSS score was 17. On diffusion-weighted imaging is an area of restricted diffusion in the right frontal lobe (**A**) with a matching area of decreased apparent diffusion coefficient (**B**) and a slightly larger area of perfusion abnormality (**C**). The fluid-attenuated inversion recovery does not show any abnormalities in the tissue yet (**D**), but the carotid flow void in the right is missing (**E**). No hemorrhages are seen on gradient echo, but a clot is noted in the right middle cerebral artery (MCA) (**F**), which corresponds to the absence of flow in one of the branches noted on magnetic resonance angiography (MRA) (**G**). The aortic arch-to-brain MRA shows absent flow in the right cervical carotid, with reconstitution in the right intracranial portion and no flow after the M1 segment of the MCA (**H**). The patient had a carotid dissection and was enrolled in a therapeutic trial.

bolus-contrast-passage method, several relative perfusion measures can be derived, including mean transit time (MTT), time to peak, regional cerebral blood volume, and regional cerebral blood flow. Methods to quantitate cerebral perfusion using an arterial input function have been proposed, but their accuracy has not been established. By identifying a penumbral pattern, PWI studies might help to select patients for therapy: a prospective, randomized clinical trial (MR and Recanalization of Clots Using Embolectomy) is underway to test this hypothesis.

GRE pulse sequences (T2*-weighted or susceptibility images) are very sensitive to the susceptibility effect of local magnetic field distortions due to unpaired electrons in the iron atom in blood breakdown products, making MRI more sensitive to ICH than CT is (24–26) and, therefore, potentially the optimal initial imaging modality in patients who might be treated with thrombolytics. In the Hemorrhage and Early MRI Evaluation study, a prospective, multicentered study that evaluated patients with stroke symptoms within 6 hr of onset, MRI was as accurate as CT for the detection of acute hemorrhage and more sensitive for the detection of chronic hemorrhage, thus refuting the early belief that MRI might be less sensitive than CT (26). In addition, MRI can detect punctate chronic hemorrhages (termed "microhemorrhages") that might indicate increased risk for bleeding complications of thrombolytic or antithrombotic therapy (Fig. 2) (27).

Cortical and periventricular lesions are very well visualized with FLAIR because the cerebrospinal fluid (CSF) signal is nearly suppressed and lesions are bright. This sequence is well suited to looking for subacute infarcts and, because extra-axial blood is hyperintense in this sequence, can identify subarachnoid and subdural hemorrhage. Hyperintense arterial signals are indicative of slow flow associated with severe occlusions or stenosis. Intracranial MRA can reliably identify intracranial and extracranial arterial occlusions in the acute setting and can identify targets for mechanical interventions.

The possibility of worse outcomes resulting from the greater time requirement for MRI is of concern. In the NINDS rtPA trial, the prospective planned analysis of the interaction of

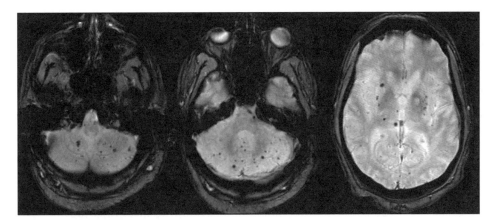

Figure 2 50-year-old patient with long-standing hypertension.

time-to-treatment and treatment assignment was not significant (28). Subsequent analyses of the NINDS trial data and the pooled data from 4 thrombolytic studies showed that the odds of a favorable outcome decreased as the time from onset to treatment increased, but in the pooled analysis the difference was only significant in the 0- to 90-min versus the 271- to 360-min cohorts (29). Time from onset is a crude approximation of the relevant variable that determines the probability of favorable response: the presence of tissue potentially salvageable by treatment. In that MRI can show that relevant variable, conclusions about the relationship of time from onset to probability of good outcome cannot be extrapolated from the CT-based trials to MRI-based clinical practice.

A randomized clinical trial is the only way to determine the optimal imaging modality in the acute phase of stroke, but such a study would require more than 1000 patients. Data from the NIH Stroke Center, however, suggest that MRI screening before intravenous thrombolysis within 3 hr of onset of symptoms is feasible, practical, and safe (30). We compared time to treatment and clinical outcome of 78 patients who were screened with MRI, 22 patients screened with CT, and data from the two largest rtPA multicenter registries: the Canadian Activase for Stroke Effectiveness Study (CASES) and the Standard Treatment with TPA to Reverse Stroke (STARS) study (Table 1) (31,32). Triage-to-treatment times in patients screened at Suburban Hospital were 31 min less if MRI was not done, but outcomes trended better for the MRI-screened subset. Time-to-treatment and CT versus MRI screening were not predictors of outcome in the multiple logistic regression analysis. Triage-to-treatment and onset-to-treatment times were similar to those described in CASES and STARS (Table 1). At our center, MRI has played a significant role in treatment decisions (27).

Table 1 Time to Treatment and Clinical Outcome of Participants in the CASES, STARS, and NSC Studies

	NSC (30) (all patients)	NSC (30) (MRI screen)	STARS (31)	CASES (32)
n	100	78	389	1132
Door-to-treatment time (min); median Interquartile range	83 (66–101)	89 (76–105)	96 (75–124)	85 (60–110)
Onset-to-treatment time (min); median Interquartile range	138 (116–167)	140 (117–165)	164 (134–176)	155 (130–175)
Percent treated within 90 min from onset (%)	9.0	6.4	4.1	N/A
mRS 0–1 (%)	39	40	35	32
mRS 0–2 (%)	47	49	43	46

Note: Times to treatment with standard rtPA therapy and outcomes at a center that uses MRI screening vs. published benchmarks from centers that do not screen with MRI.

Abbreviations: NSC, NIH Stroke Center at Suburban Hospital; STARS, Standard Treatment with TPA to Reverse Stroke; CASES, Canadian Activase for Stroke Effectiveness Study; mRS, modified Rankin Scale.

MRI IN STROKE RESEARCH

New imaging techniques, especially MRI, can provide a translational link between experimental advances in acute stroke research and clinical applications (33). MRI can identify markers of "tissue at risk" (to link therapy to tissue pathobiology); demonstrate the effects of cerebral reperfusion on the underlying vascular pathology, cerebral blood flow, and blood-brain barrier (BBB) integrity; and establish parameters for dose, duration, and time window to optimize drug delivery to the ischemic area. New knowledge in these areas and the use of MRI in therapeutic studies can lead to improved patient selection and evaluation of drug activity in clinical trials.

MRI to Study Stroke Pathophysiology

Identification of "Tissue at Risk"
The use of thrombolytic agents is currently limited to patients who meet rigid time criteria, but a more rational approach to select patients for treatment and to study pathophysiology in individual patients is to use physiologic measurements that reflect the vascular and cellular pathobiology (34). Because it can measure physiologic variables in a short time, MRI can be used to investigate the pathologic features that best identify "tissue at risk" and clinical outcomes in response to therapies; these findings can be used for the design of clinical trials and for routine clinical care.

The Use of MRI to Predict Tissue Outcome
The use of DWI and PWI to make prognoses in individual patients is an active area of research (11,16,35,36). Data from natural history studies and clinical trials show significant correlations between the volume of abnormality on acute DWI and clinical severity; they also show that a combination of clinical factors (NIHSS score and time in hours from stroke onset to DWI) and DWI volume measurements is a better predictor of stroke outcome than the use of a single factor at acute or chronic times (11,12,16,17,19,37). Several studies have analyzed early MR characteristics that, in untreated stroke patients, predict the final infarct volume. We previously used a logistic regression model to differentiate regions of ultimate infarction versus noninfarction, based on baseline perfusion measures, and to operationally define the ischemic penumbra (36). Other groups have employed a variety of statistical and empirical approaches, such as generalized linear model algorithms, multiparametric ISODATA techniques, and other automated strategies, to predict final tissue outcome. In addition, thresholds for infarct progression and risk of hemorrhagic transformation (HT) might be identified by quantitative diffusion or perfusion MRI (36,38–42). However, these thresholds are not absolute and depend on the technique of measurement and analysis, the time from onset, the therapeutic intervention, and interactions with other physiologic and clinical variables (43–45). These and other approaches are accurate but are based on small and heterogeneous samples, and the validation, accuracy, reliability, and feasibility of these models in the clinic have not been reported.

MRI as a Marker of Ischemic Lesion Recurrence
Recurrent stroke is a major cause of morbidity and mortality, and the identification of effective interventions to prevent it is a research priority. The cumulative rate of clinical stroke recurrence within a few weeks after the initial ischemic event is <5%, but as it is not easy to clinically differentiate worsening from a new ischemic event, it is probably that the true incidence rate is higher (46,47). Several groups have used DWI to study the prevalence of multiple acute ischemic lesions in patients with stroke and found that the lesions are common; their prevalence varies from 17% in patients imaged within 24 hr to 29% in the patients imaged within 4 days, and up to 83% in patients with high-grade carotid stenosis imaged within 1 week of onset (48–50).

 To test the hypothesis that risk for recurrent ischemic lesions continued in the weeks following the clinically symptomatic stroke, we analyzed 2 cohorts of acute stroke patients. The first cohort involved 99 consecutive patients who had an MRI within 6 hr of symptom onset; 1 week after stroke, 34% had a recurrent infarct (in 15%, the new lesion was outside; in 16%, the new lesion was within the original area of perfusion abnormality; in 3%, a baseline PWI was not available). Initial multiple DWI lesions were associated with lesion recurrence (hazard ratio, HR, 2.8; 95% confidence interval (CI), 1.7–10.3; $p=0.002$) and with distant lesion recurrence

(HR, 6.0; 95% CI, 4.1–64.1; $p<0.0001$). Large-artery atherosclerosis was the most frequent stroke subtype associated with lesion recurrence ($p=0.026$) (51).

In a second cohort of 80 patients, the initial MRI was performed within 48 hr of onset and follow-up MRI was done at 5, 30, and 90 days; late lesion recurrence occurred in 26% of patients and was more frequently observed on the 30-day MRI than it was on the 90-day MRI ($p=0.016$). Early-lesion recurrence (HR, 3.0; 95% CI, 1.4–8.6; $p=0.0095$), distant early-lesion recurrence (HR, 3.6; 95% CI, 1.6–26.5; $p=0.0088$), and initial multiple DWI lesions correlating with early-lesion recurrence (HR, 3.6; 95% CI, 1.6–9.4; $p=0.003$) were associated with late-lesion recurrence. These early MRI markers and a history of hypertension remained significant, independent predictors of late-lesion recurrence. The frequency of early-lesion recurrence and late-lesion recurrence on MRI was significantly higher than that of early (2%) and late (4%) clinical recurrences ($p<0.001$) (52). These data suggest that, in some stroke patients, risk of recurrent ischemic lesions continues into the weeks following the clinically symptomatic stroke. If this is the case, MRI-defined ischemic lesion recurrence is potentially a useful surrogate endpoint in clinical trials of stroke prevention therapies. If studies establish the validity of this biomarker, it can be used in future clinical trials, requiring substantially fewer patients and shorter follow-up periods than do studies that exclusively rely on clinical outcome measures, with the ultimate benefit of enormous cost and time savings in evaluating preventive therapies.

MRI to Evaluate the Effects of Cerebral Reperfusion

The most effective therapy for acute stroke in humans is the recanalization of occluded arteries enabling tissue reperfusion (28,53). The effect of reperfusion, however, can lead to injury due to activation of the endothelium, excess production of oxygen free radicals, leukocyte recruitment, increases in cytokine production, enhanced inflammatory response, and edema formation. These changes damage the microvascular structure of the BBB, a prerequisite for HT (54,55). Several animal models focus on thrombolytic-related reperfusion injury and microvascular damage, and studies of animal models of stroke report parenchymal enhancement on MRI with BBB disruption (56–58). Until recently, the relevance of these findings to the pathology and treatment of acute stroke in humans was unknown. The discovery of a new MRI marker—hyperintense acute reperfusion marker (HARM)—allows the study of BBB disruption in stroke pathophysiology (59). HARM refers to delayed gadolinium enhancement of the CSF space on FLAIR that is due to disruption of the BBB (60). The BBB opening indicated by HARM is distinct from enhancement of the leptomeninges (61–63) and from the parenchymal enhancement that is observed during the later stage (days to weeks) of cerebral ischemia (Fig. 3) (61,64,65). In a recent study on a prospective cohort of 144 patients, we found HARM in 47 (33%), with a mean time from symptom onset to the observation of BBB disruption being 12.9 hr (SD=10.3). However, based on the pharmacokinetics of gadolinium (66), it is likely that the opening of the BBB occurred before or soon after the administration of the contrast agent, at a median of 3.8 hr from onset. The timing and features of HARM are suggestive of the early BBB opening described in animals (67). The marker was focal in the sulcal space in the vascular territory of the acute stroke in 21 patients, diffuse within the ventricles in 6, and local and diffuse in 20. HARM was associated with reperfusion, subsequent HT, and poor clinical outcome (59). HT and BBB disruption were more common in patients treated with rtPA (31% and 55%) than in those not treated (14% and 25%; $p=0.057$ and 0.001, respectively). The association of HARM with HT was even greater in the subgroup of patients receiving rtPA, supporting the hypothesis that the proteolytic action of rtPA might contribute to extracellular matrix degradation and HT (68).

In collaboration with the University of California Los Angeles Stroke Center, we observed HARM in 62% of intra-arterial thrombolysis patients but only in 33% of patients treated with mechanical clot removal (69), suggesting that rapid reperfusion plays a causal role in early BBB disruption and that rtPA could exacerbate this condition. We believe that the pathophysiology indicated by HARM might present an opportunity for intervention prior to a failure of the BBB. Recent studies have implicated matrix metalloproteinases (MMPs), which attack the basal lamina and ultimately result in damage to the ultrastructure of the microvasculature (70). High plasma concentrations of MMP-9 are independent predictors of HT in treated and untreated patients. In the treated patients, however, it is unclear if high MMP levels are the direct result of the exogenous rtPA or reperfusion (71,72). Early results using the MMP inhibitor BB-94 have shown a reduction in the hemorrhage rates, providing evidence that pharmacologic intervention might limit damage to the microvasculature and suggesting that MMP inhibition as a

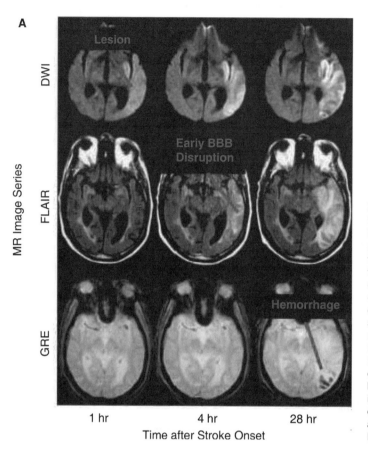

Figure 3 Magnetic resonance images from a patient undergoing hemorrhagic transformation. (A) Aligned and registered diffusion-weighted imaging (DWI), fluid-attenuated inversion recovery (FLAIR), and gradient recalled echo (GRE) images acquired at 3 different times after onset of acute symptoms. DWI of initial examination 1 hr after onset depicts ischemic lesion as hyperintense. FLAIR images acquired 4 hr after onset exhibit evidence of blood–brain barrier disruption. GRE images at 28 hr show evidence of hemorrhagic transformation as a region of hyperintensity. *Source:* From Ref. 59.

promising target for reducing the hemorrhagic complications of thrombolytic therapy. HARM might have the potential as an imaging marker to evaluate those therapies. In that, as discussed above, the BBB is permeable close to the time window of acute thrombolytic therapy, this event is relevant to the development of therapies to prevent HT and improve outcome after thrombolysis and other reperfusion therapies.

MRI in Clinical Trials

Few efficacious experimental therapeutic interventions have led to successful human clinical trials. Although the barriers to the translation of experimental findings into clinical advances are many, the adoption of innovative clinical trial designs; the development of combination neuroprotective therapies based on molecular and cellular pathways of injury; the development of new approaches to achieve reperfusion more quickly, completely, and safely; and the identification of imaging markers of disease definition, therapeutic targets, and outcomes can bridge the basic science-clinical gap, and MRI can help to achieve this objective (33,73,74).

Patient Selection

Clinical trials must enroll a sufficiently homogeneous sample to reduce the statistical variance of the data and optimize the sensitivity of the design to detect a therapeutic response, while remaining representative of the population of interest. Ischemic stroke trials have traditionally limited the range of disease studied to one or more clinical dimensions (severity, duration, or prognosis of the clinical deficits) and relied on noncontrast CT scan for exclusion of cerebral hemorrhage or other nonischemic pathology. Reliance on clinical criteria, however, can be misleading, and CT scanning has poor sensitivity for the diagnosis of early ischemic changes (75). Because MRI can detect early ischemic pathology, rule out ICH, and visualize the vasculature, it can identify the pathologic subtype and allow the appropriate use of treatment-congruent criteria for patient selection (76). Using MRI-based pathologic criteria rather than clinical assessment and CT scans for patient selection and outcome measurement is a more powerful approach to demonstrate efficacy in stroke trials (77).

MRI as a Surrogate Outcome

A surrogate endpoint in a clinical trial is "a laboratory measurement or a physical sign used as a substitute for a clinically meaningful endpoint that measures directly how a patient feels, functions, or survives. Changes induced by a therapy on a surrogate endpoint are expected to reflect changes in a clinically meaningful endpoint" (78,79). Validated surrogate markers are those for which evidence has established that a drug-induced effect on the surrogate predicts the desired effect on the clinical outcome of interest (78,79). MRI markers of ischemia recurrence can be used for selecting and screening interventions in Phase 2 trials, and if the surrogate is a correlate of the true clinical outcome and fully captures the net effect of treatment, it can be used in Phase 3 studies (79,80). One promise of MRI as a marker of outcome is that it will permit Phase 2 proof-of-principle trials using a relatively small sample size.

The citicoline MRI stroke trial illustrates the value of MRI in clinical trials. In this study, the primary outcome variable was a relative reduction in lesion growth. Although citicoline had an effect on lesion growth, the difference with placebo was not significant, perhaps because of a small sample size (80 patients). Post hoc power calculations revealed that 116 patients—a sample typical for Phase 2 studies, but an order of magnitude smaller than Phase 3 trials, which depend only on clinical variables for inclusion and as outcome—would have been sufficient to demonstrate a neuroprotective effect (12); this was confirmed by a subsequent randomized, controlled trial with approximately 60 patients per group, which showed a significant difference (23). These citicoline trials confirmed the value of MRI as a marker of disease severity and progression and indicated that the change in MRI lesion size is likely to predict clinical improvement, an essential feature of a surrogate outcome measure. Pooled analysis of the citicoline trials suggests a clinical benefit of this treatment (81), evidence that diffusion lesion volume change might be a predictor of therapeutic response.

Before MRI can be used as an outcome in stroke trials, its utility as a surrogate measure must be validated. The first step is to demonstrate that the early pathologic changes, and changes induced by treatment, can predict clinical outcome. Data discussed below suggest that this is the case.

Lesion Volume Reduction as a Predictor of Clinical Response to rtPA

In experimental models, reduction of infarct growth or reversal of ischemic injury is necessary and sufficient evidence of an effective treatment. These indicators of target drug effect have been proposed for early Phase 2 proof-of-principle clinical trials because it is likely that drugs that beneficially modify the evolution of infarction would have a therapeutic clinical effect. Four randomized clinical trials have confirmed that the acute-to-chronic change in lesion volume is a good marker of clinical change: lesion volume decrease or a lesser degree of lesion growth was strongly associated with good clinical outcome (12,16,23,76,82,83). None of those trials, however, were positive on the primary clinical endpoint, so the question of whether lesion volume change predicts response to a clinically proven therapy has not been answered. Lesion volume change has been studied following rtPA therapy, but not with a pretreatment assessment in the approved 3-hr time window (22,84–86). We tested the hypothesis that pre- to posttreatment lesion volume change would predict clinical benefit in 25 consecutive rtPA-treated stroke patients who had pretreatment DWI and follow-up FLAIR, and observed a highly significant ($p<0.0001$) difference in volume change between the patients who had very favorable recovery (modified Rankin scale, mRS=0–1) and those who did not. A 30% or greater decrease in volume had a positive predictive value (PPV) for a very favorable outcome of 100% with an accuracy of 84% ($p<0.002$), and a 30% or greater increase in volume had a 93% PPV of unfavorable outcome with an accuracy of 89% ($p<0.0001$) (87). These results suggest that lesion volume change is a good predictor of clinical outcome with standard thrombolytic therapy. Whether these markers distinguish treatment effects in a placebo-controlled trial of a thrombolytic drug will need to be tested prospectively.

Reperfusion After rtPA as a Predictor of Clinical Recovery

Ischemic changes on DWI and PWI in the first few hours after intravenous rtPA administration might predict clinical outcome. We analyzed data from 42 ischemic stroke patients treated with rtPA who had pretreatment and 2-hr posttreatment scans. Change in volume on DWI and MTT, recanalization rate on MRA, and HT on GRE were the outcomes of interest. Clinical and MRI variables were compared between those with very favorable outcome, defined as 3-month mRS of 0 to 1, and those with incomplete recovery (mRS>1); we used multiple logistic regression analysis to identify independent predictors for recovery. The median times from onset to rtPA and from rtPA to follow-up scan were 131 and 123 min, respectively. The median time between scans was 161 min. HT did not occur. By 2 hr, only 2 patients (5%) had complete recanalization and reperfusion. In univariate and multivariate analysis of 37 patients with complete data, the most powerful predictor for very favorable outcome was MTT lesion volume decrease >30% from pretreatment to 2-hour scan ($p=0.009$; odds ratio, 20.7; 95% CI: 2.1–203.9). Age (<70 years) was also an independent predictor for complete recovery ($p=0.036$). Pretreatment and posttreatment DWI and MTT lesion volumes, and pre- to post-DWI volume changes were predictors of outcome in the univariate, but not in the multivariate analysis, supporting the hypothesis that pre- to posttreatment changes have greater statistical power in predicting clinical outcome than a single time point value. We propose this degree of change as an early marker of long-term clinical benefit of thrombolytic therapy. Multicenter placebo-controlled clinical trials of thrombolytic therapy using MRI assessments are in progress at other institutions and could provide a prospective test of these early and late markers of response as discriminators of therapeutic response to thrombolytics.

REFERENCES

1. Hjort N, Butcher K, Davis SM, et al. Magnetic resonance imaging criteria for thrombolysis in acute cerebral infarct. Stroke 2005; 36(2):388–397.
2. Lattimore SU, Chalela J, Davis L, et al. Impact of establishing a primary stroke center at a community hospital on the use of thrombolytic therapy: the NINDS Suburban Hospital Stroke Center experience. Stroke 2003; 34(6):e55–e57.
3. van Everdingen KJ, van der Grond J, Kappelle LJ, Ramos LM, Mali WP. Diffusion-weighted magnetic resonance imaging in acute stroke. Stroke 1998; 29:1783–1790.
4. Lövblad KO, Laubach HJ, Baird AE, et al. Clinical experience with diffusion-weighted MR in patients with acute stroke. Am J Neuroradiol 1998; 19(6):1061–1066.
5. Gonzalez RG, Schaefer PW, Buonanno FS, et al. Diffusion-weighted MR imaging: diagnostic accuracy in patients imaged within 6 hours of stroke symptom onset. Radiology 1999; 210(1):155–162.
6. Barber PA, Darby DG, Desmond PM, et al. Identification of major ischemic change. Diffusion-weighted imaging versus computed tomography. Stroke 1999; 30(10):2059–2065.
7. Lansberg MG, Albers GW, Beaulieu C, Marks MP. Comparison of diffusion-weighted MRI and CT in acute stroke. Neurology 2000; 54(8):1557–1561.
8. Perkins CJ, Kahya E, Roque CT, Roche PE, Newman GC. Fluid-attenuated inversion recovery and diffusion- and perfusion-weighted MRI abnormalities in 117 consecutive patients with stroke symptoms. Stroke 2001; 32(12):2774–2781.
9. Mullins ME, Schaefer PW, Sorensen AG, et al. CT and conventional and diffusion-weighted MR imaging in acute stroke: study in 691 patients at presentation to the emergency department. Radiology 2002; 224(2):353–360.
10. Kelly PJ, Hedley-Whyte ET, Primavera J, He J, Gonzalez RG. Diffusion MRI in ischemic stroke compared to pathologically verified infarction. Neurology 2001; 56(7):914–920.
11. Baird AE, Benfield A, Schlaug G, et al. Enlargement of human cerebral ischemic lesion volumes measured by diffusion-weighted magnetic resonance imaging. Ann Neurol 1997; 41(5):581–589.
12. Warach S, Pettigrew LC, Dashe JF, et al. Effect of citicoline on ischemic lesions as measured by diffusion-weighted magnetic resonance imaging. Citicoline 010 Investigators. Ann Neurol 2000; 48(5):713–722.
13. Lansberg MG, O'Brien MW, Tong DC, Moseley ME, Albers GW. Evolution of cerebral infarct volume assessed by diffusion-weighted magnetic resonance imaging. Arch Neurol 2001; 58(4):613–617.
14. Schwamm LH, Koroshetz WJ, Sorensen AG, et al. Time course of lesion development in patients with acute stroke: serial diffusion- and hemodynamic-weighted magnetic resonance imaging. Stroke 1998; 29(11):2268–2276.
15. Beaulieu C, de Crespigny A, Tong DC, Moseley ME, Albers GW, Marks MP. Longitudinal magnetic resonance imaging study of perfusion and diffusion in stroke: evolution of lesion volume and correlation with clinical outcome. Ann Neurol 1999; 46:568–578.
16. Warach S, Dashe JF, Edelman RR. Clinical outcome in ischemic stroke predicted by early diffusion-weighted and perfusion magnetic resonance imaging: a preliminary analysis. J Cereb Blood Flow Metab 1996; 16(1):53–59.

17. Lovblad KO, Baird AE, Schlaug G, et al. Ischemic lesion volumes in acute stroke by diffusion-weighted magnetic resonance imaging correlate with clinical outcome. Ann Neurol 1997; 42(2):164–170.
18. Barber PA, Darby DG, Desmond PM, et al. Prediction of stroke outcome with echoplanar perfusion- and diffusion-weighted MRI. Neurology 1998; 51(2):418–426.
19. Baird AE, Dambrosia J, Janket S, et al. A three-item scale for the early prediction of stroke recovery. Lancet 2001; 357(9274):2095–2099.
20. Davis D, Ulatowski J, Eleff S, et al. Rapid monitoring of changes in water diffusion coefficients during reversible ischemia in cat and rat brain. Magn Reson Med 1994; 31(4):454–460.
21. Minematsu K, Li L, Sotak CH, Davis MA, Fisher M. Reversible focal ischemic injury demonstrated by diffusion-weighted magnetic resonance imaging in rats. Stroke 1992; 23(9):1304–1310; discussion 1310–1311.
22. Kidwell CS, Saver JL, Mattiello J, et al. Thrombolytic reversal of acute human cerebral ischemic injury shown by diffusion/perfusion magnetic resonance imaging. Ann Neurol 2000; 47(4):462–469.
23. Warach S, Sabounjian LA. ECCO 2000 study of citicoline for treatment of acute ischemic stroke: Effects on infarct volumes measured by MRI. Stroke 2000; 31(1):42.
24. Patel MR, Edelman RR, Warach S. Detection of hyperacute primary intraparenchymal hemorrhage by magnetic resonance imaging. Stroke 1996; 27(12):2321–2324.
25. Linfante I, Llinas RH, Caplan LR, Warach S. MRI features of intracerebral hemorrhage within 2 hours from symptom onset. Stroke 1999; 30(11):2263–2267.
26. Kidwell CS, Chalela JA, Saver JL, et al. Comparison of MRI and CT for detection of acute intracerebral hemorrhage. Jama 2004; 292(15):1823–1830.
27. Chalela JA, Kang DW, Warach S. Multiple cerebral microbleeds: MRI marker of a diffuse hemorrhage-prone state. J Neuroimaging 2004; 14(1):54–57.
28. National Institute of Neurological Disorders and Stroke rt-PA Stroke Study Group. Tissue plasminogen activator for acute ischemic stroke. N Engl J Med 1995; 333(24):1581–1587.
29. Hacke W, Donnan G, Fieschi C, et al. Association of outcome with early stroke treatment: pooled analysis of ATLANTIS, ECASS, and NINDS rt-PA stroke trials. Lancet 2004; 363(9411):768–774.
30. Kang D, Chalela J, Warach S. Screening MRI prior to alteplase therapy is feasible and safe. Stroke 2004; 35(1):236–237.
31. Albers GW, Bates VE, Clark WM, Bell R, Verro P, Hamilton SA. Intravenous tissue-type plasminogen activator for treatment of acute stroke: the Standard Treatment with Alteplase to Reverse Stroke (STARS) study. JAMA 2000; 283(9):1145–1150.
32. Hill M, Buchan AM. For the CASES Investigators. The Canadian Activase for Stroke Effectiveness Study (CASES). J Cereb Blood Flow Metab 2003; 23(suppl 1):552.
33. NINDS Stroke Progress Review Group. http://www.ninds.nih.gov/funding/neural_environment/stroke_prg/StrokePRGreport-4-23–02.cd.pdf. Accessed Might 25, 2005.
34. Warach S. Thrombolysis in stroke beyond three hours: targeting patients with diffusion and perfusion MRI. Ann Neurol 2002; 51(1):11–13.
35. Schlaug G, Siewert B, Benfield A, Edelman RR, Warach S. Time course of the apparent diffusion coefficient (ADC) abnormality in human stroke. Neurology 1997; 49(1):113–119.
36. Schlaug G, Benfield A, Baird AE, et al. The ischemic penumbra: operationally defined by diffusion and perfusion MRI. Neurology 1999; 53(7):1528–1537.
37. Baird AE, Lovblad KO, Dashe JF, et al. Clinical correlations of diffusion and perfusion lesion volumes in acute ischemic stroke. Cerebrovasc Dis 2000; 10(6):441–448.
38. Wu O, Koroshetz WJ, Ostergaard L, et al. Predicting tissue outcome in acute human cerebral ischemia using combined diffusion- and perfusion-weighted MR imaging. Stroke 2001; 32(4):933–942.
39. Tong DC, Adami A, Moseley ME, Marks MP. Prediction of hemorrhagic transformation following acute stroke: role of diffusion- and perfusion-weighted magnetic resonance imaging. Arch Neurol 2001; 58(4):587–593.
40. Thijs VN, Adami A, Neumann-Haefelin T, Moseley ME, Marks MP, Albers GW. Relationship between severity of MR perfusion deficit and DWI lesion evolution. Neurology 2001; 57(7):1205–1211.
41. Fiehler J, Knab R, Reichenbach JR, Fitzek C, Weiller C, Rother J. Apparent diffusion coefficient decreases and magnetic resonance imaging perfusion parameters are associated in ischemic tissue of acute stroke patients. J Cereb Blood Flow Metab 2001; 21(5):577–584.
42. Grandin CB, Duprez TP, Smith AM, et al. Which MR-derived perfusion parameters are the best predictors of infarct growth in hyperacute stroke? Comparative study between relative and quantitative measurements. Radiology 2002; 223(2):361–370.
43. Warach S. Tissue viability thresholds in acute stroke: the 4-factor model. Stroke 2001; 32(11):2460–2461.

44. Rose SE, Chalk JB, Griffin MP, et al. MRI based diffusion and perfusion predictive model to estimate stroke evolution. Magn Reson Imaging 2001; 19(8):1043–1053.

45. Jacobs MA, Mitsias P, Soltanian-Zadeh H, et al. Multiparametric MRI tissue characterization in clinical stroke with correlation to clinical outcome: part 2. Stroke 2001; 32(4):950–957.

46. Saxena R, Lewis S, Berge E, Sandercock PA, Koudstaal PJ. Risk of early death and recurrent stroke and effect of heparin in 3169 patients with acute ischemic stroke and atrial fibrillation in the International Stroke Trial. Stroke 2001; 32(10):2333–2337.

47. Petty GW, Brown RD Jr., Whisnant JP, Sicks JD, O'Fallon WM, Wiebers DO. Ischemic stroke subtypes: a population-based study of functional outcome, survival, and recurrence. Stroke 2000; 31(5):1062–1068.

48. Baird AE, Lovblad KO, Schlaug G, Edelman RR, Warach S. Multiple acute stroke syndrome: marker of embolic disease? Neurology 2000; 54(3):674–678.

49. Kang DW, Chu K, Ko SB, Kwon SJ, Yoon BW, Roh JK. Lesion patterns and mechanism of ischemia in internal carotid artery disease: a diffusion-weighted imaging study. Arch Neurol 2002; 59(10):1577–1582.

50. Roh JK, Kang DW, Lee SH, Yoon BW, Chang KH. Significance of acute multiple brain infarction on diffusion-weighted imaging. Stroke 2000; 31(3):688–694.

51. Kang DW, Latour LL, Chalela JA, Dambrosia J, Warach S. Early ischemic lesion recurrence within a week after acute ischemic stroke. Ann Neurol 2003; 54(1):66–74.

52. Kang DW, Latour LL, Chalela JA, Dambrosia JA, Warach S. Early and late recurrence of ischemic lesion on MRI: evidence for a prolonged stroke-prone state? Neurology 2004; 63(12):2261–2265.

53. Furlan A, Higashida R, Wechsler L, et al. Intra-arterial prourokinase for acute ischemic stroke. The PROACT II study: a randomized controlled trial. Prolyse in Acute Cerebral Thromboembolism [In Process Citation]. JAMA 1999; 282(21):2003–2011.

54. del Zoppo GJ, von Kummer R, Hamann GF. Ischaemic damage of brain microvessels: inherent risks for thrombolytic treatment in stroke. J Neurol Neurosurg Psychiatry 1998; 65(1):1–9.

55. Hamann GF, Okada Y, del Zoppo GJ. Hemorrhagic transformation and microvascular integrity during focal cerebral ischemia/reperfusion. J Cereb Blood Flow Metab 1996; 16(6):1373–1378.

56. Knight RA, Barker PB, Fagan SC, Li Y, Jacobs MA, Welch KM. Prediction of impending hemorrhagic transformation in ischemic stroke using magnetic resonance imaging in rats. Stroke 1998; 29(1):144–151.

57. Neumann-Haefelin T, Kastrup A, de Crespigny A, et al. Serial MRI after transient focal cerebral ischemia in rats: dynamics of tissue injury, blood-brain barrier damage, and edema formation. Stroke 2000; 31(8):1965–72; discussion 1972–1973.

58. Neumann-Haefelin C, Brinker G, Uhlenkuken U, Pillekamp F, Hossmann K-A, Hoehn M. Prediction of hemorrhagic transformation after thrombolytic therapy of clot embolism: an MRI investigation in rat brain. Stroke 2002; 33(5):1392–1398.

59. Latour LL, Kang DW, Ezzeddine MA, Chalela JA, Warach S. Early blood-brain barrier disruption in human focal brain ischemia. Ann Neurol 2004; 56(4):468–477.

60. Latour LL, Kang D, Chalela JA, Ezzeddine MA, Warach S. Evidence of early blood brain barrier disruption following acute stroke in humans: an imaging marker of reperfusion injury? 28th International Stroke Conference 2003, Phoenix, AZ, 12.

61. Elster AD, Moody DM. Early cerebral infarction: gadopentetate dimeglumine enhancement. Radiology 1990; 177(3):627–632.

62. Sze G, Soletsky S, Bronen R, Krol G. MR imaging of the cranial meninges with emphasis on contrast enhancement and meningeal carcinomatosis. Am J Neuroradiol 1989; 10(5):965–975.

63. Komiyama M, Nakajima H, Nishikawa M, Yasui T, Kitano S, Sakamoto H. Leptomeningeal contrast enhancement in moyamoya: its potential role in postoperative assessment of circulation through the bypass. Neuroradiology 2001; 43(1):17–23.

64. Virapongse C, Mancuso A, Quisling R. Human brain infarcts: Gd-DTPA-enhanced MR imaging. Radiology 1986; 161(3):785–794.

65. Imakita S, Nishimura T, Yamada N, et al. Magnetic resonance imaging of cerebral infarction: time course of Gd-DTPA enhancement and CT comparison. Neuroradiology 1988; 30(5):372–378.

66. Weinmann HJ, Laniado M, Mutzel W. Pharmacokinetics of GdDTPA/dimeglumine after intravenous injection into healthy volunteers. Physiol Chem Phys Med NMR 1984; 16(2):167–172.

67. Kuroiwa T, Ting P, Martinez H, Klatzo I. The biphasic opening of the blood-brain barrier to proteins following temporary middle cerebral artery occlusion. Acta Neuropathol 1985; 68(2):122–129.

68. Pfefferkorn T, Rosenberg GA. Closure of the blood-brain barrier by matrix metalloproteinase inhibition reduces rtPA-mediated mortality in cerebral ischemia with delayed reperfusion. Stroke 2003; 10.

69. Warach S, Latour LL, Saver JL, Alger JR, Kidwell CS. HARM: a potential marker of reperfusion injury in human stroke following intra-arterial thrombolysis. J Cereb Blood Flow Metab 2003:579.

70. Rosenberg GA. Matrix metalloproteinases in neuroinflammation. Glia 2002; 39(3):279–291.

71. Castellanos M, Leira R, Serena J, et al. Plasma metalloproteinase-9 concentration predicts hemorrhagic transformation in acute ischemic stroke. Stroke 2003; 34(1):40–46.

72. Montaner J, Molina CA, Monasterio J, et al. Matrix metalloproteinase-9 pretreatment level predicts intracranial hemorrhagic complications after thrombolysis in human stroke. Circulation 2003; 107(4):598–603.

73. Stroke Therapy Academic Industry Roundtable. Recommendations for standards regarding preclinical neuroprotective and restorative drug development. Stroke 1999; 30(12):2752–2758.
74. Stroke Therapy Academic Industry Roundtable II (STAIR-II). Recommendations for clinical trial evaluation of acute stroke therapies – Stroke Therapy Academic Industry Roundtable II (STAIR-II). Stroke 2001; 32(7):1598–1606.
75. Bryan RN, Levy LM, Whitlow WD, Killian JM, Preziosi TJ, Rosario JA. Diagnosis of acute cerebral infarction: comparison of CT and MR imaging. Am J Neuroradiol 1991; 12(4):611–620.
76. Warach S. Use of diffusion and perfusion magnetic resonance imaging as a tool in acute stroke clinical trials. Curr Control Trials Cardiovasc Med 2001; 2(1):38–44.
77. Warach S. New imaging strategies for patient selection for thrombolytic and neuroprotective therapies. Neurology 2001; 57(5 suppl 2):S48–S52.
78. Temple R. A regulatory authority's opinion about surrogate end points. In: Nimmo W, Tucker GT, eds. Clinical measurement in drug evaluation. New York: John Wiley, 1995.
79. Fleming TR, DeMets DL. Surrogate end points in clinical trials: are we being misled? Ann Intern Med 1996; 125(7):605–613.
80. Prentice RL. Surrogate endpoints in clinical trials: definition and operational criteria. Stat Med 1989; 8:431–440.
81. Davalos A, Castillo J, Alvarez-Sabin J, et al. Oral citicoline in acute ischemic stroke: an individual patient data pooling analysis of clinical trials. Stroke 2002; 33(12):2850–2857.
82. Warach S, Kaste M, Fisher M. The effect of GV150526 on ischemic lesion volume: The GAIN Americas and GAIN International MRI Substudy. Neurology 2000; 54(suppl 3): A87–A88.
83. Warach S, Hacke W, Hsu C, et al. Effect of MaxiPost on ischemic lesions in patients with acute stroke: The POST-010 MRI Substudy. Stroke 2002; 33:383.
84. Schellinger PD, Jansen O, Fiebach JB, et al. Monitoring intravenous recombinant tissue plasminogen activator thrombolysis for acute ischemic stroke with diffusion and perfusion MRI. Stroke 2000; 31(6):1318–1328.
85. Marks MP, Tong DC, Beaulieu C, Albers GW, de Crespigny A, Moseley ME. Evaluation of early reperfusion and i.v. tPA therapy using diffusion- and perfusion-weighted MRI. Neurology 1999; 52(9):1792–1798.
86. Parsons MW, Barber PA, Chalk J, et al. Diffusion- and perfusion-weighted MRI response to thrombolysis in stroke. Ann Neurol 2002; 51(1):28–37.
87. Chalela JA, Ezzeddine M, Latour L, Warach S. Reversal of perfusion and diffusion abnormalities after intravenous thrombolysis for a lacunar infarction. J Neuroimaging 2003; 13(2):152–154.
88. Sorensen AG, Copen WA, Ostergaard L, et al. Hyperacute stroke: simultaneous measurement of relative cerebral blood volume, relative cerebral blood flow, and mean tissue transit time. Radiology 1999; 210(2):519–527.
99. Oppenheim C, Grandin C, Samson Y, et al. Is there an apparent diffusion coefficient threshold in predicting tissue viability in hyperacute stroke? Stroke 2001; 32(11):2486–2491.
90. Parsons MW, Yang Q, Barber PA, et al. Perfusion magnetic resonance imaging maps in hyperacute stroke: relative cerebral blood flow most accurately identifies tissue destined to infarct. Stroke 2001; 32(7):1581–1587.
91. Rohl L, Ostergaard L, Simonsen CZ, et al. Viability thresholds of ischemic penumbra of hyperacute stroke defined by perfusion-weighted MRI and apparent diffusion coefficient. Stroke 2001; 32(5):1140–1146.
92. Staroselskaya IA, Chaves C, Silver B, et al. Relationship between magnetic resonance arterial patency and perfusion-diffusion mismatch in acute ischemic stroke and its potential clinical use. Arch Neurol 2001; 58(7):1069–1074.
93. Shih LC, Saver JL, Alger JR, et al. Perfusion-weighted magnetic resonance imaging thresholds identifying core, irreversibly infarcted tissue. Stroke 2003; 34(6):1425–1430.
94. Oppenheim C, Samson Y, Dormont D, et al. DWI prediction of symptomatic hemorrhagic transformation in acute MCA infarct. J Neuroradiol 2002; 29(1):6–13.

19 | Thrombolytic Therapy for Acute Ischemic Stroke

Christopher V. Fanale, MD, Associate Stroke Program Director
Colorado Neurological Institute–Swedish Medical Center,
Englewood, Colorado, USA

Patrick D. Lyden, MD, FAAN, Professor[a] and Director[b]
[a] *Department of Neurosciences, University of California–San Diego,*
[b] *UCSD Stroke Center, San Diego, California, USA*

INTRODUCTION

Before the Food and Drug Administration (FDA) approved the use of intravenous (IV) recombinant tissue plasminogen activator (rtPA) for acute ischemic stroke in 1996, most of the more than 700,000 strokes that occurred annually were not acutely treated. Due to this fact, stroke is the leading cause of disability in this country and costs the health-care system an estimated $53.6 billion per year (1). Over the last 10 years, groundbreaking research and advancements have occurred in the diagnosis and care of this population. However, delivering this potentially lifesaving therapy to all appropriate patients still meets with significant roadblocks.

EARLY CLINICAL CONSIDERATIONS

Basic Science Rationale

The vast majority of acute strokes are ischemic in nature. Either an embolus or an *in situ* thrombosis causes a cessation of blood flow, which triggers multiple pathways that cause ischemia and eventual cell death—events of a cascade that occurs in a time-dependent fashion. At the time of clinical significance, a core of tissue is already infarcted. However, surrounding tissue, called the ischemic penumbra, is at risk for future infarction. If blood flow is not restored to this vascular territory, the area of the ischemic penumbra will also become infarcted. Research thus far has mainly focused on investigating methods of reperfusing this "at-risk tissue" as quickly as possible, while decreasing the risk of hemorrhage transformation. Thus, significant emphasis has been placed on understanding the coagulation pathway and intervening in it as a strategy for improving early poststroke reperfusion. In short, vascular injury initiates the extrinsic pathway, which, along with the intrinsic pathway, activates factor X, eventually leading to thrombin activation, which, in turn, stimulates fibrin-clot formation and platelet aggregation (Fig. 1).

Physiologic dissolution of a fibrin clot is mediated by the activation of the circulating and fibrin-bound zymogen plasminogen to the active serine protease plasmin. The manipulation of this natural, fibrinolytic pathway is at the core of current acute stroke care. The traditional thrombolytics that have been used in acute stroke research (rtPA, streptokinase, and urokinase) work by potentiating conversion of plasminogen to plasmin.

Mechanism of Action of Thrombolytics

Urokinase is a serine protease that directly converts plasminogen to plasmin (2). It has no fibrin specificity; therefore, it has no clot specificity. Although urokinase has historical merit, it is not currently used clinically. However, its precursor—recombinant prourokinase (rpro-UK)—has been used in intra-arterial (IA) clinical trials.

Streptokinase is a secreted product of beta-hemolytic streptococci, which works by forming a complex with plasminogen, and this complex proteolytically converts plasminogen to plasmin (3). Streptokinase has been used in multiple clinical trials, but it is not currently on the market for thrombolytic therapy.

rtPA is a naturally occurring enzyme that is made by the endothelial cells in response to arterial wall injury and potentiates the conversion of plasminogen to plasmin. Unlike other thrombolytics, rtPA has high specificity for fibrin and is therefore clot specific (4). Fibrin stimulates the activity of rtPA, which minimizes the probability of hemorrhage due to decreased

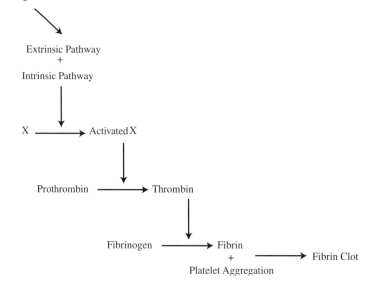

Figure 1 Fibrin-clot formation.

degradation of fibrinogen. This, along with a short half-life of 4 to 6 min, provides a marked clinical advantage over the other thrombolytics. rtPA (and its variants) is now the main lytic medication used in clinical research.

Early Clinical Work

From the late 1950s, manipulation of the thrombolytic pathway has been used to increase the levels of plasmin inside the body and, therefore, increase the likelihood of clot dissolution. In 1958, Moser first used plasmin in humans for the treatment of intravascular thrombosis (5,6). The first attempt to treat ischemic stroke with a thrombolytic agent was reported by Sussman and Fitch (7). As a group, these trials did not show any clinically significant improvement in patients treated with thrombolytics for stroke. In addition, the increased number of intracranial hemorrhages that resulted after therapy appeared to make administration of these agents prohibitive.

In retrospect, these early trials were flawed in many ways. In most of them, a surrogate marker of blood in the cerebrospinal fluid was used instead of CT scan to rule out preexistent intracranial hemorrhage. The type, dosage, route of administration, and time from onset of symptoms to treatment with thrombolytics were not standardized.

In the mid-1980s, interest in thrombolysis for ischemic stroke was renewed when Zivin et al. demonstrated improved neurologic outcome in rabbits that were administered rtPA within 45 min after ischemic stroke. Perhaps equally important, they demonstrated no increase in intracerebral hemorrhage (ICH) with rtPA administration that began up to 4 hr after vessel occlusion (8,9). Another group demonstrated improved neurologic outcome and reduced infarct size in baboons after 3 hr of proximal middle cerebral artery (MCA) occlusion and subsequent intracarotid urokinase administration (10).

A lingering question was whether rtPA would increase the risk of ICH to such an extent that its use would not be efficacious in clinical applications in stroke. Slivka and Pulsinella tested the risk of ICH after the administration of rtPA (200,000 U) or streptokinase (10,000–32,000 U/kg) in rabbits. When administered at both 1 and 24 hr after occlusion, streptokinase did not significantly increase ICH rate. However, they did report a significant increase in macroscopic ICH in animals administered rtPA after 24 hr of occlusion (11). In another study, no differences were noted in ICH rates in the rabbit embolic stroke model when rtPA (3 or 5 mg/kg) was administered up to 24 hr after emboli were introduced (12). Based on promising data in animal studies and several small, randomized trials with IV rtPA, large-scale randomized trials were launched to test thrombolytics in acute ischemic stroke.

INTRAVENOUS THROMBOLYTICS IN ACUTE STROKE THERAPY

Tissue Plasminogen Activator

European Cooperative Acute Stroke Study I
The European Cooperative Acute Stroke Study (ECASS) I was the first large-scale prospective, multicenter, double-blinded, randomized clinical trial of rtPA in the treatment of acute ischemic stroke (13). Eligible patients were between 18 and 80 years of age and presented within 6 hr of onset of a moderate-to-severe acute ischemic stroke. Patients with strokes severe enough to cause an impaired level of consciousness or forced head and eye deviation were excluded. Patients with rapidly improving symptoms or mild strokes were also excluded. Importantly, patients with CT scans that showed ICH, hypoattenuation exceeding a third of the MCA territory, or diffuse sulcal effacement of one entire brain hemisphere were excluded. Eligible patients received either 1.1 mg/kg of alteplase or placebo over 60 min (10% as a bolus).

The study sought to address two primary hypotheses: (i) a difference would be observed between the two groups in respect to activities of daily living (defined as a 15-point difference on the Barthel Index) at three months, and (ii) a difference would be observed in the global clinical conditions (defined as a difference of one grade on the Modified Rankin Scale, mRS) at three months, with a secondary endpoint of 30-day mortality.

The study enrolled 620 patients (the intent-to-treat population) at 75 centers in 14 European countries. The median time to treatment was 4 hr. The investigators also prospectively felt that a fair number of major protocol violators might be randomized. They therefore designated a target population who met all of the inclusion and exclusion criteria. Of a total of 109 (17%) protocol violators, 66 had abnormal CT scans before treatment.

In the intent-to-treat population, no significant differences were noted in 3-month means of the Barthel Index or mRS. The 30-day mortality was not significantly higher in the rtPA group versus placebo. The parenchymal hematoma rate and deaths associated with hemorrhage were significantly higher in the target group versus placebo group. When excluding major protocol violators and analyzing the prospectively designated target population, a significant decrease was reported in the mRS (2 vs. 3), as well as a significant increase in subjects with an mRS of 0 to 1 in the treatment versus placebo groups.

European Cooperative Acute Stroke Study II
Because of the conflicting results from the two populations in ECASS I and the fact that the 1995 study by the National Institute of Neurological Disorders and Stroke (NINDS) showed efficacy of rtPA within 3 hr of stroke onset, ECASS II was undertaken (14). In ECASS II, 800 patients were enrolled and assigned to rtPA or placebo, with stratification for time from onset of stroke symptoms (0 to 3 hr or 3 to 6 hr). The primary endpoint was the mRS at 90 days, dichotomized for favorable outcome (score 0–1) and unfavorable outcome (score 2–6). Another difference in ECASS II was an rtPA dose of 0.9 mg/kg. The CT scan exclusions were stricter than in ECASS I: If more than a third of the MCA territory showed signs of brain swelling, patients were excluded. A training course was also implemented to improve the quality of CT-scanning procedures and assessment.

Measurement of the trial's primary endpoints did not show significant differences. A favorable outcome was seen in 165 (40.3%; 95% confidence interval, CI: 35.6–45.4) of the rtPA-treated group versus 143 (36.6%; 95% CI: 31.8–41.6). The absolute difference was 3.7% ($p = 0.277$) in favor of rtPA. The rate of parenchymal hemorrhage was higher in the rtPA group (11.8%) than in the placebo group (3.8%). However, the 30- and 90-day mortality rates were not significantly different.

National Institute of Neurological Disorders and Stroke Recombinant Tissue
Plasminogen Activator Stroke Study
The NINDS rtPA Stroke Study was conducted at the same time as ECASS I. The NINDS trial was the first large, randomized, double-blinded trial to show benefit of a thrombolytic in acute stroke (15). Patients were enrolled if they presented within 3 hr of an acute ischemic stroke and had a deficit [as measured by the National Institute of Health (NIH) Stroke Scale, (NIHSS)], and a CT scan that showed no evidence of hemorrhage. Noteworthily, no patients were excluded due to

signs of early ischemic change, as in the ECASS trials. Table 1 contains a complete list of inclusion and exclusion criteria. Once patients were randomized, they were either administered IV rtPA at a total dose of 0.9 mg/kg (10% as bolus, remainder over 1 hr) or placebo. No patients were administered anticoagulants or antiplatelets for 24 hr after infusion of study drug, and blood pressure was strictly maintained at <185/110. The trial was split into two parts. Part 1 was designed to test if rtPA had early clinical effect. Part 2 was designed to test if rtPA improved clinical outcome at three months. Excellent protocol adherence was reported for both parts of the trial, with at least 90% of patients receiving the full dose of study drug.

Part 1 enrolled 291 patients, and by a predetermined randomization scheme, patients were stratified into two blocks according to length of time from onset of stroke to start of treatment, i.e., either 0 to 90 min or 91 to 180 min. The primary hypothesis of early clinical improvement was defined as a complete resolution of symptoms or an improvement from baseline NIHSS score of 4 or more points at 24 hr after the onset of stroke. Of the 144 patients who received rtPA, 67 (47%) showed an early clinical improvement, whereas of the 147 patients who received placebo, 57 (39%) showed an early clinical improvement ($p = 0.21$). Symptomatic ICH occurred in eight (6%) of patients treated with rtPA, and none occurred in the placebo group.

In the interim analysis of the results from Part 1, the Data and Safety Monitoring Board determined that the prospectively determined secondary outcome favored the rtPA group. A new trial was recommended, which exactly replicated the first trial, but with a primary hypothesis that a consistent and persuasive difference would be observed between the two groups in terms of improvement to little or no deficit three months after the treatment.

Part 2 enrolled 333 patients. Primary outcome was measured by the Barthel Index (score 95 or 100), the mRS (grade 0–1), the Glasgow Coma Scale (grade 1), and the NIHSS (score 0 or 1). The proportion of patients with improved clinical outcome was significantly higher in the rtPA group than in the placebo group. Symptomatic ICH occurred in 12 (7%) patients treated with rtPA and 2 (1%) patients in the placebo group.

Combining the two parts of the NINDS trial, a significant benefit was revealed for rtPA at 3 months, measured by all four functional outcome scales. The aggregate rate of symptomatic ICH was 6.4% in the rtPA-treated group and 0.6% in the placebo group ($p < 0.001$). However, no significant difference in mortality was reported between the rtPA group (17%) and the placebo

Table 1 Intravenous Tissue Plasminogen Activator Administration Inclusion/Exclusion Criteria for Ischemic Stroke

---

Inclusion
1. Clinical diagnosis of ischemic stroke with measurable deficit
2. Clear onset of symptoms <3 hr
3. CT scan shows no intracranial hemorrhage or mass

Absolute contraindications
1. CT scan showing intracranial hemorrhage
2. Prior intracranial hemorrhage that would increase the risk of recurrent intracranial hemorrhage
3. Stroke, intracranial surgery, or serious head trauma in the prior 3 mo
4. Active internal bleeding
5. Sustained systolic blood pressure >185 mm of Hg or Diastolic blood pressure >110 mm of Hg
6. Aggressive treatment to lower BP
7. Heparin during the preceding 48 hr associated with elevated PTT
8. Pregnant female
9. Currently taking oral anticoagulants with international normalized ratio > 1.7
10. Clinical presentation consistent with subarachnoid hemorrhage

Relative contraindications
1. Rapidly improving or minor deficit
2. Major surgery or trauma in the prior 2 wk
3. Blood glucose < 50 mg/dL or > 400 mg/dL
4. History of gastrointestinal or genitourinary bleeding within 21 days
5. Arterial puncture at noncompressible site within 7 days
6. Seizure at onset of symptoms
7. Clinical presentation suggesting pericarditis or myocardial infarction
8. Platelet count <100,000 mm^3

---

group (21%; $p=0.30$). Although certain rtPA-treated subgroups had worse clinical outcomes than the overall treatment group, all subgroups responded favorably to rtPA therapy when compared to their matched placebo groups (16). This trial was also the first large randomized trial that did not exclude any subtype of ischemic stroke (i.e., large vessel vs. small vessel or thrombotic vs. embolic).

Alteplase Thrombolysis for Acute Noninterventional Therapy in Stroke Study

The alteplase thrombolysis for acute noninterventional therapy in stroke (ATLANTIS) study was double-blinded, randomized, multicentered, and placebo controlled (17). It initially began in August 1991, with a goal to test the efficacy and safety of IV administration of rtPA in patients with acute ischemic stroke within a 0- to 6-hr window. This company-sponsored trial was to run concurrently with the NINDS trial. However, in December 1993, safety concerns arose concerning the 5- to 6-hr time window. Enrollment was halted, and the trial was restarted as "Part B." In February 1996, after data from the NINDS trial was available, the protocol of the ATLANTIS study was amended to include only patients in the 3- to 5-hr window. The primary outcome measure was percentage of patients at 90 days with an excellent neurologic recovery, defined as a score of 0 or 1 on the NIHSS. The rtPA dosage was the same as in the NINDS trial (0.9 mg/kg). In Part B, 613 patients were randomized at 140 sites. The trial was halted in July 1998 due to nonefficacy of the treatment arm. By that time, 31 patients had received study drug in 3 hr or less, 547 had received study drug between 3 and 5 hr. It was reported that 32% of placebo and 34% of the rtPA group had an excellent recovery at day 90 ($p=50.65$). In the 547 patients in the target population, the mean time to treatment was approximately 4.5 hr.

This trial effectively ruled out the IV use of rtPA in the 3- to 5-hr window for acute ischemic stroke. The study group later published the data on the 61 patients who received study drug within 3 hr of stroke onset. The proportion of patients with a NIHSS of <1 was significantly higher in the rtPA group (60.9%) than in the placebo group (26.3%; $p=0.01$) (18).

Streptokinase

Streptokinase for Acute Ischemic Stroke with Relationship to Time of Administration (ASK Trial)

The Australian Streptokinase (ASK) trial, conducted in Australia, was a double-blinded, randomized, placebo-controlled trial to determine whether administration of 1.5 MU of streptokinase intravenously within 4 hr of the onset of acute ischemic stroke would reduce morbidity and mortality at 3 months, and whether outcomes would be better for those receiving therapy within 3 hr of stroke onset, as compared with those receiving it after 3 hr (19). A total of 340 patients with moderate-to-severe strokes were randomized from June 1992 to November 1994. Using the outcome measure of combined death and disability score (Barthel index <60) 3 months after the stroke, no significant difference was seen between the two groups. This study was stopped early due to an increase in mortality in the treatment group (36.2%) versus the placebo group (20.5%). An excessive amount of symptomatic hematomas was also seen in the treated group (12.6%) versus the placebo group (2.4%; $p<01$). The trial did demonstrate that patients treated in <3 hr had better outcome and less mortality than those treated between 3 and 4 hr.

Multicenter Acute Stroke Trial (I and E)

Conducted in Italy in 1995, the multicenter acute stroke trial (MAST)-I was a randomized, controlled, multicenter, open trial of 622 patients who had stroke onset within 6 hr (20). The subjects were randomized to 1 of 4 groups: 1-hr IV infusion of 1.5 MU streptokinase, 300 mg/day buffered aspirin for 10 days, both streptokinase and aspirin, or neither. Streptokinase (alone or with aspirin) was associated with numerous 10-day case fatalities (odds ratio: 2.7; $p<0.001$). Comparison of groups that received streptokinase with those who did not revealed increased rates of symptomatic ICH. Due to the above results, this trial was also stopped early.

The following year, MAST-E was published (21). This was a double-blinded, controlled trial of 310 patients in France and England that assessed the efficacy and safety of administration of streptokinase within 6 hr of ischemic stroke. Noteworthily, the use of anticoagulants or antiplatelets was allowed during the first 24 hr. The primary outcome endpoint was mortality and severe disability (mRS≥3) at 6 months. Almost an equal number of patients (124 vs. 126) in the streptokinase and placebo groups were either dead or severely disabled, respectively. Again, this trial showed that a 10-day mortality rate was higher in the streptokinase group than in the placebo group (34.0% vs. 18.2%; $p = 0.002$). The results of the MAST-E trial mirrored the MAST-I trial, and it was also halted early.

Summary

Based largely on NINDS trial data, the FDA approved rtPA as the first drug therapy for acute stroke in June 1996. The FDA did limit approval of its use to patients who present within 3 hr of ischemic stroke. Deviation from the current guidelines for IV administration of rtPA in acute stroke (Table 1) has shown higher rates of symptomatic hemorrhagic complications (22). Importantly, the FDA did not limit its use in acute ischemic stroke based on age, sex, ethnicity, severity, or subtype. This approval signaled a paradigm shift in the care of stroke patients. Acute strokes would now be treated as neurologic emergencies and, therefore, need the health-care infrastructure to provide expeditious diagnosis and treatment.

INTRA-ARTERIAL THROMBOLYTICS IN ACUTE STROKE THERAPY

The trials discussed above demonstrated either a nonsignificant or negative effect of treatment of ischemic strokes beyond the 3-hr window. Relatively few patients were able to present to the emergency room, undergo a CT scan, and receive evaluation and treatment by a neurologist within 3 hr. In the NINDS rtPA trial, 16,000 patients were screened for the total study population of 624 patients (15). This time-constraint problem, along with the advent of more advanced radiographic technologies, warranted questioning whether the time window for treatment of acute stroke could be expanded by local application of IA thrombolytics to the causative clot. IA application theoretically would increase the effectiveness of thrombolytics by increasing the local concentration at the site of the clot while decreasing the total amount used, thereby decreasing the hemorrhagic complication rate. This methodology appeared especially enticing for large strokes that were caused by occlusion of major cerebral vessels.

Starting in the early 1980s, many case series provided anecdotal evidence that IA application of thrombolytics could recanalize an occluded cerebral vessel (23–25), providing the groundwork for the first randomized clinical trial to test the efficacy and safety of IA thrombolytics.

Prolyse in Acute Cerebral Thromboembolism Trials (I and II)

Prolyse in acute cerebral thromboembolism trials (PROACT) I was a Phase 2, randomized, blinded trial that compared the safety and recanalization frequency in patients who presented in <6 hr of a clinically symptomatic MCA occlusion (26). After a CT scan excluded hemorrhage, all patients were taken for cerebral angiography. Patients demonstrating an occlusion in the M1 or M2 segment of the MCA were randomized in a 2:1 fashion to receive either a placebo or rpro-UK (6 mg) over 2 hr into the proximal-third of the thrombus face. All patients received IV heparin (bolus followed by infusion) for 4 hr after occlusion was confirmed. The primary efficacy endpoint was recanalization of the M1 or M2 at 120 min after initiation of infusion. The primary safety outcome was hemorrhagic transformation that caused neurologic deterioration within 24 hr. Out of 1314 patients screened, 40 were treated (26 with rpro-UK, 14 with placebo). During the study, the hemorrhage rate that caused neurologic worsening was 72.7% in the rpro-UK group and 20.0% in the placebo group. Consequently, the trial was continued with a decreased heparin dose. The recanalization rate for all patients receiving rpro-UK was 57.7% versus 14.3% ($p = 0.017$) for the placebo group. Although the numbers were too small for statistical significance, there appeared to be a 10% to 12% absolute increase in excellent neurologic outcome at 90 days in the rpro-UK group against placebo. The rate of mortality in the rpro-UK group was 26.9% versus 42.9% in the placebo group ($p = 0.48$).

In PROACT II, patient selection was similar, but the protocol differed from PROACT I in the following ways: more patients treated (180), higher rpro-UK dose (9 mg), and all patients were placed on low-dose heparin (2000 U bolus followed by a 4-hr infusion of 500 U). The primary outcome was based on the proportion of patients with slight or no neurologic disability at 90 days (mRS≥2). Although the hemorrhage rate with neurologic deterioration within 24-hr was higher in the rpro-UK group than in the placebo (10% vs. 2%; $p = 0.06$), patients in the rpro-UK group did better at three months. Forty percent of rpro-UK patients and 25% of placebo patients achieved an mRS of <2 ($p=0.04$). The recanalization rates were 66% for the rpro-UK group and 18% for the control group ($p<0.001$). The difference in mortality was insignificant (27).

Combined Intravenous and Intra-arterial Therapies

The median time from stroke onset to treatment for the PROACT trials was approximately 5.5 hr, highlighting the problem with IA management of acute stroke. The time needed to assemble all of the components required to perform the procedure is substantial. Based on data from the NINDS trial, it would be unethical to withhold IV rtPA therapy in qualified patients presenting within 3 hr of stroke onset. However, certain subgroups of patients (hyperdense artery signs, more severe deficit, and older age) benefit from IV thrombolytics to a lesser degree than the general target population. No randomized, controlled study has compared the rates of recanalization of IV versus IA thrombolysis. Wolpert et al. reported that 32 out of 93 (34%) patients had recanalization of their MCAs after the administration of IV rtPA, with most recanalizations taking place in distal occlusions (28). In PROACT I and II, the recanalization rate was between 57.7% and 66%.

Emergency Management of Stroke: EMS-Bridging Trial

Based on the results cited and other anecdotal evidence (and before publication of the NINDS stroke trial), the EMS-bridging trial was initiated to combine the purported advantages of both IV rtPA (timeliness and relative ease of administration) and IA administration (higher recanalization rates and decreased dose) (29). This was a Phase 1 pilot study of IV rtPA or placebo followed by immediate cerebral arteriography and local IA administration of rtPA. The goal was to test the feasibility, efficacy, and safety of this combined therapy in acute stroke within 3 hr of onset. Thirty-five patients were enrolled. The 17 patients who received IV rtPA were given a dose of 0.6 mg/kg (maximum of 60 mg), 10% bolus, with remainder administered over 30 min. Of the 35 patients enrolled, 34 were taken for cerebral angiography. If an occlusion was found, a very specific protocol was followed for attempted recanalization: 1 mg of rtPA was administered beyond the thrombus and then 1 mg was infused directly into the thrombus, followed by infusion at the rate of 10 mg/hr until complete recanalization or 2 hr.

Of the 22 patients who had an occlusion on angiography, those who received combined therapy (IV/IA) had better recanalization rates (54%) versus those who received only IA therapy (10%; $p=0.03$). However, essentially no difference in clinical outcomes was observed between the two groups. The rates of symptomatic ICH were similar also.

Interventional Management of Stroke Study

Using the data from the EMS bridging trial, the interventional management of stroke (IMS) investigators wanted to explore the use of combined therapy in patients with relatively severe strokes (NIHSS≥10). They performed a multicentered, open-label, nonrandomized pilot study (30). The goal of the study was the same as the EMS-bridging trial. As the trial started after FDA approval of rtPA for stroke within 3 hr, all patients received IV rtPA at a dose of 0.6 mg/kg (maximum of 60 mg), with 15% as a bolus and the remainder over 30 min. To maximize early treatment, at least 2 out of 7 patients at each center were required to be treated within 2 hr. After IV administration, patients were to undergo an immediate cerebral angiogram. If occlusion was found, the same protocol as in the EMS-bridging trial was used, with the exception of the use of 2 mg boluses instead of 1 mg. Also, a maximum IA dose of 22 mg was allowed, with an 82 mg total rtPA dose (combined IV and IA).

Of the 80 enrolled patients, 62 underwent combined therapy. For the primary safety measure of life-threatening bleeding complications during the initial 36-hr post-treatment, the overall mortality rate was not significantly lower in the IMS study group (13/80; 16%), when compared to the NINDS rtPA group (39/182; 21%; $p=0.33$). Rates of ICH were similar among treatment groups in both trials, and no difference existed between the IMS study group and the NINDS rtPA group in the secondary outcome measures of Rankin, NIHSS, Barthel, and GCS scores at 90 days.

Currently, enrollment is underway in IMS-II to identify risks and benefits of combined IV/IA rtPA plus low-energy ultrasound in patients with ischemic stroke.

OTHER THROMBOLYTICS FOR ACUTE STROKE

Ancrod

Ancrod, a purified venom extract from the Malaysian pit viper, induces rapid defibrinogenation, which, in turn, may increase local thrombolysis by stimulating plasminogen activators. In 1994, a study was undertaken in the United States and Germany to test the safety and efficacy of this treatment in ischemic stroke patients who present within 6 hr. A nonsignificant improvement in outcome was noted at 3 months, with no symptomatic hemorrhages in the ancrod group (31). The Stroke Treatment with Ancrod trial studied ancrod in acute stroke using a 3-hr window (32). Using the primary efficacy endpoint of Barthel Index ≥ 95 at 90 days revealed a statistically significant difference in outcome between ancrod and placebo groups (42.2% vs. 34.4%; $p=0.01$). This effect was proportional to the rate of defibrinogenation. A nonsignificant trend toward increased symptomatic hemorrhages in the ancrod group was also reported.

Tenecteplase

Tenecteplase (TNK) is a biogenetic variant of wild-type rtPA that can be given as a single bolus injection and has an eightfold higher affinity for fibrin and a longer half-life. In the ASSENT-2 trial, TNK was compared to rtPA in terms of incidence of bleeding events after acute myocardial infarction (33). Almost 17,000 patients were randomized into the trial. Fewer patients (4.66%) in the TNK group had major noncerebral bleeding compared to the rtPA group (5.94%; $p=0.0002$). However, the mortality rates and rate of ICH were similar between groups (94% vs. 93%).

Starting in July 2000, a pilot dose-escalation safety study of TNK in acute ischemic stroke was undertaken. Patients presenting within 3 hr were offered traditional therapy (rtPA) or enrollment in the pilot study. Patients who received between 0.1 and 0.4 mg/kg of TNK had no symptomatic intracranial hemorrhages. Of 75 patients who received these doses, between 32% and 36%, had minimal disability (mRS ≤ 1) at 24 hr. In the NINDS stroke study, 36% of patients who received rtPA had this outcome. A dose-finding Phase 2b trial is about to commence that will compare TNK to IV rtPA.

Desmoteplase

Desmoteplase is another plasminogen activator that is an isolate of saliva from vampire bats. It has high fibrin specificity and a long half-life (34). The Desmoteplase in acute ischemic stroke trial (DIAS) was undertaken to study the safety and efficacy of desmoteplase in patients with ischemic stroke and an magnetic resonance imagining (MRI) perfusion/diffusion mismatch at between 3 and 9 hr from stroke onset (35). Using initial doses of between 25 and 50 mg, the rates of symptomatic ICH within 72 hr were high (23.5–30.8%). After a protocol amendment, the trial was continued using a body-weight adjusted dose-escalation design (Part 2). Of the 45 desmoteplase-treated patients in this portion of the trial, one (2.2%) experienced symptomatic ICH. A greater improvement in reperfusion was observed in the desmoteplase-treated patients (20 of 42; 47.6%), as compared to patients in the placebo group (2 of 10; 20%). In a comparison of treatment groups from Part 2 of the trial, the patients who received a dose of 125 µg/kg of desmoteplase had a more favorable outcome at 90 days (60.0%) than did patients in the placebo group (18.2%, $p=0.009$). However, in a comparison of all patients, the difference between placebo and desmoteplase was not significant. Currently, DIAS-2 is underway. Patients will be randomized to receive either placebo, or one of two doses (90 or 125 µ/kg) of desmoteplase.

EMERGING TECHNOLOGIES

In addition to more powerful, but safer, thrombolytics, other modalities are currently under study to treat a greater number of ischemic stroke patients. Among the goals of some of these modalities are as follows: better patient selection for IA therapy, manual clot retrieval, and discernment of patients who would safely benefit from thrombolytic therapy from those who would be injured.

Transcranial Ultrasonography

Currently, no standard, rapid method is available to functionally image the cerebral vasculature for recanalization after thrombolysis administration in suspected large vessel ischemic strokes. Taking the patient outside of the emergency room or ICU setting to undergo a CT scan, MRI, or angiography is potentially dangerous. With the advancement of ultrasound technology, the use of transcranial-Doppler ultrasonography (TCD) is being researched. The advantage of TCD is that it is a rapid, bedside assessment that can continuously monitor the offending vessel and provide valuable data about its morphology. If recanalization and clinical improvement are not seen with standard therapy, other available modalities (e.g., IA therapy) can potentially be considered more rapidly. TCD has been shown to be sensitive and specific in determining arterial occlusion in acute stroke (36). Continuous TCD monitoring has also shown clot lysis during and immediately following rtPA administration (37). Moreover, the Combined Lysis of Thrombus in Brain ischemia using transcranial Ultrasound and Systemic TPA trial has shown promising results, suggesting that continuous 2-MHz TCD of a cerebral vessel occlusion augments rtPA-induced arterial recanalization (38). The ongoing Microbubbles and Ultrasound in Stroke trial is using focused, 2-MHz, low-intensity ultrasound combined with IV microbubbles in patients with acute MCA stem occlusion, who have also received IV rtPA.

Manual Clot Retrieval

Due to the well-documented risks of thrombolytic therapy in stroke patients who present outside of the 3-hr time window, or other exclusions from standard therapy, manual thrombolectomy devices are being tested. One of the more promising of these is the concentric clot retriever device. Data was published in December 2004 from a Phase 1 trial that used this device specifically designed for intracranial embolectomy (39). Twenty-eight patients who presented within 8 hr, with a median NIHSS of 22, were treated. Successful recanalization with mechanical embolectomy was achieved in 12 (43%) patients. With the addition of IA rtPA, a total of 18 (64%) patients were recanalized. No symptomatic ICH occurred. At 1 month, 9 of 18 revascularized patients and none of the nonrevascularized patients had achieved significant recovery. However, a 7% complication rate, caused from either the device or the procedure, was reported. The mortality rate at 90 days was 39%.

At present, there is presently lack of clinical experience with the use of manual clot retriever devices for treatment of acute stroke. To further determine if this device should be added to the armamentarium of acute stroke treatment, the NINDS-funded MR and recanalization of stroke clots using embolectomy (MR-RESCUE) trial is currently enrolling stroke patients, randomizing (with the assistance of MRI perfusion and diffusion studies) those who present within 8 hr to either thrombectomy (with a modified Merci Retriever system) or medical management. The primary outcome will be functional outcome at 3 months.

CONTROVERSIES IN THE USE OF INTRAVENOUS rtPA

Exclusion from Therapy

Although rtPA has been shown to be beneficial in all properly selected patients, it has shown marginal positive impact in specific subgroups: the elderly, those with severe strokes, patients with extensive early ischemic changes on CT scan, and those with hyperdense artery signs. It has been suggested that the relative risk-to-benefit ratio of thrombolysis might vary among patient subgroups (40). To address these concerns, a post hoc subgroup analysis was completed using the data from the NINDS trial (16). All subgroups treated with IV rtPA had a better functional outcome at three months, including patients >75 years of age, those with early CT findings of ischemia, and those with a visible thrombus on CT scan.

Although the proportion of patients with basilar artery occlusion is much less than those with anterior circulation strokes, the functional outcome rates are much worse. Death is almost certain if recanalization is not achieved (41). Due to the uniformly poor prognosis of these patients, no placebo-controlled trial has been conducted using thrombolytics. However, some case reports do support the use of IA fibrinolytics in achieving recanalizations (24,42). Due to the high rate of rethrombosis, postprocedure anticoagulation is widely used. However, relatively few centers have the extremely specialized personnel and equipment required for this procedure. With the approval of IV use of alteplase for all ischemic strokes presenting within 3 hr, some have used this method in treating basilar artery occlusion patients (43,44). Currently, no "standard of care" in treating these complex patients has been established. The decision algorithm is based on available personnel, personal experience, severity of illness, and time of onset. A comparative trial in this subpopulation is needed to determine the best way to manage these patients.

Patients Outside the 3-hr Window

Although little controversy exists over the care of stroke patients presenting within 3 hr of symptom onset, patients beyond this window have increased rates of complications that bring into question the benefit of thrombolytics. Desmoteplase is the only intravenously administered thrombolytic to show improved functional outcome in patients who present >3 hr after onset of symptoms. The failure of the ECASS and ATLANTIS trials to show benefit has been largely attributed to the >3-hr time limit to administer thrombolytics. These findings beg the question: Should the 3-hr window be an absolute ceiling for administration of IV thrombolysis? A pooled analysis of ECASS I and II, the NINDS, and ATLANTIS trials, which addresses this issue, was recently published (45). Results of this analysis again clearly verified the safety and efficacy of thrombolysis within 3 hr from onset of symptoms and, in fact, showed possible efficacy up to 4.5 hr (Fig. 1), in addition to demonstrating a strong association between rapid treatment and favorable outcome.

One key to treating patients outside of the 3-hr window is to distinguish those who would benefit from reperfusion from those with no salvageable tissue who would only be exposed to the detrimental effects of administration of thrombolytics. Of these patients, better patient characterization is necessary to determine which method of revascularization would be best. The goal of the ongoing EPITHET trial is to determine whether the extent of the ischemic penumbra apparent on perfusion–diffusion MRI can be used to identify patients who would respond positively and safely to IV rtPA beyond 3 hr of stroke onset.

STROKE CENTERS

Due to the growing complexity in the decisions required to safely and effectively treat stroke patients, the efficacy of administering thrombolytic therapy outside of the confines of a tertiary academic center is a valid concern. As long as administration protocol is strictly adhered to, clinical experiences have been similar to those of the NINDS trial (46), and they have been reproduced in Europe (47). However, the adoption of IV thrombolytics in acute stroke has been slow, with possible reasons cited as the following: poor patient and family education, inexperience of personnel triaging stroke patients as nonurgent, delays in neuroimaging, inefficient delivery of in-hospital emergency stroke care, and physicians' uncertainty about administering thrombolysis (48). Therefore, loosely organized stroke centers (both academic and community based) with interested neurologists, advancing technologies, and educated hospital staff have come into existence. Although they are well meaning, the level of acute stroke care is widely variable.

Recommendations based on the trauma center model for establishing primary stroke centers have been recently published (49). These guidelines aim to define and standardize a stroke center's function. The Joint Commission on Accreditation of Health-Care Organizations now bases its accreditation of hospitals as primary stroke centers based largely on these recommendations. These centers will be able to rapidly assess and safely administer thrombolytic therapy to qualified patients, while educating the population and hospital staff. Eventually, complex patients will be transferred to a select few comprehensive stroke centers. Here, the most sophisticated technologies, medications, and health-care professionals will be brought together to synergistically deliver state-of-the-art stroke care.

REFERENCES

1. American Heart Association. Heart and Stroke Statistical Update, Dallas, Texas, 2002.
2. Lijnen HR, Stump DC, Collen DC. Single-chain urokinase-type plasminogen-activator-mechanism of action and thrombolytic properties. Semin Thromb Hemost 1987; 13(2):152–159.
3. Brogden RN, Speight TM, Avery GS. Streptokinase-review of its clinical pharmacology, mechanism of action and therapeutic uses. Drugs 1973; 5(5–6):357–445.
4. Garabedian HD, Gold HK, Leinbach RC, et al. Pharmacokinetics, hemostatic effects, and thrombolytic properties of recombinant tissue plasminogen-activator produced on an industrial-scale. Clin Res 1986; 34(2):A302.

5. Moser KM. Effects of intravenous administration of fibrinolysin (Plasmin) in Man. Circulation 1959; 20(1):42–55.
6. Moser KM. Thrombolysis with fibrinolysin (plasmin)-new therapeutic approach to thromboembolism. JAMA 1958; 167(14):1695–1704.
7. Sussman BJ, Fitch TSP. Thrombolysis with fibrinolysin in cerebral arterial occlusion. JAMA 1958; 167(14):1705–1709.
8. Zivin JA, Fisher M, DeGirolami U, Hemenway CC, Stashak KA. Tissue plasminogen activator reduces neurological damage after cerebral embolism. Science 1985; 230:1289–1292.
9. Zivin JA, Lyden PD, DeGirolami U, et al. Tissue plasminogen activator. Reduction of neurologic damage after experimental embolic stroke. Arch Neurol 1988; 45:387–391.
10. del Zoppo G, Copeland BR, Harker LA, et al. Experimental acute thrombotic stroke in baboons. Stroke 1986; 17:1254–1265.
11. Slivka A, Pulsinelli WA. Hemorrhagic complications of thrombolytic therapy in experimental stroke. Stroke 1987; 18:1148–1156.
12. Lyden PD, Zivin JA, Clark WA, et al. Tissue plasminogen activator mediated thrombolysis of cerebral emboli and its effect on hemorrhagic infarction in rabbits. Neurology 1989; 39:703–708.
13. Hacke W, Kaste M, Fieschi C, et al. Intravenous thrombolysis with recombinant tissue plasminogen activator for acute hemispheric stroke: The European Cooperative Stroke Study (ECASS). JAMA 1995; 274(13):1017–1025.
14. Hacke W, Kaste M, Fieschi C, et al. Randomised double-blind placebo-controlled trial of thrombolytic therapy with intravenous alteplase in acute ischaemic stroke (ECASS II). Lancet 1998; 352:1245–1251.
15. NINDS rt-PA Stroke Study Group. Tissue plasminogen activator for acute ischemic stroke. N Engl J Med 1995; 333(24):1581–1587.
16. The NINDS t-PA Stroke Study Group. Generalized efficacy of t-PA for acute stroke. Subgroup analysis of the NINDS t-PA stroke trial. Stroke 1997; 28:2119–2125.
17. Clark W, Wissman S, Albers GW, et al. Recombinant tissue-type plasminogen activator (Alteplase) for ischemic stroke 3 to 5 hours after symptom onset. JAMA 1999; 282(21):2019–2024.
18. Albers GW, Clark W, Madden K, Hamilton S. ATLANTIS trial-results for patients treated within 3 hr of stroke onset. Stroke 2002; 33:493–496.
19. Donnan GA, Davis SM, Chambers BR, et al. Streptokinase for acute ischemic stroke with relationship to time of administration: Australian Streptokinase (ASK) Trial Study Group. JAMA 1996; 276:961–966.
20. Multicentre Acute Stroke Trial-Italy (MAST-I) Group. Randomised controlled trial of streptokinase, aspirin, and combination of both in treatment of acute ischaemic stroke. Lancet 1995; 346:1509–1514.
21. Multicenter Acute Stroke Trial-Europe Study Group (MAST-E). Thrombolytic therapy with streptokinase in acute ischemic stroke. N Engl J Med 1996; 335:145–150.
22. Tanne D, Bates VE, Verro P, et al. Initial clinical experience with IV tissue plasminogen activator for acute ischemic stroke: a multicenter survey. The t-PA Stroke Survey Group. Neurology 1999; 53:424–427.
23. del Zoppo GJ, Ferbert A, Otis S, et al. Local intra-arterial fibrinolytic therapy in acute carotid territory stroke. A pilot study. Stroke 1988; 19(3):307–313.
24. Hacke W, Zeumer H, Ferbert A, Bruckmann H, del Zoppo G. Intra-arterial thrombolytic therapy improves outcome in patients with acute vertebrobasilar occlusive disease. Stroke 1988; 19:1216–1222.
25. Nenci GG, Gresele P, Taramelli M, Agnelli G, Signorini E. Thrombolytic therapy for thromboembolism of vertebrobasilar artery. Angiology 1983; 34(9):561–571.
26. del Zoppo GJ, Higashida RT, Furlan A, et al. PROACT: A Phase II randomized trial of recombinant pro-urokinase by direct arterial delivery in acute middle cerebral artery stroke. Stroke 1998; 29:4–11.
27. Furlan AJ, Higashida RT, Wechsler L, et al. Intra-arterial prourokinase for acute ischemic stroke. The PROACT II study: a randomized controlled trial. JAMA 1999; 282:2003–2011.
28. Wolpert SM, Bruckmann H, Greenlee R, et al. Neuroradiologic evaluation of patients with acute stroke treated with recombinant tissue plasminogen activator. AJNR Am J Neuroradiol 1993; 14:3–13.
29. Lewandowski C, Frankel M, Tomsick T, et al. Combined intravenous and intra-arterial r-tpa versus intra-arterial therapy of acute ischemic stroke. Stroke 1999; 30(2598):2605.
30. Broderick J. Combined intravenous and intra-arterial recanalization for acute ischemic stroke: The interventional management of stroke study. Stroke 2004; 35(4):904–911.
31. The Ancrod Stroke Study Investigators. Ancrod for the treatment of acute ischemic brain infarction. Stroke 1994; 25:1755–1759.
32. Sherman DG, Atkinson RP, Chippendale T, et al. Intravenous ancrod for treatment for acute ischemic stroke. JAMA 2000; 283(18):2395–2403.
33. Van de Werf F, Adgey J, Ardissino D, et al. Single-bolus tenecteplase compared with front-loaded alteplase in acute myocardial infarction: the ASSENT-2 double-blind randomised trial. Lancet 1999; 354(9180):716–722.
34. Liberatore GT, Samson A, Bladin CF, Schleuning WD, Medcalf RL. Vampire bat salivary plasminogen activator (Desmoteplase)-A fibrinolytic enzyme that does not promote neurodegeneration. Stroke 2003; 34(1):303.

35. Hacke W, Albers G, Al Rawi Y, et al. The Desmoteplase in acute ischemic stroke trial (DIAS)—A phase II MRI-based 9-hour window acute stroke thrombolysis trial with intravenous desmoteplase. Stroke 2005; 36(1):66–73.
36. Alexandrov AV, Demchuk A, Wein TH, Grotta JC. Yield of transcranial doppler in acute cerebral ischemia. Stroke 1999; 30:1604–1609.
37. Alexandrov AV, Burgin WS, Demchuk AM, El Mitwalli A, Grotta JC. Speed of intracranial clot lysis with intravenous tissue plasminogen activator therapy-Sonographic classification and short-term improvement. Circulation 2001; 103(24):2897–2902.
38. Alexandrov AV, Molina CA, Grotta JC, et al. Ultrasound-enhanced systemic thrombolysis for acute ischemic stroke. NEJM 2004; 351(21):2170–2178.
39. Gobin YP, Starkman S, Duckwiler GR, et al. MERCI 1–A phase 1 study of mechanical embolus removal in cerebral ischemia. Stroke 2004; 35(12):2848–2853.
40. Furlan A, Kanoti G. When Is thrombolysis justified in patients with acute ischemic stroke? A bioethical perspective. Stroke 1997; (28):214–218.
41. Brandt T, vonKummer R, MullerKuppers M, Hacke W. Thrombolytic therapy of acute basilar artery occlusion-variables affecting recanalization and outcome. Stroke 1996; 27(5):875–881.
42. Becker KJ, Monsein LH, Ulatowski J, et al. Intraarterial thrombolysis in vertebrobasilar occlusion. Am J Neuroradiol 1996; 17(2):255–262.
43. Grond M, Rudolf J, Schmulling S, et al. Early intravenous thrombolysis with recombinant tissue-type plasminogen activator in vertebrobasilar ischemic stroke. Arch Neurol 1998; 55:466–469.
44. Lindsberg PJ, Soinne L, Tatlisumak T, et al. Long-term outcome after intravenous thrombolysis of basilar artery occlusion. JAMA 2004; 292(15):1862–1866.
45. Hacke W, Donnan G, Fieschi C, et al. Association of outcome with early stroke treatment: pooled analysis of ATLANTIS, ECASS, and NINDS rt-PA stroke trials. Lancet 2004; 363(9411):768–774.
46. Bravata DM, Kim N, Concato J, Krumholz HM, Brass LM. Thrombolysis for acute stroke in routine clinical practice. Archives of Internal Medicine 2002; 162(17):1994–2001.
47. Wahlgren NG, Fieschi C, Grond M, et al. First safety and efficacy results on broad implementation of stroke thrombolysis in the European Union after regulatory approval (SITS-MOST). Stroke 2004; 35(1):240.
48. Kwan J, Hand P, Sandercock P. A systematic review of barriers to delivery of thrombolysis for acute stroke. Age Ageing 2004; 33(2):116–121.
49. Alberts MJ, Hademenos G, Latchaw RE, et al. Recommendations for the establishment of primary stroke centers. brain attack coalition. JAMA 2000; 283:3102–3109.

20 | Medical Management of Acute Ischemic Stroke

Kyra J. Becker, MD, Associate Professor

Departments of Neurology and Neurological Surgery, Harborview Medical Center, University of Washington School of Medicine, Seattle, Washington, USA

INTRODUCTION

The approach to stroke therapy has changed dramatically in the past few years from that of mere supportive care to aggressive intervention aimed at limiting ischemic brain injury. Although prompt recanalization of an occluded vessel can prevent cerebral infarction, attention to medical details may help to salvage tissue at risk. The only therapy shown to improve outcome from acute ischemic stroke is recombinant tissue plasminogen activator (rtPA) administered intravenously within three hours of stroke onset, which is discussed in Chapter 19. In this chapter, a rational approach to the medical management of patients with acute ischemic stroke based on data from experimental studies and observational trials, is presented.

THE ISCHEMIC PENUMBRA

The ischemic penumbra can be thought of as brain tissue in which the cerebral blood flow (CBF) is reduced to the point at which electrical failure occurs but is still above the point of energy failure and ion-pump failure (1). Theoretically, this underperfused tissue can be salvaged from infarction. A number of physiologic and metabolic variables that affect the ability to save this tissue from infarction have been identified, and medical therapies to manipulate them are discussed below.

BLOOD PRESSURE AND STROKE

The most important risk factor for stroke is hypertension, and aggressive treatment of hypertension can significantly reduce the risk of stroke (2–4). In the setting of acute ischemic stroke, however, interventions that reduce blood pressure (BP) can be detrimental (5–7). Spontaneous BP fluctuations are also predictive of outcome; both extreme hypotension and extreme hypertension after stroke onset are associated with worse outcome (8–14). Marked hypertension is associated with severe stroke, and appears to contribute to the development of cerebral edema (13,14). Whether treatment of extreme hypertension will improve outcome or limit the formation of cerebral edema has not been rigorously studied in prospective randomized, controlled trials.

Given the tight regulation of CBF, the relationship between BP and stroke outcome might seem difficult to reconcile. Blood flow to the brain is independent of mean arterial blood pressure and cerebral perfusion pressure (CPP) within the normal physiologic range, a phenomenon known as cerebral autoregulation (Fig. 1). In normotensive individuals, CBF in gray matter is maintained at approximately 50 mL/100 g tissue/min at CPP between 50 and 150 mmHg; patients with chronic hypertension autoregulate CBF at a higher CPP range. In ischemic brain, however, the ability to autoregulate is lost, and CBF becomes passively dependent on BP (15). It is this loss of cerebral autoregulation following stroke that likely accounts for the relationship between BP extremes and outcome from stroke. The loss of autoregulation also suggests that lowering BP in patients with acute stroke might further decrease CBF to already ischemic tissue (e.g., tissue in the penumbra) and threaten its survival. Given that BP directly influences CBF in ischemic tissue, BP should not be lowered in acute stroke unless signs indicate hypertensive urgency or the patient is to be treated with a thrombolytic. Failure to adequately treat hypertension prior to thrombolysis is associated with an increased risk of hemorrhagic transformation (16–19).

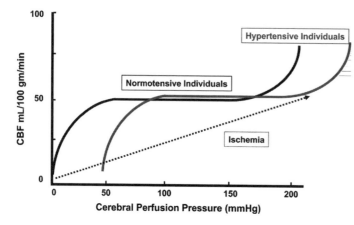

Figure 1 Cerebral autoregulation to pressure. Patients with chronic hypertension autoregulate CBF at higher cerebral perfusion pressure than normotensive individuals; the ability to autoregulate is lost in ischemic brain tissue. *Source: From Refs.* 159, 160. *Abbreviation:* CBF, cerebral blood flow.

The loss of autoregulation in ischemic brain also suggests that increasing BP could improve CBF and help salvage tissue within the ischemic penumbra. In experimental models of stroke, elevating BP decreases infarct volume; clinical data from small pilot trials also suggest that neurologic symptoms can be improved in patients by pharmacologically elevating BP (20–23). The benefits of induced hypertension, however, have not yet been proven in prospective, randomized, controlled trials; the decision to raise the BP, therefore, must be weighed against the possibility that hypertension will induce cerebral hemorrhage and exacerbate cerebral edema. Therefore, until further data are available, prudence dictates that BP not be lowered following acute stroke unless there are extenuating circumstances (i.e., desire to give thrombolytics or signs/symptoms of hypertensive urgency/emergency). However, it may be very difficult to clinically differentiate worsening ischemia (requiring maintenance of elevated BP) from hypertension-induced cerebral edema (requiring aggressive lowering of BP). If BP is to be lowered, intravenous drugs with a short half-life that do not directly affect the cerebral vasculature are preferred because the response to these drugs is predictable and easy to titrate. In general, labetalol, an $\alpha > \beta$ blocker, is the antihypertensive of choice for patients with stroke and other intracranial pathologies (24). Intravenous nicardipine can be used to lower BP in patients who are unresponsive to, or intolerant of, labetalol. For patients with relative hypotension, intravascular volume should be optimized with isotonic fluids; the use of vasopressors (e.g., phenylephrine) can be considered if BP goals cannot be met in volume-replete individuals.

Vascular tone, and thus CBF, are also regulated by the arterial content of carbon dioxide ($PaCO_2$) and oxygen (PaO_2). Reduction in $PaCO_2$ leads to vasoconstriction and decreased CBF, whereas reduction in PaO_2 leads to vasodilatation and increased CBF (Fig. 2). The response to $PaCO_2$ is much more robust than that to PaO_2; CBF increases 1 to 2 mL/100 g/min for 1 mmHg increase in $PaCO_2$ and decreases 1 to 2 mL/100 g/min for 1 mmHg decrease in $PaCO_2$ (25). In ischemic brain, the ability to autoregulate blood flow in response to changes in perfusion pressure is clearly impaired; whether an appropriate response to CO_2 occurs in ischemic brain is less clear. Within the ischemic core, CBF does not change normally in response to changes in CO_2; the response to CO_2 within the penumbra, however, may be preserved (26,27). If the CBF response to changes in $PaCO_2$ is impaired in ischemic tissue, but maintained in normal brain, the vasodilatory response to hypercapnia in the nonischemic tissue could lead to a "steal phenomenon" and exacerbate ischemia where blood flow is already impaired. Given that a significant decrease in $PaCO_2$ leads to vasoconstriction and thus decreases blood flow, hyperventilation can exacerbate ischemia in already ischemic tissue and even precipitate ischemia in previously nonischemic tissue. Hyperventilation should, therefore, be avoided in stroke patients unless it is being used as a temporizing measure in patients experiencing transtentorial herniation. The vascular response to PaO_2 is relatively weak in comparison to that for $PaCO_2$,

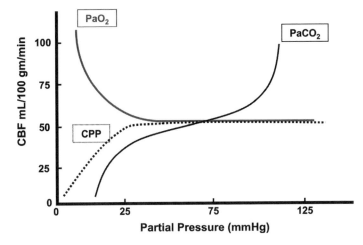

Figure 2 Changes in CBF in response to $PaCO_2$ and PaO_2. Patients with chronic hypertension autoregulate CBF at higher CPP than normotensive individuals; the ability to autoregulate is lost in ischemic brain tissue. *Source*: From Refs. 160. *Abbreviations*: CBF, cerebral blood flow; CPP, cerebral perfusion pressure.

and no data suggest that oxygen supplementation in adequately oxygenated patients improves outcome from stroke (28). Similarly, no convincing evidence supports a role for hyperbaric oxygen in the treatment of patients with acute stroke (29).

GLUCOSE AND ISCHEMIC BRAIN INJURY

Animal studies consistently show that hyperglycemia worsens ischemic brain injury and increases the risk of hemorrhagic transformation after cerebral infarction (30–32). Observational studies show that patients with hyperglycemia at the time of stroke onset have increased morbidity and mortality and that hyperglycemia is associated with more pronounced infarct growth (33–37). Patients with hyperglycemia are also at higher risk of hemorrhagic transformation after stroke, which can occur spontaneously or following the use of anticoagulants and fibrinolytics (38,39). Independent of the occurrence of hemorrhagic transformation, hyperglycemia is also associated with an increased risk of clinical deterioration in the days after stroke onset (40). Experimental data suggest that hyperglycemia might contribute to ischemic brain injury by several mechanisms, including increases in lactic acidosis, in blood–brain barrier (BBB) breakdown (and hence, cerebral edema), and in the release of excitotoxic amino acids (41,42).

Whether strict maintenance of euglycemia with infusion of insulin can improve stroke outcome has not yet been proven. A seminal study showed that aggressive insulin therapy in the intensive care unit setting could improve mortality, but the study included very few patients with brain injury (43). Pilot studies that address the role of insulin therapy in patients with acute stroke are underway (44,45). Furthermore, it is unclear whether normalization of glucose prior to administration of a thrombolytic will decrease the risk of hemorrhagic transformation. Appropriate clinical trial data are required before comprehensive recommendations about glucose management in stroke can be made, but it seems reasonable to target normoglycemia.

In experimental studies in which animals are pretreated with drugs that sensitize them to insulin [such as peroxisome proliferator–activated receptor (PPAR)-gamma agonists], outcome from stroke can be improved (46). The mechanism of action responsible for this neuroprotective effect is not yet fully understood. Trials of PPAR-gamma agonists for stroke prevention are underway, but it is too early to suggest that patients be started on PPAR-gamma agonists at stroke onset.

TEMPERATURE AND BRAIN INJURY

Hyperthermia in the immediate poststroke period is common and is associated with increased morbidity and mortality (47–51). Ironically, ischemic brain temperature tends to be higher than core body temperature (52). Hyperthermia might contribute to increased cerebral injury through several different mechanisms. First, temperature is the major determinant of the brain's metabolic rate of oxygen consumption ($CMRO_2$). For every degree centigrade above normothermia (36.8°C), $CMRO_2$ increases by approximately 5% to 10%; conversely, for every degree centigrade below normothermia, the $CMRO_2$ decreases by approximately 5% to 10% (53–55). Hyperthermia is also associated with increased inflammation and an increased release of excitotoxic amino acids; conversely, hypothermia reduces the release of excitotoxic amino acids (56–60).

Hypothermia is potently neuroprotective in animal models of stroke (61–63). Anecdotal evidence suggests that hypothermia might improve outcome from malignant cerebral infarction (64). Hypothermia improves neurologic outcome in patients who experience cardiac arrest, but prospective, randomized, controlled trials of hypothermia in stroke have not yet been completed (65,66). Given the consistent relationship between hyperthermia and poor stroke outcome, it seems reasonable to target normothermia in patients with acute stroke. Until the benefit of hypothermia can be proven in a prospective, randomized, controlled trial, it should only be used in the research setting.

INFECTION

One potential cause of fever following stroke is infection. Urinary tract infections and aspiration pneumonia are common after stroke, each occurring in up to 25% of all patients (67–70). Irrespective of the effect on body temperature, developing an infection in the immediate poststroke period is associated with increased morbidity and mortality (71–73). Whether infection itself worsens outcome from stroke or is only a marker for persons with more severe strokes cannot be determined by observational studies, but several lines of evidence suggest that it is the infection that is deleterious. First, a clinical trial that investigated the therapeutic benefit of a *murine* monoclonal antibody to intracellular adhesion molecule-1 in acute ischemic stroke showed that patients who received the monoclonal antibody experienced increased morbidity and mortality (67). In retrospect, this result might have been anticipated, as the antibody used actually activates neutrophils, complement, and the microvasculature (74,75). The premise of this trial was that inflammation contributes to cerebral ischemic injury and that limiting the inflammatory response would improve outcome. The trial offered resounding support for this premise. Second, fever is a cardinal feature of the immune response, and, as previously mentioned, hyperthermia is associated with worse neurologic outcome after stroke. In fact, experimental studies show that small increases in body temperature, even several days after the ischemic insult, are detrimental (76,77). Hyperthermia exacerbates the ischemic impairment of the BBB and enhances lymphocyte responses (56,78). Finally, cytokines that are secreted by leukocytes during the effector phase of an immune response compromise the integrity of the BBB and might be toxic to neurons and glia (79–83).

Increasing data suggest that systemic immunosuppression occurs following stroke and predisposes to infection (84). Patients with stroke might be prone to infection for obvious reasons; the use of indwelling urinary catheters predisposes to urinary tract infections, whereas a decrease in the level of consciousness, dysphagia, and impaired airway reflexes predispose to aspiration pneumonia. Further, experimental data show that outcome can be improved with prophylactic antibiotic treatment (85). Unfortunately, a recent prospective, randomized, controlled trial of levofloxacin versus placebo in patients with acute stroke failed to show any benefit to prophylactic antibiotic therapy for preventing infection; in fact, patients who received levofloxacin experienced worse stroke outcome (86). Further trials of prophylactic antibiotic therapy are ongoing. To prevent urinary tract infections, urinary catheters should be avoided. To prevent aspiration, patients should not be allowed to eat until swallow evaluations are performed; ventilated patients should be positioned with their heads elevated to prevent passive regurgitation.

VISCOSITY AND RED BLOOD CELL MASS IN STROKE

CBF falls as the hematocrit rises; as the hematocrit falls, so does the oxygen-carrying capacity of the blood. The optimal hematocrit for oxygen delivery is therefore determined by a balance of these two variables (87). Early studies suggested improved outcome with hemodilution, but these findings have not been replicated (88–97). The only situations in which venesection and hemodilution can be recommended are in patients with polycythemia vera (98,99).

MISCELLANEOUS DRUGS AND THERAPEUTIC INTERVENTIONS

Two large studies that included more than 40,000 patients investigated the benefits of aspirin administered within 48 hours of acute stroke onset. In the Chinese Aspirin Stroke Trial, the dose of aspirin was 160 mg/day; in the International Stroke Trial, it was 300 mg/day (100,101). Collectively, these trials showed that, for every 1000 patients treated with aspirin after stroke onset, death or disability could be prevented in about 10 and that there were fewer recurrent strokes. The benefit of aspirin in these trials might have been related to its antiplatelet effects and its ability to prevent recurrent stroke, but it is also possible that acute administration of aspirin produces other beneficial effects.

To date, no study has shown a benefit for acute anticoagulation in patients with stroke; in fact, most studies show an excess of hemorrhagic complications (101–107). The lack of benefit for anticoagulation in acute stroke is true even for patients with atrial fibrillation (108). Thus, anticoagulation is not indicated for treatment of the average stroke patient. Low-dose anticoagulation, however, can prevent deep venous thrombosis and pulmonary embolism in patients with stroke (107). Moreover, despite a lack of rigorous data to support its use, anticoagulation might be the best therapy for patients with cerebral vein thrombosis (109,110).

Observational studies show that magnesium levels drop in injured brain (111). Experimental data suggest that magnesium is neuroprotective (112,113). The potential benefits of magnesium could be related to its effects on ionotropic N-methyl-D-aspartate receptors or to the fact that magnesium might function as a vasodilator (114,115). Unfortunately, an initial prospective, randomized, controlled trial of magnesium administration within 12 hours of ischemic stroke failed to show any benefit (116). Another trial in which magnesium is administered by paramedics within one to two hours of symptom onset is underway (117).

The results of a Phase III European study of the neuroprotective agent NXY-059 were recently announced (118). This drug, which is thought to act as a free radical scavenger, improved neurologic outcome at three months in patients who received it within six hours of stroke onset. Approximately 30% of treated patients also received rtPA. A similar trial is ongoing in North America. Pending the results of this trial, approval to market the drug will be sought.

INTRACRANIAL PRESSURE AND MALIGNANT CEREBRAL EDEMA

The Monro-Kellie Doctrine states that the skull is a rigid box and that its contents (brain, cerebrospinal fluid, and blood) are incompressible (119). An increase in any one of the components will, therefore, displace another component, increase the pressure within the cranium, or cause a combination of the two. The relationship between intracranial pressure (ICP) and intracranial volume is often referred to as the intracranial "compliance" curve (Fig. 3). In that the relationship is really defined as the change in pressure for a given change in volume (dP/dV), the curve would more appropriately be referred to as the intracranial or "elastance" curve (120). The "compliance" curve illustrates the fact that the body is able to compensate for changes in intracranial volume without a concomitant change in pressure, to a degree; once the capacity to compensate for the change in volume is exceeded, the pressure begins to increase. It is at the high-end of intracranial volume that even small increases in volume lead to large increases in ICP.

Patients who experience large strokes that involve the entire territory of the middle cerebral artery (MCA) or internal carotid artery (ICA) are at risk for developing cerebral edema, especially with delayed reperfusion. When the amount of edema exceeds a critical level, cerebral herniation and death can occur (121–123). To decrease the risk of edema formation, occluded vessels should be recanalized early after stroke onset. Predictors of massive brain edema following hemispheric infarction include recanalization, National Institutes of Health Stroke Scale (NIHSS)≥20 for left hemispheric strokes, NIHSS≥15 for right hemispheric strokes, a history of hypertension or heart failure, increased baseline white blood cell count, major early computed tomography hypodensity involving >50% of the MCA territory and involvement of additional vascular territories (124,125).

Cerebral edema can be attenuated by a number of medical interventions, including administration of mannitol, glycerol, and hypertonic saline. These drugs increase the osmolality of the blood and facilitate the exchange of free water from the interstitial to the intravascular space; they produce their effect primarily in regions of the brain where the BBB is intact. When the BBB is impaired, the drugs can "leak" into ischemic brain tissue and theoretically lead to intracranial compartmental shift and increased risk of herniation, although these fears do not seem to be borne out clinically (126). Despite the fact that mannitol, glycerol, and hypertonic saline all decrease ICP, no data suggest that their use improves outcome in large hemispheric stroke (127–131). The benefit of corticosteroids in acute stroke is unproven, and corticosteroids do not attenuate edema associated with cerebral infarction; their use should, therefore, be avoided (132). Hypothermia might attenuate cerebral edema or, at least, delay its onset (64,133). The role of hypothermia in acute stroke therapy is discussed in Chapter 30. Finally, indomethacin is unique among the nonsteroidal antiinflammatory agents, in that it causes cerebral vasoconstriction and can decrease ICP (134–137).

Despite the presence of cerebral edema and the risk of herniation in malignant MCA/ICA infarcts, no clear role for ICP monitoring has been established for the treatment of stroke (138). Transtentorial herniation is the major risk associated with hemispheric infarction, and it is possible for the temporal lobe to slip over the tentorium without a documented increase in ICP. Thus, close and frequent neurologic examination is imperative (139). For patients who progress to herniation or are at risk of imminent herniation, emergent intubation for control of the airway and ventilation is necessary. Prolonged hyperventilation can worsen cerebral ischemia by causing arterial vasoconstriction, and prolonged hyperventilation was associated with worse clinical outcome in patients with traumatic brain injury; therefore, indefinite hyperventilation cannot be recommended in patients with stroke (140). Transient hyperventilation in the setting of acute herniation, however, might be a lifesaving measure. Mannitol at a dose of 1 g/kg is also an effective acute therapy for reversing herniation. Aggressive medical intervention for transtentorial herniation might produce reasonable clinical outcomes and should be pursued when more definitive therapy is available (141). One such therapy, early decompressive hemicraniectomy, might be lifesaving, but clinical data to support an effect on functional outcome are lacking (142–149).

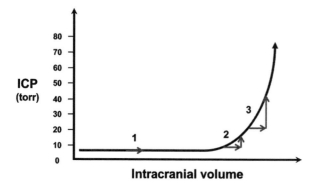

Figure 3 Intracranial "compliance" curve. For a given change in intracranial volume, the changes in ICP can be very different, depending upon the position within the compliance curve. *Abbreviation*: ICP, intracranial pressure.

STROKE UNITS

Numerous studies have demonstrated improved outcome in patients cared for in dedicated stroke units (150–158), which have staff who receive specialized training in stroke care and are aware of the medical issues that influence outcome from stroke. In addition, protocols to minimize medical complications are generally in place. Patients treated in stroke units experience a decreased rate of complications, such as deep vein thrombosis, urinary tract infection, and pneumonia. Early institution of physical therapy, speech, and language therapy, and early use of physiatry helps to speed transition from the acute inpatient medical service to rehabilitation setting.

SUMMARY

Currently, little data exist to suggest that early medical intervention, short of rtPA or aspirin administration, improves outcome after acute ischemic stroke. An organized approach to preventing complications, as demonstrated by the use of stroke units, does seem to produce better clinical outcomes. Numerous trials are underway to assess the safety and effectiveness of several different interventions, such as induced hypertension, hypothermia, aggressive insulin therapy, and administration of neuroprotective agents. Until they are completed, it seems reasonable to suggest that, in the treatment of acute ischemic stroke, measures be taken to prevent hypotension, hyperthermia, and hyperglycemia.

REFERENCES

1. Astrup J, Siesjo BK, Symon L. Thresholds in cerebral ischemia—the ischemic penumbra. Stroke 1981; 12:723–725.
2. Lawes CM, Bennett DA, Feigin VL, Rodgers A. Blood pressure and stroke: an overview of published reviews. Stroke 2004; 35:776–785.
3. Lewington S, Clarke R, Qizilbash N, Peto R, Collins R. Age-specific relevance of usual blood pressure to vascular mortality: a meta-analysis of individual data for one million adults in 61 prospective studies. Lancet 2002; 360:1903–1913.
4. Heart Disease and Stroke Statistics—2005 Update. American Heart Association, 2004.
5. Ahmed N, Wahlgren NG. Effects of blood pressure lowering in the acute phase of total anterior circulation infarcts and other stroke subtypes. Cerebrovasc Dis 2003; 15:235–243.
6. Ahmed N, Nasman P, Wahlgren NG. Effect of intravenous nimodipine on blood pressure and outcome after acute stroke. Stroke 2000; 31:1250–1255.
7. Fischberg GM, Lozano E, Rajamani K, Ameriso S, Fisher MJ. Stroke precipitated by moderate blood pressure reduction. J Emerg Med 2000; 19:339–346.
8. Vemmos KN, Tsivgoulis G, Spengos K, et al. U-shaped relationship between mortality and admission blood pressure in patients with acute stroke. J Intern Med 2004; 255:257–265.
9. Castillo J, Leira R, Garcia MM, Serena J, Blanco M, Davalos A. Blood pressure decrease during the acute phase of ischemic stroke is associated with brain injury and poor stroke outcome. Stroke 2004; 35:520–526.
10. Vlcek M, Schillinger M, Lang W, Lalouschek W, Bur A, Hirschl MM. Association between course of blood pressure within the first 24 hours and functional recovery after acute ischemic stroke. Ann Emerg Med 2003; 42:619–626.
11. Oliveira-Filho J, Silva SC, Trabuco CC, Pedreira BB, Sousa EU, Bacellar A. Detrimental effect of blood pressure reduction in the first 24 hours of acute stroke onset. Neurology 2003; 61:1047–1051.
12. Semplicini A, Maresca A, Boscolo G, et al. Hypertension in acute ischemic stroke: a compensatory mechanism or an additional damaging factor? Arch Intern Med 2003; 163:211–216.
13. Leonardi-Bee J, Bath PM, Phillips SJ, Sandercock PA. Blood pressure and clinical outcomes in the international stroke trial. Stroke 2002; 33:1315–1320.
14. Vemmos KN, Tsivgoulis G, Spengos K, et al. Association between 24-h blood pressure monitoring variables and brain oedema in patients with hyperacute stroke. J Hypertens 2003; 21:2167–2173.
15. Novak V, Chowdhary A, Farrar B, et al. Altered cerebral vasoregulation in hypertension and stroke. Neurology 2003; 60:1657–1663.
16. Gilligan AK, Markus R, Read S, et al. Baseline blood pressure but not early computed tomography changes predicts major hemorrhage after streptokinase in acute ischemic stroke. Stroke 2002; 33:2236–2242.

17. Tanne D, Kasner SE, Demchuk AM, et al. Markers of increased risk of intracerebral hemorrhage after intravenous recombinant tissue plasminogen activator therapy for acute ischemic stroke in clinical practice: the multicenter rt-PA stroke survey. Circulation 2002; 105:1679–1685.

18. Gurwitz JH, Gore JM, Goldberg RJ, et al. Risk for intracranial hemorrhage after tissue plasminogen activator treatment for acute myocardial infarction. Participants in the national registry of myocardial infarction 2. Ann Intern Med 1998; 129:597–604.

19. Aylward PE, Wilcox RG, Horgan JH, et al. Relation of increased arterial blood pressure to mortality and stroke in the context of contemporary thrombolytic therapy for acute myocardial infarction. A randomized trial. Gusto-i investigators. Ann Intern Med 1996; 125:891–900.

20. Chileuitt L, Leber K, McCalden T, Weinstein PR. Induced hypertension during ischemia reduces infarct area after temporary middle cerebral artery occlusion in rats. Surg Neurol 1996; 46:229–234.

21. Smrcka M, Ogilvy CS, Crow RJ, Maynard KI, Kawamata T, Ames A 3rd. Induced hypertension improves regional blood flow and protects against infarction during focal ischemia: time course of changes in blood flow measured by laser Doppler imaging. Neurosurgery 1998; 42:617–624; discussion 624–615.

22. Rordorf G, Koroshetz WJ, Ezzeddine MA, Segal AZ, Buonanno FS. A pilot study of drug-induced hypertension for treatment of acute stroke. Neurology 2001; 56:1210–1213.

23. Hillis AE, Ulatowski JA, Barker PB, et al. A pilot randomized trial of induced blood pressure elevation: effects on function and focal perfusion in acute and subacute stroke. Cerebrovasc Dis 2003; 16:236–246.

24. Adams H, Adams R, Del Zoppo G, Goldstein LB. Guidelines for the early management of patients with ischemic stroke: 2005 guidelines update. A Scientific Statement from the Stroke Council of the American Heart Association/American Stroke Association. Stroke 2005; 36:916–923.

25. Sato M, Pawlik G, Heiss WD. Comparative studies of regional CNS blood flow autoregulation and responses to CO_2 in the cat. Effects of altering arterial blood pressure and $PACO_2$ on RCBF of cerebrum, cerebellum, and spinal cord. Stroke 1984; 15:91–97.

26. Dettmers C, Young A, Rommel T, Hartmann A, Weingart O, Baron JC. CO_2 reactivity in the ischaemic core, penumbra, and normal tissue 6 hours after acute MCA-occlusion in primates. Acta Neurochir (Wien) 1993; 125:150–155.

27. Olsen TS, Larsen B, Herning M, Skriver EB, Lassen NA. Blood flow and vascular reactivity in collaterally perfused brain tissue. Evidence of an ischemic penumbra in patients with acute stroke. Stroke 1983; 14:332–341.

28. Ronning OM, Guldvog B. Should stroke victims routinely receive supplemental oxygen? A quasi-randomized controlled trial. Stroke 1999; 30:2033–2037.

29. Rusyniak DE, Kirk MA, May JD, et al. Hyperbaric oxygen therapy in acute ischemic stroke: results of the hyperbaric oxygen in acute ischemic stroke trial pilot study. Stroke 2003; 34:571–574.

30. Kawai N, Keep RF, Betz AL. Hyperglycemia and the vascular effects of cerebral ischemia. Stroke 1997; 28:149–154.

31. Sieber FE, Traystman RJ. Special issues: glucose and the brain. Crit Care Med 1992; 20:104–114.

32. De Courten-Myers GM, Kleinholz M, Holm P, et al. Hemorrhagic infarct conversion in experimental stroke. Ann Emerg Med 1992; 21:120–126.

33. Bruno A, Biller J, Adams HP Jr., et al. Acute blood glucose level and outcome from ischemic stroke. Trial of ORG 10172 in Acute Stroke Treatment (TOAST) investigators. Neurology 1999; 52:280–284.

34. Bruno A, Levine SR, Frankel MR, et al. Admission glucose level and clinical outcomes in the NINDS rt-PA stroke trial. Neurology 2002; 59:669–674.

35. Baird TA, Parsons MW, Phanh T, et al. Persistent poststroke hyperglycemia is independently associated with infarct expansion and worse clinical outcome. Stroke 2003; 34:2208–2214.

36. Parsons MW, Barber PA, Desmond PM, et al. Acute hyperglycemia adversely affects stroke outcome: a magnetic resonance imaging and spectroscopy study. Ann Neurol 2002; 52:20–28.

37. Weir CJ, Murray GD, Dyker AG, Lees KR. Is hyperglycaemia an independent predictor of poor outcome after acute stroke? Results of a long-term follow up study. Br Med J 1997; 314:1303–1306.

38. Demchuk AM, Morgenstern LB, Krieger DW, et al. Serum glucose level and diabetes predict tissue plasminogen activator- related intracerebral hemorrhage in acute ischemic stroke. Stroke 1999; 30:34–39.

39. Kase CS, Furlan AJ, Wechsler LR, et al. Cerebral hemorrhage after intra-arterial thrombolysis for ischemic stroke: the PROACT II trial. Neurology 2001; 57:1603–1610.

40. Grotta JC, Welch KM, Fagan SC, et al. Clinical deterioration following improvement in the NINDS rt-PA stroke trial. Stroke 2001; 32:661–668.

41. Berger L, Hakim AM. The association of hyperglycemia with cerebral edema in stroke. Stroke 1986; 17:865–871.

42. Li PA, Shuaib A, Miyashita H, He QP, Siesjo BK, Warner DS. Hyperglycemia enhances extracellular glutamate accumulation in rats subjected to forebrain ischemia. Stroke 2000; 31:183–192.

43. van den Berghe G, Wouters P, Weekers F, et al. Intensive insulin therapy in the critically ill patients. N Engl J Med 2001; 345:1359–1367.

44. Gray CS, Hildreth AJ, Alberti GK, O'Connell JE. Poststroke hyperglycemia: natural history and immediate management. Stroke 2004; 35:122–126.

45. Bruno A, Saha C, Williams LS, Shankar R. IV insulin during acute cerebral infarction in diabetic patients. Neurology 2004; 62:1441–1442.

46. Sundararajan S, Gamboa JL, Victor NA, Wanderi EW, Lust WD, Landreth GE. Peroxisome proliferator-activated receptor-gamma ligands reduce inflammation and infarction size in transient focal ischemia. Neuroscience 2005; 130:685–696.

47. Azzimondi G, Bassein L, Nonino F, et al. Fever in acute stroke worsens prognosis. A prospective study. Stroke 1995; 26:2040–2043.

48. Castillo J, Davalos A, Marrugat J, Noya M. Timing for fever-related brain damage in acute ischemic stroke. Stroke 1998; 29:2455–2460.

49. Hajat C, Hajat S, Sharma P. Effects of poststroke pyrexia on stroke outcome: a meta-analysis of studies in patients. Stroke 2000; 31:410–414.

50. Kammersgaard LP, Jorgensen HS, Rungby JA, et al. Admission body temperature predicts long-term mortality after acute stroke: the Copenhagen stroke study. Stroke 2002; 33:1759–1762.

51. Reith J, Jorgensen HS, Pedersen PM, et al. Body temperature in acute stroke: relation to stroke severity, infarct size, mortality, and outcome. Lancet 1996; 347:422–425.

52. Schwab S, Schwarz S, Aschoff A, Keller E, Hacke W. Moderate hypothermia and brain temperature in patients with severe middle cerebral artery infarction. Acta Neurochir Suppl 1998; 71:131–134.

53. Hagerdal M, Harp J, Nilsson L, Siesjo BK. The effect of induced hypothermia upon oxygen consumption in the rat brain. J Neurochem 1975; 24:311–316.

54. Klementavicius R, Nemoto EM, Yonas H. The Q10 ratio for basal cerebral metabolic rate for oxygen in rats. J Neurosurg 1996; 85:482–487.

55. Michenfelder JD, Milde JH. The relationship among canine brain temperature, metabolism, and function during hypothermia. Anesthesiology 1991; 75:130–136.

56. Huang YH, Haegerstrand A, Frostegard J. Effects of in vitro hyperthermia on proliferative responses and lymphocyte activity. Clin Exp Immunol 1996; 103:61–66.

57. Wang WC, Goldman LM, Schleider DM, et al. Fever-range hyperthermia enhances l-selectin-dependent adhesion of lymphocytes to vascular endothelium. J Immunol 1998; 160:961–969.

58. Castillo J, Davalos A, Noya M. Aggravation of acute ischemic stroke by hyperthermia is related to an excitotoxic mechanism. Cerebrovasc Dis 1999; 9:22–27.

59. Li PA, He QP, Miyashita H, Howllet W, Siesjo BK, Shuaib A. Hypothermia ameliorates ischemic brain damage and suppresses the release of extracellular amino acids in both normo- and hyperglycemic subjects. Exp Neurol 1999; 158:242–253.

60. Berger C, Schabitz WR, Georgiadis D, Steiner T, Aschoff A, Schwab S. Effects of hypothermia on excitatory amino acids and metabolism in stroke patients: a microdialysis study. Stroke 2002; 33:519–524.

61. Corbett D, Hamilton M, Colbourne F. Persistent neuroprotection with prolonged postischemic hypothermia in adult rats subjected to transient middle cerebral artery occlusion. Exp Neurol 2000; 163:200–206.

62. Dietrich WD, Busto R, Valdes I, Loor Y. Effects of normothermic versus mild hyperthermic forebrain ischemia in rats. Stroke 1990; 21:1318–1325.

63. Kawai N, Okauchi M, Morisaki K, Nagao S. Effects of delayed intraischemic and postischemic hypothermia on a focal model of transient cerebral ischemia in rats. Stroke 2000; 31:1982–1989; discussion 1989.

64. Schwab S, Schwarz S, Spranger M, Keller E, Bertram M, Hacke W. Moderate hypothermia in the treatment of patients with severe middle cerebral artery infarction. Stroke 1998; 29:2461–2466.

65. Bernard SA, Gray TW, Buist MD, et al. Treatment of comatose survivors of out-of-hospital cardiac arrest with induced hypothermia. N Engl J Med 2002; 346:557–563.

66. The Hypothermia After Cardiac Arrest Study Group. Mild therapeutic hypothermia to improve the neurologic outcome after cardiac arrest. N Engl J Med 2002; 346:549–556.

67. Enlimomab Acute Stroke Trial Investigators. Use of anti-ICAM-1 therapy in ischemic stroke: results of the Enlimomab acute stroke trial. Neurology 2001; 57:1428–1434.

68. Davenport RJ, Dennis MS, Wellwood I, Warlow CP. Complications after acute stroke. Stroke 1996; 27:415–420.

69. Hilker R, Poetter C, Findeisen N, et al. Nosocomial pneumonia after acute stroke: implications for neurological intensive care medicine. Stroke 2003; 34:975–981.

70. Langhorne P, Stott DJ, Robertson L, et al. Medical complications after stroke: a multicenter study. Stroke 2000; 31:1223–1229.

71. Georgilis K, Plomaritoglou A, Dafni U, Bassiakos Y, Vemmos K. Aetiology of fever in patients with acute stroke. J Intern Med 1999; 246:203–209.

72. Grau AJ, Buggle F, Schnitzler P, Spiel M, Lichy C, Hacke W. Fever and infection early after ischemic stroke. J Neurol Sci 1999; 171:115–120.

73. Johnston KC, Li JY, Lyden PD, et al. Medical and neurological complications of ischemic stroke: experience from the RANTTAS trial. RANTTAS investigators. Stroke 1998; 29:447–453.

74. Furuya K, Takeda H, Azhar S, et al. Examination of several potential mechanisms for the negative outcome in a clinical stroke trial of Enlimomab, a murine anti-human intercellular adhesion molecule-1 antibody: a bedside-to-bench study. Stroke 2001; 32:2665–2674.

75. Vuorte J, Lindsberg PJ, Kaste M, et al. Anti-ICAM-1 monoclonal antibody r6.5 (Enlimomab) promotes activation of neutrophils in whole blood. J Immunol 1999; 162:2353–2357.

76. Baena RC, Busto R, Dietrich WD, Globus MY, Ginsberg MD. Hyperthermia delayed by 24 hours aggravates neuronal damage in rat hippocampus following global ischemia. Neurology 1997; 48:768–773.

77. Kim Y, Busto R, Dietrich WD, Kraydieh S, Ginsberg MD. Delayed postischemic hyperthermia in awake rats worsens the histopathological outcome of transient focal cerebral ischemia. Stroke 1996; 27:2274–2280; discussion 2281.

78. Dietrich WD, Busto R, Halley M, Valdes I. The importance of brain temperature in alterations of the blood-brain barrier following cerebral ischemia. J Neuropathol Exp Neurol 1990; 49:486–497.

79. Barone FC, Arvin B, White RF, et al. Tumor necrosis factor-alpha. A mediator of focal ischemic brain injury. Stroke 1997; 28:1233–1244.

80. Claudio L, Kress Y, Factor J, Brosnan CF. Mechanisms of edema formation in experimental autoimmune encephalomyelitis. The contribution of inflammatory cells. Am J Pathol 1990; 137:1033–1045.

81. Touzani O, Boutin H, Chuquet J, Rothwell N. Potential mechanisms of interleukin-1 involvement in cerebral ischaemia. J Neuroimmunol 1999; 100:203–215.

82. Jeohn GH, Kim WG, Hong JS. Time dependency of the action of nitric oxide in lipopolysaccharide-interferon-gamma-induced neuronal cell death in murine primary neuron-glia co-cultures. Brain Res 2000; 880:173–177.

83. Hanisch UK, Neuhaus J, Quirion R, Kettenmann H. Neurotoxicity induced by interleukin-2: involvement of infiltrating immune cells. Synapse 1996; 24:104–114.

84. Prass K, Meisel C, Hoflich C, et al. Stroke-induced immunodeficiency promotes spontaneous bacterial infections and is mediated by sympathetic activation reversal by poststroke T helper cell type 1-like immunostimulation. J Exp Med 2003; 198:725–736.

85. Meisel C, Prass K, Braun J, et al. Preventive antibacterial treatment improves the general medical and neurological outcome in a mouse model of stroke. Stroke 2004; 35:2–6.

86. Chamorro A, Obach V, Vargas M, et al. The early systemic prophylaxis of infection after stroke study: final results (abstr). Stroke 2005; 36:420.

87. Dexter F, Hindman BJ. Effect of haemoglobin concentration on brain oxygenation in focal stroke: a mathematical modelling study. Br J Anaesth 1997; 79:346–351.

88. The Hemodilution in Stroke Study Group. Hypervolemic hemodilution treatment of acute stroke. Results of a randomized multicenter trial using pentastarch. Stroke 1989; 20:317–323.

89. Koller M, Haenny P, Hess K, Weniger D, Zangger P. Adjusted hypervolemic hemodilution in acute ischemic stroke. Stroke 1990; 21:1429–1434.

90. Strand T, Asplund K, Eriksson S, Hagg E, Lithner F, Wester PO. A randomized controlled trial of hemodilution therapy in acute ischemic stroke. Stroke 1984; 15:980–989.

91. Scandinavian Stroke Study Group. Multicenter trial of hemodilution in acute ischemic stroke. I. Results in the total patient population. Stroke 1987; 18:691–699.

92. Italian Acute Stroke Study Group. The Italian hemodilution trial in acute stroke. Stroke 1987; 18:670–676.

93. Italian Acute Stroke Study Group. Haemodilution in acute stroke: results of the Italian haemodilution trial. Lancet 1988; 1:318–321.

94. Scandinavian Stroke Study Group. Multicenter trial of hemodilution in acute ischemic stroke. Results of subgroup analyses. Stroke 1988; 19:464–471.

95. Rudolf J. Hydroxyethyl starch for hypervolemic hemodilution in patients with acute ischemic stroke: a randomized, placebo-controlled phase II safety study. Cerebrovasc Dis 2002; 1433–41.

96. Aichner FT, Fazekas F, Brainin M, Polz W, Mamoli B, Zeiler K. Hypervolemic hemodilution in acute ischemic stroke: the multicenter Austrian hemodilution stroke trial (MAHST). Stroke 1998; 29:743–749.

97. Asplund K. Haemodilution for acute ischaemic stroke. Cochrane Database Syst Rev 2002:CD000103.

98. Kwaan HC, Wang J. Hyperviscosity in polycythemia vera and other red cell abnormalities. Semin Thromb Hemost 2003; 29:451–458.

99. Lahtinen R, Kuikka J. Cerebral blood flow in polycythaemia vera. Ann Clin Res 1983; 15:200–202.

100. CAST (Chinese Acute Stroke Trial) Collaborative Group. Randomised placebo-controlled trial of early aspirin use in 20,000 patients with acute ischaemic stroke. Lancet 1997; 349:1641–1649.

101. International Stroke Trial Collaborative Group. The International Stroke Trial (IST). A randomised trial of aspirin, subcutaneous heparin, both, or neither among 19435 patients with acute ischaemic stroke. Lancet 1997; 349:1569–1581.

102. Counsell C, Sandercock P. Low-molecular-weight heparins or heparinoids versus standard unfractionated heparin for acute ischemic stroke (cochrane review). Stroke 2002; 33:1925–1926.

103. The Publications Committee for the Trial of Org 10172 in Acute Stroke Treatment (TOAST) Investigators. Low molecular weight heparinoid, org 10172 (danaparoid), and outcome after acute ischemic stroke: a randomized controlled trial. JAMA 1998; 279:1265–1272.

104. Bath PM, Lindenstrom E, Boysen G, et al. Tinzaparin in acute ischaemic stroke (TAIST): a randomised aspirin-controlled trial. Lancet 2001; 358:702–710.

105. Diener HC, Ringelstein EB, von Kummer R, et al. Treatment of acute ischemic stroke with the low-molecular-weight heparin certoparin: results of the TOPAS trial. Therapy of Patients with Acute Stroke (Topas) Investigators. Stroke 2001; 32:22–29.

106. Haley EC Jr, Kassell NF, Torner JC. Failure of heparin to prevent progression in progressing ischemic infarction. Stroke 1988; 19:10–14.

107. Gubitz G, Sandercock P, Counsell C. Anticoagulants for acute ischaemic stroke. Cochrane Database Syst Rev 2004:CD000024.

108. Hart RG, Palacio S, Pearce LA. Atrial fibrillation, stroke, and acute antithrombotic therapy: analysis of randomized clinical trials. Stroke 2002; 33:2722–2727.

109. de Bruijn SF, Stam J. Randomized, placebo-controlled trial of anticoagulant treatment with low-molecular-weight heparin for cerebral sinus thrombosis. Stroke 1999; 30:484–488.

110. Brucker AB, Vollert-Rogenhofer H, Wagner M, et al. Heparin treatment in acute cerebral sinus venous thrombosis: a retrospective clinical and MR analysis of 42 cases. Cerebrovasc Dis 1998; 8:331–337.

111. Helpern JA, Vande Linde AM, Welch KM, et al. Acute elevation and recovery of intracellular $[Mg^{2+}]$ following human focal cerebral ischemia. Neurology 1993; 43:1577–1581.

112. Izumi Y, Roussel S, Pinard E, Seylaz J. Reduction of infarct volume by magnesium after middle cerebral artery occlusion in rats. J Cereb Blood Flow Metab 1991; 11:1025–1030.

113. Lin JY, Chung SY, Lin MC, Cheng FC. Effects of magnesium sulfate on energy metabolites and glutamate in the cortex during focal cerebral ischemia and reperfusion in the gerbil monitored by a dual-probe microdialysis technique. Life Sci 2002; 71:803–811.

114. Zarei MM, Dani JA. Ionic permeability characteristics of the n-methyl-d-aspartate receptor channel. J Gen Physiol 1994; 103:231–248.

115. Wang Y, Santini F, Qin K, Huang CY. A Mg(2+)-dependent, Ca(2+)-inhibitable serine/threonine protein phosphatase from bovine brain. J Biol Chem 1995; 270:25607–25612.

116. Muir KW, Lees KR, Ford I, Davis S. Magnesium for acute stroke (intravenous magnesium efficacy in stroke trial): randomised controlled trial. Lancet 2004; 363:439–445.

117. Saver JL, Kidwell C, Eckstein M, Starkman S. Prehospital neuroprotective therapy for acute stroke: results of the field administration of stroke therapy-magnesium (FAST-MAG) pilot trial. Stroke 2004; 35:e106–e108.

118. Lees KR, Zivin JA, Ashwood T. et al. NXY-059 for acute ischemic stroke N Engl. J. Med. 2006; 354:588–600.

119. Stern WE. Intracranial fluid dynamics: the relationship of intracranial pressure to the monro-kellie doctrine and the reliability of pressure assessment. J R Coll Surg Edinb 1963; 168:18–36.

120. Sklar FH, Elashvili I. The pressure-volume function of brain elasticity. Physiological considerations and clinical applications. J Neurosurg 1977; 47:670–679.

121. Derouesne C, Cambon H, Yelnik A, Duyckaerts C, Hauw JJ. Infarcts in the middle cerebral artery territory. Pathological study of the mechanisms of death. Acta Neurol Scand 1993; 87:361–366.

122. Hacke W, Schwab S, Horn M, Spranger M, De Georgia M, von Kummer R. A 'malignant' middle cerebral artery territory infarction: clinical course and prognostic signs. Arch Neurol 1996; 53:309–315.

123. Wijdicks EF, Diringer MN. Middle cerebral artery territory infarction and early brain swelling: progression and effect of age on outcome. Mayo Clin Proc 1998; 73:829–836.

124. Kasner SE, Demchuk AM, Berrouschot J, et al. Predictors of fatal brain edema in massive hemispheric ischemic stroke. Stroke 2001; 32:2117–2123.

125. Cruz-Flores S, Thompson DW, Boiser JR. Massive cerebral edema after recanalization post-thrombolysis. J Neuroimaging 2001; 11:447–451.

126. Sakamaki M, Igarashi H, Nishiyama Y, et al. Effect of glycerol on ischemic cerebral edema assessed by magnetic resonance imaging. J Neurol Sci 2003; 209:69–74.

127. Bereczki D, Liu M, do Prado GF, Fekete I. Mannitol for acute stroke. Cochrane Database Syst Rev 2001:CD001153.

128. Schwarz S, Schwab S, Bertram M, Aschoff A, Hacke W. Effects of hypertonic saline hydroxyethyl starch solution and mannitol in patients with increased intracranial pressure after stroke. Stroke 1998; 29:1550–1555.

129. Berger C, Sakowitz OW, Kiening KL, Schwab S. Neurochemical monitoring of glycerol therapy in patients with ischemic brain edema. Stroke 2005; 36:e4–e6.

130. Bhardwaj A, Ulatowski JA. Hypertonic saline solutions in brain injury. Curr Opin Crit Care 2004; 10:126–131.

131. Zuliani G, Cherubini A, Atti AR, et al. Prescription of anti-oedema agents and short-term mortality in older patients with acute ischaemic stroke. Drugs Aging 2004; 21:273–278.

132. Qizilbash N, Lewington SL, Lopez-Arrieta JM. Corticosteroids for acute ischaemic stroke. Cochrane Database Syst Rev 2002:CD000064.

133. Milhaud D, Thouvenot E, Heroum C, Escuret E. Prolonged moderate hypothermia in massive hemispheric infarction: clinical experience. J Neurosurg Anesthesiol 2005; 17:49–53.

134. Forderreuther S, Straube A. Indomethacin reduces CSF pressure in intracranial hypertension. Neurology 2000; 55:1043–1045.

135. Schwarz S, Bertram M, Aschoff A, Schwab S, Hacke W. Indomethacin for brain edema following stroke. Cerebrovasc Dis 1999; 9:248–250.

136. Harrigan MR, Tuteja S, Neudeck BL. Indomethacin in the management of elevated intracranial pressure: a review. J Neurotrauma 1997; 14:637–650.

137. Jensen K, Ohrstrom J, Cold GE, Astrup J. The effects of indomethacin on intracranial pressure, cerebral blood flow and cerebral metabolism in patients with severe head injury and intracranial hypertension. Acta Neurochir (Wien) 1991; 108:116–121.

138. Schwab S, Aschoff A, Spranger M, Albert F, Hacke W. The value of intracranial pressure monitoring in acute hemispheric stroke. Neurology 1996; 47:393–398.

139. Frank JI. Large hemispheric infarction, deterioration, and intracranial pressure. Neurology 1995; 45:1286–1290.

140. Muizelaar JP, Marmarou A, Ward JD, et al. Adverse effects of prolonged hyperventilation in patients with severe head injury: a randomized clinical trial. J Neurosurg 1991; 75:731–739.

141. Qureshi AI, Geocadin RG, Suarez JI, Ulatowski JA. Long-term outcome after medical reversal of transtentorial herniation in patients with supratentorial mass lesions. Crit Care Med 2000; 28:1556–1564.

142. Schwab S, Steiner T, Aschoff A, et al. Early hemicraniectomy in patients with complete middle cerebral artery infarction. Stroke 1998; 29:1888–1893.

143. Georgiadis D, Schwarz S, Aschoff A, Schwab S. Hemicraniectomy and moderate hypothermia in patients with severe ischemic stroke. Stroke 2002; 33:1584–1588.

144. Curry WT Jr., Sethi MK, Ogilvy CS, Carter BS. Factors associated with outcome after hemicraniectomy for large middle cerebral artery territory infarction. Neurosurgery 2005; 56:681–692; discussion 681–692.

145. Fandino J, Keller E, Barth A, Landolt H, Yonekawa Y, Seiler RW. Decompressive craniotomy after middle cerebral artery infarction. Retrospective analysis of patients treated in three centres in Switzerland. Swiss Med Wkly 2004; 134:423–429.

146. Foerch C, Lang JM, Krause J, et al. Functional impairment, disability, and quality of life outcome after decompressive hemicraniectomy in malignant middle cerebral artery infarction. J Neurosurg 2004; 101:248–254.

147. Gupta R, Connolly ES, Mayer S, Elkind MS. Hemicraniectomy for massive middle cerebral artery territory infarction: a systematic review. Stroke 2004; 35:539–543.

148. Leonhardt G, Wilhelm H, Doerfler A, et al. Clinical outcome and neuropsychological deficits after right decompressive hemicraniectomy in MCA infarction. J Neurol 2002; 249:1433–1440.

149. Holtkamp M, Buchheim K, Unterberg A, et al. Hemicraniectomy in elderly patients with space occupying media infarction: improved survival but poor functional outcome. J Neurol Neurosurg Psychiatr 2001; 70:226–228.

150. Organised inpatient (stroke unit) care for stroke. Cochrane Database Syst Rev 2002:CD000197.

151. Rudd AG, Hoffman A, Irwin P, Lowe D, Pearson MG. Stroke unit care and outcome: results from the 2001 National Sentinel Audit of Stroke (England, Wales, and Northern Ireland). Stroke 2005; 36:103–106.

152. Cadilhac DA, Ibrahim J, Pearce DC, et al. Multicenter comparison of processes of care between stroke units and conventional care wards in Australia. Stroke 2004; 35:1035–1040.

153. Sulter G, Elting JW, Langedijk M, Maurits NM, De Keyser J. Admitting acute ischemic stroke patients to a stroke care monitoring unit versus a conventional stroke unit: a randomized pilot study. Stroke 2003; 34:101–104.

154. Evans A, Harraf F, Donaldson N, Kalra L. Randomized controlled study of stroke unit care versus stroke team care in different stroke subtypes. Stroke 2002; 33:449–455.

155. Indredavik B, Bakke F, Slordahl SA, Rokseth R, Haheim LL. Stroke unit treatment. 10-year follow-up. Stroke 1999; 30:1524–1527.
156. Indredavik B, Bakke F, Slordahl SA, Rokseth R, Haheim LL. Treatment in a combined acute and rehabilitation stroke unit: which aspects are most important? Stroke 1999; 30:917–923.
157. Jorgensen HS, Kammersgaard LP, Nakayama H, et al. Treatment and rehabilitation on a stroke unit improves 5-year survival. A community-based study. Stroke 1999; 30:930–933.
158. Ronning OM, Guldvog B. Stroke units versus general medical wards. I. Twelve- and eighteen-month survival: a randomized, controlled trial. Stroke 1998; 29:58–62.
159. Lassen NA Cerebral blood flow and oxygen consumption in man. Physical Rev. 39:183–238, 1959.
160. Symon L, Held K, Dorsch NWC. A study of regional autoregulation in the cerebral circulation to increase perfusion pressure in normocapnia and hypercapnia. Stroke 4:139–147, 1973.

21 | Clinical Neuroprotective Trials in Ischemic Stroke

Wayne M. Clark, MD, Professor[a] and Director[b]
Helmi L. Lutsep, MD, Associate Professor[a] and Co-Director[b]

[a] Department of Neurology, [b] Stroke Program, Oregon Stroke Center, Oregon Health & Science University, Portland, Oregon, USA

INTRODUCTION

Stroke occurs in over 700,000 Americans each year and is the third leading cause of death in the United States. Many survivors are left disabled, causing economic losses exceeding $30 billion annually (1).

An ischemic stroke occurs when cerebral blood flow is interrupted by a thrombus that either forms locally in the vessel or embolizes from a distant source, such as a proximal vessel or the heart. Stroke therapies might potentially reduce ischemic injury via 3 general mechanisms. The first and most obvious approach is to rapidly restore blood flow. The only currently approved medical stroke therapy, recombinant tissue plasminogen activator, is a thrombolytic that restores blood flow by recanalizing the occluded vessel (2). Thrombolytic stroke therapies are discussed in Chapter 19. The second approach involves protecting the neurons from injury during ischemia via therapies referred to as *neuroprotective agents*, which target the neurons in the surrounding (penumbra) region of the infarct. By slowing the activity of the neurons at various steps in the ischemic cascade, these agents can improve cell survival in the penumbra. The final approach involves limiting the effects of reperfusion injury. Even with successful blood flow return, several detrimental processes often occur that potentiate ischemic injury, including leukocyte adhesion, free radical release, and neuronal membrane breakdown (3). Various agents designed to target these processes are currently being studied.

In this chapter, we will review the results of clinical trials that tested the second approach—neuroprotective and antireperfusion injury agents in stroke. The mechanisms, safety concerns, and future directions for stroke treatment will also be discussed.

NEUROPROTECTION

Ischemia leads to excessive activation of excitatory amino acid receptors and accumulation of intracellular calcium, which cause cellular injury. Rather than dissolving the thrombus, neuroprotective agents use a variety of mechanisms to attempt to save ischemic neurons in the brain from irreversible injury. These therapies target the neurons in the penumbra region, or rim, of the infarct, which are less likely to be irreversibly injured at early time points than are the neurons in the infarct core. Because they do not directly affect clotting and blood flow, neuroprotective agents are not expected to exhibit the risk of hemorrhage seen with the use of thrombolytic agents.

Despite the completion of multiple clinical trials to investigate neuroprotective agents, no drug has yet been proven to be efficacious in the treatment of acute clinical stroke. In fact, several studies have shown adverse treatment effects. We will review the results of the major neuroprotective trials in clinical stroke, highlighting the factors that could be changed to improve outcome in future studies. Two such factors include modification of drugs in classes associated with prominent side effects, and improvement of patient selection criteria to target those groups that are most likely to respond to individual therapies.

NMDA Antagonists

The most commonly studied neuroprotective agents in human stroke patients are those that prevent the excessive activation of excitatory amino acid receptors. Agents that block the NMDA receptor have held particular interest as therapies for limiting excitatory neurotransmitter release and subsequent cellular injury. Dextrorphan, a noncompetitive NMDA antagonist and phencyclidine-like metabolite of dextromethorphan, was the first NMDA antagonist to be studied in a human stroke treatment trial (4). Dextrorphan caused hallucinations and agitation, as well as more serious hypotension, which limited its use.

Despite their promise as therapeutic agents in animal stroke models, the competitive NMDA ion channel antagonists have also been plagued by side effects. These agents have a similar mechanism of action as have phencyclidine and, not surprisingly, mimic the hallucinations and agitation it causes. A large, randomized trial using the competitive NMDA receptor antagonist selfotel was stopped prematurely due to a trend toward higher mortality within treated patients (5). Investigators also terminated a trial of the NMDA receptor antagonist aptiganel HCl (Cerestat) because of concerns regarding benefit-to-risk ratios (6).

Magnesium is an agent that acts on the NMDA receptor but with a low incidence of side effects. It might reduce ischemic injury by increasing regional blood flow, antagonizing voltage-sensitive calcium channels, and blocking the NMDA receptor. In myocardial infarction and small stroke studies, patients tolerated the drug. A Phase 3 trial that investigated the efficacy of magnesium in stroke [Intravenous (IV) Magnesium Efficacy Study] was completed recently. Patients (2589) were randomized within 12 hr of acute stroke to receive 16 nmol mgSo4 IV over 15 min, then 65 nmol or volume-matched placebo over 24 hr. Unfortunately, mortality was slightly higher in the treatment group, and no difference was seen on any of the primary or secondary outcome measures (7). The ongoing Field Administration of Stroke Therapy—Magnesium (FAST-Mag) stroke trial is assessing the very early (<2 hr) administration of magnesium by paramedics in the field (8).

To avoid the phencyclidine-like effects seen with direct NMDA antagonists, indirect NMDA receptor antagonists that work at the glycine site of the receptor were developed. These agents prevent glycine from being bound, which, in turn, is a required cofactor for glutamate activation of the receptor. Early findings suggested that these agents might have fewer side effects (9,10). A large (1367 patients) efficacy trial with the agent GV150526 was completed in 2000 (GAIN Americas; Glaxo, Inc.). Although the drug was safe and well tolerated, no improvement was seen on any of the 3-month outcome measures (11). No further trials are planned.

Modulation of Non-NMDA Receptors

Nalmefene
Nalmefene is a narcotic NMDA receptor antagonist that reduces the excitatory neurotransmitter release, which contributes to cellular injury in early ischemia. Unlike the NMDA receptor antagonists, this drug causes minimal side effects. Post hoc analyses in early Phase 2 trials suggested that nalmefene (Cervene, Baker Norton) might have greater efficacy in younger patients (<70 years of age) than in older patients (12). However, results of a Phase 3 clinical trial, in which the drug was administered intravenously within 6 hr of symptom onset in patients <70 years, showed no clinical benefit on any of the outcome measures (13). No further trials are planned.

Lubeluzole
The exact mechanism of action of lubeluzole, a drug effective in animal models, is unclear. It might block sodium channels in cells, and it might reduce the release of nitric oxide, a neurotransmitter generated by activation of the NMDA receptor. Post hoc analysis suggested that the drug was beneficial in certain age and stroke severity groups in initial Phase 2 clinical trials. However, a Phase 3 confirmatory trial did not show that lubeluzole was efficacious in this subset of acute stroke patients, and further stroke research with this drug has been abandoned (14), illustrating the danger in placing too much emphasis on subgroups analyses.

Clomethiazole
Clomethiazole, a gamma-aminobutyric acid agonist, decreases excitatory neurotransmission by increasing activity of inhibitory pathways. In Europe, clomethiazole's central nervous system inhibitory properties have been used for anticonvulsant and sedative effects. The potential efficacy of clomethiazole as a neuroprotective agent in ischemia was first investigated in Europe as part of the Clomethiazole Acute Stroke Study (15). Patients received a 24-hr IV infusion of either 75 mg/kg of clomethiazole or placebo within 12 hr of symptom onset. As predicted by its original medicinal uses, the drug's primary side effect was sedation. Overall, clomethiazole

did not show improved functional outcome compared to placebo at 3 months, which was the study's primary endpoint. However, a subgroup of patients with large strokes did show a 37% relative improvement. Patients with these large strokes were classified as having total anterior circulation syndrome (TACS), defined by higher cortical dysfunction, limb weakness, and visual field disturbances. A large (1198 patients) Phase 3 trial to evaluate the efficacy of this agent was then conducted, focusing on patients with large strokes—those with TACS. The results were negative, with 42% of the clomethiazole group and 46% of the placebo group showing a good outcome (16).

Calcium Channel Blockers

As excessive cellular calcium influx contributes to neuronal ischemic injury, calcium channel blockers have been evaluated in acute stroke. Although these agents were not efficacious in the majority of animal trials, numerous clinical studies of calcium channel blockers in acute stroke were conducted using long treatment windows. None of these trials have shown efficacy. The most recent clinical trial, which assessed the usefulness of oral nimodipine given within 6 hr of symptom onset, was terminated early after analysis of the first 439 patients predicted no beneficial effect of the drug (17).

Serotonin Agonist

Serotonin agonists have been shown to hyperpolarize glutaminergic neurons, an event that acts to inhibit glutamate release. Repinotan, or Bay x3702, is a potent 5-hydroxytryptamine 1A agonist that has shown therapeutic benefit in several preclinical stroke models. Safety and tolerability at doses up to 5 mg/day were shown in a 240-patient Phase 3 trial (18). A large Phase 3 trial with 680 patients has just been completed. In this study, a 72-hr infusion of repinotan was started within 4.5 hr of onset, and it was well balanced for baseline variables. In the repinotan treatment group, 127 patients (37%) had a successful recovery (Barthel Index>85), compared with 42% in the placebo group [nonsignificant (NS)] (19), with no safety concerns. No further trials are planned.

Bristol-Myers Squibb (BMS-204352) has a novel mechanism of action. It modulates ion flow across the maxiK channel (a transmembrane potassium channel), an action that might help to restore ion balance and cellular integrity. Two international Phase 3 clinical trials have been completed, both of which assessed the efficacy of the drug in stroke patients who received treatment within 6 hr of symptom onset and who had cortical signs on examination. Efficacy was measured at 90 days using the Barthel Index, modified Rankin Scale (mRS), and NIHSS. Neither trial showed a statistical difference between BMS-204352 and placebo for efficacy, safety, or tolerability (20).

YM-872

YM-872 (Yamanouchi Pharmaceutical Co.) is an α-amino-3-(3-hydroxy-5-methylisoxazole-4-yl)-propanoic acid antagonist. A dose-finding trial with this agent was completed without any safety concerns. A Phase 2 trial has been completed, in which patients were randomized to a 24-hr IV infusion of YM-872 or placebo within 6 hr of symptom onset. Patients with brain stem or cerebellar infarcts were excluded. Magnetic resonance imaging, including diffusion-weighted imaging and perfusion-weighted imaging, was performed prior to the randomization of each patient and again after 1 month. Although no significant safety concerns were noted, no significant treatment benefits were detected (Company press release, Yamanouchi Pharmaceutical).

ONO-2506

A novel neuroprotectant that inhibits astrocyte activation, ONO-2506 (arundic acid), has recently been tested in several large clinical trials and has been shown to prevent delayed infarct expansion in animal models. It appears to inhibit astrocytic overexpression of S100B, to inhibit the expression of inducible nitric oxide synthase, and possibly help to restore the activity of astroglial glutamate transporters post ischemia. Several small Phase 2a acute stroke trials were completed in the United States and Japan that showed that the drug was well tolerated (Investigator's Brochure. Ono Pharmaceuticals, 2004). A 1500-patient Phase 3 trial was recently in progress in North America, with the goal to test two different doses of ONO-2506 or placebo in patients presenting within 6 hr of stroke. Patients had to have "cortical" signs and an NIHSS between 11 and 22. Unfortunately, the study was discontinued after a futility analysis of the first approximately 700 patients suggested that it was very unlikely that any efficacy would be found.

Antioxidants

One final target of neuroprotective therapy in acute ischemic stroke is the generation of free radicals, resulting in further release of calcium and excitatory neurotransmitters. The free radical scavenger tirilazad did not show benefit in an acute stroke trial. The drug also was investigated in subarachnoid hemorrhage and in traumatic brain injury, without convincing evidence of benefit (21).

Another antioxidant with a novel, free radical–trapping mechanism is currently being evaluated in ischemic and hemorrhagic stroke. NXY-059 is the first neuroprotectant to meet the rigorous Stroke Therapy Academic Industry Roundtable (STAIR) preclinical evaluation criteria (22). Safety has been shown in clinical trials that achieve animal study plasma drug levels (23). The results of a Phase 3 NXY-059 trial [SAINT I-Astra Zeneca (a double blind randomized, placebo controlled, parallel group, multicenter Phase IIb/III study to assess the efficacy and safety of intravenous NXY-059 treatment in acute ischemic stroke)] were recently presented (24). The trial randomized 1722 acute stroke patients (<6 hr) to either 72 hr of NXY-059 or placebo. The trial was positive on one of its primary outcome measures, total shift in mRS ($p=0.04$), but not on any of the other outcome measures, including NIHSS and Barthel Index. Considering the percent of patients with good outcomes (mRS 0–2), the drug appears to have a very modest effect: NXY, 45%; placebo, 43%. This 2% absolute improvement rate compares to 13% seen in the National Institute of Neurological Disorders and Stroke recombinant tissue plasminogen activator trial, 15% seen in the Prolyse in Acute Cerebral Thromboembolism Trial (25), and 7% seen in the citicoline studies (discussed below), all of which used similar outcome measures. A second confirmatory Phase 3 ischemic trial (SAINT II) and an intracerebral hemorrhage trial [Cerebral Hemorrhage and NXY-059 Treatment (CHANT)] are currently in progress.

INVESTIGATIONAL AGENTS: REPERFUSION INJURY AGENTS

With the return of blood flow, several detrimental processes can occur to potentiate ischemic injury; these include leukocyte adhesion, free radical release, and neuronal membrane breakdown (3). In addition, the cell membrane itself could breakdown, which produces further free radicals. Various agents that prevent these processes from occurring are currently being studied.

Antileukocyte Adhesion Antibodies

Anti-intracellular Adhesion Molecule-1 (Enlimomab)

Returning blood flow carries white blood cells (leukocytes) to small vessels. In this process, the leukocytes can occlude the vessels and cause additional ischemia. The leukocytes also release toxic products that directly injure endothelial cells and cause the formation of free radicals and cytokines. An agent, such as a monoclonal antibody (mab) to intracellular adhesion molecule-1 (ICAM-1), which inhibits leukocyte adhesion to vessel walls, prevents leukocyte adhesion and infiltration and, in animal models, limits the extent of reperfusion injury (4).

The treatment efficacy of anti-ICAM-1 was assessed in a large, multicentered trial in which more than 600 patients received IV boluses of murine mab to ICAM-1 (enlimomab) or placebo for 5 days, beginning 6 hr or less after symptom onset (26). The study showed a significant treatment effect—unfortunately, an adverse one, revealing higher mortality and worse outcomes in the treated patients. Interestingly, the treatment group showed a marked increase in fevers. Elevated temperatures have previously been found to worsen stroke outcome (27). A viable explanation for the adverse effects seen in the anti-ICAM-1 trial is that the patients who were treated developed an immune response to the murine antibody. Although enlimomab was not clinically useful in the treatment of stroke, it is hoped that its mechanism of action still could have a role in limiting neuronal injury.

Hu23F2G

A Phase 3 trial was conducted using the human antileukocyte antibody Hu23F2G, developed by ICOS Corporation. Because it is a human antibody and not a murine antibody, it was hoped that this agent would avoid the unwanted immune effects of enlimomab. Hu23F2G did not appear to produce the immune response seen with enlimomab. However, no clinical benefit was seen on any of the planned measures (28). No further studies with this agent are planned, although smaller antibodies that target specific leukocyte receptors might still have potential.

Abciximab (Reopro)

Another antiadhesion antibody strategy in stroke therapy targets platelets. By impeding platelet aggregation, antibodies to platelets could have a role in preventing additional ischemic injury during reperfusion, as well as in potentiating thrombolytic action. Such an antiplatelet drug, abciximab (Reopro; Eli Lilly and Company), is currently in clinical stroke treatment trials. This drug is already in use in association with Phase 3 coronary angioplasty and stenting. A 400-patient Phase 2 randomized trial, with treatment started within 6 hr of stroke onset, was recently completed. A trend was observed toward higher symptomatic hemorrhage rates in the Reopro group (4%) versus placebo (1%), $p=0.09$ (29). No significant differences were seen in efficacy outcome measures. A Phase 3 trial is planned.

Growth Factors

Another agent recently studied, Fiblast (Wyeth-Ayerst Research), is a basic fibroblast growth factor that was found to promote neuronal healing after ischemia in animal studies. In a Phase 2 safety trial (Scios, Inc.), Fiblast was administered intravenously for up to 24 hr in acute stroke patients (30). Although it was associated with a transient leukocytosis, the drug was well tolerated and safe. However, a large Phase 3 trial using Fiblast with a 6-hr treatment window (Wyeth-Ayerst Research) was stopped prematurely due to a higher mortality in the treatment group (31). No further studies are planned.

Membrane Stabilization: Citicoline

Citicoline (Interneuron Pharmaceuticals) is an exogenous form of cytidine-5'-diphosphocholine (CDP-choline), used in membrane biosynthesis. Citicoline appears to reduce ischemic injury, both by stabilizing membranes and by decreasing free radical formation. Citicoline is an approved stroke treatment medication in several countries. A Phase 2 United States trial found improved outcome in stroke patients treated with 500 mg of citicoline (32). A Phase 3 trial was then conducted to confirm efficacy. This trial randomized patients in a 2:1 fashion to receive either 500 mg of citicoline ($n=267$) or placebo ($n=127$) orally in capsule form every day for 6 weeks (33). Treatment was started within 24 hr of symptom onset. Overall, no significant differences were seen between the groups on any of the planned assessments of functional outcome at 3 months. Citicoline was well tolerated, with few, if any, side effects. However, a post hoc subgroup analysis did suggest that patients with more severe strokes (NIHSS >8) might have had better functional outcome when treated with citicoline. A second 900-patient Phase 3 trial was then conducted that involved only moderate to large strokes. Unfortunately, the company chose a novel endpoint (NIHSS score improvement ≥points), and the trial was negative. Had they used more conventional endpoints (NIHSS=0 or 1, mRS=0 or 1, etc.), the trial would have been positive (34). A meta-analysis of all US citicoline trials was performed. For the 1372 patients treated within 24 hr, with NIHSS≥8, the chance of excellent recovery (global outcome measure) at 3 months was 27.2%, citicoline, versus 20.2%, placebo ($p<0.001$) (35), a 7% absolute and 35% relative improvement over placebo.

No further trials are planned, which is unfortunate, as it appears to have a modest benefit and no side effects. Interestingly, CDP-choline is available as a supplement (Jarrow Formulas, Inc.), available through the Internet. The cost is approximately $40 per month for a suggested 1000 mg/day dose.

CONCLUSION

The recent history of neuroprotective clinical trials in stroke reveals multiple agents that demonstrated efficacy in preclinical studies failed to achieve expected results in clinical trials. Although the exact reasons for this are unknown, possibilities include: longer time window in clinical trials than in animal studies, lower tolerated drug levels, a more heterogeneous variety of strokes compared to "pure" middle cerebral artery (MCA) stroke animal studies, the majority of clinical strokes involving "permanent" ischemia compared to transient reperfusion MCA filament animal studies, insensitive clinical endpoints, and inadequately powered studies. In an effort to improve the ability of preclinical trials to predict clinical success, a more rigorous preclinical evaluation program is advocated (STAIR criteria). Development of neuroprotective agents unhampered by side effects might involve modifications in structure to improve benefit-to-risk ratios and allow for improved central nervous system levels. Currently, the most promising area involves anti–free radical agents, and it is hoped that the results of the SAINT II trial will confirm the efficacy seen in SAINT I. Finally, novel agents that have not yet completed clinical trials hold the promise of potential efficacy in such areas as targeting gene and protein expression following stroke.

In the future, optimal therapy might be achieved by combining neuroprotective agents with reperfusion mechanisms to produce additive benefits. Alternatively, they might be used prior to recombinant tissue plasminogen activator therapy in an effort to "slow the brain down," so the time window for thrombolysis can be extended. Because these drugs will most likely not display adverse effects in those patients with hemorrhagic stroke, ambulance crews could begin administering this "stroke cocktail."

REFERENCES

1. American College of Physicians and the Investigators of the PORT Study, 1994. Guidelines for medical treatment for stroke prevention. Ann Intern Med 1994; 121:54–44.
2. The National Institute of Neurological Disorders and Stroke rt-PA Stroke Study Group. Tissue plasminogen activator for acute ischemic stroke. N Engl J Med 1995; 333:1581–1587.
3. Hallenbeck J, Dutka A. Background review and current concepts of reperfusion injury. Arch Neurol 1990; 47:1245–1254.
4. Clark W, Madden K, Rothlein R, et al. Reduction of central nervous system ischemic injury by monoclonal antibody to intercellular adhesion molecule. J Neurosurg 1991; 75:623–627.
5. Albers G, Atkinson R, Kelley R, et al. Safety, tolerability, and pharmacokinetics of the N-methyl-D-aspartate antagonist dextrorphan in patients with an acute stroke. Stroke 1995; 26:254–258.
6. Davis SM, Albers G, Diener H, et al. Termination of acute stroke studies involving selfotel treatment. Lancet 1997; 349:32.
7. The Intravenous magnesium Efficacy in Stroke Trial Investigators. Magnesium for acute stroke: randomized controlled trial. Lancet 2004; 363:439–445.
8. Saver J. The field administration of stroke therapy—magnesium phase III trial. Ongoing clinical trials abstracts. International Joint Conference on Stroke and Cerebral Circulation, Feb 4, 2005.
9. Lesko L for Boehringer Ingelheim Pharmaceuticals, Inc., and the Cerestat Stroke Study Group. A pivotal phase III efficacy and safety study of Cerestat (apotiganel HCl/CNS 1102) in acute stroke patients: 1996 update. Presented at the 22nd International Joint Conference on Stroke and Cerebral Circulation, Anaheim, CA, Feb 8, 1997.
10. Albers G, Clark W, Atkinson R, et al. Dose escalation study of the NMDA glycine-site antagonist ACEA 1021 in acute ischemic stroke. Presented at the 22nd International Joint Conference on Stroke and Cerebral Circulation, Anaheim, CA, Feb 8, 1997.
11. Sacco R, DeRosa J, Haley E, et al. Glycine antagonist in neuroprotection for patients with acute stroke: GAIN Americas: a randomized controlled trial. JAMA 2001; 285(13):1760–1761.
12. Clark W, Ertag W, Orecchio E, et al. Cervene in acute ischemic stroke: results of a double-blind, placebo-controlled, dose-comparison study. J Stroke Cerebrovasc Dis 1999; 8:224–230.
13. Clark W, Raps E, Tong D, et al. Cervene in acute ischemic stroke. Final results of a phase III efficacy study. Stroke 2000; 31:1234–1239.
14. Hantson L, Wessel T. Therapeutic benefits of lubeluzole in ischemic stroke. Presented at the 23rd International Joint Conference on Stroke and Cerebral Circulation, 1998.
15. Wahlgren N. The clomethiazole acute stroke study (CLASS): efficacy results in a subgroup of 545 patients with total anterior circulation syndrome. Presented at the 23rd International Joint Conference on Stroke and Cerebral Circulation, Orlando, FL, Feb 7, 1998.
16. Lyden P, Shuaib A, Ng K, et al. Clomethiazole Acute Stroke Study in ischemic stroke (CLASS-I): final results. Stroke 2002; 33(1):122–128.
17. Horn J, Haan R, Vermeulen M. VENUS—very early nimodipine use in stroke: preliminary trial results. 24th American Heart Association International Conference on Stroke and Cerebral Circulation, Nashville, TN, 1999.
18. Teal P, Rombout F, Rodriquez M, et al. Repinotan in acute ischemic stroke: a randomized exposure controlled trial. Presented at the 26th International Stroke Conference, San Antonio, TX, Feb 2001.

19. Teal P, Lyden P, Kaste M, et al. Effects of Repinotan in patients with acute ischemic stroke. (mRECT). Presented at 14th European Stroke Conference, Bologna, Italy, May 2005.
20. From the quarterly conference calls. MaxiPost-mortem. FDC Reports Pink Sheet 2001; 63(18):22.
21. STIP AS investigators. Safety study of tirilazad mesylate in patients with acute ischemic stroke (STIPAS). Stroke 1994; 25(2):418–423.
22. Stroke Therapy Academic Industry Roundtable. Recommendations for standards regarding preclinical neuroprotective drug development. Stroke 1999; 30:2752–2758.
23. Lees K, Sharma A, Barer D, et al. Tolerability and pharmacokinetics of the Nitrone NXY-059 in patient with acute stroke. Stroke 2001; 32:675–680.
24. Lees K, Zivin J, Davalos A, et al. Preliminary results of SAINT I. Presented at the European Stroke Conference, May 2005.
25. Furlan A, Higashida R, Wechsler L, et al. PROACT II: a randomized trial of intra-arterial prourokinase for acute ischemic stroke of less than 6 hour duration due to middle cerebral artery occlusion. JAMA 1999; 282:2003–2011.
26. The Enlimomab Trial Investigators. Use of anti-CAM-1 therapy in ischemic stroke: results of the Enlimomab acute stroke trial. Neurology 2001; 57:1428–1434.
27. Ginberg MD, Busto R. Combating hyperthermia in acute stroke: a significant clinical concern. Stroke 1998; 29:529–534.
28. Becher K. Anti-leukocyte antibodies: LeukArrest (Hu23F2G) and Enlimomab (R6.5) in acute stroke. Curr Med Res Opin 2002; 18 (suppl 2):s18–s22.
29. Abciximab Emergent Stroke Treatment Trial (AbESTT) Investigators. Emergency administration of abciximab for treatment of patients with acute ischemic stroke: results of a randomized phase 2 trial. Stroke 2005; 36(4):880–890.
30. The Fiblast Safety Study Group. Clinical safety trial of intravenous basic fibroblast growth factor (bFGF, Fiblast) in acute stroke. Presented at the 23rd International Joint Conference on Stroke and Cerebral Circulation, Orlando, FL, Feb 7, 1998.
31. Clark W, Schim J, Kasner S, Victor S. Trafermin in acute ischemic stroke: results of a phase II/III randomized efficacy study. Neurology 2000; 54:A88.
32. Clark W, Warach S, Pettigrew L, et al. A randomized dose response trial of citcoline in acute ischemic stroke patients. Neurology 1997; 49:671–678.
33. Clark W, Williams B, Selzer K, et al. For the Citicoline Stroke Study Group. A randomized efficacy trial of citicoline in acute ischemic stroke patients. Stroke 1999; 30:2592–2597.
34. Clark W, Wechsler L, Sabounjian L, Schwiderski U. A phase III randomized efficacy trial of 2000 mg Citicoline in acute ischemic stroke patients. Neurology 2001; 57:1595–1602.
35. Davalos A, Castillo J, Sabin J, Clark W. Oral citicoline in acute ischemic stroke. Stroke 2002; 33:2850–2866.

22 | Prognosis and Outcomes Following Ischemic Stroke

L. Creed Pettigrew, MD, MPH, Professor[a], Director[b]

[a] *Department of Neurology,* [b] *University of Kentucky Stroke Program,*
University of Kentucky Chandler Medical Center, Lexington, Kentucky, USA

INTRODUCTION

Stroke can be defined as any physical disorder that alters global or regional blood flow to the brain that results in hemorrhage, infarction, vasospasm, or inflammation. It remains the third most common cause of adult mortality in the United States, accounting for 1 of every 15 deaths from any cause (~273,000 stroke-related deaths) or 17% of all cardiovascular deaths in 2003 (1). Every year, as many as 730,000 new cases of stroke occur in the American population (2). With nearly 4.5 million surviving victims, stroke is the most frequently encountered source of long-term disability in our society. Estimates of the national cost of this disease vary depending on the reference, but most authorities agree that at least $50 billion are spent annually to cover all expenses associated with the care of stroke victims (1,3). The average direct cost per case, including all illness-related expenses, is approximately $50,000 (4). In 2006, the total lifetime cost of an ischemic stroke is estimated to be $140,048 per person, as calculated in 1999 (1).

This chapter will review outcome in ischemic stroke by focusing on prognosticative medical risk factors and identification of abnormal features on CT and MRI that predict clinical severity of neurological deficit. Thrombolytic treatments, such as systemic administration of recombinant tissue plasminogen activator (rtPA), have had not only the most favorable impact on stroke outcome but also carry the greatest risk of intracerebral hemorrhage (ICH). To achieve a balanced view of benefit versus risk in thrombolytic treatment of acute stroke, recent clinical trials of intravenous or intra-arterial thrombolysis will be reviewed, with special attention to clinical or radiographic risk factors that predicted outcome in each study.

MEDICAL RISK FACTORS FOR PROGRESSING STROKE

The terms *progressing stroke, evolving stroke, stroke in evolution,* and *stroke in progression* have all been used to define worsening of neurologic function within the first 24 hr after stroke onset. However, observed deterioration of neurologic function is not synonymous with progression of ischemia or expanding tissue necrosis in brain, because worsening deficit might occur as a result of systemic causes not directly related to the progression of the cerebral ischemic injury. Neither the temporal profile nor the qualitative and quantitative changes in neurologic function of progressing stroke have been standardized. Previous studies have shown that at least half of all cases of ischemic stroke progression occur within 24 hr of symptom onset and 90% occur within 3 days (5). Among systemic factors, elevated serum glucose (6,7), high body temperature (8,9), elevated fibrinogen levels in plasma (9), and high (6) and low (10) systolic blood pressure have been related to stroke progression. All of these factors (except for iatrogenically induced hypotension) might occur during the first 8 to 12 hr after the onset of thromboembolic stroke, as part of an acute phase response. Cardiovascular disorders that exist concomitantly in the acute stroke patient might also contribute to early neurological deterioration. Preexisting diabetes and coronary artery disease (CAD) predict early (within 24–36 hr), but not late, stroke progression (10,11). Diabetic microangiopathy that leads to chronic impairment of cerebral autoregulation in preexisting diabetes and poor collateral blood supply due to extra- or intracranial atherosclerotic disease in CAD have been proposed as likely mechanisms of neurologic progression during the first hours of ischemia (11). In comparison, older age and severity of neurologic deficit on admission have been recognized as independent predictors of delayed, but not early, stroke progression, due to anticipated comorbidities in elderly individuals (10,11).

RADIOGRAPHIC INDICATORS OF PROGRESSING STROKE

CT and MRI performed early during the evaluation of the stroke patient have become useful in the identification of risk factors for progressing stroke. In a series of 152 consecutive patients with acute ischemic stroke who were hospitalized within 5 hr of stroke onset, extended focal hypodensity on CT involving cortical or corticosubcortical areas increased the risk of neurologic worsening by a factor of 8.9 and predicted subsequent deterioration with a probability of 60% (7). The same relationship was found between early (<8 hr) CT findings of brain infarction, ischemic edema, and mass effect, which predicted the risk of progressing stroke in a prospective study of 128 subjects (9). In this study, early signs of infarction on CT were observed in 81% of progressing stroke, but in only 49% of nonprogressing stroke, correlating with the appearance of mass effect in 26% and 2.4%, respectively ($p<0.001$). Analysis of the CT images obtained from patients enrolled in the first European Cooperative Acute Stroke Study (ECASS; see below) confirmed several radiographic features that are now accepted as hallmark indicators of early neurologic deterioration. Early CT focal hypodensity [odds ratio (OR): 1.9; 95% confidence interval (CI): 1.3–2.9] and hyperdensity of the middle cerebral artery (HMCA) sign (OR: 1.8; 95% CI: 1.1–3.1) were independent prognostic factors for early progressing stroke (within 24 hr of onset), whereas brain swelling at the initial CT, obtained within 6 hr of onset, predicted delayed progression (between 24 hr and 7 days) (11). Figure 1 shows representative

(A)   **(B)**

(C)   **(D)**

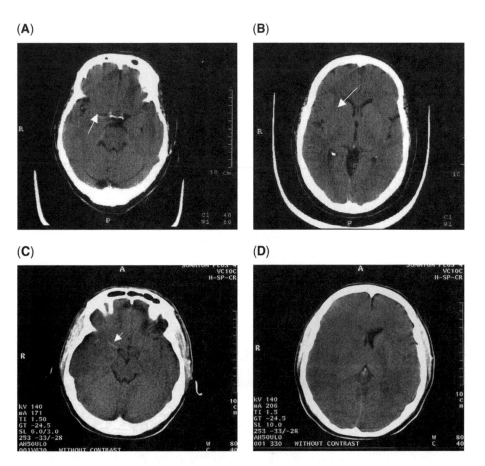

Figure 1   Computed tomography (CT) of acute cerebral infarction. (**A**) and (**B**) were selected from a CT scan performed 90 min after the acute onset of left hemiplegia in a 52-year-old woman. The arrow in (**A**) identifies fresh thrombus lodged in the right middle cerebral artery [hyperdense middle cerebral artery (MCA) sign]. In (**B**), the arrow indicates subtle hypodensity affecting the right lenticular nuclei and blurring of the adjacent insular ribbon. (**C**) and (**D**) were selected from a CT scan performed 7 hr after the onset of left hemiplegia in a 48-year-old man. The arrow in (**C**) again indicates the hyperdense MCA sign. Note large hypodensity representing acute infarction within the vascular territory of the right MCA in (**C**) and (**D**); the sulcal indentations in the right frontotemporal region have been obliterated by gyral edema and the anatomical landmarks defining the right basal ganglia have been obscured.

examples of early focal hypodensity, HMCA, and brain swelling. The association between early hypodensity, HMCA sign, and progressing stroke is in agreement with angiographic and ultrasonographic studies that show that MCA occlusion with little or no collateral blood supply is responsible for the early development of intracellular edema and stroke progression (7,12).

MRI includes a variety of techniques that can be employed to predict outcome of progressing stroke and are described in detail in Chapter 18. Diffusion-weighted imaging (DWI) permits the *in vivo* measurement of the translational mobility of water in tissue and was first reported as a marker of acute ischemic brain injury in 1990 (13,14). The image intensity on DWI is dependent on the apparent diffusion coefficient (ADC), measuring the mobility of water molecules in tissue and the transverse relaxation time (T2) that might represent prior distortion of tissue architecture ("T2 shine-through"). In ischemic brain tissue, ADC values decline, leading to a region of hyperintensity on a gray-scale derived image. The ADC probably reflects the accumulation of intracellular water (cytotoxic edema) caused by disruption of energy metabolism and loss of ion homeostasis (15). These ADC changes do not occur uniformly throughout the ischemic lesion. Serial studies performed in experimental stroke models show that the most severe perfusion deficit has the earliest and correspondingly most severe drop in ADC value (16). Reversal of initial ADC changes after early reperfusion does not necessarily predict tissue salvage. In rats that were subjected to focal cerebral ischemia and reperfused up to 30 min afterward, ADC values completely reverted to normal within 90 min, but histopathology examination 3 days later demonstrated heterogeneous cell injury directly related to the severity of the initial decline in cerebral blood flow (17).

In clinical imaging of ischemic stroke, DWI will indicate the volume of injured brain within as early as 1 hr after the onset of perfusion arrest (Fig. 2). Several studies are being conducted to assess the relationships between MR-derived lesion volumes and clinical measures of outcome at acute and chronic time points to determine the efficacy of establishing MRI as a surrogate marker of injury severity. In one of the first studies evaluating DWI and a companion technique, perfusion-weighted imaging (PWI), as predictors of stroke outcome, DWI or PWI lesion volumes obtained within 6.5 hr of ischemic stroke onset were correlated to performance on the NIHSS at 24 hr (18). A high correlation was noted between 24-hr NIHSS score and lesion volumes as determined by PWI (Pearson's $r = 0.96$; $p < 0.001$) or DWI ($r = 0.67$; $p = 0.03$). Furthermore, a similar high correlation was noted between lesion size on routine T2-weighted (T2W) imaging and initial DWI and PWI size ($r = 0.99$; $p < 0.00001$). Serial DWI and PWI were performed within 24 hr, subacutely within 5 days, and after a delay of 84 days in 18 patients with acute ischemic stroke (19). Acute PWI lesion volumes correlated with acute neurologic state, clinical outcome, and final infarct volume on T2W. Serial MRIs/DWIs were performed on 50 patients

(A)   **(B)**

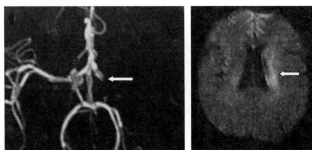

(C)

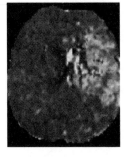

Figure 2 Magnetic resonance (MR) imaging of acute cerebral infarction. **(A)** A selected view from a three-dimensional, time-of-flight MR angiogram performed 2 hr after the onset of acute left cerebral infarction. The arrow indicates the location of an embolus occluding the left middle cerebral artery. **(B)** A diffusion-weighted image obtained on the same subject and at the same time as the MR angiogram in **(A)**. The arrow indicates a well-defined area of restricted diffusion representing the developing core of the infarct. **(C)** A mean transit-time map obtained after bolus administration of gadolinium contrast to define a perfusion-imaging deficit. The large, wedge-shaped area of lighter gray coloration represents hypoperfused brain tissue. Subtracting the smaller area of restricted diffusion in **(A)** from the much larger area of hypoperfusion shown in **(B)** will derive the perfusion–diffusion mismatch.

with ischemic stroke in the MCA territory, beginning within 24 hr after symptom onset and repeated at a median interval of 7.5 weeks (20). Acute DWI lesion volumes correlated with NIHSS ($r=0.56$), Barthel index ($r=-0.60$), and chronic lesion volumes ($r=0.80$). Considered in aggregate, these studies support the conclusion that DWI lesion volumes predict the eventual severity of ischemic brain injury, thereby defining the potential for DWI as a surrogate marker of clinical efficacy in experimental studies that test new stroke treatments.

The combination of DWI and PWI is necessary for MRI to be fully predictive of injury progression after acute ischemic stroke. The need to assess perfusion–diffusion "mismatch" is driven by a dynamic balance between zones of ischemic tissue in brain that are at different levels of metabolic function, as affected by regional heterogeneity of blood flow (Fig. 2). Tissue within the developing infarct core that is subject to severe perfusion deficits ($\leq 15 \, mL/100 \, g$ brain/ min) that lead to failure of Na^+/K^+-ATPase ion pumps in the neuronal plasma membrane are encompassed within early DWI lesion volumes. However, tissue within the peri-infarct zone, which includes the ischemic penumbra, has perfusion at intermediate levels ($15–25 \, mL/100 \, g$ brain/min) that produces transient metabolic arrest in neurons, thereby causing a neurologic deficit that could be reversed with timely reperfusion. The resulting volume of hypoperfused, but potentially salvageable, tissue that surrounds the developing infarct core is described as the perfusion–diffusion mismatch, a functional definition of "tissue-at-risk" for conversion to infarct. Baird et al. (21) were among the first to suggest the potential value of the perfusion–diffusion mismatch as an indicator of stroke outcome in 13 patients who underwent DWI/PWI within the acute to subacute phase of cerebral infarction (2–53 hr after symptom onset) and after prolonged survival for up to 725 days later. These investigators found that eventual lesion volume increased by $230\pm95\%$ when the initial PWI volume was greater than the DWI volume but decreased by $47\pm8\%$ when the PWI volume was smaller than, or equivalent to, the DWI volume. Several confirmatory studies that show the perfusion–diffusion mismatch as a predictor of tissue at risk for stroke progression have been published (18,19,22–24). Recently, attempts have been made to define tissue viability thresholds, as quantified by cerebral blood volume or mean transit time of a blood flow tracer moving through the ischemic region, to predict rate of growth of the DWI lesion to fill the original "mismatch" volume (25,26), although this approach has yet to be confirmed in a prospective study that incorporates voxel-based, serial imaging. In another variant of multimodal prediction of stroke lesion progression, a "clinical-DWI mismatch" (CDM) has been described that incorporates quantification of neurologic deficit by standardized physical examination with DWI (NIHSS ≥ 8 and ischemic volume $\leq 25 \, mL$ on DWI) (27). These investigators found that patients with CDM were at greater risk for early neurological deterioration, defined as an increase in NIHSS ≥ 4 points between acute (≤ 12 hr) and subacute (72 ± 12 hr) examination times, although again, this concept awaits validation in a prospective study that incorporates a large number of subjects.

THROMBOLYSIS, RISK OF HEMORRHAGE, AND MODIFICATION OF OUTCOME IN ACUTE ISCHEMIC STROKE

The most important advance that has emerged from the last 25 years of clinical research in stroke is cerebral reperfusion therapy by intravenous or intra-arterial thrombolysis. Although this important topic is covered extensively in Chapter 19, the present review will consider how long-term outcome has been affected by major thrombolysis trials to determine the resilience of this treatment.

European Cooperative Acute Stroke Study I
The first major trial to suggest potential efficacy of the systemically administered thrombolytic drug, rtPA, in acute ischemic stroke was the ECASS (28). Designated as ECASS I, this placebo-controlled, randomized, prospective trial was designed to test the efficacy and safety of 1.1 mg/kg rtPA given intravenously in acute ischemic stroke. All patients were enrolled within 6 hr of symptom onset at 75 centers distributed among 14 countries. Cerebral angiography was not required for randomization or confirmation of arterial occlusion. Patients could not be treated with full-dose intravenous heparin or antiplatelet agents during the first 24 hr after randomization, but use of low-dose subcutaneous heparin was permitted to prevent deep-vein thrombosis and pulmonary thromboembolism.

The ECASS I investigators enrolled 620 subjects, but only 511 remained eligible for statistical analysis after exclusion of protocol violations. The rate of symptomatic ICH was higher in the treated patients (19.8% vs. 6.5% in the placebo group), but no significant difference was observed in the mortality rate at 1 month. Intent-to-treat analysis of data from all 620 patients showed no difference in outcome between the treatment and placebo groups. After 109 patients were excluded because of protocol violations pertaining to misinterpreted CT scans or entry criteria, the treatment group showed an absolute increase of 11.7% in the number of patients with favorable modified Rankin Scale (mRS) measured at 90 days.

Although the intent-to-treat analysis of the ECASS I trial was negative, *post hoc* evaluation of the results of this study yielded many important observations on the impact of systemic thrombolysis on stroke outcome. By the ECASS study protocol, a baseline CT was required at randomization and was repeated between 24 and 36 hr and again between days 4 and 10. In 1999, subtypes of hemorrhagic infarction (HI) or parenchymal hemorrhage (PH) on CT performed at the scheduled follow-up intervals were analyzed to determine which predicted early neurological deterioration, death, or severe disability among survivors at 3 months (29). By adapting previously established criteria (30) to the ECASS I protocol, HI was defined as a petechial infarction without space-occupying effect, and PH was described as a confluent hemorrhage with mass effect. The designation of HI was further subdivided into 2 types by severity of petechial transformation, and PH was subclassified into (i) ≤ 30% infarcted volume, with mild space-occupying effect (PH1) and (ii) greater 30% infarct volume with significant space-occupying effect or hemorrhage remote from the infarcted area (PH2). Although PH2 lesions were significantly more frequent in the rtPA-treated group, rtPA or placebo allocation had no statistically significant effect on the relationship between subtype of hemorrhagic transformation and clinical evolution. ORs calculated on the pooled active and placebo treatment groups, after adjustment for age of patient and extent of ischemic injury on baseline CT (none, lesser than 33%, or greater than 33% of MCA territory), showed that PH2 lesions on 24-hour post-treatment CTs had strongly increased risk of 24-hr deterioration (OR: 32.3; 95% CI: 13.4–77.7) and of death at 3 months (OR: 18.0; 95% CI: 8.05–40.1). In contrast to the outcomes of other subtypes of bleeding, PH2 significantly increased the risk of early deterioration and death, even after adjustment for possible confounders, thereby validating the clinical presumption that only large, confluent hematomas that cause local mass effect that influences survival after thrombolytic therapy.

Another *post hoc* analysis of the ECASS I database was conducted to focus on predictors of early or late neurologic deterioration in acute ischemic stroke (11). In ECASS I, stroke severity was determined by the Scandinavian Stroke Scale (SSS) (31), which consists of seven domains used to describe consciousness, speech, motor performance, and gait, and was assessed at baseline and periodically up to 7 days after randomization. Early (randomization to 24 hr) and late (postrandomization from 24 hr to 7 days) progressing stroke was defined by advanced impairment of speech or loss of consciousness or motor capacity by prespecified intervals on the SSS. Of 615 patients enrolled in ECASS I with data sets usable for this *post hoc* analysis, 231 (37.5%) worsened during the first 24 hr: 112 in the placebo group (37%) and 119 in the rtPA-treated group (38%; p=NS). After controlling for baseline risk factors, logistical regression modeling applied to the pooled treatment and placebo groups demonstrated that size of infarct involving greater than 33% of the MCA territory (OR: 2.5; 95% CI: 1.6–4.0; p<0.001) and brain swelling (OR: 1.8; 95% CI: 1.1–3.2; p=0.023) seen on baseline CT were the only factors independently associated with early progressing stroke. Late progressing stroke was predicted by older age, low SSS score, and brain swelling on CT at baseline. In controlled logistical regression modeling applied to the pooled groups, hyperdense MCA sign (OR: 3.0; 95% CI: 1.3–6.6), all types of hemorrhagic transformation (OR: 1.8; 95% CI: 1.1–3.0), low SSS score at baseline (OR: 0.98; 95% CI: 0.96–0.99), and no treatment with intravenous heparin during the first week after stroke (OR: 0.55; 95% CI: 0.3–0.96) were factors that independently predicted late progressing stroke. It is noteworthy that brain edema was the most consistently identified risk factor for both early and late progressing stroke in ECASS I, underscoring its development within the first 5 days in patients with large infarctions exceeding 33% of the MCA territory.

National Institute of Neurological Disorders and Stroke Stroke Study
The National Institute of Neurological Disorders and Stroke (NINDS) rtPA Stroke Study Group published its historic findings in December of 1995, <1 year after the ECASS report. The

NINDS investigators had also published 2 open-label, dose-escalation studies that showed doses of <0.95 mg/kg of rtPA could be administered in relative safety and resulted in early neurologic improvement (32,33). Based upon the encouraging results of these open-label studies, the NINDS group proceeded with a randomized, double-blinded, placebo-controlled, prospective trial that was conducted in 2 parts. Part 1 assessed changes in neurologic deficits 24 hr after the onset of stroke. Part 2 was conducted as a pivotal efficacy trial to determine whether treatment with rtPA resulted in sustained clinical benefit at three months. To prevent bias, the investigators remained unaware of the results of Part 1 until Part 2 had been completed. The primary hypothesis for Part 2 was that there would be a "consistent and persuasive difference between the rtPA and placebo groups in terms of the proportion of patients who recovered with minimal or no deficit 3 months after treatment." Each patient was treated intravenously with placebo or rtPA in a dose of 0.9 mg/kg, 10% of which was given as a bolus, followed by delivery of the remaining 90% as a constant infusion over 60 min. It was required that all patients be enrolled and treated within 3 hr of the onset of symptoms. To detect intracranial hemorrhage, CT scans were performed at 24 hr, between 7 and 10 days after the onset of stroke, and if neurologic deterioration occurred at any time after treatment. Four outcome measures, including the Barthel index, the mRS, the Glasgow outcome scale, and the NIHSS, were fashioned into a global test statistic applied to the primary hypothesis of Part 2.

Eight centers in the United States enrolled 624 patients in the NINDS study between 1991 and 1994. In Part 1, no difference was observed between the treatment and placebo groups in the primary outcome measure completed at 24 hr (NIHSS improvement by at least 4 points or complete resolution of neurological deficit). In Part 2, the number of patients with favorable scores on each of the 4 outcome measures after 3 months was higher in the treatment group than in the placebo arm. As evaluated by the global test statistic, the OR for a favorable outcome with administration of rtPA was 1.7 (95% CI, 1.2–2.6; $p=0.008$), 30% higher than would be seen in placebo-treated patients. As compared with the placebo group, a 12% absolute increase was noted in the number of patients with Barthel scores of 95 or 100 in the rtPA group. Additionally, an 11% absolute increase was seen in the number of treated patients with an NIHSS of 0 or 1. Similar results that demonstrated the benefit of active treatment were seen with the mRS and Glasgow outcome scales. These beneficial effects were so robust that they occurred despite stratification of the patients according to age, stroke subtype or severity, and presymptomatic use of aspirin. Furthermore, the NINDS investigators published follow-up data that showed that the 30% greater likelihood of favorable outcome noted 3 months after treatment persisted to 6 and 12 months (34). They also conducted a cost-benefit analysis that demonstrated net savings in treatment cost and improved quality of life for patients treated with rtPA (35).

Although patients treated with rtPA fared better than those given placebo, no significant difference in mortality between the 2 groups at 3, 6, or 12 months was reported (34,36) Symptomatic ICH occurred during the first 36 hr in 6.4% of the rtPA-treated patients, compared to only 0.6% of patients in the placebo arm ($p<0.001$). Of the 20 symptomatic hemorrhages that developed in the rtPA patients during the first 36 hr, 9 were fatal. Minor external bleeding during the first 10 days was also more common with rtPA than with placebo (23% vs. 3%). Greater severity of the initial neurologi deficit and evidence of edema or mass effect on the baseline CT scan were associated with higher risk of symptomatic ICH in patients treated with rtPA (37). Considering the added burden of mortality and long-term morbidity associated with the ICH that affected patients given rtPA, it is all the more remarkable that this treatment remained significantly effective over placebo up to 12 months later. After Food and Drug Administration (FDA) approval of rtPA in 1996, the Stroke Council of the American Heart Association (AHA) and the American Academy of Neurology (AAN) issued practice guidelines formally adapting its use in acute ischemic stroke (38,39).

Adherence to the guidelines for thrombolytic therapy is mandatory, as shown by a report on community use of rtPA at hospitals in the Cleveland, Ohio, area. An in-hospital mortality rate of 15.7% and ICH occurrence of 22% was found in 70 patients treated with rtPA (40). These authors found deviations from the national guidelines in 50% of cases, including use of antithrombotic drugs within 24 hr of rtPA administration in 37.1% and treatment beyond 3 hr in 12.9%. Hemorrhage and mortality rates approximate those observed with the NINDS rtPA Stroke Study when the drug is used by well-trained stroke therapists following the guidelines written in the AHA and AAN statements (41,42).

European Cooperative Acute Stroke Study II

In the wake of the NINDS rtPA Stroke Study, ECASS II was undertaken to determine if rtPA could be effective even when administered more than 3 hr after the onset of stroke symptoms. ECASS II is the largest randomized trial of thrombolytic therapy that has been conducted in acute stroke to date, enrolling 800 patients in 108 centers throughout Europe, Australia, and New Zealand, randomly assigning them to rtPA, using the NINDS Stroke Study dosing regimen versus placebo (43). To prevent the large number of protocol violations observed in ECASS I, the steering committee for ECASS II undertook more rigorous training of investigators to improve interpretation of CT scans and treat hypertension appropriately. The primary endpoint was a favorable outcome on the mRS, using the dichotomized method of analysis employed in the NINDS study. Only 158 (19.8%) of the 800 patients were enrolled, randomized, and treated within 3 hr of stroke symptom onset. A favorable outcome of no more than 1 point on the mRS was seen in 40.3% of patients in the rtPA group and 36.6% in the placebo group, but this was not statistically significant. *Post hoc* analysis based on a dichotomized mRS that represented physical independence (0–2) uncovered a statistically significant benefit to treatment with rtPA, with 54.3% of treated patients returning to independence, compared to 46% of placebo patients ($p=0.024$). Symptomatic ICH occurred more frequently in the rtPA-treated group (8.8%), compared to 3.4% in the placebo group, but no difference in mortality at 30 or 90 days was observed. The ECASS investigators concluded that their data failed to support the use of rtPA beyond 3 hr.

As in ECASS I and the NINDS rtPA Stroke Study, risk factors for hemorrhagic transformation of infarct were identified in *post hoc* analysis of the ECASS II data set. In ECASS I, screening for risk factors associated with postthrombolytic hemorrhage was focused on radiographic criteria for ICH. In the NINDS study, hemorrhagic transformation was classified into symptomatic or asymptomatic hemorrhage, regardless of appearance on CT. In ECASS II, as in ECASS I, analysis of risk factors for ICH relied on categorization of HI and PH, but investigators surveyed clinical criteria to address symptomatic expression of ICH (SICH). Similar to ECASS I, the study protocol in ECASS II required a baseline CT scan to determine eligibility, a second CT at 22 to 36 hr, and a third scan on day 7 postrandomization. Review of post-thrombolytic brain hemorrhage in ECASS II showed that HIs occurred in 283 (35.7%), PHs in 60 (7.6%), and SICHs in 49 (6.2%) of the aggregated sample (44). HIs were no more frequent in the rtPA group than in the placebo group, as in ECASS I, whereas PHs and SICHs were associated with active thrombolysis. Logistic regression analyses showed significant interactions for poor outcome—defined as mRS 5 (severely disabled and dependent on nursing care) or 6 (death)—between rtPA exposure and PH (OR: 4.8; 95% CI: 1.2–24.7) and between rtPA use and SICH (OR: 6.9; 95% CI: 1.8–30.3), suggesting that both categories of hemorrhagic transformation were not only more common but were also more severe in rtPA-treated patients. Significant risk factors for PH were exposure to rtPA, extent of parenchymal hypoattenuation on baseline CT scan, history of congestive heart failure, increased age, and baseline systolic blood pressure. However, logistic regression analysis showed that interactions between rtPA exposure and any of the remaining factors were significant only for increased age and prior aspirin exposure, suggesting that PHs that resulted from rtPA use in ECASS II were more frequent in older patients and in those who used aspirin before stroke. Significant risk factors for SICH included exposure to rtPA, history of congestive heart failure, extent of parenchymal hypoattenuation on baseline CT, and increased age, with no interaction detected on subsequent regression analysis. This secondary analysis of hemorrhagic risk in ECASS II confirmed the importance of the volume of hypoattenuated brain seen on baseline CT as a risk factor for serious ICH and suggested, but could not confirm, that older patients and those with prior use of aspirin are at higher risk. As with the hemorrhagic risk factors identified in the ECASS I and NINDS rtPA Stroke Studies, these variables would have to be confirmed in independent trials before they could be applied to risk stratification for rtPA use in daily practice.

Alteplase Thrombolysis for Acute Noninterventional Therapy in Ischemic Stroke

The second attempt to extend the time window of rtPA administration was the Alteplase Thrombolysis for Acute Noninterventional Therapy in Ischemic Stroke (ATLANTIS) study (45). Like ECASS II, ATLANTIS was originally designed to show if the benefits of systemic thrombolysis could extend up to 6 hr. After the publication of the NINDS study in 1995, the time window for enrollment was changed to encompass 3 to 5 hr. The primary endpoint for the modified study was good outcome, defined as an NIHSS score of 0 or 1 at 90 days. After 761 patients had been enrolled in ATLANTIS, the trial was terminated prematurely because of projected lack of benefit with active treatment. Again, no difference in mortality was observed between the 2 treatment groups, suggesting that "delayed" administration of rtPA was safe. The ATLANTIS investigators followed the precedent observed in ECASS II by concluding that the use of rtPA for acute ischemic stroke should not be undertaken after 3 hr.

Intra-arterial Thrombolysis

Recombinant prourokinase (rpro-UK; Prolyse), the inactive, single-chain precursor of uro-kinase that has greater fibrin specificity, has been used in 2 randomized trials of intra-arterial thrombolysis in acute ischemic stroke. The Prolyse in Acute Cerebral Thromboembolism Trial (PROACT) was a Phase 2 study that enrolled patients who presented within 6 hr of symptom onset and had acute occlusion of the MCA on angiography (46). Forty-six patients who displayed Thrombolysis in Acute Myocardial Infarction (TIMI) grade 0 or 1 of the M1 or M2 portions of the MCA were randomized 2:1 to receive intra-arterial rpro-UK (6 mg) or placebo over 120 min into the proximal face of the thrombus. All patients received intravenous heparin. Recanalization efficacy was evaluated at the end of the 120-min infusion, and ICH that caused neurologic deterioration was assessed at 24 hr. Partial (TIMI 2) or complete (TIMI 3) reperfusion through the occluded MCA segment was observed in 58% of the rpro-UK group and in only 14% of the placebo-treated patients ($p=0.017$). Hemorrhagic transformation that caused neurologic deterioration within 24 hr of treatment occurred in 15.4% of the rpro-UK–treated patients and 7.1% of the placebo group, but this finding was not significant due to the small numbers of subjects. Based upon the encouraging results of the original PROACT study, PROACT II was designed as a Phase 3 trial and conducted in 54 university and community hospitals in the United States and Canada (47). One hundred eighty patients with the same clinical and angiographic character-istics as those enrolled in the original PROACT study were randomized 2:1 to receive 9 mg of intra-arterial rpro-UK over 120 min plus intravenous heparin, or heparin only. Recanalization efficacy was again determined at the end of the 120 min. The primary endpoint of PROACT II was the percentage of patients who achieved an mRS of 2 or less at 90 days following initial therapy. For this primary analysis, 40% of rpro-UK patients and 25% of control patients met this criteria ($p=0.04$). There was no significant difference in mortality observed between the rpro-UK (25%) and control (27%) patients. The recanalization rate was 66% for the rpro-UK group and 18% for controls ($p<0.001$). ICH with neurologic deterioration within 24 hr occurred in 10% of rpro-UK patients and 2% of control patients ($p=0.06$).

A *post hoc* analysis of PROACT II confirmed, in a multivariate regression model, that age, baseline NIHSS score, and hypodensity were the most important prognostic variables for good outcome (48). After dividing all subjects treated in PROACT II into quartiles based on calculated risk scores, the probability of good outcome was observed uniformly across all quartiles, with no differential treatment effect defined by type of stroke. Although the PROACT studies demonstrated that intra-arterial thrombolysis can be performed effectively in patients with occlusion of major intracranial vessels, the high rate of ICH associated with intra-arterial clot lysis in PROACT II prevented FDA approval of rpro-UK.

Alternative Agents for Systemic Thrombolysis

Other trials of systemic thrombolytic therapy in acute ischemic stroke have failed to meet the standard set by the NINDS rtPA Stroke Study, possibly because treatment was delayed beyond 3 hr (49). Three large, randomized, double-blinded, placebo-controlled trials of streptokinase given within 6 hr after the onset of stroke symptoms showed no benefit before being terminated prematurely because of increased rates of ICH and mortality in treated patients (50–52). Because of these drawbacks, streptokinase has been abandoned as therapy for acute ischemic stroke. In the Multi-Center Acute Stroke Trial—Italy, patients who took aspirin before exposure to streptokinase were at significantly greater risk for hemorrhagic transformation, as in ECASS II (53,54).

Ancrod, a defibrinogenating agent extracted from the venom of the Malayan pit viper, was tested in a Phase 3 trial that required drug administration within 6 hr of ischemic stroke onset. This study showed no benefit to ancrod treatment, perhaps because fibrinogen levels remained higher than desired (55). In the more recently completed Stroke Treatment with Ancrod Trial (STAT), 500 patients were randomly assigned to receive ancrod or placebo as a continuous 72-hr intravenous infusion, beginning within 3 hr of stroke onset and followed by 1-hr infusions at 96 and 120 hr (56). The ancrod regimen was designed to reduce plasma fibrinogen levels to 1.18 to 2.03 µmol/L. The primary endpoint was functional status, defined as survival to 90 days with a Barthel index score of 95 or more, or at least the estimated pre-morbid value. A larger proportion of patients in the ancrod group (42.2%) finished the trial at the targeted Barthel range than in the placebo group, 34.4% ($p=0.04$). No difference in mortality was observed at 90 days (25.4% for ancrod and 23% for placebo). A trend toward a higher rate of symptomatic ICH in the ancrod group versus placebo (5.2% vs. 2.0%; $p=0.06$) and a significant increase in asymptomatic ICH (19.0% vs. 10.7%; $p=0.01$) were noted. The authors concluded that ancrod could be administered effectively with an acceptable margin of safety. Clinical effi-cacy was enhanced by more rapid defibrinogenation. However, the complexity of titrating the dose of ancrod to serial fibrinogen levels makes this therapeutic approach more complex than that already available with rtPA at a similar level of hemorrhagic complications.

The most promising alternative to rtPA in the thrombolytic treatment of stroke is des-moteplase, a unique thrombolytic protein isolated from the saliva of South American vampire bats and mass-produced by recombinant technology. Desmoteplase has several technical advan-tages over rtPA in that it is highly specific and selective for fibrin, can be administered rapidly by bolus, minimizes systemic and cerebral bleeding by preservation of whole-blood fibrinogen, and has no recognized neurotoxicity. In a novel Phase 2 trial, Desmoteplase in Acute Stroke (DIAS), patients were selected for treatment with desmoteplase or placebo after MRI to con-firm the presence of a perfusion–diffusion mismatch (57). In this approach, viable candidates for delayed reperfusion therapy were identified by imaging that revealed a target volume of poorly perfused, but viable, tissue surrounding an infarct core. The trial was conducted at 44 centers in 12 countries, excluding the United States. The safety endpoint of DIAS was symp-tomatic ICH. Efficacy endpoints included the rate of reperfusion on MRI obtained 4 to 8 hr after treatment and clinical outcome as assessed by NIHSS, mRS, and Barthel index at 90 days. The first 47 patients were randomized to fixed doses of desmoteplase (25, 37.5, or 50 mg) or placebo without adjustment for body weight. Symptomatic ICH occurred within 24 hr of drug administration in 8 of 30 desmoteplase-treated patients (26.7%), causing this dosing regimen to be abandoned in favor of a weight-adjusted strategy (62.5, 90, or 125 µg/kg vs. placebo). After the weight-adjusted regimen was implemented and another 57 patients were enrolled, the overall symptomatic ICH rate fell to 2.2%, the MRI reperfusion rate in the 125 µg/kg-dose tier rose to 71.4% ($p=0.0012$, in comparison to placebo), and favorable 90-day outcome observed with this dose climbed to 60% ($p=0.009$, in comparison to placebo). An identically designed trial conducted in the United States has been reported to show no symptomatic ICH in actively treated patients and no growth of the ischemic lesion on MRI after treatment with 125 µg/kg desmoteplase. In 2005, a Phase 3 efficacy trial of desmoteplase versus placebo was inaugurated at more than 100 international centers, using CT or MRI perfusion studies to recruit patients who present within 3 and 9 hr of ischemic stroke onset.

CONCLUSIONS AND FUTURE DIRECTIONS

The acceptance and use of systemic thrombolysis for treatment of acute ischemic stroke in the United States, Canada, and most European countries is predicated upon accurate risk stratifica-tion and careful patient selection. CT remains the most commonly used and widely available tool for identification of patients at high risk for hemorrhagic complications of systemic thrombolysis. However, the insensitivity of CT in prediction of the total volume of brain tissue susceptible to ischemic injury or hemorrhagic transformation is well recognized. The recent incorporation of CT perfusion imaging, CT angiography, and easily performed, reproducible paradigms for estimation of ischemic injury volume may overcome the limitations of static CT imaging in pre-dicting stroke outcome (58,59). MRI, when performed in a multimodality format that includes DWI and PWI, has already shown potential to identify candidates for delayed treatment with experimental thrombolytic drugs (57).

One approach to diagnosis of acute ischemic stroke and prediction of outcome that was not considered in this review is the use of blood-borne proteins or nucleic acids as biomarkers. Although still in its infancy, the development of biomarkers to confirm the diagnosis of stroke and to prognosticate short-term outcome has made promising advances. Future use of bio-markers may be in "point-of-care" laboratory panels developed for early diagnosis of ischemic brain injury in the absence of, or to complement, radiographic imaging. Reynolds *et al.* tested a point-of-care laboratory panel of 50 target molecules and found that elevated plasma levels of S-100β (a calcium-binding protein expressed by astroglial cells), von Willebrand factor, and other markers of neural injury or vascular occlusion were 92% sensitive for brain infarction within 6 hr of symptom onset (60). Tang *et al.* recently reported the use of oligonucleotide microarrays to characterize rapid changes in peripheral white blood cell populations in acute stroke patients treated with systemic thrombolysis (61). Use of a highly sensitive biomarker in the setting of acute stroke could facilitate rapid referral of patients to hospitals specializing in acute stroke care, guide medical management, supplement or augment diagnostic imaging, and determine effectiveness of experimental therapy in future clinical trials (62).

ACKNOWLEDGMENTS

Financial support was provided by NIH M01 RR02602 (University of Kentucky General Clinical Research Center). Sherry Chandler Williams, E. L. S., prepared and edited this chapter.

REFERENCES

1. American Heart Association Statistics Committee and Stroke Statistics Subcommittee. Heart disease and stroke statistics—2006 update. Circulation 2006 (published online at http://circ.ahajournals.org; accessed January 28, 2006).
2. Broderick J, Brott T, Kothari R, et al. The Greater Cincinnati/Northern Kentucky Stroke Study: preliminary first-ever and total incidence rates of stroke among blacks. Stroke 1998; 29:415–421.
3. Matchar DB, Samsa GP, Matthews JR, et al. The Stroke Prevention Policy Model: linking evidence and clinical decisions. Ann Int Med 1997; 127:704–711.
4. Taylor TN, Davis PH, Torner JC, et al. Lifetime cost of stroke in the United States. Stroke 1996; 27:1459–1466.
5. Rödén-Jüllig A. Progressing stroke: epidemiology. Cerebrovasc Dis 1997; 7:2–5.
6. Dávalos A, Cendra E, Teruel J, et al. Deteriorating ischemic stroke: risk factors and prognosis. Neurology 1990; 40:1865–1869.
7. Toni D, Fiorelli M, Gentile M, et al. Progressing neurological deficit secondary to acute ischemic stroke. A study on predictability, pathogenesis, and prognosis. Arch Neurol 1995; 52:670–675.
8. Castillo J, Dávalos A, Noya M. Progression of ischaemic stroke and excitotoxic amino acids. Lancet 1997; 349:79–83.
9. Dávalos A, Castillo J, Pumar JM, Noya M. Body temperature and fibrinogen are related to early neurological deterioration in acute ischemic stroke. Cerebrovasc Dis 1997; 7:64–69.
10. Jørgensen HS, Nakayama H, Raaschou HO, Olsen TS. Effect of blood pressure and diabetes on stroke in progression. Lancet 1994; 344:156–159.
11. Dávalos A, Toni D, Iweins F, et al. Neurological deterioration in acute ischemic stroke: potential predictors and associated factors in the European cooperative acute stroke study (ECASS) I. Stroke 1999; 30:2631–2636.
12. Toni D, Fiorelli M, Zanette EM, et al. Early spontaneous improvement and deterioration of ischemic stroke patients. A serial study with transcranial Doppler ultrasonography. Stroke 1998; 29:1144–1148.
13. Moseley ME, Kucharczyk J, Mintorovitch J, et al. Diffusion-weighted MR imaging of acute stroke: correlation with T2-weighted and magnetic susceptibility-enhanced MR imaging in cats. Am J Neuroradiol 1990; 11:423–429.
14. Moseley ME, Cohen Y, Mintorovitch J, et al. Early detection of regional cerebral ischemia in cats: comparison of diffusion- and T2-weighted MRI and spectroscopy. Magn Reson Med 1990; 14:330–346.
15. Mintorovitch J, Yang GY, Shimizu H, et al. Diffusion-weighted magnetic resonance imaging of acute focal cerebral ischemia: comparison of signal intensity with changes in brain water and Na+,K(+)-ATPase activity. J Cereb Blood Flow Metab 1994; 14:332–336.
16. Pierce AR, Lo EH, Mandeville JB, et al. MRI measurements of water diffusion and cerebral perfusion: their relationship in a rat model of focal cerebral ischemia. J Cereb Blood Flow Metab 1997; 17:183–190.
17. Li F, Han SS, Tatlisumak T, et al. Reversal of acute apparent diffusion coefficient abnormalities and delayed neuronal death following transient focal cerebral ischemia in rats. Ann Neurol 1999; 46:333–342.
18. Tong DC, Yenari MA, Albers GW, et al. Correlation of perfusion- and diffusion-weighted MRI with NIHSS score in acute (<6.5 hr) ischemic stroke. Neurology 1998; 50:864–870.

19. Barber PA, Darby DG, Desmond PM, et al. Prediction of stroke outcome with echoplanar perfusion- and diffusion-weighted MRI. Neurology 1998; 51:418–426.
20. Lövblad KO, Baird AE, Schlaug G, et al. Ischemic lesion volumes in acute stroke by diffusion-weighted magnetic resonance imaging correlate with clinical outcome. Ann Neurol 1997; 42:164–170.
21. Baird AE, Benfield A, Schlaug G, et al. Enlargement of human cerebral ischemic lesion volumes measured by diffusion-weighted magnetic resonance imaging. Ann Neurol 1997; 41:581–589.
22. Darby DG, Barber PA, Gerraty RP, et al. Pathophysiological topography of acute ischemia by combined diffusion-weighted and perfusion MRI. Stroke 1999; 30:2043–2052.
23. Sorenson AG, Buonanno FS, Gonzalez RG, et al. Hyperacute stroke: evaluation with combined multisection diffusion-weighted and hemodynamically weighted echo-planar MR imaging. Radiology 1996; 199:391–401.
24. Warach S, Pettigrew LC, Dashe JF, et al. Effect of citicoline on ischemic lesions as measured by diffusion-weighted MRI. Ann Neurol 2000; 48:713–722.
25. Røhl L, Østergaard L, Simonsen CZ, et al. Viability thresholds of ischemic penumbra of hyperacute stroke defined by perfusion-weighted MRI and apparent diffusion coefficient. Stroke 2001; 32:1140–1146.
26. Thijs VN, Adami A, Neumann-Haefelin T, et al. Relationship between severity of MR perfusion deficit and DWI lesion evolution. Neurology 2001; 57:1205–1211.
27. Dávalos A, Blanco M, Pedraza S, et al. The clinical-DWI mismatch: a new diagnostic approach to the brain tissue at risk of infarction. Neurology 2004; 62:2187–2192.
28. Hacke W, Kaste M, Fieschi C et al. Intravenous thrombolysis with recombinant tissue plasminogen activator for acute hemispheric stroke: The European Cooperative Stroke Study (ECASS). JAMA 1995; 274(13):1017–1025.
29. Fiorelli M, Bastianello S, von Kummer R, et al. Hemorrhagic transformation within 36 hours of a cerebral infarct: relationships with early clinical deterioration and 3-month outcome in the European Cooperative Acute Stroke Study I (ECASS I) cohort. Stroke 1999; 30:2280–2284.
30. del Zoppo GJ, Poeck K, Pessin MS, et al. Recombinant tissue plasminogen activator in acute thrombotic and embolic stroke. Ann Neurol 1992; 32:78–86.
31. Lindenstrøm E, Boysen G, Christiansen LW, et al. Reliability of Scandinavian Stroke Scale. Cerebrovasc Dis 1991; 1:103–107.
32. Brott TG, Haley ECJ, Levy DE, et al. Urgent therapy for stroke. Part I. Pilot study of tissue plasminogen activator administered within 90 minutes. Stroke 1992; 23:632–640.
33. Haley EC Jr., Levy DE, Brott TG, et al. Urgent therapy for stroke. Part II. Pilot study of tissue plasminogen activator administered 91–180 minutes from onset. Stroke 1992; 23:641–645.
34. Kwiatkowski TG, Libman RB, Frankel M, et al. Effects of tissue plasminogen activator for acute ischemic stroke at one year. National Institute of Neurological Disorders and Stroke Recombinant Tissue Plasminogen Activator Stroke Study Group. New Engl J Med 1999; 340:1781–1787.
35. Fagan SC, Morgenstern LB, Petitta A, et al. Cost-effectiveness of tissue plasminogen activator for acute ischemic stroke. NINDS rtPA Stroke Study Group. Neurology 1998; 50:883–890.
36. The National Institute of Neurological Disorders and Stroke rtPA Stroke Study Group. Tissue plasminogen activator for acute ischemic stroke. New Engl J Med 1995; 333:1581–1587.
37. The NINDS t-PA Stroke Study Group. Intracerebral hemorrhage after intravenous t-PA therapy for ischemic stroke. Stroke 1997; 28:2109–2118.
38. Adams HP Jr., Brott TG, Furlan AJ, et al. Guidelines for thrombolytic therapy for acute stroke: a supplement to the guidelines for the management of patients with acute ischemic stroke. A statement for healthcare professionals from a Special Writing Group of the Stroke Council, American Heart Association. Stroke 1996; 27:1711–1718.
39. Practice advisory: thrombolytic therapy for acute ischemic stroke—summary statement. Report of the Quality Standards Subcommittee of the American Academy of Neurology. Neurology 1996; 47:835–839.
40. Katzan IL, Furlan AJ, Lloyd LE, et al. Use of tissue-type plasminogen activator for acute ischemic stroke: the Cleveland area experience. JAMA 2000; 283:1151–1158.
41. Albers GW, Bates VE, Clark WM, et al. Intravenous tissue-type plasminogen activator for treatment of acute stroke: the Standard Treatment with Alteplase to Reverse Stroke (STARS) study. JAMA 2000; 283:1145–1150.
42. Buchan AM, Barber PA, Newcommon N, et al. Effectiveness of t-PA in acute ischemic stroke: outcome relates to appropriateness. Neurology 2000; 54:679–684.
43. Hacke W, Kaste M, Fieschi C, et al. Randomised double-blind placebo-controlled trial of thrombolytic therapy with intravenous alteplase in acute ischaemic stroke (ECASS II). Second European-Australasian Acute Stroke Study Investigators. Lancet 1998; 352:1245–1251.
44. Larrue V, von Kummer R, Muller A, Bluhmki E. Risk factors for severe hemorrhagic transformation in ischemic stroke patients treated with recombinant tissue plasminogen activator. Stroke 2001; 32:438.

45. Clark WM, Wissman S, Albers GW, et al. Recombinant tissue-type plasminogen activator (Alteplase) for ischemic stroke 3 to 5 hours after symptom onset. The ATLANTIS Study: a randomized controlled trial. Alteplase Thrombolysis for Acute Noninterventional Therapy in Ischemic Stroke. JAMA 1999; 282:2019–2026.

46. del Zoppo GJ, Higashida RT, Furlan AJ, et al. PROACT: a phase II randomized trial of recombinant pro-urokinase by direct arterial delivery in acute middle cerebral artery stroke. PROACT Investigators. Prolyse in Acute Cerebral Thromboembolism. Stroke 1998; 29:4–11.

47. Furlan A, Higashida R, Wechsler L, et al. The PROACT II study: a randomized controlled trial. JAMA 1999; 282:2003–2011.

48. Wechsler LR, Roberts R, Furlan AJ, et al. Factors influencing outcome and treatment effect in PROACT II. Stroke 2003; 34:1224–1229.

49. del Zoppo GJ, Ferbert A, Otis S, et al. Local intra-arterial fibrinolytic therapy in acute carotid territory stroke. A pilot study. Stroke 1988; 19:307–313.

50. Multicentre Acute Stroke Trial—Italy (MAST-I) Group. Randomised controlled trial of streptokinase, aspirin, and combination of both in treatment of acute ischaemic stroke. Lancet 1995; 346:1509–1514.

51. Donnan GA, Davis SM, Chambers BR, et al. Streptokinase for acute ischemic stroke with relationship to time of administration: Australian Streptokinase (ASK) Trial Study Group. JAMA 1996; 271:961–966.

52. Thrombolytic therapy with streptokinase in acute ischemic stroke. The Multicenter Acute Stroke Trial—Europe Study Group. New Engl J Med 1996; 334:145–150.

53. Ciccone A, Motto C, Aritzu E, Piana A, Candelise L. Risk of aspirin use plus thrombolysis after acute ischaemic stroke: a further MAST-I analysis. MAST-I Collaborative Group. Multicentre Acute Stroke Trial—Italy. Lancet 1998; 352:880.

54. Levy DE, Brott TG, Haley EC Jr., et al. Factors related to intracranial hematoma formation in patients receiving tissue-type plasminogen activator for acute ischemic stroke. Stroke 1994; 25:291–297.

55. The Ancrod Stroke Study Investigators. Ancrod for the treatment of acute ischemic brain infarction. Stroke 1994; 25:1755–1759.

56. Sherman DG, Atkinson RP, Chippendale T, et al. Intravenous ancrod for treatment of acute ischemic stroke: the STAT study: a randomized controlled trial. Stroke Treatment with Ancrod Trial. Stroke 2000; 283:2395–2403.

57. Hacke W, Albers G, Al-Rawi Y, et al. The Desmoteplase in Acute Ischemic Stroke Trial (DIAS): a phase II MRI-based 9-hour window acute stroke thrombolysis trial with intravenous desmoteplase. Stroke 2005; 36:66–73.

58. Parsons MW, Pepper EM, Chan V, et al. Perfusion computed tomography: prediction of final infarct extent and stroke outcome. Ann Neurol 2005; 58:672–679.

59. Scharf J, Brockmann MA, Daffertshofer M, et al. Improvement of sensitivity and interrater reliability to detect acute stroke dynamic perfusion computed tomography and computed tomography angiography. J Comput Assist Tomogr 2006; 30:105–110.

60. Reynolds MA, Kirchick HJ, Dahlen JR, et al. Early biomarkers of stroke. Clin Chem 2003; 49:1733–1739.

61. Tang Y, Xu H, Lit L, et al. Gene expression in blood changes rapidly in neutrophils and monocytes after ischemic stroke in humans: a microarray study. J Cereb Blood Flow Metab advance online publication, 04 January 2006.

62. Lynch JR, Blessing R, White WD, et al. Novel diagnostic test for acute stroke. Stroke 2004; 35:57–63.

23 | Venous Strokes and Venous Sinus Thrombosis

Izabella Rozenfeld, MD, Resident
Madeline C. Fields, MD, Resident
Department of Neurology, Mount Sinai School of Medicine,
New York, New York, USA

Steven R. Levine, MD, Professor
The Stroke Center, Department of Neurology, Mount Sinai School of Medicine, New York, New York, USA

INTRODUCTION

The scientific understanding of the problem of cerebral venous thrombosis (CVT) and venous stroke and their treatment is based upon several factors, including cerebral venous anatomy, physiology of venous circulation, underlying genetic and/or environmental/acquired factors that influence clotting and circulation, and the use of rigorous, well-controlled clinical trials. Timely and accurate diagnosis of CVT depends on an understanding of the myriad of clinical presentations in the proper setting and the urgent use of appropriate, sensitive diagnostic studies. In this chapter, we review several clinically important aspects of CVT (in both adults and children), focusing on the scientific basis for clinical presentation, risk factors, pathogenesis, natural history and prognosis, diagnostic imaging, and treatment.

CLINICAL PRESENTATION

The most common clinical feature of CVT is the nonfocal syndrome of intracranial hypertension, characterized by headache and papilledema. The classic description of headache associated with nausea, emesis, visual blurring, and horizontal diplopia (due to the false localizing sign of abducens nerve palsy), without focal signs or altered consciousness, occurs in 37% of CVT patients (1). The initial presentation might be acute, such as in puerperal women and when infection is the etiology. Headache might be the only early complaint in 70% of patients, especially in puerperal women, but it is a major one, regardless of etiology. Seizures occur in 40% of patients (2). Focal deficits and altered consciousness will develop in less than half of patients. Clot propagation is more gradual and fluctuant than in arterial occlusions (in part due to the extensive collateralization of the venous and sinus drainage), and delay in hospital presentation often results. In one case series, 28% of patients presented within 48 hr of symptom onset, 42% presented between 48 hr and 30 days, and 30% presented after 30 days (3).

Initially, symptoms of superior sagittal sinus (SSS) thrombosis resemble the pseudotumor cerebri syndrome; however, extension into rolandic and parietal veins is common, with subsequent development of focal neurologic signs and seizures. These signs can be transient, resembling a transient ischemic attack, and/or they can be bilateral. In approximately two-thirds of patients, occlusion involves more than one venous channel (4). Occlusion of the deep veins is less common than occlusion of the dural sinus.

Deep CVT presents with headache, typically followed by confusion, reduced level of consciousness, vertical gaze palsy, rigidity, and decerebrate posturing. Apathy, abulia, attention deficits, and poor memory might be observed at presentation or upon recovery. Seizures are the major presentation of cortical vein thrombosis. Headache, focal or generalized seizures, and focal signs, such as a hemiparesis or aphasia, are common. Patients with deep CVT present with a decreased level of consciousness and increased intracranial pressure (ICP) less commonly than do patients with dural sinus thrombosis.

Septic thrombosis preferentially involves the lateral and cavernous sinuses (5). Cavernous sinus thrombosis is most commonly caused by *Staphylococcus aureus* infections. Pneumococci,

Streptococcal species, gram-negative bacteria, and Aspergillus have also been implicated (6). Nonseptic cavernous sinus thrombosis usually develops after head trauma, facial surgery, and in the setting of prothrombotic states (7). The earliest symptoms are headache, facial pain, and fever. The physical findings include proptosis of the eye with periorbital edema, chemosis, ptosis, ophthalmoplegia, pupillary abnormalities, facial edema, erythema, and decreased sensation. Retinal hemorrhages and a swollen optic disc might also be present. Further, unilateral thrombosis can spread via the intracavernous sinus, located around the cell turcica, to become bilateral.

Widespread use of antibiotics has decreased the occurrence of septic lateral sinus thrombosis, the major signs and symptoms of which include fever, neck pain, and tenderness over the mastoid process and behind the ear. Patients might complain of diffuse, severe, persistent headache localized to the frontotemporal area, vertigo, nausea, vomiting, diplopia (sixth-nerve palsy), or retro-orbital pain (fifth-nerve irritation). The combination of fifth- and sixth-nerve involvement is known as Gradenigo's syndrome and indicates involvement of the petrous bone. Because blood from the inferior portions of the temporal lobe and cerebellum drains into the lateral sinuses, aphasia, agitation, and right hemianopia or superior quadrantanopia will be seen with left lateral sinus thrombosis, whereas right temporal lobe involvement causes an agitated state with left visual field defects (7). Nystagmus and gait ataxia correlate with cerebellar involvement. Spread of the thrombosis into the jugular vein rarely is complicated by pulmonary embolism.

EPIDEMIOLOGY AND RISK FACTORS

In that no prospective, population-based, epidemiologic studies have been conducted to specifically examine CVT, the current incidence in the general population is not known. Most studies are from autopsy series (7–13). However, in the last decade an increase in diagnosis and survival of patients with CVT can be attributed to improved knowledge of hypercoagulable states, better detection via magnetic resonance imaging (MRI), which includes magnetic resonance venography (MRV), (Fig. 1) and increased use of intravenous anticoagulation as treatment. The ratio of CVT to arterial stroke is approximately 1:62.5 but only 1:8.5 in patients aged 15 to 45. CVT is more common in children (7 in 1,000,000/yr) than in adults (3 to 4 in 1,000,000/yr) and is reported in 7 out of 100,000 hospitalized adults (14,15).

Table 1 contains a list of risk factors for CVT. Approximately 75% to 85% of adult patients with CVT are women (2). The frequency of CVT was equal among men and women until the 1970s, when the widespread use of oral contraceptive (OC) pills came into use (2). Currently,

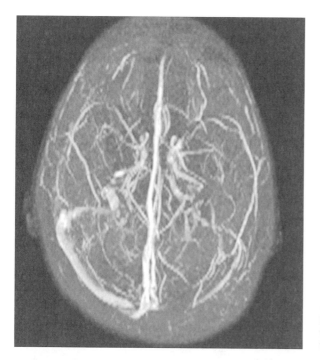

Figure 1 Magnetic resonance venography (MRV). Currently, many cerebral venous thromboses can be diagnosed noninvasively with the use of MRI and MRV, obviating the need to perform invasive catheter angiography.

75% of female cases present with CVT during pregnancy, during puerperium, or while they are taking OC pills. The prevalence of CVT associated with pregnancy or pueperium ranges from 2 to 500 per 100,000 deliveries, depending upon the country (1). During the last trimester and first 2 weeks postpartum, the risk of CVT is increased (16,17). Hormonal changes in males using androgens might also increase the risk of CVT. In 85% of people with CVT, a cause or prothrombotic risk factor can be identified.

Hypercoaguable states can be either inherited or acquired. Deficiencies of protein C, protein S, and antithrombin III can be inherited as autosomal-dominant conditions or acquired via inflammatory states, liver disease, disseminated intravascular coagulation, L-asparaginase therapy, and vitamin K deficiency. Deficiency of one of these anticoagulants is found in 2% to 12% of CVT patients (15,18,19). Activated protein C resistance can be inherited or acquired and is most commonly caused by factor V Leiden mutation (20). Factor V Leiden and prothrombin G20210A mutations are the most common inherited hypercoagulable states associated with CVT (10–20% of CVT patients) (15). Women who take OCs and who have genetic hypercoaguable predisposition, (e.g., factor V Leiden or prothrombin gene mutation) have an increased risk of developing CVT, compared to women of the same age who do not take OCs and do not have the factor V defect (21). An increased risk of CVT has also been reported in pregnant or puerperal women with factor V Leiden or prothrombin gene mutations (21). Abnormal recombinant plasminogen activator inhibitor-1 or lipoprotein(a) might also contribute to CVT because of decreased fibrinolysis. Prolonged elevation of clotting factors, such as fibrinogen and factor VIII, can increase the risk of venous thrombosis (22). Additionally, hyperhomocysteinemia and antiphospholipid antibodies, such as lupus anticoagulant and anticardiolipin antibodies,

Table 1 Risk Factors, Predisposing Conditions, and Causes of Cerebral Venous Thrombosis

Genetic hypercoagulable states
Factor V Leiden mutation
Antithrombin deficiency
Protein C and protein S deficiency
Prothrombin 20210A mutation
Hyperhomocysteinemia (gene mutations in methylenetetrahydrofolate reductase), homocystinuria
Plasminogen deficiency
Thrombomodulin gene mutation
Sickle cell anemia and traits
Hereditary dysfibrinogenemia
β-Thalassemia
Acquired prothrombotic states/hematologic conditions
Thrombocythemia (primary or secondary)
Nephrotic syndrome
Antiphospholipid antibodies
Hyperhomocysteinemia
Pregnancy
Puerperium
Increased resistance to activated protein C
Paroxysmal nocturnal hemoglobinuria
Leukemia, cancer
Anemia (posthemorrhagic, iron deficiency, hemolytic)
Polycythemia
Heparin- or heparinoid-induced thrombocytopenia
Disseminated intravascular coagulation
Cryofibrinogenemia
Elevated coagulation factors VII, VIII
Protein C and protein S deficiency
Infections
Otitis, mastoiditis, sinusitis
Meningitis
Systemic infectious disease (parasitic, fungal, viral, bacterial)
Intracranial infection

(Continued)

Table 1   Risk Factors, Predisposing Conditions, and Causes of Cerebral Venous Thrombosis (*Continued*)

Inflammatory disease
  Systemic lupus erythematosus
  Wegener's granulomatosis
  Sarcoidosis
  Inflammatory bowel disease (Crohn's disease, ulcerative colitis)
  Temporal arteritis
  Sjogren's syndrome
  Behcet's disease
Drugs
  Oral contraception
  L-Asparaginase
  ε-Aminocaproic acid
  Tamoxifen
  Epoetin alfa
  Lithium
  Androgen therapy
  "Ectasy"
  Thyrotoxicosis
Mechanical causes, trauma
  Head injury
  Injury to sinuses of jugular vein, jugular catheterization
  Neurosurgical procedures
  Dural puncture
  Lumbar puncture
  Electrical injury
  Any surgical procedure
Miscellaneous
  Dehydration, especially in children
  Dural arteriovenous malformations
  Tumors
  Arachnoid cysts
  Congenital heart disease
  Congestive heart failure
  Pacemaker
  Carcinoid syndrome
  Cirrhosis
  Ovarian hyperstimulation syndrome
  Severe exfoliative dermatitis

have been detected in patients with CVT from 27% to 40% and 8% to 53%, respectively (15). Antiphospholipid antibodies are the most commonly acquired type of thrombophilia, although the mechanism in this setting remains unknown. Direct causes of sinus thrombosis include head injury or manipulation of the vasculature from neurosurgical procedures (i.e., catheterizations). Additionally, lumbar puncture can sometimes cause CVT from traction and deformation of the vessels.

Infections were the leading cause of CVT until the development of antibiotics. Otitis and mastoiditis can cause thrombosis via direct seeding to the adjacent sigmoid and transverse sinuses (Table 1).

PATHOGENESIS

Typically, a triggering event or combination of events/predisposing factors initiate clotting in a cerebral vein or sinus. When coagulation is activated and thrombosis occurs, the vein, sinus, or frequently both structures become obstructed, with increased resistance to normal venous return to the heart, which leads to a rise in venous and tissue pressure. Most of the consequences of CVT are directly related to some combination of brain edema (tissue congestion), increased ICP, and hemorrhagic infarction.

Venous Thrombosis

When a cerebral vein is unable to return blood, normally due to thrombosis, the tissue pressure can increase due to continued normal arterial flow. The brain then swells, as do the neighboring venous structures (compensatory), with a tendency for tissue ischemia and hemorrhage (hemorrhagic infarction or confluent petechial hemorrhages that can appear as a large parenchymal hematoma). Autopsy studies reveal dilated veins, tissue edema, ischemic neurons, and hemorrhagic changes (of varying sizes and degrees). The final pathology depends on the site and completeness of thrombosis and the timing of thrombosis to death.

As with other venous clots, fibrin and erythrocytes with a paucity of platelets comprise the majority of fresh thromboses, and fibrous tissue is seen within older clots. Thrombus formation generally originates from venous stasis, procoagulant states, and changes in the vessel wall. As many patients with CVT survive and are left without clinical or imaging evidence of permanent tissue damage (infarction), the pathophysiologic process is mostly consistent with temporary ischemia and edema.

The International Study on Cerebral Vein and Dural Sinus Thrombosis (ISCVT) (13) studied the frequency of thrombosis. The transverse sinus was the most commonly thrombosed structure (86%), followed by the SSS (62%), straight sinus (18%), cortical veins (17%), jugular veins (12%), and vein of Galen/internal cerebral veins (11%). With adequate collateral circulation, the level of tissue ischemia might be insufficient to cause permanent tissue damage or infarction.

Sinus Thrombosis

With sinus occlusion and continued pressure to return flowing blood out of the head, venous pressure increases, which can lead to intracranial hypertension from impaired cerebrospinal fluid (CSF) absorption. A distinct lack of development of hydrocephalus is associated with CVT because the CSF obstruction occurs at the end of its transport pathway, such that no pressure gradient occurs between the subarachnoid spaces at the surface of the brain and ventricles (2). Intracranial hypertension without evidence of CVT occurs in approximately 20% of patients with sinus thrombosis (13).

Occlusion of one of the larger venous sinuses generally does not result in localized permanent tissue injury unless retrograde propagation of thrombosis with obstruction of the cortical veins is involved. When a thrombus extends into the sinus, as well as into some of its tributaries or into the galenic venous system, generally, important and serious disruption of cerebral venous drainage occurs. When hemorrhage occurs, it is typically in the white matter and can range from petechial to large with mass effect, with extension to the subarachnoid space.

NATURAL HISTORY/PROGNOSIS

Scientifically reliable data on the natural history and prognosis of CVT are lacking due to the generally small sample sizes of patients (typically <80) from single-center reports. Because of improvements in timely diagnosis, more sensitive diagnostic imaging tools, supportive hospitalized care and management, and treatment of CVT, the natural history of CVT has likely improved over time in the industrialized world. It has been estimated that >80% of all patients with CVT currently have a good outcome (2).

Prognosis is based on the location, extent, and mechanism of the occlusive process. Generally, involvement of the deep venous structures portends a worse prognosis (higher mortality rate) than does involvement of the superficial venous system. The ISCVT (13) collected 624 adult patients (from 21 countries and 89 centers) with CVT to determine prognosis. Follow-up was for a median of 1.25 years. More than half (57%) had a modified Rankin Scale score (mRS) of 0 (no signs or symptoms), 22% had minor residual symptoms (mRS = 1), and 7.5% had mild impairments (mRS=2). Moderate impairment (mRS = 3) was seen in 2.9%, and 2.2% were severely disabled (mRS = 4 or 5). CVT was fatal in 8.3%. The 30-day fatality rate was 3.4%. Independent predictors of death or dependence using a cynooxyginase regression analysis are listed in Table 2.

Patients who presented with isolated intracranial hypertension had better outcomes (7% death–dependency rate) than those who did not (13.6% death–dependency rate); hazard ratio, 0.45; 95% confidence interval (CI) 0.23–0.87. Recurrence rate for sinus thrombosis was 2.2% (95% CI, 1.3–3.7), whereas other thrombotic events occurred in 4.3% (95% CI, 3.0–6.2). Seizures occurred in 10.6% (95% CI, 8.4–13.2). Severe headaches during follow-up occurred

Table 2 Outcome of Cerebral Venous Thrombosis Based on 624 Patients from the International Study on Cerebral Vein and Dural Sinus Thrombosis

Predictor	Death or dependency		Hazard ratio	95% Confidence interval
	n/N	Percentage		
Age > 37 yr	26/312	8.3	2.00	1.23–3.27
Male gender	32/159	20.1	1.59	1.01–2.52
Mental status disorder	37/137	27.0	1.95	1.23–2.09
Glasgow Coma Scale <9	12/31	38.7	2.65	1.41–4.55
Deep venous system involvement	20/68	29.4	2.92	1.70–5.00
Intracranial hemorrhage	47/245	19.2	1.88	1.17–3.03
Any malignancy	15/46	32.6	2.90	1.60–5.08
Central nervous system infection	4/13	30.8	3.34	1.98–17.24

Note: *n*, number of patients with the outcome (death or dependency) and the predictor; *N*, total patients with the predictor.
Source: Adapted from Ref. 13.

in 14.1% (95% CI, 11.6–17.1), and median hospitalization duration was 17 days (mean, 20 days). This recent, large prospective data set (largest to date with only 1.3% lost to follow-up after discharge) supports the observation that outcome from CVT is better than previously reported. Prior prospective studies (*n* = 6) had limited statistical power and generalizability, but had suggested that coma, intracerebral hemorrhage (ICH), and malignancy were important prognostic indicators for death or dependence. Further, except for miscarriages, complications rarely occurred during or after new pregnancies (13), strongly supporting the evidence that history of a prior CVT (including puerperal CVT) is not a contraindication to pregnancy (23,24).

Patients with CVT and poor prognostic indicators should be more closely monitored, preferably in an intensive care unit setting, and consideration should be given to more aggressive treatment strategies (e.g., local thrombolysis, reduction of ICP, etc.) (13). The occluded sinus might remain occluded, partially or totally recanalize, stimulate alterative drainage pathways, cause persistent increased ICP, or more uncommonly, develop into a dural arteriovenous malformation. Causes of death are primarily transtentorial herniation due to unilateral focal mass effect or diffuse cerebral edema with multple parenchymal lesions (25).

CEREBRAL VENOUS THROMBOSIS IN CHILDREN

Clinical presentation of CVT in neonates and infants differs in some respects from adults. Children with CVT often have underlying serious systemic disease, involvement of the deep venous system, and a poorer prognosis than adults.

When the cranial sutures have not completely closed, the clinical syndrome might include a tense fontanel, dilated scalp veins, and scalp edema. The neonate/infant might have a depressed level of consciousness, seizures, respiratory distress, fever, and decreased oral intake (26). The older the child is at the time of presentation, the more likely the clinical presentation will mimic that of an adult (27). Older children often have seizures and intracranial hypertension (as manifested by papilledema, emesis, and abducens nerve palsy).

Intraventricular hemorrhage might be seen in neonates with either superficial or deep CVT. Neonatal CVT is often associated with shock, dehydration, or acidosis but can remain idiopathic in up to 40% of cases (26,27). Seizures are the presenting feature in 71% to 80% of cases, and the first neurologic assessment is normal in 40%. Focal neurologic signs are seen in 29%. The deep venous system is involved in 60%. The prognosis is worse in older children who more often present with deep cerebral infarctions. Developmental delay is more commonly seen than hemiparesis or other focal deficits as long-term sequelae of untreated (no anticoagulation) children.

IMAGING/DIAGNOSIS

Improvements in neuroimaging have made the diagnosis of CVT less complicated. Knowledge of the cerebral sinovenous anatomy, as well as direction of blood flow, aids in interpretation of imaging studies. Venous blood flows in the axial plane, forehead to occiput, perpendicular to arterial flow that flows in the coronal plane from skull base. Flow images are acquired in the plane perpendicular to the direction of blood flow. MRI and MRV are the most sensitive techniques in diagnosing intracranial venous thrombosis because they show abnormalities in the normal flow signals, nonopacification of the sinuses, and evidence of collateral venous channels (2,28).

The flow-dependent signal changes and the chemical transformation of hemoglobin occur from periphery of the thrombus inward. During the first 5 days, the signal appears homogenous and, therefore, isointense on T1-weighted scans and hypointense on T2-weighted images. With the appearance of deoxyhemoglobin and extracellular methemoglobin, the thrombus becomes strongly hyperintense on both T1 and T2 images. After a month, the sinus appears isointense on T1-weighted images and gradient echo and hyperintense on T2-weighted images. When the sinus completely recanalizes, the signals return to normal.

The distribution of edema and parenchymal hemorrhages on noncontrast CT that does not conform to a typical arterial territory should make one suspicious of CVT. However, CT might be normal in 4% to 25% of patients, especially those presenting with only isolated intracranial hypertension (2). Bilateral and ill-defined hemorrhagic infarctions in the thalami and basal ganglia are indirect signs of deep venous occlusion. The cord sign, a cerebral cortical vein visualized as a high-density, thin, cylindrical structure, is rarely seen on noncontrast CT, but it is specific for venous thrombosis. If present, it is short-lived, as the thrombus becomes isodense in 1 to 2 weeks (2).

The empty delta or triangle sign on contrast-enhanced CT scans suggests sagittal sinus thrombosis and represents the nonenhanced thrombosed lumen surrounded by enhancing collateral channels. Unfortunately, this sign is seen in only approximately 25% of patients and usually in the second week after the onset of symptoms. False-positive empty delta signs have been seen in subarachnoid hemorrhages and small subdural hematomas. Similar findings can be observed in lateral and straight sinuses and vein of Galen thromboses. Likewise, the nonpacification of the vein of Galen and straight sinus, as well as prolonged retention of contrast in thalamostriate veins and basal veins of Rosenthal suggest occlusion of the deep venous system. In cavernous sinus thrombosis, a postcontrast CT scan demonstrates heterogeneous filling defects.

Catheter angiography remains the gold standard in diagnosis. When angiography is performed, anteroposterior and lateral views are needed. An oblique view is needed if sagittal sinus thrombosis is suspected. Delay in venous filling or emptying and presence of dilated collateral veins extending away from the thrombosis are consistent with venous occlusion. Angiography is less reliable in the diagnosis of cavernous sinus and isolated cortical vein thrombosis and in distinguishing between lateral sinus hypoplasia and thrombosis. MRI is better at distinguishing between hypoplastic and thrombosed sinuses (28). The former are smaller, asymmetric structures on parasagittal MRI without abnormal signal intensities along the course. Occluded sinuses show increased intraluminal signals. The left lateral sinus can fail to opacify in 1 in 7 patients on normal angiograms.

By measuring the increase in flow velocities in the veins of Labbe and Rosenthal, which serve as collateral channels, transcranial Doppler ultrasonography has been utilized in the diagnosis of dural sinus thrombosis. Venous signals can be detected from the vein of Galen, which lies close to the second section of PCA, as well as straight sinus and superior and inferior sagittal sinuses. Transcranial Doppler ultrasonography might be useful in monitoring changes in venous flow and documenting the effect of treatment; however, these data are still preliminary.

ANATOMY

The superficial sinovenous system consists of cortical veins, the SSS, the inferior sagittal sinus, the torcular Herophili (also known as confluence of sinuses), and the transverse and sigmoid sinuses. The straight sinus is functionally and clinically included with the deep sinuses, as it serves as the main outlet for the deep cerebral veins. The dural sinuses contain arachnoid villi and granulations for CSF uptake and communicate via emissary veins with meningeal veins and with extracranial veins in the scalp.

Both superior and inferior sagittal sinuses run within the falx cerebri. The SSS terminates directly into the right transverse sinus, while the inferior terminates into the straight sinus. Occasionally, SSS enters the confluence located at the internal occipital protuberance rather than transverse sinus. Within the confluence, the SSS and the straight sinus join the 2 transverse sinuses. The SSS increases progressively in caliber. In anatomic variations, the rostral SSS might be absent and replaced by 2 superior cerebral veins. The inferior sagittal sinus receives flow from corpus collosum and medial cerebral hemispheres. It might be too narrow to be visualized on MRI.

The transverse sinuses run laterally and anteriorly within the attached margin of the tentorium cerebelli. They originate at the occipital protuberance of the torcular Herophili, and, at the base of the petrous portion of the temporal bone, transverse sinuses curve to form the sigmoid sinuses. The transverse sinuses are of unequal size—the larger has direct connection with the SSS. In 20% of people, one of the transverse sinuses, usually the left, is hypoplastic.

Cavernous sinuses lie on either side of the sphenoid bone, extending superior and lateral to the sphenoid sinuses from the superior orbital fissure to dorsum sellae. Blood flow from facial, ophthalmic, retinal, cerebral, and meningeal veins terminates in the cavernous sinuses, which in turn drain into the petrosal sinuses. The superior petrosal sinus empties into the transverse or sigmoid sinuses, while the inferior drains into the sigmoid sinus or the internal jugular vein.

The straight sinus runs from the splenium of the corpus collosum to the occipital protuberance within the junction of the falx cerebri and the tentorium cerebelli. It is really an extension of the Great vein of Galen as it joins the inferior sagittal sinus. The straight sinus receives cerebellar veins and is often visualized superior to the cerebellum on midsagittal MRI.

Superficial cerebral veins receive blood from superficial medullary veins that begin a few centimeters below the cortex and drain the cortex and adjacent white matter. The superficial cerebral veins are divided into 3 groups—dorsomedial, posterior–inferior, and anterior—based on the sinus into which they empty. The superficial venous system is variable; any of the 3 components might be absent or hypoplastic.

The deep venous system is less variable and includes internal cerebral veins, which receive flow from septal and thalamostriate veins, the basal veins of Rosenthal, the Great vein of Galen, and, functionally, the straight sinus. The deep venous system drains the deep white matter, periventricular regions, corpus collosum, and structures of the diencephalon. The basal veins of Rosenthal drain the inferior aspect of lentiform nuclei, midbrain, medial temporal, and occipital lobes. The internal cerebral veins course posteriorly in the roof of the third ventricle, beneath the corpus collosum, and around the splenium to join the basal veins of Rosenthal, forming the Great vein of Galen, which is often seen on midsagittal MRI. Blood flow within the vein of Galen runs posteriorly in the coronal plane, perpendicular to the flow in other veins, so it might not be well visualized on MRV. Venous drainage of posterior fossa structures is highly variable. The vein of Galen receives flow from dorsal cerebellum, vermis, and upper brainstem. The petrosal system and straight and transverse sinuses all receive drainage from the posterior fossa veins.

Cerebral veins and venous sinuses have no valves; therefore, blood can flow in either direction, depending on the pressure gradient. Extensive anastomosis exists among cortical veins, allowing for collateralization when a sinus is occluded. The vein of Trolad on the lateral surface of the hemisphere serves as a connection between the SSS and the superficial sylvian vein. The vein of Labbe connects the superficial sylvian vein to the transverse sinus.

TREATMENT

Initially, stabilization of the patient is prioritized. If an underlying cause of CVT can be established, it should be treated next. Discontinuing possible causative medications (i.e., OCs, androgen therapy, etc.), treating infectious etiologies with antibiotics and treating underlying medical conditions (i.e., hyperhomocysteinemia, inflammatory bowel disease, nephrotic syndrome, Behcet's disease) should be considerations in first-line management.

Preventing or reversing cerebral herniation can be accomplished by intravenous mannitol, by neurosurgical procedures, such as removal of hemorrhagic clot, or by decompressive hemicraniectomy (2). Treatment of intracranial hypertension by administration of mannitol, acetazolamide, and lumbar punctures may be used when appropriate for the underlying condition. Lumbar puncture is the first step toward measuring pressure and draining CSF. Next, oral acetazolamide is administered. If increased ICP continues despite use of repeat lumbar punctures and azetazolamide, surgical drainage via lumboperitoneal shunt might be necessary. Isolated elevations in ICP can be treated with lumbar puncture and acetazolamide. If visual acuity worsens, a dehydrating agent, such as mannitol, should be administered or optic nerve fenestration performed. Anticonvulsants should be used to treat seizures, but not necessarily prophylactically, as antiepileptic drugs interact with warfarin.

Anticoagulants

Treatment with anticoagulants has been controversial due to the propensity of venous infarcts to bleed. In fact, approximately 40% of patients with CVT have a hemorrhagic infarct prior to any treatment (13). However, the risk of intracranial hemorrhage seems to be greater in CVT patients who do not receive anticoagulation (15). Currently, it is acceptable to administer heparin when radiologic evidence demonstrates a hemorrhagic lesion (7). The efficacy of heparin in CVT is based on case reports, retrospective series, and 3 randomized clinical trials, which compared the effect of intravenous heparin, high-dose subcutaneous nadroparin, and intravenous unfractionated heparin with placebo (29–31). The 3 trials demonstrated a nonsignificant benefit of anticoagulation treatment over placebo. These trials included patients who already had hemorrhagic infarcts prior to treatment and who, during the trial, did not demonstrate new ICH after treatment was initiated. Another argument for the use of heparin is the prevention of pulmonary embolism, a common complication seen in patients with CVT.

Animal models of CVT have also shown that rats that receive anticoagulation clinically do better than those that do not. Additionally, such treatments as inhibitors of platelet glycoprotein IIb/IIIa appear to have benefit in rats and might eventually prove to be beneficial in humans as well.

No controlled data on the duration of oral anticoagulation post-CVT is established, but most treatment is given for 3 to 6 months (2). Recurrent CVT occurs in 2% of patients, and 4% have extracranial thrombotic events within 1 year (13). Longer or indefinite anticoagulation is recommended in patients with thrombophilia, recurrent CVT, inflammatory disease, malignancy, or immobilization (7). Arguments against the use of heparin include the risk of larger hemorrhage into a venous sinus that has resulted in infarction with hemorrhagic transformation, and the high incidence of spontaneous recovery seen in patients with CVT.

Thrombolytics

Thrombolytics aim at rapid restoration of venous outflow by clot destruction. Local thrombolysis restores flow more often and faster than heparin by itself. Multiple cases with administration of urokinase or recombinant tissue-type plasminogen activator (rtPA) plus heparin have been reported. No randomized trials have been reported, only case reports and small series of thrombolysis administration in patients with CVT (level IV evidence). In a review of all published information regarding thrombolytics ($n = 169$ patients, 76% treated with urokinase; dependency at discharge in 7%, 95% CI, 3–12%; 5% mortality, 95% CI, 2–9%; ICH in 17%), the treatment appears safe with relatively few serious hemorrhagic complications (32). However, as no controlled studies have been reported, no good scientific evidence exists to strongly endorse routine use in standard clinical practice.

In one study (33), intrathrombus rtPA and intravenous heparin combined in patients with CVT demonstrated rapid flow restoration and improved clinical outcome in the majority of patients who did not have ICH prior to treatment. In patients with hemorrhagic CVT, the risk of bleeding is high with this therapy. Thrombolysis seems useful in patients with no ICH resulting from treatment, but the numbers of patients treated until now is still much less than the number of patients treated with heparin (2,7). Additionally, the location of the ICH, whether it is deep or on a convexity, influences the efficiency of thrombolytic treatment. The use of local thrombolysis is currently indicated if the patient worsens after medical and heparin therapy (7). No randomized trials have been reported showing that the clinical outcome is better with the use of thrombolytics compared to anticoagulants; however, thrombolytics appear to restore flow faster than heparin alone.

A few cases have been reported in which direct thrombectomy was used within the cerebral venous sinuses (15). In experimental SSS thrombosis in rats, abciximab, a GPIIb/IIIa platelet antagonist, resulted in the best clinical outcomes (residual sinus occlusion of 36% at 1 week), although the highest recanalization rates were seen with rtPA (34). A randomized clinical trial of thrombolysis for CVT is urgently needed (35) and would probably have to be multicentered and international to obtain an adequate sample size.

SUMMARY AND CONCLUSIONS

CVT, a condition frequently underdiagnosed in clinical practice is caused by a disturbed balance between endogenous thrombogenic and fibrinolytic factors. Clinical presentation may be varied from headaches and focal neurologic deficits to rapidly progressive decline in level of consciousness accompanied by bilateral long-tract symptoms. Cranial CT coupled with angiography or MRI and magnetic resonance angiography are studies of choice to confirm the clinical diagnosis. The mainstay of therapy is effective anticoagulation with heparin, even in the presence of intraparenchymal hemorrhage. In select few patients local fibrinoylsis may be considered.

REFERENCES

1. Mas JL, Meder JF. Cerebral venous thrombosis. In: Bogousslavsky J, Ginsberg M, eds. Cerebrovascular Disease: Pathology, Diagnosis and Management. 1st ed. Blackwell Publishers, 1998:1487–1501.
2. Stam J. Thrombosis of the cerebral veins and sinuses. N Engl J Med 2005; 352(17):1791–1798.
3. Bousser MG, Barnett HJM. Cerebral venous thrombosis. In: Mohr JP, Choi DW, Grotta JC, Weir B, Wolf PA, eds. Stroke. Pathophsiology, Diagnosis, and Management. 4th ed. Philadelphia, PA: Churchill Livingstone, 2004:301–325.
4. Breteau G, Mounier-Vehier F, Godefroy O, et al. Cerebral venous thrombosis: 3-year clinical outcome in 55 consecutive patients. J Neurol 2003; 250:29–35.
5. Dinubile MJ. Septic thrombosis of the cavernous sinuses. Arch Neurol 1988; 45(5):567–572.
6. Lefkowitz D. Cortical thrombophlebitis and sinovenous disease. In: Toole JF, ed. Handbook of Clinical Neurology; 10(54): Vascular Diseases Part II. Amsterdam: Elsevier Science Publishers, 1989:395–423.
7. Bousser MG, Russell RR. Cerebral venous thrombosis. In: Warlow CP, Van Gijn J, eds. Major Problems in Neurology. London UK: WB Saunders; 1997:27–29.
8. Ehlers H, Courville CB. Thrombosis of internal cerebral veins in infancy and childhood: review of the literature and report of five cases. J Pediatr 1936; 8:600–623.
9. Barnett HJM, Hyland HH. Non-infective intracranial venous thrombosis. Brain 1953; 76:36–49.
10. Kalbag RM, Woolf AL. Cerebral Venous Thrombosis. London: University Press, 1967.
11. Towbin A. The syndrome of the lateral cerebral venous thrombosis: its frequency and relation to age and congestive heart failure. Stroke 1973; 4:419–430.
12. Averback P. Primary cerebral venous thrombosis in yound adults: the diverse manifestations of an underrecognized disease. Ann Neurol 1978; 3:81–86.
13. Ferro JM, Canhao P, Stam J, Bousser MG, Barinagarrementeria F (for the ISCVT Investigators). Prognosis of cerebral vein and dural sinus thrombosis. Results of the International Study of Cerebral Vein and Dural Sinus Thrombosis (ISCVT). Stroke 2004; 35:664–670.
14. Daif A, Awada A, et al. Cerebral venous thrombosis in adults. A study of 40 cases from Saudi Arabia. Stroke 1995; 26(7):1193–1195.
15. Gordon DL. The diagnosis and management of cerebral venous thrombosis. In: Adams HP Jr., ed. Handbook of Cerebrovascular Diseases; 2nd ed. Revised and Expanded. Series: Neurological Disease and Therapy. New York: Marcel Dekker, 2005; 66:605–636.
16. Cantu C, Barinagarrementeria F. Cerebral venous thrombosis associated with pregnancy and puerperium. Review of 67 cases. Stroke 1993; 24:1880–1884.
17. Helms AK, Kittner SJ. Pregnancy and stroke. CNS Spectrums 2005; 10(7):580–587.
18. de Bruijn SF, de Haan RF, et al. Clinical features and prognostic factors of cerebral venous sinus thrombosis in a prospective series of 59 patients. The Cerebral Venous Sinus Thrombosis Study Group. J Neurol Neurosurg Psych 2001; 70:105–108.
19. Deschiens MA, Conard J. Coagulation studies, factor V Leiden, and anticardiolipin antibodies in 40 cases of cerebral venous thrombosis. Stroke 1996; 27:1724–1730.
20. Levine SR. Hypercoagulable states and stroke: a selective review. CNS Spectrums 2005; 10(7): 567–578.
21. Martinelli I, Sacchi E, Landi G, Taioli E, Duca F, Mannucci PM. High risk of cerebral-vein thrombosis in carriers of a prothrombin-gene mutation and in users of oral contraceptives. N Engl J Med 1998; 338:1793–1797.
22. Seligson U, Lubetsky A. Genetic susceptibility to venous thrombosis. New Engl J Med 2001; 344:1222–1231.
23. Lamy C, Hamon JB, Cose J, et al. Ischemic stroke in young women: risk of recurrence during subsequent pregnancies. French Study Group on Stroke in Pregnancy. Neurology 2000; 55:269–275.
24. Lanska DJ, Kryscio RJ. Risk factors for peripartum and postpartum stroke and intracranial venous thrombosis. Stroke 2000; 31:1274–1282.

25. Canhão P, Ferro JM, Lindgren AG, Bousser M-G, Stam J, Barinagarrementeria F (for the ISCVT Investigators). Causes and predictors of death in cerebral venous thrombosis. Stroke 2005; 36:1720–1725.
26. Carvalho KS, Bodensteiner JB, Connolly PJ, Garg BP. Cerebral venous thrombosis in children. J Child Neurol 2001; 16:574–580.
27. Sébire G, Tabarki B, Saunders DE, et al. Cerebral venous sinus thrombosis in children: risk factors, presentation, diagnosis and outcome. Brain 2005; 128:477–489.
28. Dormont D, Anxionnat R, Evrad S, Louaille C, Chiras J, Marsault C. MRI in cerebral venous thrombosis. J Neuroradiol 1994; 21:81–99.
29. Einhaupal KM, Villringer A, Meister W, et al. Heparin treatment in sinus venous thrombosis. Lancet 1991; 338:597–600. [Erratum Lancet 1991; 338:958.]
30. de Bruijn SF, Stam J. Randomized, placebo-controlled trial of anticoagulant treatment with low-molecular-weight heparin for cerebral sinus thrombosis. Stroke 1999; 30:484–488.
31. Nagaraja D, Rao BSS, Taly AB, Subhash MN. Randomized controlled trial of heparin in puerperal cerebral venous/sinus thrombosis. Nimhans J 1995; 13:111–115.
32. Canhão P, Falcão F, Ferro JM. Thrombolytics for cerebral sinus thrombosis. A systematic review. Cerebrovasc Dis 2003; 15:159–166.
33. Frey JL, Muro GJ, McDougall CG, Dean BL, Jahnke HK. Cerebral venous thrombosis. Combined intrathrombus rtPA and intravenous heparin. Stroke 1999; 30:489–494.
34. Röttger C, Madlener K, Heil M, et al. Is heparin treatment the optimal management for cerebral venous thrombosis? Effect of abciximab, recombinant tissue plasminogen activator, and enoxaparin in experimentally induced superior sagittal sinus thrombosis. Stroke 2005; 36:841–846.
35. Ciccone A, Canhão P, Falcão F, Ferro JM, Sterzi R. Thrombolysis for cerebral vein and dural sinus thrombosis. Cochrane corner. Stroke 2004; 35:2428.

24 | Animal Models of Global Cerebral Ischemia

Thaddeus S. Nowak, Jr., PhD, Professor

Department of Neurology, University of Tennessee, Memphis, Tennessee, USA

INTRODUCTION

Animal models of global cerebral ischemia are designed to replicate consequences of cardiac arrest and resuscitation in humans. As such, they typically involve short insult durations (min to tens of min) that are below the temporal threshold for overt brain infarction. Their relevance to the focal injury that occurs in stroke lies in elucidating intrinsic differences in regional- and cell type-specific vulnerability to ischemia. These models, therefore, provide insight into the continuum of injury that results following transient ischemic events, upon which consequences of longer insults will be superimposed. In this chapter, we will briefly review the pathologies recognized to occur following global cerebral ischemia and consider in detail the optimal use of commonly accepted adult rodent models for their study.

HISTOPATHOLOGY OF GLOBAL ISCHEMIA

The spectrum of brain pathology observed following global ischemic insults has been extensively studied in a range of clinical and experimental conditions (1). Neuron populations throughout the brain represent the major cell type at risk, illustrated in Figure 1 by the distribution of stress response gene induction in a rat model of cardiac arrest (2). A comparatively small subset of these neurons exhibits histopathologic evidence of vulnerability under the experimental conditions of commonly used experimental models.

Loss of hippocampal CA1 neurons is evident in patients who are resuscitated following cardiac arrest (3), and this has long been the most common endpoint examined in rodent studies of transient global ischemia (4–8). The experimental methods have largely evolved to meet the requirements for reproducible study of injury to this cell population. The well-defined and densely packed cell layers in the hippocampus permit straightforward anatomic identification, and the short temporal threshold for CA1 neuronal injury (typically 5–10 min) permits the use of brief experimental insults with low mortality. The most notable feature of this loss is its substantial delay, with the lesion evolving over an interval of several days (5,6). CA1 neuron vulnerability is largely restricted to the dorsal hippocampus, with greater sensitivity of medial CA1/subiculum and decreasing vulnerability more lateral to these structures. (7,9,10). However, the small CA2 region at the CA1/CA3 transition appears to be anatomically contiguous with subiculum (11) and can exhibit comparable vulnerability (9,11,12). A subset of neurons in the dentate hilus is recognized to be impacted earlier (8,13) and at a still lower threshold (7,14,15), sometimes showing loss after even the short 2- to 3-min ischemic insults used to induce CA1 neuronal protection in studies of ischemic preconditioning (14,16). Septal neurons with anatomic connections to CA1 are also vulnerable (8,17), whereas dentate granule (DG) cells and CA3 neurons typically become involved only under severe insult conditions (7).

The thalamic reticular nucleus is another region of recognized pathology in human brain following brief intervals of cardiac arrest (18), with parallels in many animal models (7,17,19–21). Lesions can occur after brief insults and progress surprisingly quickly, showing evidence of irreversible damage within minutes of recirculation (20,22). However, factors that determine the marked variability of reticular nucleus involvement in either clinical or experimental ischemia remain undefined (18).

Cortical neurons become progressively involved with increasing insult duration in animal models (5,7), although the observed injury threshold can vary markedly with experimental conditions (8,23). Injury occurs with a laminar distribution in layers 3, 5, and 6 of the somatosensory

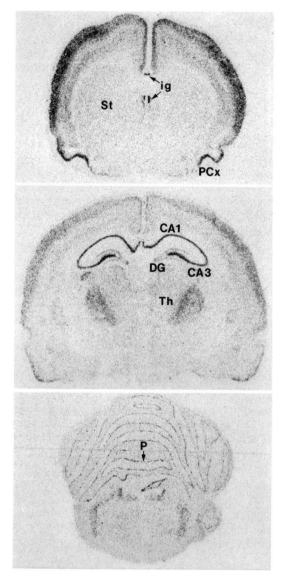

Figure 1 Potential neuron vulnerability identified by a persistent stress response after transient global ischemia. Induction of mRNA encoding the stress protein, hsp72, was detected by *in situ* hybridization in rat brain following 10-min cardiac arrest and 6-hr survival. Sustained expression of hsp72 mRNA is evident in hippocampal CA1 neurons that will undergo subsequent degeneration, as well as in more resistant CA3 neurons (*middle panel*). The mRNA was only transiently expressed in still less vulnerable dentate granule cells, which no longer display robust expression at this time point. Strong expression remains evident in outer layers of the cortical mantle, in which scattered neuronal loss is expected, particularly evident in frontal sections (*upper panel*). Signal is particularly evident in the densely packed cells of prepiriform cortex (PCx) and induseum griseum (ig), the frontal extension of CA3. Insults of this duration remain below the threshold for injury to striatum (St), which shows only weak expression. The Purkinje cell layer (P) exhibits foci of intense signal, consistent with the recognized vulnerability of this neuron population (*lower panel*) (Th, thalamus). *Source*: Adapted from Ref. 2.

cortex (5,8), suggested to be in anatomic relationship with vulnerable regions of striatum (8). Injury to striatum typically occurs after still longer insults (7) but progresses rapidly with a time course of only a few hours (5,8). The vulnerable cells in the striatum include the "medium spiny" projection neurons that comprise as much as 90% of the population in this region (24,25). This component of global ischemic injury is particularly relevant to studies of experimental stroke, as focal ischemia produced by intraluminal filaments often involves comparatively short occlusion times to reduce mortality. Resulting striatal lesions in such cases can reflect the selective loss of these abundant neurons rather than tissue infarction (26,27) and clearly arise via distinct pathophysiologic mechanisms. Delayed damage in the substantia nigra can occur in the weeks following striatal injury (28).

Although not widely evaluated experimentally, postischemic injury to cerebellar Purkinje cells is recognized clinically (1) and was identified in early experimental studies (29). A hindbrain ischemia model specifically targeting cerebellum and brainstem structures identified acute vulnerability of additional cerebellar nuclei prior to any identifiable impact on Purkinje cells (30,31).

Apart from reactive glial responses in regions of neuronal injury, involvement of non-neuron cell types is rarely considered after global ischemia. However, oligodendrocyte injury has been quite extensively studied in developing brain (32,33). Evidence now suggests that oligodendrocytes may constitute the majority of cells that undergo histologically identifiable apoptosis after moderate durations of global ischemia in the adult rat (34,35), accounting for a wave of apoptotic cell death that peaks at 18 to 24 hr that was originally interpreted as neuronal in origin (36). This pathology should receive increasing attention in future studies.

Regions of infarction sometimes appeared in early experimental studies after long durations of global ischemia (7), particularly under conditions of elevated blood glucose (37). Partial ischemia has the potential to produce more severe pathology than a similar duration of complete ischemia, generally considered to reflect the consequences of sustained anaerobic metabolism supported by continued glucose delivery, ultimately resulting in higher lactate production and lower tissue pH (38). Watershed areas can become involved under conditions of globally impaired perfusion during recovery from cardiac arrest (1). Prolonged ischemia was also found in some early studies to result in a "no reflow" phenomenon (39,40), typically associated with more complete stasis during occlusion (41) or reduced blood pressure during early reperfusion (42,43). Even microinfarcts should not be detected after the short insults encountered in current models and, if they do appear, could be considered indicative of poor reperfusion.

GLOBAL ISCHEMIA MODELS

Gerbil Carotid Artery Occlusion

The Mongolian gerbil provides, in principle, the technically simplest global ischemia model. Most gerbils lack robust communication between the carotid and vertebral arteries (44,45), and a significant proportion of the animals shows limited anastomoses between anterior cerebral arteries (46,47). This combination of vascular configurations permits production of unilateral forebrain ischemia by occlusion of a single common carotid artery (47–49), albeit at a success rate of only approximately 40%. Efficacy of unilateral occlusion can be predicted at the time of surgery by the reduction of arterial caliber distal to the occlusion site (50,51) or by behavioral observations after recovery from anesthesia in the case of longer occlusions (45). Study of such unilateral ischemia led to an initial description of the more rapid "maturation" of postischemic neuropathology with increasing insult duration (4). However, this model of hemispheric focal ischemia is now rarely applied. Rather, occlusion of both carotid arteries achieves severe bilateral forebrain ischemia in perhaps 90% of animals, and this has evolved into a widely used model of transient global ischemia (6). Conversely, although little studied, the vascular anatomy of the gerbil also permits production of selective hindbrain ischemia by bilateral occlusion of the vertebral arteries (30,31). Early dye perfusion studies sometimes demonstrated residual filling of forebrain vasculature after carotid artery occlusions (52), but quantitative cerebral blood flow (CBF) estimates are typically at the lower limit of the methodologies (53,54). Therefore, as is the intended result for most contemporary surgical occlusions in rodents, the gerbil is considered to model "severe incomplete" ischemia.

The carotid arteries of the gerbil are more accessible than those of the rat and the surgery itself can be completed in a matter of minutes, but this procedural simplicity is counterbalanced by several complications. A long recognized but sometimes still ignored feature of the gerbil model is the pronounced hyperthermic response (to 39°C or more) that can emerge in postischemic animals during the initial hours of recovery from anesthesia (55), presumably because of effects on hypothalamic signaling. Although sufficiently long insults can produce robust CA1 neuronal loss in the absence of hyperthermia (56,57), amplification of insult severity is apparent after short occlusions (55,58). This almost certainly contributes to the striking neuronal injury sometimes reported following very brief (e.g., 3 min) insults under conditions of aggressive, unmonitored postischemic warming (59). This makes the gerbil model particularly sensitive to artifacts that arise from intervention-induced hypothermia, as treated animals maintained at 37°C could still experience significant cooling relative to an untreated ischemic group. Such hyperthermia can be avoided if animals are maintained under anesthesia through approximately 90-min recirculation (58). The additional effort clearly lessens the convenience of the model, but it is a practical necessity if results in the gerbil are to be compared with those obtained in other species. Temperature issues in model control will be considered more generally below.

Successful ischemia in the gerbil model is determined entirely by the vascular anatomy, which varies considerably among animals (52). Unilateral lesions occur with appreciable frequency (58,60), although such inconsistencies can be identified using electrophysiologic recording approaches (60). Seizure susceptibility has been raised as an issue in this species (61) but is largely a property of specific substrains independent of variations in vascular anatomy that impact ischemia (49). In addition, it has been argued that those seizures observed following forebrain ischemia involve spinal cord, rather than the cortical circuitry implicated in spontaneous seizures (62). A more fundamental disadvantage is that the genomic sequence information and related tools that are increasingly available for mouse and rat remain lacking for the gerbil, which restricts the utility of the model for basic research. Commercially available gerbils are not inbred, although it should be noted that most commonly used rats are also outbred strains. Importantly, with proper temperature control, there appears to be no intrinsic difference in hippocampal CA1 neuronal vulnerability between rats and gerbils (Fig. 2), and the gerbil should therefore continue to be considered a reliable screening tool for intervention studies.

Rat 4-Vessel Occlusion

Unlike gerbils, rats exhibit robust communication between carotid and vertebral arterial supplies to the brain. Therefore, one surgical approach to selective forebrain ischemia in the rat involves permanent cauterization of both vertebral arteries at the level of the first cervical

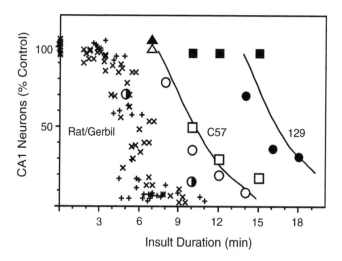

Figure 2 Insult thresholds for hippocampal CA1 neuronal injury in rodent models of global ischemia. The proportion of surviving neurons is plotted against insult duration. Data for rat (x) and gerbil (+) are derived from recent studies that monitored ischemic depolarization to define insult severity for individual hippocampi (60,80), and they demonstrate the comparability of results for the two species. Mice typically exhibit longer insult thresholds, the C57Bl/6 strain (*open symbols*) showing greater vulnerability than the SV129 strain (*closed symbols*). Compatible results have been obtained for insults produced by cardiac arrest (*triangles*) (99), 2-vessel occlusion (VO) (*squares*) (114), and 3-VO (*circles*) (116). One early 3-VO study in mice indicated a threshold consistent with rat and gerbil studies (*half-open circles*) (115), perhaps reflecting more aggressive control of head temperature. Except for the cardiac arrest study, for which data were available on mean depolarization time, mouse results are plotted as group averages, using insult duration defined by occlusion times.

vertebra, followed later by bilateral carotid artery occlusion (63). This 4-vessel occlusion (VO) is typically performed as a 2-stage procedure, allowing a day for recovery following the initial surgery for vertebral cauterization and preparatory isolation of the carotid arteries. Occluding devices are left in place around the carotid arteries to permit their rapid retrieval and occlusion. An early modification of the method led to additional routing of a suture line around the neck musculature, but behind the trachea and major vessels, to be tightened at the time of occlusion to further limit collateral perfusion (64). The standard model involved carotid occlusion in unanesthetized animals under brief restraint, permitting early behavioral evaluation. Criteria for successful occlusion included prompt loss of righting reflex, bilateral pupil dilation, and unresponsiveness to tail pinch. The original 4-VO methodology with described modifications can result in reproducible ischemia, with a success rate of up to 90% of operated animals from the Wistar colony employed (65).

Generally comparable results were noted in a modified method in which carotid occlusions were performed under initial halothane anesthesia (66). However, technical challenges can be associated with vertebral artery cauterization and inconsistencies have been reported (67,68). Alternative approaches have been suggested to improve visual confirmation of vessel disruption (69,70). A 3-VO model has also been developed in which the basilar artery is occluded in place of the vertebral arteries (71). Inter- and intrastrain heterogeneity impact model reproducibility (63,68,72,73), presumably reflecting variations in collateral perfusion, but supplemental neck ligatures have not been systematically applied across laboratories. Some studies in anesthetized animals have alternatively included systemic hypotension (67,74,75), or at least avoidance of pressure increases after carotid artery occlusion (76), to improve insult uniformity. A completely surgical extension of this approach involves a 7-vessel procedure (77) with permanent basilar artery cauterization, temporary clamping of bilateral external carotid, and pterygopalatine arteries to attenuate collateral perfusion, and, finally, carotid artery occlusions.

Long occlusions were initially required to produce a given extent of brain injury after 4-VO (5), undoubtedly reflecting unrecognized protective effects of incidental head cooling (74). Recent applications have used anesthetized animals with epidural temperature control and electrophysiologic monitoring of ischemic depolarization to verify successful occlusion (78–80), considered in detail below. This implementation of the model exhibits a threshold for CA1 neuronal injury identical to that observed in the gerbil (Fig. 2).

Rat 2-Vessel Occlusion

Another widely used approach to an effective global ischemia model in rats combines carotid artery occlusion with systemic hypotension (81,82). An early study that used this method produced what remains one of the more comprehensive histopathologic assessments of ischemic brain injury in the rat (7). The method can be applied in any strain, but most investigators have used Wistar or Sprague-Dawley rats. The main advantage of this approach over the 4-VO model is the relatively straightforward surgery required for carotid artery occlusion and release. However, as originally described, additional procedures are necessary to insert cannulae into the jugular vein and tail artery for blood withdrawal and blood pressure monitoring, respectively, and animals are routinely heparinized, paralyzed, and ventilated. Temperature control of the withdrawn blood is essential to avoid incidental cooling upon reinfusion.

It is relatively easy to achieve reproducible insult severity across rat strains using the 2-VO approach, as the depth of ischemia is dependent on successful blood pressure reduction rather than surgical attenuation of collateral perfusion. Effective ischemia in some animals may require more severe hypotension than initially reported, with 30 mmHg identified as optimal in 2 independent evaluations (83,84). Increasing the halothane level has been suggested by several investigators as an alternative to hypovolemic hypotension (85–87), although this clearly also impacts metabolic rate (88–90). Another noninvasive approach to blood pressure reduction has been proposed, in which external suction is applied to pool blood in the lower body (91), which also avoids the need for heparin administration.

The comparatively robust pathology initially reported after brief insults in the 2-VO model (7) was subsequently attributed to aggressive head warming in the earlier experiments (92) and has been a consistent finding under such conditions (23). However, repeated rectal temperature measurements in this model also demonstrated a prolonged hyperthermia during 1 to 3 days of reperfusion, followed by a gradual recovery of the diurnal temperature rhythm (93). Although delayed, this phenomenon is much more persistent than the response noted in the gerbil and appears to be of pathophysiologic significance. Pharmacologic intervention to blunt the delayed temperature increase was required to maintain long-term protection after an interval of early postischemic hypothermia (93). If this hyperthermic phase should emerge as a general feature of the 2-VO model as applied across laboratories, it must be considered a significant contributor to insult severity and recognized as a potential source of increased sensitivity to interventions that influence temperature regulation.

Cardiac Arrest and Other Methods

Conceptually, the most straightforward approach to global ischemia is cardiac arrest itself, and this is the requisite model if all issues that relate to resuscitation after systemic ischemia are to be investigated. With respect to the study of brain pathology per se, the one advantage of cardiac arrest is that complete and homogeneous ischemia is guaranteed. However, insult durations compatible with survival are short and will vary with the timing of successful resuscitation in individual animals. Nevertheless, it is possible to define the interval of effective ischemia quite precisely with appropriate monitoring approaches (see below). Injection of potassium chloride is a commonly used method to stop the heart, sometimes followed by infusion of donor blood at the time of resuscitation (17). Simultaneous mechanical obstruction of all major cardiac vessels with a hooked device inserted into the chest has been used to induce arrest in a few studies (20,94), with resuscitation accomplished by subsequent ventilation and external chest massage. A similar but less invasive method relies solely on external chest compression to both deflate the lungs and stop the heart (95).

A comprehensive overview of rodent models is included in an earlier review (96). Worth further mention in the present context are those approaches developed to improve occlusion efficacy and reliability. The 3-vessel (71) and 7-vessel occlusions (77) were noted above as conceptual extensions of the 4-VO model. More recently, a 9-VO model has been described (97), which involves initial permanent occlusion of the basilar artery, as well as bilateral pterygopalatine, external carotid, and occipital arteries, with placement of balloon occluders to initiate ischemia by subsequent common carotid artery occlusion. Increased intracranial pressure has been combined with systemic hypotension to produce more complete ischemia during 2-VO (85). Such models can have applications in specific studies that require more profound reductions in CBF (41,98).

Mouse Models

The technical challenges of surgery and physiologic monitoring and control in mice have limited global ischemia studies in this species, but mouse equivalents of the common rodent models have been described. Complete global ischemia can be produced by cardiac arrest, but, in normothermic animals, it fails to result in hippocampal damage (99) or produces only slight injury (100) after insult durations compatible with long-term survival. Another study noted more than 50% CA1 injury after cardiac arrest in Balb/c mice, but comparable loss of the usually resistant DG cells was also reported (101). Very recent work combined body cooling with normothermic or even hyperthermic head temperature during cardiac arrest in an attempt to increase brain injury, while avoiding systemic complications (102,103), but only partial CA1 loss could be achieved.

Bilateral carotid artery occlusion results in strikingly strain-dependent effects (104–108), with greater susceptibility of C57BL/6 and BALB/c strains that, like the gerbil, show frequent insufficiency in communication between carotid and posterior circulations. However, long insults are required to observe neuronal injury in these mouse models, and increasing insult duration produces surprisingly little impact on the extent of hippocampal damage, even with progressive injury to striatum and cortex (106,109), which may be suggestive of incomplete ischemia and/or significant postischemic brain cooling, as will be considered in detail below. Robust CA1 damage has been reported for individual C57BL/6 mice subjected to relatively long (15 min) occlusions that resulted in documented severe perfusion deficits under conditions of maintained head temperature (107). Generally comparable results have been obtained in ventilated animals of the same strain (110,111). An inverse correlation was also noted between histopathologic damage and the extent of posterior communicating artery development for individual hemispheres in CD-1 mice (112).

A model of 2-VO with hypotension has also been established in mice (113,114). Histopathology was strain dependent, with significant damage in C57Bl/6, but not in SV129 mice, despite severe and equivalent CBF reduction demonstrated autoradiographically (114). Surprisingly, the efficacy of carotid artery occlusion alone was identical in the 2 strains, and it was suggested that a smaller caliber basilar artery could have restricted perfusion in the SV129 strain.

The functional equivalent of the rat 4-VO model is a 3-VO method, combining bilateral carotid artery occlusion with targeting of the basilar artery to disrupt the posterior circulation (115,116). An initial study noted striking vulnerability of hippocampal CA1 neurons, essentially equivalent to that occurring in rat and gerbil models, with no difference between C57Bl/6 and SV129 strains (115). More recent results indicate a requirement for longer insult durations and evident strain differences (116), remarkably consistent with reported 2-VO results in mice. Figure 2 shows the comparison of insult thresholds for CA1 damage identified in representative mouse studies with those of rat and gerbil.

Significant inconsistencies in outcome remain among mouse global ischemia models, as well as notable differences in histopathology in comparison with rat and gerbil. For example, in contrast to most other models, cardiac arrest with head hyperthermia results in somewhat more severe damage in SV129 than in C57Bl/6 mice (102). These strains differ in pial vasomotor responses (117), which could conceivably influence brain heat exchange. The greater vulnerability of striatum relative to hippocampus, a frequent finding in mice (102,106,109), precludes straightforward comparison with other rodent models. Mortality is high in many studies, and histology is often assessed at survival times of only a few days. Whether this relative lack of CA1 vulnerability reflects a fundamental biologic difference or a modeling issue (e.g., temperature control or survival time) remains to be determined, but the latter remains likely.

Comparisons with Other Species

The above-described rodent models were an extension of earlier experiences in larger animals, and many such models continue to be used, as recently reviewed (118). Suffice it to point out here that the technical capabilities of large animal models with respect to physiologic monitoring and control (and, more recently, access to *in vivo* imaging) are increasingly applicable to rodent models. Stringent standards of model control, historically more routine in large animals, are recognized to be at least as critical in rodents. The lower cost of purchasing and maintaining small animals, and, in most cases, their greater genetic homogeneity remain important advantages, but the experimental complexity of rodent studies must rival that of large animal experiments to meet rising standards in data reliability.

CONTROL OF MODEL VARIABILITY

Insult Duration

The severity of an ischemic insult is determined by the depth and duration of the perfusion deficit. Because, under optimal conditions, the various rodent models produce severe reductions in forebrain CBF (54,119,120), injury thresholds are almost universally measured with respect to the duration of global ischemia produced. However, even with reproducible surgical occlusions, differences in vascular anatomy can lead to varied efficacy of flow disruption within a given model. Although this is less an issue for ischemia produced by cardiac arrest, the timing of flow restoration upon resuscitation becomes more difficult to assess. Independent measures of insult severity become particularly critical in the context of very short insults, such as those used to induce preconditioning effects (see Chapter 29).

Laser-Doppler perfusion estimates are not sufficiently quantitative to reliably assess whether intraischemic CBF falls below the threshold for energy failure. Electroencephalographic (EEG) assessment of spontaneous neuronal activity, although often applied as an index of successful occlusion, is also an inappropriate measure. The EEG flattens within seconds as tissue oxygen levels fall (121), independent of maintained ATP production by anaerobic glycolysis

(122), and therefore does not discriminate ischemia severity in the range relevant to global ischemia studies. An increasingly applied method relies on the duration of ischemic depolarization as an index of insult severity, as this parameter is closely linked to ATP depletion (123). This approach has been successfully applied in rodent hippocampus (60,78–80,124–129), as well as in striatum (130) and cortex (131,132). As shown for rat hippocampus experiencing 4-VO ischemia (Fig. 3), considerable differences can exist between occlusion and depolarization durations, including extreme cases of hippocampi failing to depolarize. In the face of such heterogeneity, ischemic depolarization provides a robust measure by which to define insult thresholds (Fig. 2).

The technical demands of this approach are substantial but straightforward. Occlusion methods must be compatible with stereotaxic positioning, and electrodes must be sufficiently small and carefully placed to avoid cortical injury, which could otherwise induce spreading depression and associated transcriptional responses (133) and potentially impact blood flow (54). Exposure of the brain surface requires rigorous attention to temperature but, at the same time, provides ready access to an epidural site for the necessary monitoring and control. Anesthesia should be kept to the minimum required, because although an elevated halothane level can reduce blood pressure during ischemia (85–87), it also influences metabolism (88–90) and is of questionable merit as a mechanism to modulate occlusion efficacy. However, the modest hypotensive effect of surgical anesthesia levels may contribute beneficially to the procedure, because a neck ligature has been found unnecessary to achieve a high success rate in the 4-VO model using this approach (80). Most studies thus far have involved spontaneously breathing animals, but ventilation is possible.

As considered below, variations in physiologic parameters, such as temperature and blood glucose, contribute to heterogeneity in all models. To a considerable extent, these variables become factored into assessments of insult severity based on depolarization measurements (134). However, one report suggests that hippocampal damage and depolarization time may become markedly dissociated during hyperglycemic ischemia (135). A converse failure of depolarization monitoring appears to arise in its attempted application to some mouse models, in that very prolonged depolarizations can persist after recirculation following 3-VO in association with only modest CA1 neuronal damage (116). The same group noted prompt repolarization during resuscitation following cardiac arrest in mice (99). It must be concluded that ischemic depolarization provides a powerful index of insult severity in global ischemia models, but it does not eliminate the requirement to monitor and control other variables.

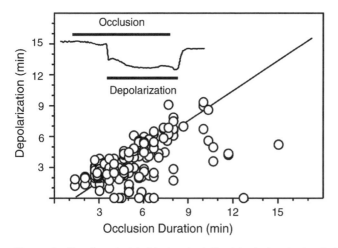

Figure 3 Duration of global ischemia defined by ischemic depolarization versus occlusion time. Rats were subjected to 4-vessel occlusion of the indicated durations, and the interval of resulting ischemic depolarization was recorded in each hippocampus. A representative tracing is illustrated in the inset. Depolarization occurs with a characteristic lag, after which the duration of depolarization is generally well correlated with occlusion time. However, for a given duration of occlusion, the depolarization interval can vary by several minutes, and occasional hippocampi fail to depolarize. *Source*: Ueda M, Nowak TS Jr., unpublished observations.

Temperature

Apart from occlusion efficacy and duration, temperature is the most important variable in studies of global ischemia. The early literature that dealt with temperature effects, particularly hypothermic protection, has been comprehensively reviewed (136). Specific consideration will be given below to the avoidance of confounding factors in rodent models due to temperature changes intrinsic to the experimental procedures. These factors arise via the opposing effects of brain heat loss during ischemia and postischemic hyperthermia that is recognized to occur in specific models, the latter potentially sensitizing the model to protective effects of drug-induced cooling. Persistent lack of attention to these parameters remains the most serious problem in experimental ischemia research (137).

Hypothermia during global ischemia is clearly protective (138–140). A critical observation is that, even with adequate control of body temperature, brain cooling that occurs during global ischemic insults in rodents can itself be sufficient to blunt the resulting injury (74,92,141). The unrecognized contributions of such effects to outcomes of earlier studies undoubtedly varied considerably, depending on the extent to which heat loss from the head had been limited by the type and geometry of any heat sources used to maintain rectal temperature. Although heating may preclude the study of prolonged occlusions (142), avoidance of heat loss is essential if rodent models are to be consistently applied among investigators and compared with studies involving larger animals. Temporalis muscle temperature measurement and control are often used for this purpose (74), but epidural probes provide a better index of brain temperature (143). An added concern is that even when superficial head temperature is maintained, deeper brain structures can lose temperature via respiratory cooling mechanisms, which can only be fully avoided by maintaining a warm, humid environment (144). Under conditions of surface warming alone, the magnitude of temperature drop in striatum was only 1°C during a 15-min interval of 2-VO ischemia (144), but a comparable decline was noted in cortex during only 5-min ischemia in the gerbil (145). Apart from the obvious impact of species mass, variations in ambient temperature could easily contribute to such differences (146). The consistent insult thresholds for rat and gerbil models obtained with epidural temperature control (Fig. 2) and the short occlusion durations required to produce hippocampal pathology argue against the practical need for more aggressive measures if large variations in ambient temperature and humidity are avoided. However, brain regions differ in their sensitivity to temperature change during ischemia (92), and it clearly becomes important to monitor and maintain deep brain temperature if consequences of long insults are to be reliably studied. Although thermocouple wires can be suitable for short-term measurements (147), telemetric methods are best suited to this purpose (145). However, both methods require chronic placement of either a guide cannula or the probe itself, and the interval required for subsequent recovery of brain blood flow and metabolism should be verified in the course of establishing this invasive procedure.

Temperature remains a critical variable following reperfusion and recovery from anesthesia. In the absence of maintained temperature control, rats cool sufficiently during this early postischemic period to influence the threshold for CA1 damage (Fig. 4). However, hippocampal pathology continues to evolve throughout a significant interval after global ischemia, during which outcome remains sensitive to temperature modulation. For example, intraischemic cooling alone was not protective when gerbils were aggressively rewarmed during early recirculation (148). Brief cooling of 20- to 30-min duration initiated at the time of recirculation was not protective in the gerbil when characteristic hyperthermia was subsequently allowed to occur (149). More prolonged postischemic hypothermia confers unequivocal long-term protection (150,151), and cooling is established as a major confound in pharmacologic protection studies that involved global ischemia models (152–154). Conversely, even delayed temperature elevation can worsen injury (155). These issues become particularly significant in view of the intrinsic hyperthermic intervals that characterize gerbil and some rat models (see above). Long-term temperature recording is therefore mandatory in any global ischemia experiment in which outcomes are to be compared between treatment groups. Deep brain temperature remains the gold standard, but the relative merits of brain versus body measurements must be weighed in a given study. Occasional discrepancies between brain and core temperatures have been reported in anesthetized gerbils (57). However, if appropriate measures are taken to minimize brain cooling and avoid substantive dissociation of these parameters during ischemia, core body temperature is probably an adequate endpoint during the postischemic phase of most studies. Repeated measurement of rectal temperature is tedious, provides limited information, and introduces

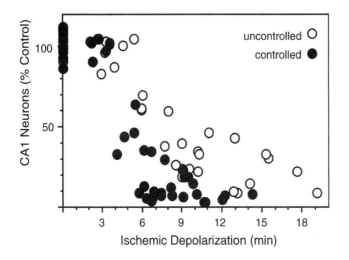

Figure 4 Postischemic temperature maintenance and insult severity. Rats were subjected to 4-vessel occlusion ischemia, producing ischemic depolarizations of varied durations, and CA1 neuronal survival was evaluated at 1 week. All rats experienced rigorous intraischemic control of brain and rectal temperature. In one group, rectal temperature control was maintained through approximately 90-min recirculation (*closed circles*), whereas another group of animals recovered from anesthesia without further temperature control, permitting spontaneous cooling (*open circles*). In the absence of sustained postischemic temperature control, some hippocampi exhibited 30% to 40% neuronal preservation after insults that produced essentially complete CA1 loss in normothermic animals. *Source*: Unpublished observations, Howard EM, Nowak TS Jr. (University of Tennessee at Memphis, Memphis, Tennessee, USA).

additional variables (156,157). Although rectal temperature monitoring may suffice to rule out gross artifact in preliminary work, continuous brain or body telemetry must be the expected standard for a definitive intervention study. Elaborate temperature control measures may become necessary should altered thermoregulation be observed in any treatment context (158).

Heat loss is a particularly critical problem in mouse models. As global ischemia studies in this species evolved comparatively recently, the need for temperature control during ischemia has been well recognized, and independent head temperature control has even been used in attempts to modulate injury (102). However, the 3-VO study in mice that identified an injury threshold comparable to rats and gerbils included brain temperature control (115) and cited the use of elevated ambient air temperature. Studies that demonstrated higher, strain-dependent injury thresholds indicated only maintained head surface temperature (114,116). Whether selective brain cooling can fully account for such differences in vulnerability remains to be established. Neither brain nor body temperature has been monitored for an extended period after global ischemia in mice, but telemetry has demonstrated profound spontaneous cooling after transient focal ischemia (159) and should prove essential in refining the use of this species in global ischemia models as well.

Glucose and Other Physiologic Variables

Elevated blood glucose can worsen global ischemic injury in a number of rodent models (37,113,160–163), and it is an established practice to minimize this potential variability by fasting animals prior to an insult. However, the impact of glucose level is dependent on both insult duration and occlusion efficacy. Hippocampal CA1 neuronal loss after insults of moderate duration in the gerbil appears to be insensitive to the physiologic range of glucose variation between fed and fasted states (138). Pathology can be largely unaffected even by profound hyperglycemia after insults of several minutes' duration in either rats (135) or gerbils (164), although other studies have noted increased striatal injury after occlusions as short as 4 min (165). Importantly, a threshold of approximately 12 mM glucose must be exceeded to exacerbate injury in a standard rat model of 10-min 2-VO plus hypotension (166). This permits the use of normally fed animals in most global ischemia studies, which is a practical necessity in preconditioning paradigms that may involve insults repeated on successive days. To the extent that glucose effects can be attributed to greater acidosis under conditions of sustained substrate delivery (38,167), its potential impact will be minimized in models that involve short, effective occlusions.

Elevated glucose sustains anaerobic metabolism and prolongs the delay in ischemic depolarization (168), which might be expected to reduce the impact of very short occlusions. However, as noted above, a quite surprising report indicated that profound hyperglycemia, sufficient to completely prevent hippocampal depolarization during brief ischemia, nevertheless permitted detectable CA1 loss to occur (135). This would imply that neuronal damage could occur in the absence of overt ion fluxes associated with ischemic depolarization. A lingering technical concern is that different groups of animals were used to generate the physiologic and pathologic data in that study, and any differential cooling that might have occurred during the brain exposure necessary for physiologic recording would not have been present in the histopathology group. Nevertheless, this remains an intriguing observation, and the extent to which differences in blood glucose may contribute to the small residual heterogeneity in outcome in depolarization-monitored studies remains to be fully investigated.

Global ischemia models are relatively insensitive to variations in blood gases. Extreme hypercapnia can worsen ischemic injury when associated with reductions in pH comparable to those observed during hyperglycemic ischemia (169). Moderately reduced oxygenation has been observed to attenuate pharmacologic protection in one study (138).

In summary, modest variations in glucose and blood gases appear to have comparatively little impact under the conditions of severe CBF reduction and short insult duration that characterize current global ischemia models. No difficulties have been encountered with the use of fed, spontaneously respiring animals to define consistent depolarization thresholds for hippocampal injury in rats and gerbils (60,79,80). Nevertheless, it remains good practice to establish the impact of physiologic variables on outcome under specific conditions of model usage.

Survival Time

It has long been recognized that neuron populations differ with respect to the time course of detectable injury, with relatively rapid progression in striatum and cortex (5) but characteristic delayed neuronal death in the CA1 region of hippocampus (4–6,170,171). Most other vulnerable neuron populations that have been examined in any detail, e.g., dentate hilus (5,7) and thalamic reticular nucleus (7,20), also show overt damage within 1 day or less. Factors affecting the timing of cell loss have therefore been extensively studied for CA1 neurons. The rate at which pathology evolves can be influenced by the severity of the initial insult, as suggested by observations that the "maturation" of CA1 neuronal damage is more rapid after ischemic insults of longer duration in the gerbil (4). A reexamination of the issue in the rat supported the same conclusion, showing maximal damage within 3 days after long occlusions (15 or 30 min), at which time animals subjected to 5-min ischemia had achieved approximately half of their eventual CA1 neuronal loss (172). Some studies have made specific use of short insults and efforts to avoid hyperthermia to produce a model that exhibits slow CA1 degeneration in the gerbil (173). However, this is not a particularly robust phenomenon, and recent experiments have identified negligible change in the depolarization threshold for CA1 injury in rats evaluated at survival times of 1 week or longer (80).

In contrast, a 1-week survival interval is not sufficient in the context of protection studies. Adrenalectomy slowed, but did not prevent, the evolution of hippocampal damage in a gerbil model (174). Similarly, an acute ischemic preconditioning protocol demonstrated protection at 3 days that was lost by 1 week (175). Brief postischemic cooling that was protective at 3-day survival (176) showed some residual attenuation of injury at 1 week that was completely lost by 2 months (177). Progressive neuronal loss was suggested to occur over many weeks in preconditioned animals (178,179), and this has been rigorously confirmed in recent depolarization-monitored studies in both gerbils (6) and rats (80). Although sustained lesion evolution between 1 and 3 months was suggested in previously preconditioned rats, injury progress occurred most markedly between 1 and 2 weeks (80). Available results therefore suggest a minimum standard of 2-week survival for future intervention studies.

Increased neurogenesis occurs in the dentate gyrus after global ischemia in gerbils (180,181), and some evidence suggests that proliferating cells can also be found in CA1 (182). However, long-term evaluations of hippocampal morphology after ischemia have typically shown either no change in the CA1 neuron population (183) or very small increases in neuronal density that may correlate with overall tissue shrinkage (184). However, one report described detectable CA1 repopulation at long survival intervals after severe ischemia in a rat model of

4-VO plus hypotension that becomes more robust with supplementary growth factor treatments (75). CA1 neuronal recovery by 3 months was also suggested in a more variable 2-VO model (185), and very recently, striking increases in CA1 neuron number were described by 90 days in a 2-VO model using halothane-induced hypotension (186). In contrast, it is certain that no such recovery occurs within the same interval after depolarization-monitored 4-VO (80). Resolution of the sources of variability underlying these conflicting observations requires a new generation of very long-term survival studies, for which highly controlled and predictable models will be essential.

CONCLUSIONS AND FUTURE DIRECTIONS

Proper application of global ischemia models requires considerable attention to procedural details. Rigorous temperature control and monitoring during both intraischemic and early postischemic intervals is essential for even the most rudimentary experiment, and continuous temperature telemetry should be the requirement for a definitive intervention study. Survival times of at least 2 weeks must be the standard for evaluations of delayed hippocampal neuronal injury in such protection experiments. Electrophysiologic assessment of ischemic depolarization, although invasive and time consuming, provides a quantitative index of insult severity that identifies model inconsistencies and markedly reduces the number of animals required to draw firm conclusions. Applying current standards of monitoring and control, widely used rat and gerbil models demonstrate strikingly concordant thresholds for hippocampal neuronal damage. However, no mouse model yet meets the standards of robust injury and reproducibility that have been achieved in other rodents, and further progress is needed on this front to take full advantage of genetic resources.

REFERENCES

1. Auer RN, Sutherland GR. Hypoxia and related conditions. In: Graham DI, Lantos PL, eds. Greenfield's Neuropathology. Vol. 1. 7th ed. Arnold: London, 2002:233–280.
2. Saito N, Kawai K, Nowak TS Jr. Reexpression of developmentally regulated MAP2c mRNA after ischemia: colocalization with hsp72 mRNA in vulnerable neurons. J Cereb Blood Flow Metab 1995; 15:205–215.
3. Petito C, Feldmann E, Pulsinelli W, et al. Delayed hippocampal damage in humans following cardio-respiratory arrest. Neurology 1987; 37:1281–1286.
4. Ito U, Spatz M, Walker JT Jr., et al. Experimental cerebral ischemia in Mongolian gerbils. I. Light microscopic observations. Acta Neuropathol (Berl) 1975; 32:209–223.
5. Pulsinelli WA, Brierley JB, Plum F. Temporal profile of neuronal damage in a model of transient forebrain ischemia. Ann Neurol 1982; 11:491–498.
6. Kirino T. Delayed neuronal death in the gerbil hippocampus following ischemia. Brain Res 1982; 239:57–69.
7. Smith M-L, Auer RN, Siesjo BK. The density and distribution of ischemic brain injury in the rat following 2–10 min of forebrain ischemia. Acta Neuropathol (Berl) 1984; 64:319–332.
8. Crain BJ, Westerkam WD, Harrison AH, et al. Selective neuronal death after transient forebrain ischemia in the Mongolian gerbil: a silver impregnation study. Neuroscience 1988; 27:387–402.
9. Hatakeyama T, Matsumoto M, Brengman JM, et al. Immunohistochemical investigation of ischemic and postischemic damage after bilateral carotid occlusion in gerbils. Stroke 1988; 19:1526–1534.
10. Iwai T, Hara A, Niwa M, et al. Temporal profile of nuclear DNA fragmentation in situ in gerbil hippocampus following transient forebrain ischemia. Brain Res 1995; 671:305–308.
11. Yoshimi K, Takeda M, Nishimura T, et al. An immunohistochemical study of MAP2 and clathrin in gerbil hippocampus after cerebral ischemia. Brain Res 1991; 560:149–158.
12. Iwai T, Niwa M, Hara A, et al. DNA fragmentation in the CA2 sector of gerbil hippocampus following transient forebrain ischemia. Brain Res 2000; 857:275–278.
13. Johansen FF, Zimmer J, Diemer NH. Early loss of somatostatin neurons in dentate hilus after cerebral ischemia in the rat precedes CA1 pyramidal loss. Acta Neuropathol (Berl) 1987; 73:110–114.
14. Matsuyama T, Tsuchiyama M, Nakamura H, et al. Hilar somatostatin neurons are more vulnerable to an ischemic insult than CA1 pyramidal neurons. J Cereb Blood Flow Metab 1993; 13:229–234.

15. Sugimoto A, Shozuhara H, Kogure K, et al. Exposure to sub-lethal ischemia failed to prevent subsequent ischemic death of dentate hilar neurons, as estimated by laminin immunohistochemistry. Brain Res 1993; 629:159–162.

16. Nishino K, Nowak TS Jr. Time course and cellular distribution of hsp27 and hsp72 stress protein expression in a quantitative gerbil model of ischemic injury and tolerance: thresholds for hsp72 induction and hilar lesioning in the context of ischemic preconditioning. J Cereb Blood Flow Metab 2004; 24:167–178.

17. Blomqvist P, Wieloch T. Ischemic brain damage in rats following cardiac arrest using a long-term recovery model. J Cereb Blood Flow Metab 1985; 5:420–431.

18. Ross DT, Graham DI. Selective loss and selective sparing of neurons in the thalamic reticular nucleus following human cardiac arrest. J Cereb Blood Flow Metab 1993; 13:558–567.

19. Ross DT, Duhaime AC. Degeneration of neurons in the thalamic reticular nucleus following transient ischemia due to raised intracranial pressure: excitotoxic degeneration mediated via non-NMDA receptors? Brain Res 1989; 501:129–143.

20. Kawai K, Nitecka L, Ruetzler CA, et al. Global cerebral ischemia associated with cardiac arrest in the rat: I. Dynamics of early neuronal changes. J Cereb Blood Flow Metab 1992; 12:238–249.

21. Kawai K, Nowak TS Jr., Klatzo I. Loss of parvalbumin immunoreactivity defines selectively vulnerable thalamic reticular nucleus neurons following cardiac arrest in the rat. Acta Neuropathol 1995; 89:262–269.

22. Kawai K, Nakayama H, Tamura A. Limited but significant protective effect of hypothermia on ultraearly-type ischemic neuronal injury in the thalamus. J Cereb Blood Flow Metab 1997; 17:543–552.

23. Kobayashi S, Harris VA, Welsh FA. Spreading depression induces tolerance of cortical neurons to ischemia in rat brain. J Cereb Blood Flow Metab 1995; 15:721–727.

24. Chesselet M-F, Gonzales C, Lin C-S, et al. Ischemic damage in the striatum of adult gerbils: relative sparing of somatostatinergic and cholinergic interneurons contrasts with loss of efferent neurons. Exp Neurol 1990; 110:209–218.

25. Meade CA, Figueredo-Cardenas G, Fusco F, et al. Transient global ischemia in rats yields striatal projection neuron and interneuron loss resembling that in Huntington's disease. Exp Neurol 2000; 166:307–323.

26. Korematsu K, Goto S, Nagahiro S, et al. Changes of immunoreactivity for synaptophysin ('protein p38') following a transient cerebral ischemia in the rat striatum. Brain Res 1993; 616:320–324.

27. Katchanov J, Waeber C, Gertz K, et al. Selective neuronal vulnerability following mild focal brain ischemia in the mouse. Brain Pathol 2003; 13:452–464.

28. Volpe BT, Blau AD, Wessel TC, et al. Delayed histopathological neuronal damage in the substantia nigra compacta (nucleus A9) after transient forebrain ischemia. Neurobiol Dis 1995; 2:119–127.

29. Diemer NH, Siemkovicz E. Regional neurone damage after cerebral ischemia in the normo- and hypoglycemic rat. Neuropathol Appl Neurobiol 1981; 7:217–227.

30. Hata R, Matsumoto M, Hatakeyama T, et al. Differential vulnerability in the hindbrain neurons and local cerebral blood flow during bilateral vertebral occlusion in gerbils. Neuroscience 1993; 56:423–439.

31. Hata R, Matsumoto M, Kitagawa K, et al. A new gerbil model of hindbrain ischemia by extracranial occlusion of the bilateral verterbral arteries. J Neurol Sci 1994; 121:79–89.

32. Kinney HC, Duncan Armstrong D. Perinatal neuropathology. In: Graham DI, Lantos PL, eds. Greenfield's Neuropathology. Vol. 1. 7th ed. Arnold: London, 2002:519–606.

33. Back SA, Han BH, Luo NL, et al. Selective vulnerability of late oligodendrocyte progenitors to hypoxia-ischemia. J Neurosci 2002; 22:455–463.

34. Petito CK, Torres-Munoz J, Roberts B, et al. DNA fragmentation follows delayed neuronal death in CA1 neurons exposed to transient global ischemia. J Cereb Blood Flow Metab 1997; 17:967–976.

35. Petito CK, Olarte J-P, Roberts B, et al. Selective glial vulnerability following transient global ischemia in rat brain. J Neuropathol Exp Neurol 1998; 57:231–238.

36. Schmidt-Kastner R, Fliss H, Hakim AM. Subtle neuronal death in striatum after short forebrain ischemia in rats detected by in situ end-labeling for DNA damage. Stroke 1997; 28:163–170.

37. Pulsinelli WA, Waldman S, Rawlinson D, et al. Moderate hyperglycemia augments ischemic brain damage: a neuropathological study in the rat. Neurology 1982; 32:1239–1246.

38. Rehncrona S, Rosén I, Siesjö BK. Brain lactic acidosis and ischemic brain damage: 1. Biochemistry and neurophysiology. J Cereb Blood Flow Metab 1981; 1:297–311.

39. Ames A III, Wright RL, Kowada M, et al. Cerebral ischemia. II. The no-reflow phenomenon. Am J Pathol 1968; 52:437–453.

40. Kågström E, Smith M-L, Siesjö BK. Local cerebral blood flow in the recovery period following complete cerebral ischemia in the rat. J Cereb Blood Flow Metab 1983; 3:170–182.

41. Dietrich WD, Busto R, Yoshida S, et al. Histopathological and hemodynamic consequences of complete versus incomplete ischemia in the rat. J Cereb Blood Flow Metab 1987; 7:300–308.

42. Ito U, Ohno K, Yamaguchi T, et al. Transient appearance of "no-reflow" phenomenon in Mongolian gerbils. Stroke 1980; 11:517–521.

43. Bottiger BW, Krumnikl JJ, Gass P, et al. The cerebral 'no-reflow' phenomenon after cardiac arrest in rats—influence of low-flow reperfusion. Resuscitation 1997; 34:79–87.

44. Levine S, Sohn D. Cerebral ischemia in infant and adult gerbils. Relation to incomplete circle of Willis. Arch Pathol 1969; 87:315–317.

45. Kahn K. The natural course of experimental cerebral infarction in the gerbil. Neurology 1972; 22:510–515.

46. Harrison MJG, Brownbill D, Lewis PD, et al. Cerebral edema following carotid artery ligation in the gerbil. Arch Neurol 1973; 28:389–391.

47. Berry K, Wisniewski HM, Svarzbein L, et al. On the relationship of brain vasculature to production of neurological deficit and morphological changes following acute unilateral common carotid artery ligation in gerbils. J Neurol Sci 1975; 25:75–92.

48. Levine S, Payan H. Effects of ischemia and other procedures on the brain and retina of the gerbil (*Meriones unguiculatus*). Exp Neurol 1966; 16:255–262.

49. Donadio MF, Kozlowski PB, Kaplan H, et al. Brain vasculature and induced ischemia in seizure-prone and non-seizure-prone gerbils. Brain Res 1982; 234:263–273.

50. Matsumoto M, Hatakeyama T, Akai F, et al. Prediction of stroke before and after unilateral occlusion of the common carotid artery in the gerbil. Stroke 1988; 19:490–497.

51. Kitagawa K, Matsumoto M, Handa N, et al. Prediction of stroke-prone gerbils and their cerebral circulation. Brain Res 1989; 479:263–269.

52. Levy DE, Brierley JB. Communications between vertebro-basilar and carotid arterial circulations in the gerbil. Exp Neurol 1974; 45:503–508.

53. Crockard A, Iannotti F, Hunstock AT, et al. Cerebral blood flow and edema following carotid occlusion in the gerbil. Stroke 1980; 11:494–498.

54. Tomida S, Wagner HG, Klatzo I, et al. Effect of acute electrode placement on regional CBF in the gerbil: a comparison of blood flow measured by hydrogen clearance, [^{3}H]nicotine, and [^{14}C]iodoantipyrine techniques. J Cereb Blood Flow Metab 1989; 9:79–86.

55. Kuroiwa T, Bonnekoh P, Hossmann K-A. Prevention of postischemic hyperthermia prevents ischemic injury of CA_1 neurons in gerbils. J Cereb Blood Flow Metab 1990; 10:550–556.

56. Welsh FA, Harris VA. Postischemic hypothermia fails to reduce ischemic injury in gerbil hippocampus. J Cereb Blood Flow Metab 1991; 11:617–620.

57. Colbourne F, Nurse SM, Corbett D. Spontaneous postischemic hyperthermia is not required for severe CA1 ischemic damage in gerbils. Brain Res 1993; 623:1–5.

58. Suga S, Nowak TS Jr. Postischemic hyperthermia increases expression of hsp72 mRNA after brief ischemia in the gerbil. Neurosci Lett 1998; 243:57–60.

59. Mitani A, Andou Y, Masuda S, et al. Transient forebrain ischemia of three-minute duration consistently induces severe neuronal damage in field CA1 of the hippocampus in the normothermic gerbil. Neurosci Lett 1991; 131:171–174.

60. Abe H, Nowak TS Jr. Induced hippocampal neuroprotection in an optimized gerbil ischemia model: Insult thresholds for tolerance induction and altered gene expression defined by ischemic depolarization. J Cereb Blood Flow Metab 2004; 24:84–97.

61. Brown AW, Levy DE, Kublik M, et al. Selective chromatolysis of neurons in the gerbil brain: a possible consequence of "epileptic" activity produced by common carotid artery occlusion. Ann Neurol 1979; 5:127–138.

62. Cohn R. Convulsive activity in gerbils subjected to cerebral ischemia. Exp Neurol 1979; 65:391–397.

63. Pulsinelli WA, Brierley JB. A new model of bilateral hemispheric ischemia in the unanesthetized rat. Stroke 1979; 10:267–272.

64. Pulsinelli WA, Duffy TE. Regional energy balance in rat brain after transient forebrain ischemia. J Neurochem 1983; 40:1500–1503.

65. Pulsinelli WA, Buchan AM. The four-vessel occlusion rat model: method for complete occlusion of vertebral arteries and control of collateral circulation. Stroke 1988; 19:913–914.

66. Schmidt-Kastner R, Paschen W, Grosse Ophoff B, et al. A modified four-vessel occlusion model for inducing incomplete forebrain ischemia in rats. Stroke 1989; 20:938–946.

67. Furlow TW Jr. Cerebral ischemia produced by four-vessel occlusion in the rat: a quantitative evaluation of cerebral blood flow. Stroke 1982; 13:852–855.

68. Blomqvist P, Mabe H, Ingvar M, et al. Models for studying long-term recovery following forebrain ischemia in the rat. 1. Circulatory and functional effects of 4-vessel occlusion. Acta Neurol Scand 1984; 69:376–384.

69. Todd NV, Picozzi P, Crockard HA, et al. Recirculation after cerebral ischemia. Simultaneous measurement of cerebral bloodflow, brain edema, cerebrovascular permeability and cortical EEG in the rat. Acta Neurol Scand 1986; 74:269–278.

70. Sugio K, Horigome N, Sakaguchi T, et al. A model of bilateral hemispheric ischemia—modified four-vessel occlusion in rats. Stroke 1988; 19:922.

71. Kameyama M, Suzuki J, Shirane R, et al. A new model of bilateral hemispheric ischemia in the rat—three vessel occlusion model. Stroke 1985; 16:489–493.
72. Pulsinelli WA, Levy DE, Duffy TE. Cerebral blood flow in the four-vessel occlusion rat model [Letter]. Stroke 1983; 14:832–833.
73. Furlow TW Jr. Cerebral blood flow in the four-vessel occlusion rat model [Letter]. Stroke 1983; 14:833–834.
74. Busto R, Dietrich WD, Globus MY-T, et al. Small differences in intraischemic brain temperature critically determine the extent of ischemic neuronal injury. J Cereb Blood Flow Metab 1987; 7:729–738.
75. Nakatomi H, Kuriu T, Okabe S, et al. Regeneration of hippocampal pyramidal neurons after ischemic brain injury by recruitment of endogenous neural progenitors. Cell 2002; 110:429–441.
76. Alps BJ, Hass WK. The potential beneficial effect of nicardipine in a rat model of transient forebrain ischemia. Neurology 1987; 37:809–814.
77. Shirane R, Shimizu H, Kameyama M, et al. A new method for producing temporary complete cerebral ischemia in rats. J Cereb Blood Flow Metab 1991; 11:949–956.
78. Xu ZC, Pulsinelli WA. Responses of CA1 pyramidal neurons in rat hippocampus to transient forebrain ischemia: an in vivo intracellular recording study. Neurosci Lett 1994; 171:187–191.
79. Halaby IA, Takeda Y, Yufu K, et al. Depolarization thresholds for hippocampal damage, ischemic preconditioning, and changes in gene expression after global ischemia in the rat. Neurosci Lett 2004; 372:12–16.
80. Ueda M, Nowak TS Jr. Protective preconditioning by transient global ischemia in the rat. Components of delayed injury progression and lasting protection distinguished by comparisons of depolarization thresholds for cell loss at long survival times. J Cereb Blood Flow Metab 2005; 25:949–958.
81. Eklöf B, Siesjö BK. The effect of bilateral carotid artery ligation upon the blood flow and energy state of the rat brain. Acta Physiol Scand 1972; 86:155–165.
82. Smith M-L, Bendek G, Dahlgren N, et al. Models for studying long-term recovery following forebrain ischemia in the rat. 2. A 2-vessel occlusion model. Acta Neurol Scand 1984; 69:385–401.
83. Gionet TX, Warner DS, Verhaegen M, et al. Effects of intra-ischemic blood pressure on outcome from 2-vessel occlusion forebrain ischemia in the rat. Brain Res 1992; 586:188–194.
84. Sugawara T, Kawase M, Lewén A, et al. Effect of hypotension severity on hippocampal CA1 neurons in a rat global ischemia model. Brain Res 2000; 877:281–287.
85. Yoshida S, Busto R, Martinez E, et al. Regional brain energy metabolism after complete versus incomplete ischemia in the rat in the absence of severe lactic acidosis. J Cereb Blood Flow Metab 1985; 5:490–501.
86. McBean DE, Winters V, Wilson AD, et al. Neuroprotective efficacy of lifarizine (RS-87476) in a simplified rat survival model of 2-vessel occlusion. Br J Pharmacol 1995; 116:3093–3098.
87. Bendel O, Alkass K, Bueters T, et al. Reproducible loss of CA1 neurons following carotid artery occlusion combined with halothane-induced hypotension. Brain Res 2005; 1033:135–142.
88. Brunner EA, Passonneau JV, Molstad C. The effect of volatile anaesthetics on level of metabolites and on metabolic rate in brain. J Neurochem 1971; 18:2301–2316.
89. Harp JR, Nilsson L, Siesjö BK. The effect of halothane anesthesia upon cerebral oxygen consumption in the rat. Acta Anesthesiol Scand 1976; 20:83–90.
90. Keykhah MM, Welsh FA, Harp JR. Cerebral energy levels during trimethaphan-induced hypotension in the rat: effects of light versus deep halothane anesthesia. Anesthesiology 1979; 50:36–39.
91. Dirnagl U, Thorén P, Villringer A, et al. Global forebrain ischemia in the rat: controlled reduction of cerebral blood flow by hypobaric hypotension and two-vessel occlusion. Neurol Res 1993; 15:128–130.
92. Minamisawa H, Nordström C-H, Smith M-L, et al. The influence of mild body and brain hypothermia on ischemic brain damage. J Cereb Blood Flow Metab 1990; 10:365–374.
93. Coimbra C, Drake M, Boris-Möller F, et al. Long-lasting neuroprotective effect of postischemic hypothermia and treatment with an anti-inflammatory/antipyretic drug. Evidence for chronic encephalopathic processes following ischemia. Stroke 1996; 27:1578–1585.
94. Pluta R, Lossinsky AS, Mossakowski MJ, et al. Reassessment of a new model of complete cerebral ischemia in rats. Acta Neuropathol 1991; 83:1–11.
95. Reid KH, Young C, Schurr A, et al. Audiogenic seizures following global ischemia induced by chest compression in Long-Evans rats. Epilepsy Res 1996; 23:195–209.
96. Ginsberg MD, Busto R. Rodent models of global ischemia. Stroke 1989; 20:1627–1642.
97. Melgar MA, Park H, Rafols JA, et al. A model of global forebrain ischemia/reperfusion in the awake rat. Neurol Res 2002; 24:97–106.
98. Phillis JW, Perkins LM, Smith-Barbour M, et al. Transmitter amino acid release from rat neocortex: complete versus incomplete ischemia models. Neurochem Res 1994; 19:1387–1392.
99. Kawahara N, Kawai K, Toyoda T, et al. Cardiac arrest cerebral ischemia model in mice failed to cause delayed neuronal death in the hippocampus. Neurosci Lett 2002; 322:91–94.
100. Böttiger BW, Teschendorf P, Krumnikl JJ, et al. Global cerebral ischemia due to cardiocirculatory arrest in mice causes neuronal degeneration and early induction of transcription factors in the hippocampus. Mol Brain Res 1999; 65:135–142.

101. Mizushima H, Zhou CJI, Dohi K, et al. Reduced postischemic apoptosis in the hippocampus of mice deficient in interleukin-1. J Comp Neurol 2002; 448:203–216.
102. Kofler J, Hattori K, Sawada M, et al. Histopathological and behavioral characterization of a novel model of cardiac arrest and cardiopulmonary resuscitation in mice. J Neurosci Meth 2004; 136:33–44.
103. Neigh GN, Kofler J, Meyers JL, et al. Cardiac arrest/cardiopulmonary resuscitation increases anxiety-like behavior and decreases social interaction. J Cereb Blood Flow Metab 2004; 24:372–382.
104. Barone FC, Knudsen DJ, Nelson AH, et al. Mouse strain differences in susceptibility to cerebral ischemia are related to vascular anatomy. J Cereb Blood Flow Metab 1993; 13:683–692.
105. Yang G, Kitagawa K, Matsushita K, et al. C57BL/6 strain is most susceptible to cerebral ischemia following bilateral common carotid artery occlusion among seven mouse strains: selective neuronal death in the murine transient forebrain ischemia. Brain Res 1997; 752:209–218.
106. Fujii M, Hara H, Meng W, et al. Strain-related differences in susceptibility to transient forebrain ischemia in SV-129 and C57Black/6 mice. Stroke 1997; 28:1805–1811.
107. Kitagawa K, Matsumoto M, Yang G, et al. Cerebral ischemia after bilateral carotid artery occlusion and intraluminal suture occlusion in mice: evaluation of the patency of the posterior communicating artery. J Cereb Blood Flow Metab 1998; 18:570–579.
108. Tsuchiya D, Hong SJ, Won Suh S, et al. Mild hypothermia reduces zinc translocation, neuronal cell death, and mortality after transient global ischemia in mice. J Cereb Blood Flow Metab 2002; 22:1231–1238.
109. Terashima T, Namura S, Hoshimaru M, et al. Consistent injury in the striatum of C57BL/6 mice after transient bilateral common carotid artery occlusion. Neurosurgery 1998; 43:900–908.
110. Olsson T, Hansson O, Nylandsted J, et al. Lack of neuroprotection by heat shock protein 70 over-expression in a mouse model of global cerebral ischemia. Exp Brain Res 2004; 154:442–449.
111. Olsson T, Wieloch T, Smith M-L. Brain damage in a mouse model of global cerebral ischemia. Effect of NMDA receptor blockade. Brain Res 2003; 982:260–269.
112. Murakami K, Kondo T, Kawase M, et al. The development of a new mouse model of global ischemia: focus on the relationships between ischemia duration, anesthesia, cerebral vasculature, and neuronal injury following global ischemia in mice. Brain Res 1998; 780:304–310.
113. Sheng H, Laskowitz DT, Pearlstein RD, et al. Characterization of a recovery global cerebral ischemia model in the mouse. J Neurosci Meth 1999; 88:103–109.
114. Wellons JC III, Sheng H, Laskowitz DT, et al. A comparison of strain-related susceptibility in two murine recovery models of global cerebral ischemia. Brain Res 2000; 868:14–21.
115. Panahian N, Yoshida T, Huang PL, et al. Attenuated hippocampal damage after global cerebral ischemia in mice mutant in neuronal nitric oxide synthase. Neuroscience 1996; 72:343–354.
116. Yonekura I, Kawahara N, Nakatomi H, et al. A model of global ischemia in C57 BL/6 mice. J Cereb Blood Flow Metab 2004; 24:151–158.
117. Meng W, Ayata C, Waeber C, et al. Neuronal NOS-cGMP-dependent Ach-induced relaxation in pial arterioles of endothelial NOS knockout mice. Am J Physiol 1998; 274:H411–H415.
118. Traystman RJ. Animal models of focal and global cerebral ischemia. ILAR J 2003; 44:85–95.
119. Pulsinelli WA, Levy DE, Duffy TE. Regional cerebral blood flow and glucose metabolism following transient forebrain ischemia. Ann Neurol 1982; 11:499–509.
120. Kågström E, Smith M-L, Siesjö BK. Recirculation in the rat brain following incomplete ischemia. J Cereb Blood Flow Metab 1983; 3:183–192.
121. Fleidervish IA, Gebhardt C, Astman N, et al. Enhanced spontaneous transmitter release is the earliest consequence of neocortical hypoxia that can explain the disruption of normal circuit function. J Neurosci 2001; 21:4600–4608.
122. Raffin CN, Harrison MA, Sick TJ, et al. EEG suppression and anoxic depolarization: Influences on cerebral oxygenation during ischemia. J Cereb Blood Flow Metab 1991; 11:407–415.
123. Ekholm A, Katsura K, Siesjö BK. Coupling of energy failure and dissipative K^+ flux during ischemia: role of preischemic plasma and glucose concentration. J Cereb Blood Flow Metab 1993; 13:193–200.
124. Xu ZC, Pulsinelli WA. Electrophysiological changes of CA1 pyramidal neurons following transient forebrain ischemia: an in vivo intracellular recording and staining study. J Neurophysiol 1996; 76:1689–1697.
125. Abe H, Nowak TS Jr. Gene expression and induced ischemic tolerance following brief insults. Acta Neurobiol Exp 1996; 56:3–8.
126. Bart RD, Takaoka S, Pearlstein RD, et al. Interactions between hypothermia and the latency to ischemic depolarization: implications for neuroprotection. Anesthesiology 1998; 88:1266–1273.
127. Sorimachi T, Abe H, Takeuchi S, et al. Neuronal damage in gerbils caused by intermittent forebrain ischemia. J Neurosurg 1999; 91:835–842.
128. Sorimachi T, Abe H, Takeuchi S, et al. Ischemic depolarization monitoring: evaluation of protein synthesis in the hippocampal CA1 after brief unilateral ischemia in a gerbil model. J Neurosurg 2002; 97:104–111.
129. Sorimachi T, Nowak TS Jr. Pharmacological manipulations of ATP–dependent potassium channels and adenosine A1 receptors do not impact hippocampal ischemic preconditioning *in vivo*: evidence in a highly quantitative gerbil model. J Cereb Blood Flow Metab 2004; 24:556–563.

130. Xu ZC. Neurophysiological changes of spiny neurons in rat neostriatum after transient forebrain ischemia: an *in vivo* intracellular recording and staining study. Neuroscience 1995; 67:823–836.

131. Kaminogo M, Suyama K, Ichikura A, et al. Anoxic depolarization determines ischemic brain injury. Neurol Res 1998; 20:343–348.

132. Li J, Takeda Y, Hirakawa M. Threshold of ischemic depolarization for neuronal injury following four-vessel occlusion in the rat cortex. J Neurosurg Anesthesiol 2000; 12:247–254.

133. Belluardo N, Mudo G, Dell'Albani P, et al. NMDA receptor-dependent and -independent immediate early gene expression induced by focal mechanical brain injury. Neurochem Int 1995; 26:443–453.

134. Katsura K, Minamisawa H, Ekholm A, et al. Changes of labile metabolites during anoxia in moderately hypothermic and hyperthermic rats: correlation to membrane fluxes of K^+. Brain Res 1992; 590:6–12.

135. Li P-A, Kristián T, Shamloo M, et al. Effects of preischemic hyperglycemia on brain damage incurred by rats subjected to 2.5 or 5 minutes of forebrain ischemia. Stroke 1996; 27:1592–1602.

136. Colbourne F, Sutherland G, Corbett D. Postischemic hypothermia. A critical appraisal with implications for clinical treatment. Mol Neurobiol 1997; 14:171–201.

137. DeBow SB, Clark DL, MacLellan CL, et al. Incomplete assessment of experimental cytoprotectants in rodent ischemia studies. Can J Neurol Sci 2003; 30:368–374.

138. Clifton GL, Taft WC, Blair RE, et al. Conditions for pharmacological evaluation in the gerbil model of forebrain ischemia. Stroke 1989; 20:1545–1552.

139. Welsh FA, Sims RE, Harris VA. Mild hypothermia prevents ischemic injury in gerbil hippocampus. J Cereb Blood Flow Metab 1990; 10:557–563.

140. Mitani A, Kataoka K. Critical levels of extracellular glutamate mediating gerbil hippocampal delayed neuronal death during hypothermia: brain microdialysis study. Neuroscience 1991; 42:661–670.

141. Freund TF, Buzsáki G, Leon A, et al. Hippocampal cell death following ischemia: effects of brain temperature and anesthesia. Exp Neurol 1990; 108:251–260.

142. Miyazawa T, Bonnekoh P, Widmann R, et al. Heating of the brain to maintain normothermia during ischemia aggravates brain injury in the rat. Acta Neuropathol 1993; 85:488–494.

143. Miyazawa T, Hossmann K-A. Methodological requirements for accurate measurements of brain and body temperature during global forebrain ischemia of rat. J Cereb Blood Flow Metab 1992; 12:817–822.

144. Minamisawa H, Mellergård P, Smith M-L, et al. Preservation of brain temperature during ischemia in rats. Stroke 1990; 21:758–764.

145. Colbourne F, Nurse SM, Corbett D. Temperature changes associated with forebrain ischemia in the gerbil. Brain Res 1993; 602:264–257.

146. Seif el Nasr M, Nuglisch J, Krieglstein J. Prevention of ischemia-induced cerebral hypothermia by controlling the environmental temperature. J Pharmacol Toxicol Meth 1992; 27:23–26.

147. Neill KH, Crain BJ, Nadler JV. A simple, inexpensive method of monitoring brain temperature in conscious rodents. J Neurosci Meth 1990; 33:179–183.

148. Nakane M, Kubota M, Nakagomi T, et al. Rewarming eliminates the protective effect of cooling against delayed neuronal death. Neuroreport 2001; 12:2439–2442.

149. Iwai T, Niwa M, Yamada H, et al. Hypothermic prevention of the hippocampal damage following ischemia in Mongolian gerbils. Comparison between intraischemic and brief postischemic hypothermia. Life Sci 1993; 52:1031–1038.

150. Colbourne F, Corbett D. Delayed and prolonged postischemic hypothermia is neuroprotective in the gerbil. Brain Res 1994; 654:265–272.

151. Colbourne F, Corbett D. Delayed postischemic hypothermia: a six month survival study using behavioral and histological assessments of neuroprotection. J Neurosci 1995; 15: 7250–7260.

152. Buchan A, Pulsinelli WA. Hypothermia but not the N-methyl-D-aspartate antagonist MK-801, attenuates neuronal damage in gerbils subjected to transient global ischemia. J Neurosci 1990; 10:311–316.

153. Corbett D, Evans S, Thomas C, et al. MK-801 reduced cerebral ischemic injury by inducing hypothermia. Brain Res 1990; 514:300–304.

154. Nurse S, Corbett D. Neuroprotection after several days of mild, drug-induced hypothermia. J Cereb Blood Flow Metab 1996; 16:474–480.

155. Baena RC, Busto R, Dietrich WD, et al. Hyperthermia delayed by 24 hours aggravates neuronal damage in rat hippocampus following global ischemia. Neurology 1997; 48:768–773.

156. Van der Heyden JA, Zethof TJ, Olivier B. Stress-induced hyperthermia in singly housed mice. Physiol Behav 1997; 62:463–470.

157. Clark DL, DeBow SB, Iseke MD, et al. Stress-induced fever after postischemic rectal temperature measurements in the gerbil. Can J Physiol Pharmacol 2003; 81:880–883.

158. Colbourne F, Sutherland GR, Auer RN. An automated system for regulating brain temperature in awake and freely moving rats. J Neurosci Meth 1996; 67:185–190.

159. Barber PA, Hoyte L, Colbourne F, et al. Temperature-regulated model of focal ischemia in the mouse. A study with histopathological and behavioral outcomes. Stroke 2004; 35:1720–1725.

160. Siemkowicz E, Hansen AJ. Clinical restitution following cerebral ischemia in hypo-, normo- and hyperglycemic rats. Acta Neurol Scand 1978; 58:1–8.

161. Kalimo H, Rehncrona S, Soderfeldt B, et al. Brain lactic acidosis and ischemic cell damage: 2. Histopathology. J Cereb Blood Flow Metab 1981; 1:313–327.

162. Dietrich WD, Alonso OF, Busto R. Moderate hyperglycemia worsens acute blood-brain barrier injury after forebrain ischemia in rats. Stroke 1993; 24:111–116.

163. Garnier P, Bertrand N, Flamand B, et al. Preischemic blood glucose supply to the brain modulates HSP(72) synthesis and neuronal damage in gerbils. Brain Res 1999; 836:245–255.

164. Kondo F, Kondo Y, Makino H, et al. Delayed neuronal death in hippocampal CA1 pyramidal neurons after forebrain iscemia in hyperglycemic gerbil: amelioration by indomethacin. Brain Res 2000; 853:93–98.

165. Warner DS, Todd MM, Dexter F, et al. Temporal thresholds for hyperglycemia-augmented ischemic brain damage in rats. Stroke 1995; 26:655–660.

166. Li P-A, Shamloo M, Katsura K, et al. Critical values for plasma glucose in aggravating ischaemic brain damage: correlation to extracellular pH. Neurobiol Dis 1995; 2:97–108.

167. Combs DJ, Reuland DS, Martin DB, et al. Glycolytic inhibition by 2-deoxyglucose reduces hyperglycemia-associated mortality and morbidity in the ischemic rat. Stroke 1986; 17:989–994.

168. Hansen AJ. The extracellular potassium concentration in brain cortex following ischemia in hypo- and hyperglycemic rats. Acta Physiol Scand 1978; 102:324–329.

169. Katsura K, Kristián T, Smith M-L, et al. Acidosis induced by hypercapnia exaggerates ischemic brain injury. J Cereb Blood Flow Metab 1994; 14:243–250.

170. Kirino T, Sano K. Selective vulnerability in the gerbil hippocampus following transient ischemia. Acta Neuropathol (Berl) 1984; 62:201–208.

171. Kirino T, Sano K. Fine structural nature of delayed neuronal death following ischemia in the gerbil hippocampus. Acta Neuropathol (Berl) 1984; 62:209–218.

172. Colbourne F, Li H, Buchan AM. Continuing postischemic neuronal death in CA1. Influence of ischemia duration and cytoprotective doses of NBQX and SNX-111 in rats. Stroke 1999; 30:662–668.

173. Morita F, Wen T-C, Tanaka J, et al. Protective effect of a prosaposin-derived, 18-mer peptide on slowly progressive neuronal degeneration after brief ischemia. J Cereb Blood Flow Metab 2001; 21:1295–1302.

174. Morse JK, Davis JN. Regulation of ischemic hippocampal damage in the gerbil: adrenalectomy alters the rate of CA_1 cell disappearance. Exp Neurol 1990; 110:86–92.

175. Pérez-Pinzón MA, Xu G-P, Dietrich WD, et al. Rapid preconditioning protects rats against ischemic neuronal damage after 3 but not 7 days of reperfusion following global cerebral ischemia. J Cereb Blood Flow Metab 1997; 17:175–182.

176. Busto R, Dietrich WD, Globus MY-T, et al. Postischemic moderate hypothermia inhibits CA_1 hippocampal ischemic neuronal injury. Neurosci Lett 1989; 102:299–304.

177. Dietrich WD, Busto R, Alonso O, et al. Intraischemic but not postischemic brain hypothermia protects chronically following global forebrain ischemia in rats. J Cereb Blood Flow Metab 1993; 13:541–549.

178. Corbett D, Crooks P. Ischemic preconditioning: a long-term survival study using behavioral and histological endpoints. Brain Res 1997; 760:129–136.

179. Dowden J, Corbett D. Ischemic preconditioning in 18- to 20-month-old gerbils. Long-term survival with functional outcome measures. Stroke 1999; 30:1240–1246.

180. Liu J, Solway K, Messing RO, et al. Increased neurogenesis in the dentate gyrus after transient global ischemia in gerbils. J Neurosci 1998; 18:7768–7778.

181. Sharp FR, Liu J, Bernabeu R. Neurogenesis following brain ischemia. Dev. Brain Res. 2002; 134:23–30.

182. Schmidt W, Reymann KG. Proliferating cells differentiate into neurons in the hippocampal CA1 region of gerbils after global cerebral ischemia. Neurosci Lett 2002; 334:153–156.

183. Beck T, Wree A, Schleicher A. Glucose utilization in rat hippocampus after long-term recovery from ischemia. J Cereb Blood Flow Metab 1990; 10:542–549.

184. Bonnekoh P, Barbier A, Oschlies U, et al. Selective vulnerability in the gerbil hippocampus: morphological changes after 5 min ischemia and long survival times. Acta Neuropathol 1990; 80:18–25.

185. Elsersy H, Sheng H, Lynch JR, et al. Effects of isoflurane anesthesia versus fentanyl-nitrous oxide anesthesia on long-term outcome from severe forebrain ischemia in the rat. Anesthesiology 2004; 100:1160–1166.

186. Bendel O, Bueters T, von Euler M, et al. Reappearance of hippocampal CA1 neurons after ischemia is associated with recovery of learning and memory. J Cereb Blood Flow Metab 2005; 25:1586–1595.

25 | Pathogenic Mechanisms of Brain Injury Following Global Cerebral Ischemia

Raymond C. Koehler, PhD, Professor

Department of Anesthesiology and Critical Care Medicine, Johns Hopkins University School of Medicine, Johns Hopkins Medical Institutions, Baltimore, Maryland, USA

SEQUENCE OF EVENTS DURING COMPLETE AND INCOMPLETE CEREBRAL ISCHEMIA

Complete global cerebral ischemia refers to situations in which cerebral blood flow (CBF) falls to zero, such as in the case of cardiac arrest. Incomplete global cerebral ischemia refers to situations in which CBF does not completely cease but falls sufficiently to impair cellular processes, metabolism, and function. Incomplete ischemia arises from various causes of arterial hypotension, shock, and intracranial hypertension. The brain requires a continuous supply of oxygen and glucose for normal function. With the sudden onset of complete cerebral ischemia, consciousness can be lost within 10 sec, and the electroencephalogram (EEG) can become isoelectric within 20 sec. The onset of isoelectric EEG is associated with (i) an efflux of potassium ions (K^+) that increases the extracellular concentration from ~3–12 mM, and (ii) a moderate increase in intracellular calcium ions (Ca^{2+}) (1,2). Because of the high rate of oxidative metabolism in the brain, phosphocreatine becomes largely depleted within 1 min, and adenosine triphosphate (ATP) becomes depleted within 2 min of the onset of complete ischemia (3,4). When ATP falls to ~30% of normal levels, the cells depolarize, causing an additional large efflux of K^+, an increase in extracellular K^+ in excess of 60 mM, and a large influx of sodium (Na^+), Ca^{2+}, and water. Consequently, the extracellular space shrinks and the cells swell. The continued consumption of ATP and anaerobic glycolysis of glycogen and glucose stores generate a large proton load in the cell. The intracellular pH gradually falls from 7.1 to ~6.2 over the first 6 min of cardiac arrest (5). The lack of clearance of CO_2 by blood flow contributes to the fall in pH. Therefore, complete lack of CBF initiates a rapid sequence of disturbances in cell homeostasis (Fig. 1).

For incomplete global cerebral ischemia, this sequence of events depends on reductions of CBF below a set of thresholds: inhibition of protein synthesis when CBF is below ~50% of normal, suppressed electrical activity and O_2 consumption when CBF is below ~40% of normal, decreased ATP when CBF is below ~25% of normal, and anoxic depolarization when CBF is below ~20% of normal (6,7). The decrease in protein synthesis and electrical activity helps to conserve ATP for maintaining ionic homeostasis. This sequence of events is also time dependent and is delayed relative to that occurring with complete ischemia. Small, incremental improvements in CBF can forestall the loss of ATP. For example, with intracranial hypertension sufficient to reduce CBF to ~15% of baseline and O_2 consumption to ~25% of baseline, ATP takes 12 min to fall to 35% of baseline and 30 min to fall to <10% (8). Thus, the time course of ATP loss can be delayed more than 10-fold compared to complete ischemia, even at "trickle" levels of blood flow. One concern is that "trickle" flow will worsen tissue acidosis by sustaining anaerobic glycolysis. However, after 30 min of CBF at 15% of baseline, intracellular pH falls to ~6.4 at 12 min and 6.2 at 30 min of normoglycemic ischemia. This fall in pH is slower than that observed during complete ischemia, where intracellular pH decreases from ~7.1 to 6.4 at 3 min and to 6.0 to 6.2 at 12 min (3,9). However, in the presence of acute or chronic hyperglycemia, the fall in intracellular pH during incomplete global ischemia is more rapid and can reach levels <6.0 by 30 min (8,10). This augmented acidosis is associated with poor metabolic, functional, and histologic outcome (8,10–12).

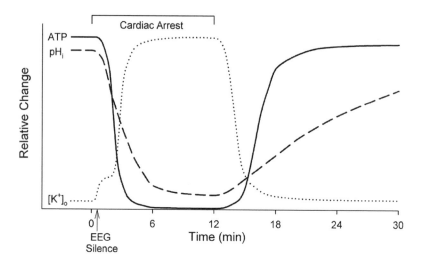

Figure 1 Schematic representation of the time course of relative changes in cerebral ATP concentration, $[K^+]_o$ concentration, and pH_i with the onset of cardiac arrest (time=0 min) and onset of full reperfusion (12 min). An initial, moderate increase in $[K^+]_o$ is associated with EEG silence, and subsequent depletion of ATP <30% of normal is associated with anoxic depolarization. Increases in intracellular Na^+ and Ca^{2+} tend to parallel changes in $[K^+]_o$, although compartmental changes in Ca^{2+} stores may persist for prolonged periods of reperfusion. Recovery of pH_i lags behind recovery of $[K^+]_o$ and ATP. *Abbreviations*: $[K^+]_o$, extracellular potassium concentration; pH_i, intracellular pH; EEG, electroencephalogram; ATP, adenosine triphosphate.

SEQUENCE OF EVENTS DURING REPERFUSION

Because of rheological factors and cellular swelling that restricts capillary diameter, restoration of CBF after complete cerebral ischemia initially requires higher perfusion pressure than that anticipated from a CBF autoregulatory curve. Thus, the low cerebral perfusion pressures typically attained during chest compressions with cardiopulmonary resuscitation are generally inadequate for restoring cerebral energy metabolism (13,14). Moreover, delaying the onset resuscitation after cardiac arrest from 0 min to 1.5, 3, 6, and 12 min progressively worsens the level of CBF attained at low reperfusion pressures (15). Once cardiac function is restored, arterial pressure may transiently increase above normal levels because of the persistent action of endogenously released and exogenously administered vasopressors during resuscitation. It has been argued that brief hypertension after resuscitation may be beneficial for the brain by washing out the poorly deformable leukocytes and reestablishing flow in all capillaries (16,17).

Full reperfusion leads to recovery of oxidative phosphorylation and ATP. Full recovery of ATP lags behind recovery of the transcellular Na^+ gradient by several minutes as additional ATP is required for enhanced ionic pump activity (3). However, complete ischemia of long durations, such as 30 min, results in incomplete recovery of ATP (9), presumably because of mitochondrial dysfunction, loss of adenine nucleotide base and nicotinamide adenine dinuclotide (NAD$^+$), and microcirculatory patches of poor reflow. A secondary delayed loss of ATP at several hours or days of reperfusion is thought to be related to opening of the mitochondrial transition pore and loss of mitochondrial membrane potential. Recovery of intracellular pH lags the initial recovery of ATP (Fig. 1), and recovery of electrical conduction as assessed by evoked potentials lags recovery of pH (9). A relationship between tissue acidosis during early reperfusion and evoked potential recovery is suggested by the observations that augmenting carbonic acidosis during reperfusion suppresses evoked potential recovery (18), while accelerating intracellular pH recovery with antioxidant treatment improves evoked potential recovery (19).

SELECTIVE VULNERABILITY

The degree of neuronal injury after cardiac arrest varies among brain regions. For example, brainstem function in cardiovascular and respiratory control regions is resistant to anoxia. Part of this resistance can be attributed to better CBF autoregulation (20), improved CBF during chest compression resuscitation (15), and less delayed hypoperfusion. However, differences in ionic conduction, neuronal connectivity, and neurochemical phenotypes may also contribute to ischemic resistance in parts of the brainstem (21,22).

Within a particular brain region, subpopulations of neurons also have differential vulnerability to ischemia. Soon after the onset of complete ischemia, ultrastructural changes, such as chromatin clumping, cytosolic swelling, and dilation of the endoplasmic reticulum (ER) and Golgi apparatus, become evident (23). Depending on ischemic duration, some of these changes are reversible (11,24). However, with continued reperfusion, subpopulations of neurons display a disruption and loss of organelles and cell shrinkage (25–27). Certain populations of neurons, such as pyramidal neurons in the CA1 region of the hippocampus and Purkinje neurons of the cerebellum, are considered to be particularly vulnerable. Cell loss in the hippocampal CA1 region can be delayed for several days when the duration of ischemia is brief, for example 5 to 15 min, although some variation among species may occur in the duration of ischemia required for hippocampal injury (28–33). In analyzing the histopathology 4 days after 5, 10, 12.5, 15, 17, or 20 min of cardiac arrest, the prevalence of necrotic neurons increased progressively with ischemic duration (34). At the shorter durations, hippocampal CA1 injury was greater than in dentate gyrus, and Purkinje cell loss was greater than granule cell loss in the cerebellum. After ischemic durations of 15 to 20 min, the prevalence of neuronal cell death became similar among hippocampal regions, and most cerebellar Purkinje and granule cells were necrotic. Injury of medium spiny neurons in striatum required 10 min of arrest, whereas magnocellular neurons were spared. Neuronal necrosis in cerebral cortex was more prominent in superior and middle gyri than in inferior gyri, cingulate gyrus, or insular cortex. With global incomplete ischemia arising from intracranial hypertension, the pattern of selective vulnerability was also observed, although neocortical neurons were more vulnerable than striatal and thalamic neurons (22).

In a neonatal swine model of asphyxic cardiac arrest, selective vulnerability of neuronal populations and brain regions was evident (35). Rapid necrotic cell death of striatal medium spiny neurons developed over the first 24 hr after resuscitation. Necrosis in cerebral cortex developed between 24 and 72 hr of recovery and was restricted to primary sensorimotor cortex, which was the most metabolically active portion of cortex at this stage of development. Delayed apoptosis in thalamic sensory nuclei can occur after 72 hr, apparently as a result of target deprivation. In contrast to mature brain, CA1 hippocampal neurons were not more vulnerable than other hippocampal regions. Therefore, neuronal cell death varies with brain maturation, duration of the insult, the phenotype of the neuronal population, and the connectivity of that population.

EXCITOTOXICITY

To understand why some neurons die while nearby neurons are spared in a nonrandom manner, much research has focused on the pattern of excitatory and inhibitory receptors on particular neuronal populations. Anoxic depolarization results in the release of excitatory and inhibitory neurotransmitters. Impaired reuptake by energy-dependent mechanisms results in large increases in intrasynaptic and extrasynaptic concentrations of neurotransmitters. In the case of the primary excitatory neurotransmitter glutamate, reuptake largely depends on transporters in astrocytes and neurons that are driven by the high extracellular-to-intracellular Na^+ gradient that is normally maintained by Na,K-ATPase. This gradient is lost during anoxic depolarization but can gradually recover during reperfusion (3). After some delay in the restoration of ATP production during reperfusion, extrasynaptic glutamate concentration measured by microdialysis is reduced (36). However, intrasynaptic glutamate concentration may not necessarily be restored uniformly because of persistent swelling in astrocyte and dendritic processes associated with incomplete and heterogeneous restoration of ionic gradients and energy metabolism. Thus, glutamate may continue to act on its excitatory ionotropic receptors, not only during ischemia but also during the reperfusion period, when other cellular processes are recovering and continued Ca^{2+} signaling could have adverse effects. Glutamate acting on the AMPA receptor would continue to enhance Na^+ entry, keep the cells in a partially depolarized state, and thereby promote Ca^{2+} entry through voltage-dependent Ca^{2+} channels. Additionally, AMPA receptors that lack the GluR2 subunit also permit direct Ca^{2+} entry. Decreased expression of GluR2 subunits has been described in hippocampus over the first few days of reperfusion (37). Glutamate acting on NMDA receptors also permits Ca^{2+} entry. Moreover, phosphorylation of NMDA receptors occurs during the reperfusion period (38,39) and thereby alters the function of the receptor and channel. Enhanced Ca^{2+} entry in neurons with excitatory receptors is thought to lead to selective vulnerability of these neurons. In that many of these neurons release gamma-aminobutyric acid (GABA) as their neurotransmitter, selective loss of neurons with inhibitory output is thought to create an imbalance of excitation and inhibition, which contributes to the secondary injury of selectively vulnerable neurons during reperfusion.

CALCIUM

Large increases in intracellular Ca^+ during ischemia have been a central focus for initiating multiple mechanisms of injury. Loss of ATP results in an inability to actively extrude Ca^{2+} or to sequester Ca^{2+} in the ER. The large increase in intracellular Na^+ causes a reversal of the Na^+/Ca^{2+} exchanger on the cell membrane and results in a net influx of Ca^{2+}. Because most neurons can survive brief periods of increased Ca^{2+}, the downstream mechanisms of cell death appear to take many minutes or hours to become fully recruited and probably depend on compartmentalization of increased Ca^{2+}. Early attempts to limit Ca^{2+} influx utilized inhibitors of voltage-dependent Ca^{2+} channels. However, these studies showed either no effect or modest protection from global ischemia (40–43). Subsequent attempts utilized antagonists of NMDA receptors. Results with these agents in models of global cerebral ischemia were generally disappointing in gerbil (44), rat (45), cat (46), dog (29,47), and monkey (48). Although these agents were effective when given early in experimental stroke, their mechanism of protection during focal ischemia appeared to depend largely on reducing spreading waves of depolarization and the associated energy cost. Areas salvaged by NMDA antagonists were in penumbral zones, where blood flow was sufficient to maintain some degree of ATP synthesis for a significant duration, in contrast to the situation in severe global cerebral ischemia. Interestingly, NMDA antagonists can protect hippocampal CA1 neurons from severe hypoglycemia but not from global ischemia (49). When hypoglycemia silences spontaneous electrical activity, intracellular pH undergoes an alkaline shift (50,51), in contrast to the acidosis present during ischemia. Because acidosis inhibits NMDA currents (52) and alkalosis promotes NMDA-dependent injury (53), NMDA antagonists are expected to be more effective in the absence of acidosis. Thus, the greater efficacy of these agents in hypoglycemia may be related to differences in tissue pH. In organotypic slice cultures of hippocampus that undergo oxygen–glucose deprivation with ischemic-like extracellular electrolyte concentrations, acidosis following the insult selectively protected the CA3 region, compared to the CA1 region, in association with delayed recovery of NMDA-mediated excitatory postsynaptic currents in CA3 neurons (54). Acidosis during ischemia and early reperfusion may protect the CA3 region selectively. The lack of efficacy of NMDA antagonists *in vivo* in hippocampus after global ischemia may be related to suppression of NMDA currents in CA3 neurons by acidosis, whereas other mechanisms appear to play a role in CA1 neurons.

Recently, acidosis itself has been shown to open large conductance calcium channels, and pretreatment of inhibitors of these channels has reduced infarct volume from focal ischemia (55). Determination of the role of these channels during global cerebral ischemia and during early reperfusion when tissue acidosis persists will be important.

Another channel that could be involved in Ca^{2+} entry during anoxia is TRPM7, a member of the transient receptor potential channel (56). This channel can be activated by reactive oxygen/nitrogen species and contribute to neuronal death from oxygen–glucose deprivation. Impaired function of the Na^+/Ca^{2+} exchanger has also been implicated in sustaining elevated intracellular Ca^{2+} (57). Thus, several pathways independent of NMDA channels appear to be involved in increasing intracellular Ca^{2+} during ischemia/reperfusion.

Calcium is involved in multiple signaling processes and activation of many enzymes. Thus, the large increase in Ca^{2+} during ischemia and its persistence during early reperfusion initiate a multitude of effects, including alterations in the phosphorylation state of various kinases and activation of calpain and other proteases, nitric oxide synthase (NOS), and phospholipase A_2.

CALPAIN

Calpain is a Ca^{2+}-dependent cysteine protease with multiple substrates, including caspases and the cytoskeletal protein fodrin. Increased calpain activity has been observed during the early hours of reperfusion after global ischemia in selectively vulnerable regions (58–60). A delayed increase in activity can also occur in hippocampus (59,61). In dendrites, calpain is associated with NMDA receptors whose activity can normally modulate cytoskeletal reorganization during synaptic plasticity (62). After ischemia, degradation of fodrin is ameliorated by NMDA receptor antagonists and calpain inhibition (58). Abnormalities in dendritic morphology and synaptic organization during reperfusion (63) might contribute to abnormal Ca^{2+} signaling and electrophysiologic function, at least temporarily, despite overall recovery of cellular energy metabolism. Calpain may play a role in (i) initially downregulating caspase-3 activity, (ii) later augmenting apoptotic signaling through actions on Bid and several downstream caspases (64), and (iii) cleaving apoptosis-inducing factor (AIF) (65). Other actions of calpain include cleavage of the Na^+/Ca^{2+} exchanger (57), which will retard extrusion of Ca^{2+} once the Na^+ gradient is restored during early reperfusion. Therefore, calpain can control the ischemic injury cascade at multiple sites.

NITRIC OXIDE

Studies of neuronal cultures have indicated a key role for NO in the excitotoxic actions of NMDA (66). The neuronal isoform of NOS (nNOS) is linked to NMDA receptors by postsynaptic density-95 protein, thereby permitting activity to be controlled by Ca^{2+} influx through the NMDA receptor–channel complex. Overexcitation of NMDA receptors during ischemia and reperfusion leads to bursts of NO production, which can alter protein function by nitrosylation of cysteine residues and nitration of tyrosine residues. Furthermore, if superoxide production is amplified during reoxygenation, increased NO and superoxide will generate toxic levels of peroxynitrite. In focal ischemia, loss of the nNOS isoform is protective, whereas loss of the endothelial NOS isoform worsens injury (67,68). The latter effect is thought to be related to the vasodilatory and antiplatelet aggregatory effects of NO. Early attempts to assess the role of NO in global ischemia models generally revealed no protection in hippocampal pyramidal neurons or cerebellar Purkinje neurons by administration of nonselective NOS inhibitors (30,69–71), although one study did find hippocampal protection with short (5 min) ischemic duration (72) and another study found decreased blood–brain barrier permeability (73). However, studies with gene deletion of nNOS or with administration of a selective nNOS inhibitor reported protection in the hippocampal CA1 region (74,75). Increases in NO production have been measured during forebrain ischemia (76) and specifically in hippocampus during reperfusion (77). The increase in hippocampal NO production persisted over a 3-hr observation period after 10 or 15 min of global ischemia and was blocked by a selective nNOS inhibitor (77). However, the inhibitor provided hippocampal protection after 5 min of ischemia but not after 10 min of ischemia. Therefore, despite the lack of efficacy of NMDA receptor antagonists and nonselective NOS inhibitors in most studies of global cerebral ischemia, neuronally derived NO appears to contribute to hippocampal injury. However, inconsistent efficacy with inhibition of the neuronal isoform after moderately prolonged ischemia indicates the importance of other mechanisms in triggering cell death.

ARACHIDONIC ACID METABOLISM

The increase in Ca^{2+} during ischemia stimulates Ca^{2+}-dependent phospholipase activity, which mobilizes arachidonic acid and other lipids from the phospholipid pool (4). Arachidonic acid is used as a substrate by cyclooxygenase (COX), lipoxygenase, and selective cytochrome P450 enzymes possessing ω-hydroxylase or epoxygenase activity. Early work with pharmacologic inhibitors implicated a greater role for COX than for lipoxygenase in hippocampal neuronal death from global ischemia (78). The anti-inflammatory epoxyeicosatrienoic acids produced by expoxygenases (79,80) and the proinflammatory 20-hydroxyeicosatetraenoic acid produced by ω-hydroxylase (81,82) have not been well studied in global cerebral ischemia. COX-1 is constitutively expressed in neurons, glia, and endothelium, whereas COX-2 is constitutively expressed in subpopulations of neurons, including some that express nNOS (83,84). After global ischemia, COX-2 is induced in various cell types, including neurons destined to die in the CA1 region (85,86). Increased expression of COX-2 is dependent on activation of AMPA receptors, rather than that of NMDA receptors (87). Gene deletion of COX-2 or administration of COX-2 inhibitors provided neuroprotection in hippocampus (86,88,89). However, brief periods of global ischemia were used to assess the effect of COX inhibitors, and efficacy with prolonged, complete ischemia is unknown. A biphasic increase in the concentration of prostaglandin E_2 (PGE_2) was reported in hippocampus after brief ischemia (89). An increase in PGE_2 seen at 2 hr of reperfusion was primarily derived from COX-1, whereas an increase seen at 24 hr was primarily derived from COX-2. Likewise, an early decrease in glutathione was attenuated by COX-1 inhibition, and a delayed decrease in glutathione was attenuated by COX-2 inhibition, thereby implicating COX-1 activity in early oxidant stress and COX-2 activity in delayed oxidant stress. When administered at 6 hr of reperfusion, both COX-1 and COX-2 inhibitors conferred partial neuroprotection associated with reduced markers of lipid peroxidation (89). Long-term protection with a COX-2 inhibitor administered as late as 24 hr after brief global ischemia has also been reported (88). Thus, both COX-1 and COX-2 activities are implicated in delayed neurodegeneration, and the role of COX-2 persists beyond 24 hr. The mechanism of injury may be related to the actions of prostaglandins and thromboxanes on specific receptors. In general, receptors coupled to increases in intracellular Ca^{2+} are thought to promote cell death, whereas those coupled to increases in cyclic adenosine monophosphate appear to promote cell survival (90–92). Interestingly, the inducible NOS (iNOS) isoform can bind directly to COX-2 and increase COX-2 activity by nitrosylation of a specific cysteine residue (93). Thus, a delayed increase in iNOS activity (94) may amplify COX-2–mediated injury.

REACTIVE OXYGEN SPECIES

Enhanced production of oxygen radicals during ischemia/reperfusion can overwhelm endogenous defense mechanisms and lead to damage of lipids, proteins, and DNA. Superoxide dismutase (SOD) isoforms located in the cytosol, mitochondria, and extracellular membrane convert the superoxide radical to hydrogen peroxide, which is then metabolized by catalase. Superoxide is a normal byproduct of mitochondrial respiration, but Ca^{2+} overload in mitochondria during ischemia leads to electron transport uncoupling and excessive superoxide production. A role for superoxide in global ischemia is supported by the observations that decreasing the expression of the cytosolic Cu,Zn-SOD augments hippocampal injury from global ischemia (95), whereas increasing expression reduces activation of proapoptotic signaling from the mitochondria and alleviates neuronal injury (96,97).

Iron can be mobilized by the action of superoxide on ferritin (98) and by the action of lactic acid on bicarbonate bridges on transferrin (99). Iron can catalyze hydroxyl radical formation by the Fenton reaction and participate in other free radical reactions (100). A role for iron-induced injury is implicated by a mobilization of iron from its storage proteins and a beneficial effect of the iron chelator deferoxamine in sustaining energy metabolism after severe acidotic ischemia (101,102).

Peroxynitrite is considered to be a major source of hydroxyl radical formation during ischemia/reperfusion (103–105). Peroxynitrite is formed in the presence of superoxide and NO, both of which are abundant during reperfusion. Protection seen with increased SOD activity and decreased nNOS activity are thought to be linked to decreased peroxynitrite formation. Free radical reactions initiated by peroxynitrite are implicated in damage to DNA, lipids, and proteins and to nitration of tyrosine residues that may alter protein function (106).

Conversion of xanthine dehydrogenase to xanthine oxidase by Ca^{2+}-activated proteases can lead to increased superoxide formation. This enzyme is enriched in endothelium and may contribute to recruitment of leukocytes and the inflammatory response. Protection by allopurinol from hypoxia-ischemia in newborn rats suggests that this pathway may be particularly important in immature brain (107). However, whether conversion of xanthine dehydrogenase to xanthine oxidase occurs in mature brain after cerebral ischemia is unclear (108,109). Beneficial effects of allopurinol and oxypurinol may be related to preventing loss of adenine nucleotides (110).

During inflammation, nicotinamide adenine dinucleotide phosphate (NADPH) oxidase in leukocytes is a major source of superoxide. More recently, superoxide generated by NADPH oxidase has been studied as a physiologic signaling molecule in endothelium (111). Impaired cerebrovascular reactivity associated with angiotensin-mediated hypertension and increased β-amyloid has been attributed to increased NADPH oxidase activity (112). The role of NADPH oxidase isoforms that are present in neurons, endothelium, microglia, and macrophages has not been well characterized in global ischemic injury. However, vascular dysfunction after global ischemia is anticipated to be augmented in patients with underlying hypertension, Alzheimer's disease, and diabetes, in part, because of elevated vascular superoxide production.

ER STRESS

The early damage to the ER and Golgi apparatus and the loss of ribosomes preceding mitochondrial damage indicate that the ER is a major target for oxidative damage during reperfusion (113,114). Folding of newly synthesized proteins requires high levels of Ca^{2+} in the ER lumen. Depletion of ER Ca^{2+} during reperfusion and oxidative damage to proteins and the ER lipid membrane result in accumulation of unfolded proteins (Fig. 2). The normal homeostatic response to accumulation of unfolded proteins is to decrease translation by regulation of eukaryotic initiation factor 2α (eIF2α) and to increase synthesis of chaperone proteins until unfolded proteins no longer accumulate (115). The chaperone protein glucose-regulated protein-78 (GRP78) binds to the unfolded proteins. With excess unfolded proteins, GRP78 dissociates from two kinases in the ER membrane: RNA-dependent protein kinase–like ER eIF2α kinase (PERK) and inositol-requiring enzyme (IRE1). As a result of GRP78 dissociation, PERK is activated and phosphorylates eIF2α,

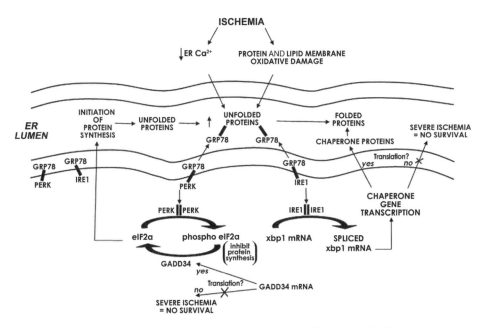

Figure 2 ER stress after cerebral ischemia results in accumulation of unfolded/misfolded proteins in the ER lumen because of oxidative damage and loss of the high intralumen Ca^{2+}. GRP78 in the ER membrane dissociates from PERK and IRE1 and binds to the excess of unfolded proteins in the lumen. Dissociated PERK forms dimers, which phosphorylate eIF2α and inhibit general protein synthesis. Restoration of protein synthesis requires dephosphorylation of eIF2α by GADD34, which, in turn, requires a minimal amount of intact translation machinery for expression of new protein after damage by ischemia. Dissociated IRE1 forms dimers that cleave X-box binding protein mRNA into a splice variant that acts as a transcription factor on chaperone genes. Proper folding of proteins requires expression of chaperone proteins, which, in turn, requires a minimal amount of intact translation machinery after damage by ischemia. Long-term survival of selective neurons depends on ability to express GADD34 and chaperone proteins. *Abbreviations*: ER, endoplasmic reticulum; PERK, protein kinase–like ER eIF2α kinase; IRE1, Inositol-requiring enzyme; eIF2α, eukaryotic initiation factor 2α; GRP78, glucose-regulated protein-78.

which shuts down translation and leads to disaggregation of polyribosomes. In addition, IRE1 is activated and cuts X-box binding protein (xbp1) mRNA, which leads to synthesis of a variant protein that acts as a transcription factor for inducing ER chaperone proteins (115).

Evidence for ER stress after global cerebral ischemia includes increased accumulation of unfolded protein in the ER lumen, decreased binding of GRP78 to PERK, phosphorylation of eIF2α by PERK, and inhibition of protein synthesis (116,117). Markers of ER stress are reduced in animals with overexpression of Cu,Zn-SOD (118,119), consistent with a key role of oxygen radicals in initiating the stress response. However, depending on the severity and duration of ischemia, the homeostatic unfolded protein response may not be fully executed, and some neurons will eventually die. For example, the variant form of processed xbp1 may not be expressed because of damage to the ER machinery (120,121). Consequently, restitution of chaperone proteins may be impaired. Moreover, eIF2α is normally dephosphorylated by GADD34, and although GADD34 mRNA is increased after ischemia, protein expression of GADD34 remained suppressed in vulnerable regions (122). Thus, oxidative damage to the ER may limit its ability to synthesize the new proteins necessary to repair the dysfunctional ER. Persistent phosphorylation of eIF2α by the lack of GADD34 and activation of mitochondrial-dependent apoptosis occur in the same neurons that are destined to die (123). In addition to inhibiting translation, phosphorylation of eIF2α also leads to induction of activating transcription factor-4 (ATF-4) and proapoptotic C/EBP-homologous protein (CHOP). Induction of ATF-4 and CHOP was reduced after ischemia in animals that overexpressed Cu,Zn-SOD (119), again emphasizing the role of reactive oxygen species in ER stress. Although blocking synthesis of specific proteins during early reperfusion might be beneficial for cell survival, persistent ER stress and suppression of overall protein synthesis will lead to dysfunction of neurons in which proteins typically turnover every 1 to 2 days. Crosstalk between ER and mitochondria probably plays an important role in controlling cell death pathways after ischemia.

APOPTOTIC PATHWAYS

Cell Morphology

Apoptosis represents an actively regulated form of cell death, whereas necrosis is considered to represent a passive form of cell death secondary to the loss of energy metabolism. Because energy metabolism usually recovers initially after reperfusion, but can decline hours later depending on ischemic duration, the role of apoptotic and necrotic mechanisms can be interrelated temporally in a complex fashion. With complete or near-complete global cerebral ischemia, most neurons that die have a necrotic appearance. Neurons that display classic apoptotic morphology are uncommon (124), unless the blood flow reduction is moderate or brief (125). Apoptotic morphology is more common in models of hypoxia-ischemia in immature rodents (126). This age-dependent pattern probably reflects the increased expression of many of the apoptosis-regulatory proteins in immature brain, which normally undergo increased baseline apoptosis (127). However, the lack of pure apoptotic morphology in mature brain after ischemia does not mean that molecular mechanisms of apoptosis are not contributing to cell death. The processing of cell death signaling proteins may be modified by disturbed energy metabolism and free radical damage to the ER, Golgi apparatus, mitochondria, and nuclear membranes. Within neuronal subpopulations, multiple mechanisms may contribute to cell death, with each mechanism operating over different time courses and modifying the cell's response to other cell death pathways. Thus, hybrids of cell death mechanisms can display different morphologies along a necrosis-apoptosis continuum (128,129). Moreover, broad-spectrum caspase inhibitors are capable of ameliorating hippocampal damage from global ischemia (130–132), thereby implicating apoptotic signaling.

Studies of excitotoxicity in neuronal cell culture indicate that AMPA-induced cell death is partially dependent on apoptotic mechanisms (133). Large, discrete, irregularly shaped clusters of chromatin appear to be a hybrid between the large, uniformly rounded shape of apoptotic bodies versus the multiple, small chromatin clumps appearing in necrotic and NMDA-induced cell death (128,129). NMDA-induced cell death also yields a sequence of ultrastructural changes, including dilation of rough ER, disaggregation of polyribosomes, Golgi vesiculation, and mitochondrial swelling (128). After global ischemia, neurons in striatum undergo rapid cell death with an appearance that resembles NMDA and non-NMDA excitotoxic cell death (128,129). Delayed degeneration of pyramidal neurons in hippocampus and of Purkinje neurons in cerebellum does not typically display classic apoptotic morphology (134–136). Interestingly, degenerating granule neurons in hippocampal dentate gyrus and granule neurons in cerebellar cortex display an apoptotic appearance at 1 day of reperfusion and often precede the necrotic appearance of pyramidal and Purkinje neurons. In immature rats and pigs subjected to hypoxia-ischemia, necrotic morphology is prominent in striatum and cerebral cortex, whereas delayed apoptotic morphology appears in thalamic sensory nuclei, apparently as a result of target deprivation (128,137,138). Thus, the mechanisms of cell death vary among specific neuronal populations with different temporal profiles and are influenced by connectivity and developmental maturity.

DNA Damage and Fragmentation

Reactive oxygen species can damage DNA. DNA strand breaks are detected at as early as 3 hr of reperfusion and increase over a 24-hr period in selectively vulnerable regions of striatum, cerebral cortex, and thalamus after global ischemia (125,139). In contrast, DNA strand breaks in CA1 hippocampus can be delayed by 72 hr, which is close to the time that the pyramidal neurons undergo cell death. These findings support the hypothesis for a different molecular mechanism of cell death in the CA1 region. Expression of apurinic/apyrimidinic endonuclease (APE/ref-1) was found to decrease 1 day prior to cell death (140). Overexpression of Cu,Zn-SOD attenuated the decrease in APE and protected CA1 neurons (141). The delayed decreased activity of this DNA repair enzyme was postulated to contribute to delayed cell death in the CA1 region.

Classic programmed cell death is associated with internucleosomal DNA fragmentation that results in a laddered pattern during electrophoresis, whereas necrosis results in DNA fragments of random size and a smeared electrophoretic pattern (142,143). After global cerebral ischemia, the laddered pattern of DNA fragmentation is not prominent, although the pattern is not completely random (136). Initially, 10-kilo-base pairs (kbp) fragments with a high proportion of 5'-OH ends and 50-kbp fragments with a high proportion of 3'-OH ends are found (143). The 50-kbp fragments are degraded into a laddered oligonucleosomal pattern. Use of ligation-mediated polymerase chain reaction (PCR) indicated that most of the DNA fragments after global cerebral ischemia have staggered ends with a 3' recess of 8 to 10 nucleotides, whereas apoptosis results in blunt-ended double-strand breaks (144). These findings imply that different sequences of endonucleases are activated in global ischemia versus classic apoptosis.

Regulators of Apoptosis

Apoptosis is regulated through extrinsic and intrinsic pathways that are dependent on activation of the caspase family of cysteine proteases (Fig. 3). In addition, extrinsic and intrinsic pathways of regulated cell death have been identified that are independent of caspase activation. Loss of neurotrophin signaling and increased activation of tumor necrosis factor-α (TNF-α) receptors produce apoptosis via the extrinsic pathway. This pathway involves recruitment of the Fas and TNF death-domain receptors, which creates the death-inducing signaling complex and leads to activation of caspase-8 and, subsequently, to execution of apoptosis by activation of caspase–3, –6, and –7. This mechanism can contribute to neuronal death after ischemia in populations of neurons undergoing target deprivation, such as in thalamic sensory nuclei in immature brain after loss of targets in cerebral cortex (137,145), and in regions where the inflammatory response causes activation of TNF-α receptors. An early increase in the Fas ligand has also been reported in thalamus of mature rats after 6 min of cardiac arrest (146). In addition, expression of activated caspase-8 in hippocampal CA1 increased at as early as 2 hr of reperfusion after 10 min of cardiac arrest in dogs (147), and expression of the Fas receptor and Fas ligand increased by 24 hr in hippocampus after forebrain ischemia (148). Together, these findings suggest that the extrinsic pathway is activated in hippocampus as well as in thalamus.

The intrinsic pathways of apoptosis involve apoptotic stimuli acting on mitochondria. Release of cytochrome c from the mitochondria triggers caspase-dependent cell death, whereas release of AIF and translocation to the nucleus causes execution of caspase-independent cell death. Release of cytochrome c into the cytosol has been reported in forebrain ischemia and cardiac arrest models (147,149,150). In rat forebrain ischemia, an early increase in cytochrome c release at 5 hr and a delayed increase at 48 hr were observed in hippocampus (132). The

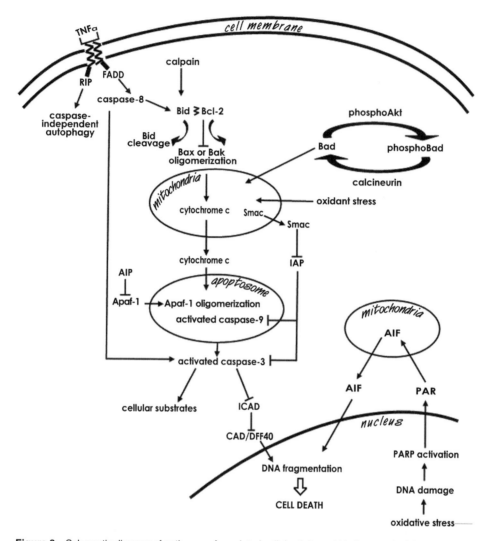

Figure 3 Schematic diagram of pathways of regulated cell death thought to be recruited during cerebral ischemia. Pathways include the extrinsic pathway, which involves recruitment of cell membrane death receptors, leading to caspase-8 activation or to a more recently described caspase-independent pathway through RIP. The intrinsic, caspase-dependent mitochondrial pathway involves cell stress signals that cause release of cytochrome c, which then triggers formation of the apoptosome complex of oligomerized Apaf-1 and activated caspase-9. Activated caspase-8 or caspase-9 cleaves procaspase-3, and the execution of DNA fragmentation and subsequent cell death are initiated by activation of caspase-3. The release of cytochrome c is facilitated by oligomerization of Bax to form channels in the mitochondrial membrane, and this process is inhibited by Bcl-2. Cytochrome c release is also promoted by dephosphorylated Bad. Mitochondria also release second mitochondrial activator of caspase, which, by inhibiting inhibitors of apoptosis, acts to disinhibit formation of activated caspase-3 and caspase-9. The intrinsic, caspase-independent pathway is primarily initiated by oxidant damage to DNA, which causes activation of PARP, which, in turn, triggers release of AIF from the mitochondria and translocation to the nucleus, where AIF binds to DNA and stimulates large-scale DNA fragmentation by an endonuclease. *Abbreviations*: TNF, tumor necrosis factor; RIP, receptor interacting protein; FADD, fes-associated death domain; Smac, second mitochondrial activator of caspase; Apaf-1, apoptotic protease activating factor–1; AIP, Apef-1–interacting protein; IAP, inhibitors of apoptosis; AIF, apoptosis inducing factor; ICAD, inhibitor of caspase-activated deoxyribonuclease; PAR, poly (ADP-ribose); PARP, poly (ADP-ribose) polymerase CAD, caspase activated deoxyribonuclease; DFF40, DNA fragmentation factor 40.

delayed increase was reduced by brief hypothermia over the first 3 hr of reperfusion, thereby indicating that events occurring in early reperfusion influence cytochrome c release and cell death 2 days later. Once in the cytosol, cytochrome c can combine with apoptotic protease activating factor-1 (Apaf-1) and deoxy-ATP to form the apoptosome, which activates caspase-9 (Fig. 3). Caspase-9 cleaves caspase-7 and caspase-3, which initiate the execution phase of apoptosis.

Activated caspase-3 cleaves ICAD, a natural inhibitor of caspase-activated deoxyribonuclease/ DNA fragmentation factor 40 (CAD/DFF40). Release of CAD/DFF40 from the ICAD complex permits internucleosomal DNA fragmentation. Expression of CAD/DFF40 in the nucleus increases progressively between 8 and 24 hr of reperfusion in the CA1 hippocampal region (151). In a canine model of cardiac arrest, expression of activated caspase-3 in the cytosol also increases progressively over the first 24 hr of reperfusion (147), but translocation of caspase-3 to the nucleus is delayed until 24 to 72 hr. Thus, the delay in translocation of activated caspase-3 to the nucleus is thought to contribute to the delayed cell death in CA1.

Apaf-1 can bind to an Apaf-1–interacting protein (AIP) and reduce apoptosome formation. Transfection of AIP into hippocampus reduces formation of activated caspase-3 and results in CA1 neuroprotection from global ischemia (152). Endogenous expression of AIP is relatively low but increases selectively in CA3 and dentate gyrus after ischemia and might help confer selective protection in these regions. The threshold for gating apoptosis is also controlled by inhibitors of apoptosis (IAP) proteins that bind caspases. The X-chromosome–linked IAP (XIAP) inhibits caspase-3, -7, and -9. XIAP, in turn, is inhibited by the second mitochondrial activator of caspase (Smac). Thus, release of Smac from the mitochondria is thought to inhibit XIAP and permit activation of caspase-3 and other caspases. In support of this concept, increased levels of Smac in the cytosol and decreased levels in the mitochondria correlate with the appearance of activated caspase-3 in hippocampus after global ischemia (153).

The mitochondrial apoptotic pathway is regulated by members of the Bcl-2 family of proteins. Release of cytochrome c depends on an increase in permeability of the outer mitochondrial membrane that is regulated by dimerization of Bax and Bak and inhibited by Bcl-2. Expression of antiapoptotic Bcl-2 and Bcl-X_L decreased, and proapoptotic Bcl-X_S, Bax, and Bak increased over a 24-hr period after resuscitation from cardiac arrest in hippocampal CA1 sector, with little change in the less vulnerable CA3 sector (147). Increased detection of smaller fragments of Bcl-2 suggested cleavage by caspases. In global ischemia, inhibitors of the mitochondrial permeability transition pore and inhibitors of Bax, which regulates outer mitochondrial membrane permeability, provide neuroprotection (154,155). Expression of Bcl-2, which acts to suppress cytochrome c release (156,157), is increased in the CA3 hippocampal region and may act to limit apoptosis in this region (158).

Further regulation of apoptotic signaling occurs by the action of kinases and phosphatases on the phosphorylation state of key signaling proteins. Inhibitors of the c-Jun-N-terminal kinase reduced the phosphorylation of c-Jun and Bcl-2, decreased cytochrome c release, decreased activation of caspase-3, and protected hippocampal neurons from global ischemia (159,160). Another example of phosphorylation regulation of apoptosis is through Akt. When the kinase Akt is phosphorylated, it maintains a phosphorylated state on some of the Bcl-2 family members, such as Bad, whereas such phosphatases as calcineurin decrease the phosphorylation state. Dephosphorylation of Bad permits calcium-dependent translocation of Bad into the mitochondria, where it can inhibit the antiapoptotic effects of Bcl-2 and Bcl-X_L and promote cytochrome c release (161). Phosphorylation of Akt has been noted to increase transiently at 24 hr of reperfusion before declining, after which the neurons die (162). The time course of Akt phosphorylation and of Akt and calcineurin interactions with Bad are thought to contribute to the timing of delayed neuronal death in the CA1 region.

Activation of caspase-8 in the extrinsic pathway also leads to truncation of Bid and stimulation of the mitochondrial pathway, thereby providing a mechanism for interaction between the extrinsic and intrinsic pathways. Calpain can also act on Bid, thereby providing one of the links between Ca^{2+} levels and the intrinsic pathway. A rapid cleavage of Bid soon after resuscitation from cardiac arrest implies an early signaling of proapoptotic signaling in hippocampal CA1 region, presumably mediated by calpain or caspases (147).

Caspase-Independent Pathways

AIF represents another component of the intrinsic cell death mechanism. However, this pathway does not require the activation of caspases. AIF normally functions as an oxidoreductase in mitochondria, and knockdown of AIF is associated with impaired oxidative phosphorylation and cerebellar granule cell degeneration during aging (163,164). Oxidative damage of DNA can cause AIF to be translocated to the nucleus, where it initiates large-scale DNA fragmentation and cell death (Fig. 3). The exact mechanism involved in the execution of AIF-induced DNA fragmentation is not known, although endonuclease G is postulated to be involved in some forms of cell death (165,166). Release of AIF can be suppressed by Bcl-2 (167), and crosstalk signaling between the AIF and the caspase-dependent cell death pathways likely occurs at various levels of signaling. Increased nuclear AIF has been reported after hypoxia-ischemia in immature rats (168), global ischemia in mature rats (169), and hypoglycemia (170). With NMDA-induced excitotoxicity in neurons, AIF translocation to the nucleus occurs rapidly and depends on activation of poly(ADP-ribose) polymerase (PARP) activity (171,172). In contrast, AMPA-induced injury is not dependent on PARP activation (173). PARP-1 normally participates in DNA repair by temporarily elongating the helical strands to permit access by other repair enzymes. However, hyperactivation of this DNA repair enzyme from excessive DNA damage leads to formation of an abundant amount of poly(ADP-ribose) (PAR) and consumption of NAD^+. Moreover, hyperactivation of PARP-1 can cause mitochondrial state 4 respiration, followed by loss of mitochondrial membrane potential and release of AIF and cytochrome c (174). Release of PAR from the nucleus is involved in triggering release of AIF from the nucleus (175). Partial neuroprotection after cardiac arrest by PARP-1 gene deletion supports a role for PARP-1 in global ischemic cell death (176), although another PARP isoform, PARP-2, may have a different functional role (177). Because some of the injury from global ischemia is dependent on AMPA receptor activation and because AMPA-mediated excitotoxicity does not depend on PARP activation, the precise role of PARP enzymes and AIF in mediating neuronal death in global cerebral ischemia *in vivo* remains to be elucidated.

A mechanism of regulated cell death with necrotic morphology has been identified in the TNF-α extrinsic pathway that is independent of caspases, mitochondria transition pore, PARP, and AIF (178). This pathway has been implicated in focal ischemic injury, but its role in global ischemia is yet to be explored.

ZINC

Zinc has been implicated in selective, delayed neuronal death (Fig. 4). Zinc is present in a variety of neuronal populations and is particularly enriched in mossy fiber projections of the hippocampus. Normally, presynaptic release of Zn^{2+} with glutamate modulates neurotransmission by inhibiting NMDA and GABA receptors and by potentiating AMPA receptors. Postsynaptic entry of Zn^{2+} can occur via voltage-gated Ca^{2+} channels and NMDA receptor channels, but entry is particularly high through AMPA receptors that lack the GluR2 subunit. Expression of the latter receptor is normally low in the CA1 region but increases by 48 hr after global ischemia (179,180). Selectively inhibiting current in Ca^{2+}- and Zn^{2+}-permeable AMPA receptors reduced Zn^{2+} accumulation in CA1 neurons and provided partial protection from ischemia (180), whereas inducing these receptors in hippocampal granule cells augmented ischemic cell death (37). Toxic accumulation of Zn^{2+} in mitochondria inhibits energy metabolism (181). The cell-impermeant chelator ethylene diamine tetra acetic acid (EDTA) retains high binding affinity for Zn^{2+} when saturated with Ca^{2+} (182). Intraventricular injection of CaEDTA reduced Zn^{2+} accumulation in CA1 neurons after global ischemia and protected these neurons, as well as neurons in cortex,

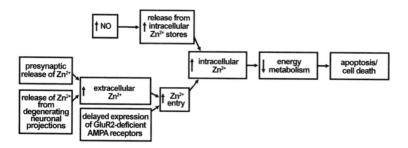

Figure 4 Increases in intracellular zinc are postulated to cause mitochondrial dysfunction and decreased energy metabolism, which lead to cell death, in part by apoptotic mechanisms. Current evidence suggests that increased nitric oxide can cause release of zinc from intracellular stores and that extracellular sources of zinc are also important, particularly in delayed death via entry through newly synthesized GluR2-deficient α-amino-3-hydroxy-5-methyl-4-isoxazole propionic acid receptors.

amygdala, and thalamic reticular nucleus (182). Global cerebral ischemia also produces a delayed increase in Zn^{2+} (182). Consequently, neuroprotection in CA1 by CaEDTA is biphasic. Pretreatment reduced downregulation of NMDA NR2, delayed increase in intracellular Zn^{2+}, release of cytochrome c and Smac into the cytosol, increased caspase-3 activity, DNA fragmentation, and cell death (179). Treatment at 3 to 6 hr after ischemia provided no protection, but treatment at 48 to 60 hr remarkably provided partial protection by inhibiting the delayed increase in Zn^{2+} accumulation and DNA fragmentation, despite the presence of GluR2-deficient AMPA receptors and activated caspase-3 at the time of administration (179). Efficacy of the cell-impermeable CaEDTA supports a transcellular source of Zn^{2+}, possibly arising from degenerating presynaptic terminals. Oxygen–glucose deprivation in hippocampal slices acutely increased extracellular Zn^{2+}, even after isolating CA1 from the rest of the hippocampus (183). The increase was dependent on NOS activity. However, intracellular Zn^{2+} can also be mobilized by NO. In primary cortical neuronal cultures, elevating NO with either an NO donor or by NMDA administration mobilized intracellular Zn^{2+}, which then accumulated in mitochondria where it inhibited respiration, generated reactive oxygen species, decreased mitochondrial membrane potential, released cytochrome c, and eventually led to apoptotic cell death that had a caspase-independent component (184). Therefore, Zn^{2+} accumulation has received attention as an important player in acute and delayed neurodegeneration after global ischemia, and further work is expected to refine insights into its mechanism of action.

CONCLUSIONS AND FUTURE DIRECTIONS

The events that lead to neuronal death after global cerebral ischemia and reperfusion are multifactorial and interrelated in a complex fashion. Many agents have been described as neuroprotectants in experimental stroke models, but fewer agents have been documented as neuroprotectants in global cerebral ischemia models. Experimental stroke models have a gradient of CBF reduction, permitting salvage of tissue, in which metabolism is only partially compromised. With uniformly severe reductions in CBF in most global ischemia models, the mechanisms of cell death are multifactorial, and manipulation of a single pathway is less likely to have a significant impact on cell survival. When an improvement in outcome can be demonstrated with a particular agent, the duration of global ischemia is typically constrained to 5 to 12 min, and efficacy may be limited to delayed neurodegeneration in hippocampus. The use of multiple agents in a "cocktail" regimen, targeting reactive oxygen species, ER stress, multiple pathways of regulated cell death signaling, and inflammatory mediators, is more likely to be required for obtaining clinically significant improvements from global ischemia, particularly for long ischemic durations. Postresuscitation hypothermia, which is one of the few therapies found to be efficacious clinically after cardiac arrest, acts to limit injury via multiple mechanisms and may be viewed as a "broad-spectrum" neuroprotectant. However, the logistic constraints of rapidly reducing brain temperature in humans during early reperfusion after cardiac arrest, particularly out-of-hospital arrests, will require the continued search for neuroprotectants that (i) can be administered early to limit the initial injury and extend the therapeutic window for hypothermia and (ii) can complement the efficacy of agents targeted at delayed mechanisms of injury that involve apoptosis and inflammation. As in the field of focal ischemic research, future work on global ischemic injury is expected to expand into cell engineering strategies for regenerating selectively vulnerable neurons.

REFERENCES

1. Hansen AJ. Effect of anoxia on ion distribution in the brain. Physiol Rev 1985; 65:101–148.
2. Silver IA, Erecinska M. Intracellular and extracellular changes of [Ca^{2+}] in hypoxia and ischemia in rat brain in vivo. J Gen Physiol 1990; 95:837–866.
3. Eleff SM, Maruki Y, Monsein LH, et al. Sodium, ATP, and intracellular pH transients during reversible complete ischemia of dog cerebrum. Stroke 1991; 22:233–241.
4. Katsura K, Rodriguez de Turco EB, Folbergrova J, et al. Coupling among energy failure, loss of ion homeostasis, and phospholipase A2 and C activation during ischemia. J Neurochem 1993; 61:1677–1684.
5. Eleff SM, Schleien CL, Koehler RC, et al. Brain bioenergetics during cardiopulmonary resuscitation in dogs. Anesthesiology 1992; 76:77–84.

6. Heiss WD. Experimental evidence of ischemic thresholds and functional recovery. Stroke 1992; 23:1668–1672.
7. Koehler RC, Backofen JE, McPherson RW, et al. Cerebral blood flow and evoked potentials during Cushing response in sheep. Am J Physiol Heart Circ Physiol 1989; 256:H779–H788.
8. Hurn PD, Koehler RC, Norris SE, et al. Dependence of cerebral energy phosphate and evoked potential recovery on end-ischemic pH. Am J Physiol Heart Circ Physiol 1991; 260:H532–H541.
9. Nishijima MK, Koehler RC, Hurn PD, et al. Postischemic recovery rate of cerebral ATP, phosphocreatine, pH, and evoked potentials. Am J Physiol Heart Circ Physiol 1989; 257:H1860–H1870.
10. Sieber FE, Koehler RC, Brown PR, et al. Diabetic chronic hyperglycemia and cerebral pH recovery following global ischemia in dogs. Stroke 1994; 25:1449–1455.
11. Kalimo H, Rehncrona S, Soderfeldt B, et al. Brain lactic acidosis and ischemic cell damage: 2. Histopathology. J Cereb Blood Flow Metab 1981; 1:313–327.
12. Pulsinelli WA, Waldman S, Rawlinson D, et al. Moderate hyperglycemia augments ischemic brain damage: a neuropathologic study in the rat. Neurology 1982; 32:1239–1246.
13. Eleff SM, Kim H, Shaffner DH, et al. Effect of cerebral blood flow generated during cardiopulmonary resuscitation in dogs on maintenance versus recovery of ATP and pH. Stroke 1993; 24:2066–2073.
14. Shaffner DH, Eleff SM, Brambrink AM, et al. Effect of arrest time and cerebral perfusion pressure during cardiopulmonary resuscitation on cerebral blood flow, metabolism, adenosine triphosphate recovery, and pH in dogs. Crit Care Med 1999; 27:1335–1342.
15. Shaffner DH, Eleff SM, Koehler RC, et al. Effect of the no-flow interval and hypothermia on cerebral blood flow and metabolism during cardiopulmonary resuscitation in dogs. Stroke 1998; 29:2607–2615.
16. Safar P, Stezoski W, Nemoto EM. Amelioration of brain damage after 12 minutes cardiac arrest in dogs. Arch Neurol 1976; 33:91–95.
17. Sterz F, Leonov Y, Safar P, et al. Hypertension with or without hemodilution after cardiac arrest in dogs. Stroke 1990; 21:1178–1184.
18. Maruki Y, Koehler RC, Eleff SM, et al. Intracellular pH during reperfusion influences evoked potential recovery after complete cerebral ischemia. Stroke 1993; 24:697–703.
19. Maruki Y, Koehler RC, Kirsch JR, et al. Effect of the 21-aminosteroid tirilazad on cerebral pH and somatosensory evoked potentials after incomplete ischemia. Stroke 1993; 24:724–730.
20. Sadoshima S, Heistad DD. Regional cerebral blood flow during hypotension in normotensive and stroke-prone spontaneously hypertensive rats: effect of sympathetic denervation. Stroke 1983; 14:575–579.
21. Haddad GG, Jiang C. O_2 deprivation in the central nervous system: on mechanisms of neuronal response, differential sensitivity and injury. Prog Neurobiol 1993; 40:277–318.
22. Sieber FE, Palmon SC, Traystman RJ, et al. Global incomplete cerebral ischemia produces predominantly cortical neuronal injury. Stroke 1995; 26:2091–2095.
23. Kalimo H, Garcia JH, Kamijyo Y, et al. The ultrastructure of "brain death." II. Electron microscopy of feline cortex after complete ischemia. Virchows Arch B Cell Pathol 1977; 25:207–220.
24. Arsenio-Nunes ML, Hossmann KA, Frakas-Bargeton E. Ultrastructural and histochemical investigation of the cerebral cortex of cat during and after complete ischemia. Acta Neuropathol 1973; 26:329–344.
25. Ginsberg MD, Graham DI, Welsh FA, et al. Diffuse cerebral ischemia in the cat: III. Neuropathological sequelae of severe ischemia. Ann Neurol 1979; 5:350–358.
26. Kawai K, Nitecka L, Ruetzler CA, et al. Global cerebral ischemia associated with cardiac arrest in the rat: I. Dynamics of early neuronal changes. J Cereb Blood Flow Metab 1992; 12:238–249.
27. Jenkins LW, Povlishock JT, Lewelt W, et al. The role of postischemic recirculation in the development of ischemic neuronal injury following complete cerebral ischemia. Acta Neuropathol (Berl) 1981; 55:205–220.
28. Blomqvist P, Wieloch T. Ischemic brain damage in rats following cardiac arrest using a long-term recovery model. J Cereb Blood Flow Metab 1985; 5:420–431.
29. Helfaer MA, Ichord RN, Martin LJ, et al. Treatment with the competitive NMDA antagonist GPI 3000 does not improve outcome after cardiac arrest in dogs. Stroke 1998; 29:824–829.
30. Kirsch JR, Bhardwaj A, Martin LJ, et al. Neither L-arginine nor L-NAME affects neurological outcome after global ischemia in cats. Stroke 1997; 28:2259–2264.
31. Kirino T. Delayed neuronal death in the gerbil hippocampus following ischemia. Brain Res 1982; 239:57–69.
32. Myers RE, Yamaguchi S. Nervous system effects of cardiac arrest in monkeys. Preservation of vision. Arch Neurol 1977; 34:65–74.
33. Pulsinelli WA, Brierley JB, Plum F. Temporal profile of neuronal damage in a model of transient forebrain ischemia. Ann Neurol 1982; 11:491–498.
34. Radovsky A, Safar P, Sterz F, et al. Regional prevalence and distribution of ischemic neurons in dog brains 96 hours after cardiac arrest of 0 to 20 minutes. Stroke 1995; 26:2127–2133.
35. Martin LJ, Brambrink A, Koehler RC, et al. Primary sensory and forebrain motor systems in the newborn brain are preferentially damaged by hypoxia-ischemia. J Comp Neurol 1997; 377:262–285.

36. Globus MY, Busto R, Dietrich WD, et al. Effect of ischemia on the in vivo release of striatal dopamine, glutamate, and gamma-aminobutyric acid studied by intracerebral microdialysis. J Neurochem 1988; 51:1455–1464.
37. Liu S, Lau L, Wei J, et al. Expression of Ca(2+)-permeable AMPA receptor channels primes cell death in transient forebrain ischemia. Neuron 2004; 43:43–55.
38. Guerguerian AM, Brambrink AM, Traystman RJ, et al. Altered expression and phosphorylation of N-methyl-D-aspartate receptors in piglet striatum after hypoxia-ischemia. Brain Res Mol Brain Res 2002; 104:66–80.
39. Takagi N, Shinno K, Teves L, et al. Transient ischemia differentially increases tyrosine phosphorylation of NMDA receptor subunits 2A and 2B. J Neurochem 1997; 69:1060–1065.
40. Brain Resuscitation Clinical Trial II Study Group. A randomized clinical study of a calcium-entry blocker (lidoflazine) in the treatment of comatose survivors of cardiac arrest. N Engl J Med 1991; 324:1225–1231.
41. Forsman M, Aarseth HP, Nordby HK, et al. Effects of nimodipine on cerebral blood flow and cerebrospinal fluid pressure after cardiac arrest: correlation with neurologic outcome. Anesth Analg 1989; 68:436–443.
42. Sakabe T, Nagai I, Ishikawa T, et al. Nicardipine increases cerebral blood flow but does not improve neurologic recovery in a canine model of complete cerebral ischemia. J Cereb Blood Flow Metab 1986; 6:684–690.
43. Steen PA, Gisvold SE, Milde JH, et al. Nimodipine improves outcome when given after complete cerebral ischemia in primates. Anesthesiology 1985; 62:406–414.
44. Buchan A, Pulsinelli WA. Hypothermia but not the N-methyl-D-aspartate antagonist, MK-801, attenuates neuronal damage in gerbils subjected to transient global ischemia. J Neurosci 1990; 10:311–316.
45. Nellgard B, Wieloch T. Postischemic blockade of AMPA but not NMDA receptors mitigates neuronal damage in the rat brain following transient severe cerebral ischemia. J Cereb Blood Flow Metab 1992; 12:2–11.
46. Fleischer JE, Tateishi A, Drummond JC, et al. MK-801, an excitatory amino acid antagonist, does not improve neurologic outcome following cardiac arrest in cats. J Cereb Blood Flow Metab 1989; 9:795–804.
47. Sterz F, Leonov Y, Safar P, et al. Effect of excitatory amino acid receptor blocker MK-801 on overall, neurologic, and morphologic outcome after prolonged cardiac arrest in dogs. Anesthesiology 1989; 71:907–918.
48. Lanier WL, Perkins WJ, Karlsson BR, et al. The effects of dizocilpine maleate (MK-801), an antagonist of the N-methyl-D-aspartate receptor, on neurologic recovery and histopathology following complete cerebral ischemia in primates. J Cereb Blood Flow Metab 1990; 10:252–261.
49. Wieloch T. Hypoglycemia-induced neuronal damage prevented by an N-methyl-D-aspartate antagonist. Science 1985; 230:681–683.
50. Pelligrino D, Almquist LO, Siesjo BK. Effects of insulin-induced hypoglycemia on intracellular pH and impedance in the cerebral cortex of the rat. Brain Res 1981; 221:129–147.
51. Sieber FE, Derrer SA, Eleff SM, et al. Hypocapnic-hypoglycemic interactions on cerebral high-energy phosphates and pH in dogs. Am J Physiol 1992; 263:H1864–H1871.
52. Giffard RG, Monyer H, Christine CW, et al. Acidosis reduces NMDA receptor activation, glutamate neurotoxicity, and oxygen-glucose deprivation neuronal injury in cortical cultures. Brain Res 1990; 506:339–342.
53. Hurn PD, Koehler RC, Traystman RJ. Alkalemia reduces recovery from global cerebral ischemia by NMDA receptor-mediated mechanism. Am J Physiol Heart Circ Physiol 1997; 272:H2557–H2562.
54. Cronberg T, Jensen K, Rytter A, et al. Selective sparing of hippocampal CA3 cells following in vitro ischemia is due to selective inhibition by acidosis. Eur J Neurosci 2005; 22:310–316.
55. Xiong ZG, Zhu XM, Chu XP, et al. Neuroprotection in ischemia: blocking calcium-permeable acid-sensing ion channels. Cell 2004; 118:687–698.
56. Aarts M, Iihara K, Wei WL, et al. A key role for TRPM7 channels in anoxic neuronal death. Cell 2003; 115:863–877.
57. Bano D, Young KW, Guerin CJ, et al. Cleavage of the plasma membrane Na+/Ca2+ exchanger in excitotoxicity. Cell 2005; 120:275–285.
58. Roberts-Lewis JM, Savage MJ, Marcy VR, et al. Immunolocalization of calpain I-mediated spectrin degradation to vulnerable neurons in the ischemic gerbil brain. J Neurosci 1994; 14:3934–3944.
59. Yokota M, Saido TC, Kamitani H, et al. Calpain induces proteolysis of neuronal cytoskeleton in ischemic gerbil forebrain. Brain Res 2003; 984:122–132.
60. Zhang C, Siman R, Xu YA, et al. Comparison of calpain and caspase activities in the adult rat brain after transient forebrain ischemia. Neurobiol Dis 2002; 10:289–305.
61. Yokota M, Saido TC, Tani E, et al. Three distinct phases of fodrin proteolysis induced in postischemic hippocampus. Involvement of calpain and unidentified protease. Stroke 1995; 26:1901–1907.
62. Hewitt KE, Lesiuk HJ, Tauskela JS, et al. Selective coupling of mu-calpain activation with the NMDA receptor is independent of translocation and autolysis in primary cortical neurons. J Neurosci Res 1998; 54:223–232.

63. Martone ME, Jones YZ, Young SJ, et al. Modification of postsynaptic densities after transient cerebral ischemia: a quantitative and three-dimensional ultrastructural study. J Neurosci 1999; 19:1988–1997.

64. Neumar RW, Xu YA, Gada H, et al. Cross-talk between calpain and caspase proteolytic systems during neuronal apoptosis. J Biol Chem 2003; 278:14,162–14,167.

65. Polster BM, Basanez G, Etxebarria A, et al. Calpain I induces cleavage and release of apoptosis-inducing factor from isolated mitochondria. J Biol Chem 2005; 280:6447–6454.

66. Dawson VL, Kizushi VM, Huang PL, et al. Resistance to neurotoxicity in cortical cultures from neuronal nitric oxide synthase-deficient mice. J Neurosci 1996; 16:2479–2487.

67. Huang Z, Huang PL, Panahian N, et al. Effects of cerebral ischemia in mice deficient in neuronal nitric oxide synthase. Science 1994; 265:1883–1885.

68. Huang Z, Huang PL, Ma J, et al. Enlarged infarcts in endothelial nitric oxide synthase knockout mice are attenuated by nitro-L-arginine. J Cereb Blood Flow Metab 1996; 16:981–987.

69. Buchan AM, Gertler SZ, Huang ZG, et al. Failure to prevent selective CA1 neuronal death and reduce cortical infarction following cerebral ischemia with inhibition of nitric oxide synthase. Neuroscience 1994; 61:1–11.

70. Sancesario G, Iannone M, Morello M, et al. Nitric oxide inhibition aggravates ischemic damage of hippocampal but not of NADPH neurons in gerbils. Stroke 1994; 25:436–443.

71. Shapira S, Kadar T, Weissman BA. Dose-dependent effect of nitric oxide synthase inhibition following transient forebrain ischemia in gerbils. Brain Res 1994; 668:80–84.

72. Caldwell M, O'Neill M, Earley B, et al. Nω-Nitro-L-arginine protects against ischaemia-induced increases in nitric oxide and hippocampal neuro-degeneration in the gerbil. Eur J Pharmacol 1994; 260:191–200.

73. Zhang J, Benveniste H, Klitzman B, et al. Nitric oxide synthase inhibition and extracellular glutamate concentration after cerebral ischemia/reperfusion. Stroke 1995; 26:298–304.

74. Nanri K, Montecot C, Springhetti V, et al. The selective inhibitor of neuronal nitric oxide synthase, 7-nitroindazole, reduces the delayed neuronal damage due to forebrain ischemia in rats. Stroke 1998; 29:1248–1253.

75. Panahian N, Yoshida T, Huang PL, et al. Attenuated hippocampal damage after global cerebral ischemia in mice mutant in neuronal nitric oxide synthase. Neuroscience 1996; 72:343–354.

76. Tominaga T, Sato S, Ohnishi T, et al. Electron paramagnetic resonance (EPR) detection of nitric oxide produced during forebrain ischemia of the rat. J Cereb Blood Flow Metab 1994; 14:715–722.

77. Lei B, Adachi N, Nagaro T, et al. Nitric oxide production in the CA1 field of the gerbil hippocampus after transient forebrain ischemia: effects of 7-nitroindazole and NG-nitro-L-arginine methyl ester. Stroke 1999; 30:669–677.

78. Nakagomi T, Sasaki T, Kirino T, et al. Effect of cyclooxygenase and lipoxygenase inhibitors on delayed neuronal death in the gerbil hippocampus. Stroke 1989; 20:925–929.

79. Alkayed NJ, Goyagi T, Joh HD, et al. Neuroprotection and P450 2C11 upregulation after experimental transient ischemic attack. Stroke 2002; 33:1677–1684.

80. Node K, Huo Y, Ruan X, et al. Anti-inflammatory properties of cytochrome P450 epoxygenase-derived eicosanoids. Science 1999; 285:1276–1279.

81. Takeuchi K, Miyata N, Renic M, et al. Hemoglobin, NO, and 20-HETE interactions in mediating cerebral vasoconstriction following SAH. Am J Physiol Regul Integr Comp Physiol 2006; 290:R84–R89.

82. Miyata N, Seki T, Tanaka Y, et al. Beneficial effects of a new 20-hydroxyeicosatetraenoic acid synthesis inhibitor, TS-011 [N-(3-chloro-4-morpholin-4-yl) phenyl-N'-hydroxyimido formamide], on hemorrhagic and ischemic stroke. J Pharmacol Exp Ther 2005; 314:77–85.

83. Breder CD, Dewitt D, Kraig RP. Characterization of inducible cyclooxygenase in rat brain. J Comp Neurol 1995; 355:296–315.

84. Wang H, Hitron IM, Iadecola C, et al. Synaptic and vascular associations of neurons containing cyclooxygenase-2 and nitric oxide synthase in rat somatosensory cortex. Cereb Cortex 2005; 15:1250–1260.

85. Maslinska D, Wozniak R, Kaliszek A, et al. Expression of cyclooxygenase-2 in astrocytes of human brain after global ischemia. Folia Neuropathol 1999; 37:75–79.

86. Sasaki T, Kitagawa K, Yamagata K, et al. Amelioration of hippocampal neuronal damage after transient forebrain ischemia in cyclooxygenase-2-deficient mice. J Cereb Blood Flow Metab 2004; 24:107–113.

87. Koistinaho J, Koponen S, Chan PH. Expression of cyclooxygenase-2 mRNA after global ischemia is regulated by AMPA receptors and glucocorticoids. Stroke 1999; 30:1900–1905.

88. Candelario-Jalil E, Alvarez D, Gonzalez-Falcon A, et al. Neuroprotective efficacy of nimesulide against hippocampal neuronal damage following transient forebrain ischemia. Eur J Pharmacol 2002; 453:189–195.

89. Candelario-Jalil E, Gonzalez-Falcon A, Garcia-Cabrera M, et al. Assessment of the relative contribution of COX-1 and COX-2 isoforms to ischemia-induced oxidative damage and neurodegeneration following transient global cerebral ischemia. J Neurochem 2003; 86:545–555.

90. Ahmad AS, Saleem S, Ahmad M, et al. Prostaglandin EP1 receptor contributes to excitotoxicity and focal ischemic brain damage. Toxicol Sci 2006; 89:265–270.

91. Kawano T, Anrather J, Zhou P, et al. Prostaglandin E(2) EP1 receptors: downstream effectors of COX-2 neurotoxicity. Nat Med 2006; 12:225–229.
92. McCullough L, Wu L, Haughey N, et al. Neuroprotective function of the PGE2 EP2 receptor in cerebral ischemia. J Neurosci 2004; 24:257–268.
93. Kim SF, Huri DA, Snyder SH. Inducible nitric oxide synthase binds, S-nitrosylates, and activates cyclooxygenase-2. Science 2005; 310:1966–1970.
94. Mori K, Togashi H, Ueno KI, et al. Aminoguanidine prevented the impairment of learning behavior and hippocampal long-term potentiation following transient cerebral ischemia. Behav Brain Res 2001; 120:159–168.
95. Kawase M, Murakami K, Fujimura M, et al. Exacerbation of delayed cell injury after transient global ischemia in mutant mice with CuZn superoxide dismutase deficiency. Stroke 1999; 30:1962–1968.
96. Murakami K, Kondo T, Epstein CJ, et al. Overexpression of CuZn-superoxide dismutase reduces hippocampal injury after global ischemia in transgenic mice. Stroke 1997; 28:1797–1804.
97. Sugawara T, Noshita N, Lewen A, et al. Overexpression of copper/zinc superoxide dismutase in transgenic rats protects vulnerable neurons against ischemic damage by blocking the mitochondrial pathway of caspase activation. J Neurosci 2002; 22:209–217.
98. Biemond P, van Eijk HG, Swaak AJ, et al. Iron mobilization from ferritin by superoxide derived from stimulated polymorphonuclear leukocytes. Possible mechanism in inflammation diseases. J Clin Invest 1984; 73:1576–1579.
99. Rehncrona S, Hauge HN, Siesjo BK. Enhancement of iron-catalyzed free radical formation by acidosis in brain homogenates: differences in effect by lactic acid and CO2. J Cereb Blood Flow Metab 1989; 9:65–70.
100. Halliwell B. Reactive oxygen species and the central nervous system. J Neurochem 1992; 59:1609–1623.
101. Komara JS, Nayini NR, Bialick HA, et al. Brain iron delocalization and lipid peroxidation following cardiac arrest. Ann Emerg Med 1986; 15:384–389.
102. Lipscomb DC, Gorman LG, Traystman RJ, et al. Low molecular weight iron in cerebral ischemic acidosis in vivo. Stroke 1998; 29:487–492.
103. Beckman JS, Beckman TW, Chen J, et al. Apparent hydroxyl radical production by peroxynitrite: implications for endothelial injury from nitric oxide and superoxide. Proc Natl Acad Sci USA 1990; 87:1620–1624.
104. Eliasson MJ, Huang Z, Ferrante RJ, et al. Neuronal nitric oxide synthase activation and peroxynitrite formation in ischemic stroke linked to neural damage. J Neurosci 1999; 19:5910–5918.
105. Fukuyama N, Takizawa S, Ishida H, et al. Peroxynitrite formation in focal cerebral ischemia-reperfusion in rats occurs predominantly in the peri-infarct region. J Cereb Blood Flow Metab 1998; 18:123–129.
106. Ischiropoulos H, Beckman JS. Oxidative stress and nitration in neurodegeneration: cause, effect, or association? J Clin Invest 2003; 111:163–169.
107. Palmer C, Towfighi J, Roberts RL, et al. Allopurinol administered after inducing hypoxia-ischemia reduces brain injury in 7-day-old rats. Pediatr Res 1993; 33:405–411.
108. Betz AL, Randall J, Martz D. Xanthine oxidase is not a major source of free radicals in focal cerebral ischemia. Am J Physiol 1991; 260:H563–H568.
109. Mink RB, Dutka AJ, Kumaroo KK, et al. No conversion of xanthine dehydrogenase to oxidase in canine cerebral ischemia. Am J Physiol Heart Circ Physiol 1990; 259:H1655–H1659.
110. Phillis JW, Perkins LM, Smith-Barbour M, et al. Oxypurinol-enhanced postischemic recovery of the rat brain involves preservation of adenine nucleotides. J Neurochem 1995; 64:2177–2184.
111. Faraci FM. Reactive oxygen species: influence on cerebral vascular tone. J Appl Physiol 2006; 100:739–743.
112. Girouard H, Iadecola C. Neurovascular coupling in the normal brain and in hypertension, stroke, and Alzheimer disease. J Appl Physiol 2006; 100:328–335.
113. Martin LJ, Brambrink AM, Price AC, et al. Neuronal death in newborn striatum after hypoxia-ischemia is necrosis and evolves with oxidative stress. Neurobiol Dis 2000; 7:169–191.
114. Rafols JA, Daya AM, O'Neil BJ, et al. Global brain ischemia and reperfusion: Golgi apparatus ultrastructure in neurons selectively vulnerable to death. Acta Neuropathol (Berl) 1995; 90:17–30.
115. Paschen W, Mengesdorf T. Cellular abnormalities linked to endoplasmic reticulum dysfunction in cerebrovascular disease—therapeutic potential. Pharmacol Ther 2005; 108:362–375.
116. DeGracia DJ, Kumar R, Owen CR, et al. Molecular pathways of protein synthesis inhibition during brain reperfusion: implications for neuronal survival or death. J Cereb Blood Flow Metab 2002; 22:127–141.
117. Hu BR, Martone ME, Jones YZ, et al. Protein aggregation after transient cerebral ischemia. J Neurosci 2000; 20:3191–3199.
118. Hayashi T, Saito A, Okuno S, et al. Oxidative damage to the endoplasmic reticulum is implicated in ischemic neuronal cell death. J Cereb Blood Flow Metab 2003; 23:1117–1128.
119. Hayashi T, Saito A, Okuno S, et al. Damage to the endoplasmic reticulum and activation of apoptotic machinery by oxidative stress in ischemic neurons. J Cereb Blood Flow Metab 2005; 25:41–53.
120. Kumar R, Krause GS, Yoshida H, et al. Dysfunction of the unfolded protein response during global brain ischemia and reperfusion. J Cereb Blood Flow Metab 2003; 23:462–471.

121. Paschen W, Aufenberg C, Hotop S, et al. Transient cerebral ischemia activates processing of xbp1 messenger RNA indicative of endoplasmic reticulum stress. J Cereb Blood Flow Metab 2003; 23:449–461.

122. Paschen W, Hayashi T, Saito A, et al. GADD34 protein levels increase after transient ischemia in the cortex but not in the CA1 subfield: implications for post-ischemic recovery of protein synthesis in ischemia-resistant cells. J Neurochem 2004; 90:694–701.

123. Page AB, Owen CR, Kumar R, et al. Persistent eIF2alpha(P) is colocalized with cytoplasmic cytochrome c in vulnerable hippocampal neurons after 4 hours of reperfusion following 10-minute complete brain ischemia. Acta Neuropathol (Berl) 2003; 106:8–16.

124. Ruan YW, Ling GY, Zhang JL, et al. Apoptosis in the adult striatum after transient forebrain ischemia and the effects of ischemic severity. Brain Res 2003; 982:228–240.

125. Schmidt-Kastner R, Fliss H, Hakim AM. Subtle neuronal death in striatum after short forebrain ischemia in rats detected by in situ end-labeling for DNA damage. Stroke 1997; 28:163–169.

126. Nakajima W, Ishida A, Lange MS, et al. Apoptosis has a prolonged role in the neurodegeneration after hypoxic ischemia in the newborn rat. J Neurosci 2000; 20:7994–8004.

127. Krajewska M, Mai JK, Zapata JM, et al. Dynamics of expression of apoptosis-regulatory proteins Bid, Bcl-2, Bcl-X, Bax and Bak during development of murine nervous system. Cell Death Differ 2002; 9:145–157.

128. Martin LJ, Al-Abdulla NA, Brambrink AM, et al. Neurodegeneration in excitotoxicity, global cerebral ischemia, and target deprivation: a perspective on the contributions of apoptosis and necrosis. Brain Res Bull 1998; 46:281–309.

129. Martin LJ. Neuronal cell death in nervous system development, disease, and injury (Review). Int J Mol Med 2001; 7:455–478.

130. Chen J, Nagayama T, Jin K, et al. Induction of caspase-3-like protease may mediate delayed neuronal death in the hippocampus after transient cerebral ischemia. J Neurosci 1998; 18:4914–4928.

131. Himi T, Ishizaki Y, Murota S. A caspase inhibitor blocks ischaemia-induced delayed neuronal death in the gerbil. Eur J Neurosci 1998; 10:777–781.

132. Zhao H, Yenari MA, Cheng D, et al. Biphasic cytochrome c release after transient global ischemia and its inhibition by hypothermia. J Cereb Blood Flow Metab 2005; 25:1119–1129.

133. Larm JA, Cheung NS, Beart PM. Apoptosis induced via AMPA-selective glutamate receptors in cultured murine cortical neurons. J Neurochem 1997; 69:617–622.

134. Deshpande J, Bergstedt K, Linden T, et al. Ultrastructural changes in the hippocampal CA1 region following transient cerebral ischemia: evidence against programmed cell death. Exp Brain Res 1992; 88:91–105.

135. Colbourne F, Sutherland GR, Auer RN. Electron microscopic evidence against apoptosis as the mechanism of neuronal death in global ischemia. J Neurosci 1999; 19:4200–4210.

136. Martin LJ, Sieber FE, Traystman RJ. Apoptosis and necrosis occur in separate neuronal populations in hippocampus and cerebellum after ischemia and are associated with differential alterations in metabotropic glutamate receptor signaling pathways. J Cereb Blood Flow Metab 2000; 20:153–167.

137. Northington FJ, Ferriero DM, Flock DL, et al. Delayed neurodegeneration in neonatal rat thalamus after hypoxia-ischemia is apoptosis. J Neurosci 2001; 21:1931–1938.

138. Northington FJ, Ferriero DM, Graham EM, et al. Early neurodegeneration after hypoxia-ischemia in neonatal rat is necrosis while delayed neuronal death is apoptosis. Neurobiol Dis 2001; 8:207–219.

139. Jin K, Chen J, Nagayama T, et al. In situ detection of neuronal DNA strand breaks using the Klenow fragment of DNA polymerase I reveals different mechanisms of neuron death after global cerebral ischemia. J Neurochem 1999; 72:1204–1214.

140. Kawase M, Fujimura M, Morita-Fujimura Y, et al. Reduction of apurinic/apyrimidinic endonuclease expression after transient global cerebral ischemia in rats: implication of the failure of DNA repair in neuronal apoptosis. Stroke 1999; 30:441–448.

141. Narasimhan P, Sugawara T, Liu J, et al. Overexpression of human copper/zinc-superoxide dismutase in transgenic animals attenuates the reduction of apurinic/apyrimidinic endonuclease expression in neurons after in vitro ischemia and after transient global cerebral ischemia. J Neurochem 2005; 93:351–358.

142. MacManus JP, Hill IE, Preston E, et al. Differences in DNA fragmentation following transient cerebral or decapitation ischemia in rats. J Cereb Blood Flow Metab 1995; 15:728–737.

143. MacManus JP, Rasquinha I, Tuor U, et al. Detection of higher-order 50- and 10-kbp DNA fragments before apoptotic internucleosomal cleavage after transient cerebral ischemia. J Cereb Blood Flow Metab 1997; 17:376–387.

144. MacManus JP, Fliss H, Preston E, et al. Cerebral ischemia produces laddered DNA fragments distinct from cardiac ischemia and archetypal apoptosis. J Cereb Blood Flow Metab 1999; 19:502–510.

145. Graham EM, Sheldon RA, Flock DL, et al. Neonatal mice lacking functional Fas death receptors are resistant to hypoxic-ischemic brain injury. Neurobiol Dis 2004; 17:89–98.

146. Padosch SA, Popp E, Vogel P, et al. Altered protein expression levels of Fas/CD95 and Fas ligand in differentially vulnerable brain areas in rats after global cerebral ischemia. Neurosci Lett 2003; 338:247–251.

147. Krajewska M, Rosenthal RE, Mikolajczyk J, et al. Early processing of Bid and caspase-6, -8, -10, -14 in the canine brain during cardiac arrest and resuscitation. Exp Neurol 2004; 189:261–279.
148. Jin K, Graham SH, Mao X, et al. Fas (CD95) may mediate delayed cell death in hippocampal CA1 sector after global cerebral ischemia. J Cereb Blood Flow Metab 2001; 21:1411–1421.
149. Sugawara T, Fujimura M, Morita-Fujimura Y, et al. Mitochondrial release of cytochrome c corresponds to the selective vulnerability of hippocampal CA1 neurons in rats after transient global cerebral ischemia. J Neurosci 1999; 19:RC39.
150. Raval AP, Dave KR, Prado R, et al. Protein kinase C delta cleavage initiates an aberrant signal transduction pathway after cardiac arrest and oxygen glucose deprivation. J Cereb Blood Flow Metab 2005; 25:730–741.
151. Cao G, Pei W, Lan J, et al. Caspase-activated DNase/DNA fragmentation factor 40 mediates apoptotic DNA fragmentation in transient cerebral ischemia and in neuronal cultures. J Neurosci 2001; 21:4678–4690.
152. Cao G, Xiao M, Sun F, et al. Cloning of a novel Apaf-1-interacting protein: a potent suppressor of apoptosis and ischemic neuronal cell death. J Neurosci 2004; 24:6189–6201.
153. Siegelin MD, Kossatz LS, Winckler J, et al. Regulation of XIAP and Smac/DIABLO in the rat hippocampus following transient forebrain ischemia. Neurochem Int 2005; 46:41–51.
154. Abe T, Takagi N, Nakano M, et al. The effects of monobromobimane on neuronal cell death in the hippocampus after transient global cerebral ischemia in rats. Neurosci Lett 2004; 357:227–231.
155. Hetz C, Vitte PA, Bombrun A, et al. Bax channel inhibitors prevent mitochondrion-mediated apoptosis and protect neurons in a model of global brain ischemia. J Biol Chem 2005; 280:42,960–42,970.
156. Yang J, Liu X, Bhalla K, et al. Prevention of apoptosis by Bcl-2: release of cytochrome c from mitochondria blocked. Science 1997; 275:1129–1132.
157. Kluck RM, Bossy-Wetzel E, Green DR, et al. The release of cytochrome c from mitochondria: a primary site for Bcl-2 regulation of apoptosis. Science 1997; 275:1132–1136.
158. Chen J, Graham SH, Nakayama M, et al. Apoptosis repressor genes Bcl-2 and Bcl-x-long are expressed in the rat brain following global ischemia. J Cereb Blood Flow Metab 1997; 17:2–10.
159. Carboni S, Antonsson B, Gaillard P, et al. Control of death receptor and mitochondrial-dependent apoptosis by c-Jun N-terminal kinase in hippocampal CA1 neurones following global transient ischaemia. J Neurochem 2005; 92:1054–1060.
160. Guan QH, Pei DS, Zhang QG, et al. The neuroprotective action of SP600125, a new inhibitor of JNK, on transient brain ischemia/reperfusion-induced neuronal death in rat hippocampal CA1 via nuclear and non-nuclear pathways. Brain Res 2005; 1035:51–59.
161. Abe T, Takagi N, Nakano M, et al. Altered Bad localization and interaction between Bad and Bcl-xL in the hippocampus after transient global ischemia. Brain Res 2004; 1009:159–168.
162. Ouyang YB, Tan Y, Comb M, et al. Survival- and death-promoting events after transient cerebral ischemia: phosphorylation of Akt, release of cytochrome C and Activation of caspase-like proteases. J Cereb Blood Flow Metab 1999; 19:1126–1135.
163. Klein JA, Longo-Guess CM, Rossmann MP, et al. The harlequin mouse mutation downregulates apoptosis-inducing factor. Nature 2002; 419:367–374.
164. Vahsen N, Cande C, Briere JJ, et al. AIF deficiency compromises oxidative phosphorylation. EMBO J 2004; 23:4679–4689.
165. Li LY, Luo X, Wang X. Endonuclease G is an apoptotic DNase when released from mitochondria. Nature 2001; 412:95–99.
166. Lee BI, Lee DJ, Cho KJ, et al. Early nuclear translocation of endonuclease G and subsequent DNA fragmentation after transient focal cerebral ischemia in mice. Neurosci Lett 2005; 386:23–27.
167. Zhao H, Yenari MA, Cheng D, et al. Bcl-2 transfection via herpes simplex virus blocks apoptosis-inducing factor translocation after focal ischemia in the rat. J Cereb Blood Flow Metab 2004; 24:681–692.
168. Zhu C, Qiu L, Wang X, et al. Involvement of apoptosis-inducing factor in neuronal death after hypoxia-ischemia in the neonatal rat brain. J Neurochem 2003; 86:306–317.
169. Cao G, Clark RS, Pei W, et al. Translocation of apoptosis-inducing factor in vulnerable neurons after transient cerebral ischemia and in neuronal cultures after oxygen-glucose deprivation. J Cereb Blood Flow Metab 2003; 23:1137–1150.
170. Ferrand-Drake M, Zhu C, Gido G, et al. Cyclosporin A prevents calpain activation despite increased intracellular calcium concentrations, as well as translocation of apoptosis-inducing factor, cytochrome c and caspase-3 activation in neurons exposed to transient hypoglycemia. J Neurochem 2003; 85:1431–1442.
171. Wang H, Yu SW, Koh DW, et al. Apoptosis-inducing factor substitutes for caspase executioners in NMDA-triggered excitotoxic neuronal death. J Neurosci 2004; 24:10,963–10,973.
172. Yu SW, Wang H, Poitras MF, et al. Mediation of poly(ADP-ribose) polymerase-1-dependent cell death by apoptosis-inducing factor. Science 2002; 297:259–263.
173. Mandir AS, Poitras MF, Berliner AR, et al. NMDA but not non-NMDA excitotoxicity is mediated by Poly(ADP-ribose) polymerase. J Neurosci 2000; 20:8005–8011.

174. Cipriani G, Rapizzi E, Vannacci A, et al. Nuclear poly(ADP-ribose) polymerase-1 rapidly triggers mitochondrial dysfunction. J Biol Chem 2005; 280:17227–17234.
175. Koh DW, Lawler AM, Poitras MF, et al. Failure to degrade poly(ADP-ribose) causes increased sensitivity to cytotoxicity and early embryonic lethality. Proc Natl Acad Sci USA 2004; 101:17,699–17,704.
176. Kofler J, Sawada M, Hattori H, Dawson VL, Hurn PD, Traystman RJ. Brain injury after cardiac arrest and cardiopulmonary resuscitation (CPR): role of poly(ADP-ribose) polymerase (PARP). In: Krieglstein J, Klumpp S, eds. Pharmacology of Cerebral Ischemia. Stuttgart: Medpharm Scientific Publishers, 2002:397–403.
177. Kofler J, Otsuka T, Zhang Z, et al. Differential effect of PARP-2 deletion on brain injury after focal and global cerebral ischemia. J Cereb Blood Flow Metab 2006; 26:135–141.
178. Degterev A, Huang Z, Boyce M, et al. Chemical inhibitor of nonapoptotic cell death with therapeutic potential for ischemic brain injury. Nat Chem Biol 2005; 1:112–119.
179. Calderone A, Jover T, Mashiko T, et al. Late calcium EDTA rescues hippocampal CA1 neurons from global ischemia-induced death. J Neurosci 2004; 24:9903–9913.
180. Noh KM, Yokota H, Mashiko T, et al. Blockade of calcium-permeable AMPA receptors protects hippocampal neurons against global ischemia-induced death. Proc Natl Acad Sci USA 2005; 102: 12,230–12,235.
181. Sheline CT, Behrens MM, Choi DW. Zinc-induced cortical neuronal death: contribution of energy failure attributable to loss of NAD(+) and inhibition of glycolysis. J Neurosci 2000; 20:3139–3146.
182. Koh JY, Suh SW, Gwag BJ, et al. The role of zinc in selective neuronal death after transient global cerebral ischemia. Science 1996; 272:1013–1016.
183. Wei G, Hough CJ, Li Y, et al. Characterization of extracellular accumulation of Zn2+ during ischemia and reperfusion of hippocampus slices in rat. Neuroscience 2004; 125:867–877.
184. Bossy-Wetzel E, Talantova MV, Lee WD, et al. Crosstalk between nitric oxide and zinc pathways to neuronal cell death involving mitochondrial dysfunction and p38-activated K+ channels. Neuron 2004; 41:351–365.

26 | Management of Brain Injury Following Cardiopulmonary Arrest

Romergryko G. Geocadin, MD, Assistant Professor[a], Director[b], Associate Director[c]

[a]Departments of Neurology, Anesthesiology/Critical Care Medicine, and Neurosurgery, Johns Hopkins University School of Medicine, [b]Neurosciences Critical Care Unit, Johns Hopkins Bayview Medical Center, and [c]Neurosciences Critical Care Division, The Johns Hopkins Medical Institutions, Baltimore, Maryland, USA

INTRODUCTION

The pioneering work of Safar et al. in 1958 (1) on airway methods of artificial respiration and of Kouwenhoven et al. in the early 1960s (2,3) on the closed cardiac massage with external defibrillation led to the development of modern basic and advanced cardiac life support for patients in cardiopulmonary arrest. Since these early works, several large clinical trials have been undertaken to improve survival and functional outcome in this patient population.

With advances in critical care, cardiopulmonary resuscitation led to increased survival, but the functional outcome continued to be poor. Many patients who were successfully resuscitated remained in persistent coma or suffered significant cognitive deficits. Realizing the importance of neurologic injury from global cerebral ischemia of cardiac arrests (CA), the American Heart Association focused on brain injury and introduced the term "cardiopulmonary-cerebral resuscitation" in the Guidelines for Cardiopulmonary Resuscitation and Emergency Cardiovascular Care of 2000 (4). The same guidelines further provide that, "The cerebral cortex, the tissue most susceptible to hypoxia, is irreversibly damaged, resulting in death or severe neurological damage. The need to preserve cerebral viability must be stressed in research endeavors and in practical interventions." (4).

Several advances have been added in the practice of resuscitation, but neurologic functional outcome, especially in comatose patients following CA, continues to be poor. Examples of these advancements include faster response time to patients with out-of-hospital CA, the use of early cardiac defibrillation, and increased public awareness of basic life-support skills (5,6). Consequently, the number of CA victims who survive with severe neurologic injury has increased (7).

However, recently, survival and functional neurologic outcomes have been significantly improved by therapeutic intervention. Two studies reported that induced hypothermia from 32 to 34°C for 12 to 24 hours resulted in improved survival and functional outcome (8,9), and these findings led the International Liaison Committee on Resuscitation (ILCOR) to recommend hypothermia in patients who are unconscious after resuscitation from CA (10). This chapter discusses the development of controlled clinical trials and management of brain injury after CA.

PATHOPHYSIOLOGIC CONSIDERATION

The field of medicine related to cardiopulmonary resuscitation deals with a hypoxic-ischemic process that involves the entire body. Although the inciting factors that lead to CA can be varied (e.g., primary ventricular fibrillation or asphyxiation), total circulatory failure with CA injures both brain and extracerebral organs. The injury stimulates complex adaptive and maladaptive responses at the levels of cells, tissues, organs, and, ultimately, the organism. The primary injury in specific organs causes secondary effects on other organs, which can worsen injury to the brain and heart. A common example of such an injury is disruption of the gastrointestinal barrier caused by ischemia, leading to bacterial toxin leakage into the bloodstream (11,12). Ischemic injury can also disrupt blood vessels, releasing a variety of mediators that potentially injure otherwise unaffected tissues and cells (13,14). This complex interplay between the heart, brain, vasculature, gastrointestinal tract, muscle, inflammatory system, coagulation system, and other organs requires intervention by a multidisciplinary team that can address multiorgan injury. Although the focus of this chapter is the management of brain injury after CA, some discussions will address the systemic injury in relation to the neurologic injury and recovery. A detailed discussion of the cellular and molecular pathophysiologic mechanisms of post cardiac arrest, ischemic brain injury, and their relevance to neuroprotective therapies is provided in Chapters 25 and 29.

CONTROLLED CLINICAL TRIALS OF BRAIN-DIRECTED THERAPIES AFTER CARDIAC ARREST

The controlled clinical trials that focus on brain injury from global ischemia in CA started with the Brain Resuscitation Clinical Trials (BRCT) in 1986 (15) and have continued with studies by the Hypothermia After Cardiac Arrest (HACA) Study Group (8) and Australian groups (9) in 2002, which studied the use of moderate hypothermia. The agents used in these studies were chosen based on results of preclinical animal experimentation that showed potential benefit. Further clinical studies using similar agents in related neurologic injuries also demonstrated efficacy. All of these therapies, with the exception of induced hypothermia, provided no significant benefit to neurologic or functional outcome. However, the failed clinical trials provided critical insight into the epidemiology, pathophysiology, and clinical trial design in this injury paradigm.

Thiopental
Thiopental was the first agent used in a well-organized, randomized, clinical study. It was successfully tested in a primate model of global ischemia (16) and in successful pilot studies in humans (17). As a barbiturate, it can ameliorate injury by reducing metabolism, edema formation, intracranial pressure (ICP), seizure activity, and damage by focal and incomplete ischemia (15). The thiopental study was also known as the BRCT 1.

The BRCT 1 included all comatose patients after return of spontaneous circulation (ROSC). Clinical parameters, such as initial cardiac rhythm, the duration of CA and resuscitation, and place of arrest (in-hospital or out-of-hospital), were not stratified or controlled. The BRCT trials (18) developed a functional outcome measure as defined by the five-point scale of the Glasgow-Pittsburgh Outcome Categories, as follows: Cerebral Performance Category (CPC) 1, conscious and normal, without disability; CPC 2, conscious with moderate disability; CPC 3, conscious with severe disability; CPC 4, comatose or vegetative state; CPC 5, death. This scale was divided into favorable outcome, defined as CPC 1 and 2, and unfavorable outcome, CPC 3, 4, and 5. For the BRCT trial, the outcome was determined at 48 and 72 hours, 10 days, and 1, 3, 6, and 12 months (18).

BRCT 1 compared a thiopental intravenous (IV) loading dose of 30 mg/kg at 10 to 50 minutes after ROSC to placebo, and both arms enrolled 131 participants (15). The primary outcome, as measured by a treatment-blinded investigator using the five-point CPC scale, showed no difference between treated and control groups. Overall good outcome with thiopental treatment was seen in 20% of patients, and good outcome in the control group was 15%. Mortality was 70% in the thiopental group and 80% in the control group. A significant factor that may have contributed to the failure of thiopental was the excess in hypotensive episodes (60%), compared to the control group (29%) (15).

Glucocorticoids
The BRCT 1 trial allowed for the addition of glucocorticoids to the study agent (thiopental or placebo) at the discretion of the treating physician. This arm of the BRCT 1 was not controlled, and the data was analyzed retrospectively (19). The inclusion criteria and the primary outcome measure were identical to the thiopental study. The choice of glucocorticoid, either dexamethazone or methylprednisolone, was dependent on the treatment preference of the center and was administered during the first 8 hours post ROSC. The glucocorticoid treatment doses were divided into no dose, low dose (1–20 mg of dexamethazone), medium dose (21–70 mg of dexamathazone), and high dose (equivalent >70 mg of dexamathazone). The percentage of patients with good outcome (CPC 1 and 2) was similar for all dose groups, which ranged from 34.0% to 37.3% (19).

Lidoflazine

As a follow-up study, the BRCT 2 compared the functional outcomes of patients treated with the calcium channel blocker lidoflazine (1 mg/kg IV) within 30 minutes after ROSC, followed by 0.25 mg/kg at 8 hours and 16 hours (n = 257) or placebo (20). The 6-month functional outcome by CPC showed no significant difference between groups, with good outcome in 15% of lidoflazine-treated patients, compared to 13% in the placebo-treated patients. The 6-month mortality was also similar, at 82% with lidoflazine treatment and 83% with placebo (20).

Despite the failure of the BRCT trials to show therapeutic benefit, many important findings were noted, especially pertaining to epidemiology and methodology of clinical trials in brain injury after CA. After the BRCT 1 trials, the American Heart Association and the European Resuscitation Council jointly sponsored a consensus meeting to facilitate research and reduce variability in methodologies. The task force published the "Utstein Style Guidelines" in 1991, which provided recommendations for the conducting, reporting, and reviewing of research on out-of-hospital CA (21); in 1997, they published guidelines for in-hospital resuscitation (22). Many of these methodologies were used in succeeding trials, especially in the HACA hypothermia trial in 2002 (8).

Nimodipine

Based on the observation that nimodipine reduced death or severe ischemic deficits in subarachnoid hemorrhage (23), several clinical trials were conducted (24,25). An open pilot study on the safety and efficacy of nimodipine in patients after out-of-hospital ventricular CA (24) was followed by a controlled, randomized clinical study. The clinical trial excluded prolonged resuscitation (>30 minutes), limited the cases to ventricular fibrillation and ventricular tachycardia (25), and used the Glasgow Outcome Score (GOS) at one year and a secondary endpoint of Glasgow Coma Score (GCS 1) at 24 hours and 1 week as outcomes. Interval functional evaluations were conducted at 3 and 12 months using the Mini-mental Examination, Barthels, and Katz ADL Scale (24).

Nimodipine was given as a bolus of 10 µg/kg followed by 0.5 µg/kg over 24 hours, and the treated group was compared to a placebo group (24). The study agent was given immediately after resuscitation, which was usually at the site of the resuscitation, with 75 patients in the nimodipine arm and 80 patients in the placebo arm. The 1-year good outcome (GOS 1) for the nimodipine-treated patients was 29%, compared to placebo with 24%. One-year mortalities were 60% in the nimodipine-treated group and 64% in the placebo group (23).

Glucose-Free Solution

The next study was conducted because of an observation that hyperglycemia was associated with poor recovery after CA (26). Undertaken primarily by the Emergency Medical Services, the study compared the effect of nondextrose (0.45% NaCl; n=377) and dextrose (5%; n=371) solution during resuscitation. Of the 748 patients randomized, 291 patients were admitted to the hospital. Of those admitted, 141 patients received the dextrose solution and 150 received the nondextrose solution. With the patient awakening as the functional endpoint, no difference was observed between the dextrose solution arm (16.7%) and the nondextrose arm (14.6%). The number of patients surviving to discharge after treatment was similar, with 15.1% in the dextrose-solution arm and 13.3% in the nondextrose-solution arm (26).

Magnesium

The search for effective therapies continued with the idea that magnesium, with its antiarrythmic effects and ability to block excitatory neurotransmitters, would be beneficial in CA victims (27). Two clinical trials were undertaken in this area, the first conducted in 1997 (27), followed by another study using magnesium in association with diazepam in 2002 (28). The inhibitory action of diazepam was hypothesized to reduce neuroexcitotoxic injury after CA.

A randomized, double-blinded, placebo-controlled study (27) compared the efficacy of empiric magnesium supplementation to placebo in patients resuscitated from in-hospital CA on successful ROSC and survival to discharge. Magnesium was administered in a 2-g IV bolus followed by 8 g over 24 hours. ROSC was the primary outcome, and survival and GCS at discharge was the secondary outcome. The observed ROSC was 54% in magnesium-treated patients, compared to 60% in the placebo group. Patient survival was 43% in the magnesium arm, and 50% in the placebo arm survived to 24 hours (27).

Diazepam

The comparative effectiveness of magnesium, diazepam, magnesium+diazepam, and placebo in patients awakening from CPR from out-of-hospital CA was studied in 2002 (28). The study agents were administered intravenously upon ROSC at the following doses: 2 g magnesium, 10 mg diazepam, 2 g magnesium+10 mg diazepam, and placebo. At three months, no significant difference was noted in the proportion of patients who awoke (magnesium: 46.7%, diazepam: 30.7%, magnesium+diazepam: 29.3%, and placebo: 37.3%). The mortality at three months was likewise similar in the four groups: magnesium: 62.7%, diazepam: 76.0%, magnesium+diazepam: 77.3%, and placebo: 68% (28).

Systemic Thrombolytics and Brain Injury in Cardiac Arrest

A significant number of patients in CA have underlying myocardial infarction or pulmonary embolism. Thrombolysis as a therapy has been a concern because of the potential increased risk of intracranial bleeding. Several uncontrolled studies found that systemic thrombolysis for acute myocardial infarction in this setting is relatively safe for the brain (29,30).

Besides the ability to promote perfusion in larger vessels affected with coronary thrombosis and pulmonary emboli, experimental data indicate that thrombolysis during CPR can improve microcirculatory reperfusion, especially in the brain (31). With this finding as the basis, a pilot study was undertaken to investigate the use of recombinant tissue plasminogen activator (rtPA) in patients in whom conventional CPR had been unsuccessful. More patients treated with rtPA (68%) had ROSC, compared with 44% in controls (32). With these findings, a multicentered trial is currently being undertaken in Europe, designed to assess the effectiveness of rtPA in improving the outcome in patients who were initially unsuccessfully resuscitated in the field.

Adverse Events Reported in Clinical Trials

The adverse events related to the agents studied must be considered. Only two complications that reached statistical significance over controls were reported in the aforementioned clinical trials. First is the excess occurrence of hypotension in the group treated with thiopental (60%), compared to the control group (29%; $p < 0.001$) in the BRCT 1 study (15). This increase in hypotensive episodes required more vasopressor use in the thiopental group. In the Roine Study (24), the group treated with nimodipine was also observed to have more hypotensive episodes, requiring dopamine infusion (73% compared to 49% for controls; $p = 0.003$) Several other adverse events did not reach statistical significance but are worth noting, such as the tendency to increase infection rates with glucocorticoid treatment in BRCT 1 (19).

CLINICAL TRIALS IN HYPOTHERMIA AND CARDIAC ARREST

The process of induced hypothermia as a therapy for acute brain injury was first described in the 1940s with the therapeutic cooling of patients (33). Several reports followed with the use of induced hypothermia during cardiac surgery in the 1950s (34) and 1960s (35). In the 1980s, researchers in Pittsburgh (36,37) and Miami (38,39) approached induced hypothermia for brain injury after CA in a more systematic manner, leading to extensive preclinical studies that showed functional and survival benefit of hypothermia in rodent (40,41) and canine models (42,43). Based on these findings, pilot hypothermia studies in human were undertaken and showed encouraging results of improved clinical outcomes (44,45).

The mechanism by which hypothermia leads to improved survival and functional recovery is not precisely understood. Numerous mechanisms have been suggested (38), including the effect of hypothermia on (i) cerebral blood flow and metabolism that retards the initial rate of ATP depletion (46,47), (ii) reduction of excitotoxic neurotransmitter release (48), (iii) alteration of intracellular messenger and mediator activity (49), (iv) blood-brain barrier breakdown (50), (v) reduction of inflammatory response (51), and (vi) alteration in gene expression and protein synthesis (52,53). Recent studies found that hypothermia-induced neuroprotection in a rodent model ameliorates cell death of hippocampal CA1 neurons via the ischemia-induced down-regulation of the AMPA-receptor subunit GluR2 (54). Neuroprotection was noted as early as two days after ischemia, with normalization of GluR2 mRNA levels in hypothermia-treated animals within one week (54). Although the brain was the primary beneficiary of hypothermia

Table 1   Checklist for Initiation of Hypothermia After Cardiac Arrest

Assessment

Initial patient assessment prior to beginning cooling

- ❏   Assess medical therapy. (Vasopressor and vasodilators might affect heat transfer, increase potential for skin injury, and contribute to adverse hemodynamic response.)
- ❏   Obtain core (rectal or bladder) temperature
- ❏   Obtain vitals and hemodynamic values
- ❏   Monitor cardiac rhythm
- ❏   Assess baseline electrolytes, glucose, ABG, coagulation labs, lactate, and CPK with MB fractions
- ❏   Assess baseline neurologic examination
- ❏   Assess ventilatory function
- ❏   Assess bowel sounds, abdomen, and GI function
- ❏   Assess skin integrity. (External cooling devices might exacerbate skin injury, especially if the patient has preexisting conditions, such as diabetes, and/or the patient is on vasopressors.)

Ongoing assessment

- ❏   Full assessment q 4 hr
- ❏   Temperature check q 1 hr
- ❏   Vitals every 15 min × 4, then every 1 hr
- ❏   Hemodynamics evaluation by pulmonary artery catheter protocol
- ❏   Assess for signs of shivering
- ❏   Cardiac rhythm every 4 hr
- ❏   If shivering occurs and no pulse oximetry available, draw ABGs every 1 hr until shivering ceases
- ❏   Maintain normal blood glucose. Use insulin as necessary

Interventions (cooling process)

- ❏   Initiate ICU sedation. (Midazolam infusion is agent of choice.)
- ❏   Vecuronium IV for signs of shivering
- ❏   Adjust cooling/warming based on established clinical target (32–34°C from 24 hr) and on method and device used for cooling/warming

Interventions (rewarming process)

- ❏   Once patient is maintained at target temperature for 24 hr, remove cooling blanket; may add warm blankets, and remove wet/damp clothing or bed linens
- ❏   Passive rewarming to normal temperature over 8 hr (not faster than 0.5°C/hr)

Abbreviations: ICU, intensive care unit; IV, intravenous; ABG, arterial blood gas; CPK, creatine phosphokinase; MB, myocardial isoenzyme (** such as in CPK-MB or creatine phosphokinase—myocardial isoenzyme); GI, gastrointestinal.
Source: Modified from Johns Hopkins Hospital – CCU Nursing Protocol, 2002.

therapy, other organ systems could have also benefited from this treatment, a consequence that might play an important role in reducing extracerebral injury and help to promote overall survival (Table 1).

European Hypothermia Study

In the multicentered European study conducted by the HACA group (8), 3551 potentially eligible patients were screened with a waiver of consent, and 273 patients were included in the study. The study randomized patients to induced hypothermia for 24 hours versus standard normothermic post-ROSC care, with 137 patients in the hypothermia arm and 138 in the normothermia arm. The patients assigned to the hypothermia group were cooled to a target temperature of 32°C to 34°C via a covered external cooling mattress cover that delivers cold air over the entire body. The goal was to reach the target temperature within four hours from ROSC. Core temperature was monitored via a sensor in the urinary bladder catheter. The temperature was maintained at 32°C to 34°C for 24 hours from the start of cooling, followed by passive rewarming over a period of 8 hours. Patients were sedated with midazolam and provided with paralytics (vecuronium) to prevent shivering, a cause of rise in temperature. This is the only study that showed a significant difference in both mortality and functional outcome. Using the 5-point CPC, 55% of patients treated with hypothermia had a favorable outcome (CPC 1 and 2), compared to 39% in the normothermia control group (relative risk of good outcome: 1.40; 95% confidence interval (CI), CI: 1.08–1.81). The hypothermia arm also had significantly lower six-month mortality, at 41% compared to 55% of the control (risk ratio: 0.74; 95% CI: 0.58–0.95) (8).

Australian Hypothermia Study

The Australian study (9) enrolled comatose patients after ROSC who presented with an initial cardiac rhythm of ventricular fibrillation. Seventy-seven patients were randomly assigned to hypothermia or normothermia, according to the day of the month, with patients assigned to hypothermia on odd-numbered days. The hypothermia arm had 43 patients, and the normothermia arm had 34 patients. Paramedics initiated hypothermia by removing the patient's clothing and applying cold packs to the head and torso. In the hospital, patients underwent vigorous cooling by means of extensive application of ice packs around the head, neck, torso, and limbs to a target core temperature of 33°C, which was monitored by tympanic or bladder thermometer. The target temperature was maintained for 12 hours, and the patient was sedated and paralyzed with small doses of midazolam and vecuronium, as needed to prevent shivering. The patients were actively rewarmed by external warming with a heated-air blanket, beginning at the 18th hour after arrival, with continued sedation and neuromuscular blockade to suppress shivering. Similar sedation and paralysis protocol was provided to patients assigned to the normothermic group, but the target core temperature was maintained at 37°C. Passive rewarming was used in these patients if they presented with mild spontaneous hypothermia.

The primary outcome measures were the places of discharge: to home, to a rehabilitation facility, or to a long-term nursing facility. Prior to discharge from the hospital, patients were evaluated by a specialist in rehabilitation medicine who was blinded to the treatment protocol. Discharge to home or to a rehabilitation facility was regarded as a good outcome, whereas death in the hospital or discharge to a long-term nursing facility, whether the patient was conscious or unconscious, was regarded as a poor outcome. The study found that 49% of patients in the hypothermia arm had good outcome, compared to 26% in the normothermia arm (relative risk for good outcome: 1.85, 95% CI: 0.97–3.49; $p = 0.046$). The overall mortality between the two groups did not reach statistical significance, with 51% for the hypothermia arm and 68% for the normothermia arm.

Based on the results of these two induced-hypothermia studies (8,9), a recommendation was made by the Task Force of the ILCOR (10,55) such that, "Unconscious adult patients with spontaneous circulation after out-of-hospital cardiac arrest should be cooled to 32°C–34°C for 12–24 hours when the initial rhythm was ventricular fibrillation (VF)." Such cooling may also be beneficial for other rhythms or in-hospital cardiac arrest.

Timing of Cooling and Rewarming

The ideal time to initiate hypothermia post-ROSC has not yet been determined, but its benefits could be maximized if it is initiated as soon as possible after ROSC. Despite a delay of 4 to 6 hours, hypothermia still provides benefit. In the European study, the interval between ROSC and attainment of target temperature had an interquartile range of 4 to 16 hours (8,10,55).

Rewarming to normothermia should be undertaken slowly to avoid worsening of neurologic injury, which has been associated with rewarming posthypothermia (56,57). The European study rewarmed patients passively over 8 hours after 24 hours of hypothermia, whereas the Australian study reported active rewarming for 6 hours at 18 hours of ROSC (8,9). The ILCOR recommended that emphasis be placed on research to determine optimal duration of therapeutic hypothermia, optimum target temperature, and rates of cooling and rewarming.

Complications of Hypothermia

The clinical use of induced hypothermia must be undertaken with its potential adverse effects in mind. Although no single complication was reported to be statistically significant over controls in the two trials, the potential risk of harm remains real. The HACA study defined complications to be any of the following: bleeding of any severity, pneumonia, sepsis, pancreatitis, renal failure, pulmonary edema, seizures, arrhythmias, and pressure sores (8). The proportion of patients reported with complications in the HACA study is provided in Figure 1. Although numerous patients were reported to have complications from therapy, the proportion of patients did not differ significantly between the two groups, with 93 of 132 patients in the normothermia group (70%) and 98 of 135 in the hypothermia group (73%; $p = 0.70$). The total number of complications was not significantly higher in the hypothermia group than in the normothermia group ($p = 0.09$).

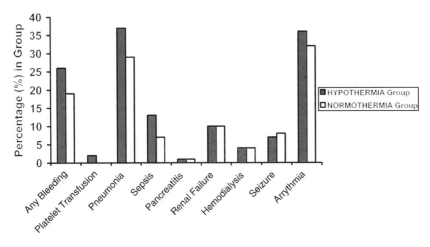

Figure 1   Complications at 0 to 7 days after cardiac arrest (European Hypothermia Study 2002).

Devices and Methods of Induced Hypothermia

As hypothermia evolves as a therapy, the types of devices used to induce it are also increasing dramatically. Generally, these methods can be classified either as surface cooling or invasive (endovascular) cooling. The two controlled studies successfully used surface cooling, with the European group using external cooling by a mattress that delivers cold air over the entire body, and the Australian study using extensive application of ice packs around the head, neck, torso, and limbs (8,9). Some devices introduced for temperature control by means of invasive (endovascular) cooling (58,59) or surface cooling (60,61) have also been used to induce hypothermia. At the time of this writing, no published study comparing any of these hypothermia methods and devices is available. Although manufacturers of these devices claim the ability to induce hypothermia, it is important several factors be considered when deciding on which methods and devices to use, including: the clinical setting where cooling is initiated [in the field, in the emergency department, or in the intensive care unit (ICU)], the ability of the first responders to initiate hypothermia, the rapidity of induction and stability of temperature while in the therapeutic range (with careful consideration to maintain temperature in the desired range), the transportability of the device and the ability to allow procedures, such as cardiac catheterization, to be undertaken, the adverse effects associated with the specific method or device, and, lastly, the user-friendly interface of the device and how it facilitates or hampers provision of care in a critical care environment.

Another means of inducing hypothermia is to infuse ice-cold IV fluid after successful resuscitation in the field (62,63). Bernard et al. showed that rapid infusion of large volume (30 mL/kg), ice-cold (4°C) IV fluid would be a safe, rapid, and inexpensive technique to induce mild hypothermia in 22 comatose survivors of out-of-hospital CA (63). The ability of this method to rapidly initiate hypothermia, especially in the field, complements the established methods of surface and endovascular cooling in the Emergency Department or in the Critical Care Unit.

Shivering and Pharmacologic Paralysis

Shivering can cause a significant disruption of therapeutic hypothermia by generation of heat, leading to increased core body temperature and oxygen consumption (10,55). The European and Australian studies used vecuronium infusion as a paralytic, with IV midazolam as an accompanying sedative (8,9). The initiation of pharmacologic paralysis with sedation will require full mechanical respiratory support. Total paralysis will also make clinical neurologic assessment very limited. Therefore, a detailed neurologic assessment is essential prior to the start and at the completion of pharmacologic paralysis and sedation. The neurologic evaluation must consist of not only the GCS, but also a careful evaluation of cranial nerve function, and sensory motor responses. A decline in neurologic function merits emergent diagnostic evaluation (such as brain imaging) and neurophysiologic assessment (such as an electroencephalography or somatosensory-evoked potential testing).

Another concern related to shivering is that the discomfort associated with shivering might also be a problem for those patients who are emerging from coma. Although no comparison studies exist that address the degree of shivering in the different methods of hypothermia, more patients have been noted to shiver with rapid surface-cooling systems (60). In studies of cases of hypothermia in other conditions, such as stroke and postoperative states without total pharmacologic paralysis and sedation, the shivering threshold was lowered by the use of meperidine (64–67). The synergistic effect of buspirone with meperidine in controlling shivering has also been reported (64). Other agents that might be helpful in controlling shivering are clonidine, ketanserin, and doxapram (67).

The induction of hypothermia in post CA patients by means of an endovascular catheter has also been reported to be safe (68,69). The endovascular catheters are inserted percutaneously into large veins, such as the femoral and subclavian, to induce hypothermia. As this is an invasive procedure, technical expertise is warranted to attenuate complications. Other concerns include venous thrombosis, infection, and bleeding.

Metabolic Considerations in Therapeutic Hypothermia

Beyond the reported possible adverse events monitored in the two clinical trials, some metabolic perturbations might occur while patients are undergoing hypothermic therapy and rewarming to normothermic range. Hypothermia has been associated with hypokalemia, metabolic acidosis, and hyperglycemia (70). Close monitoring and appropriate correction of these conditions is essential for patient safety. Other electrolytes, such as magnesium and phosphates, must be monitored as well. Rebound of these abnormalities with rewarming must be considered when actively normalizing temperature to normothermia.

Limitations in the Widespread Use of Hypothermia

A recent study by Abella et al. (71) surveyed 265 randomly selected physicians from emergency medicine, critical care, and cardiology as to whether they treated patients with hypothermia. The majority (87%) had not used hypothermia for patients after CA. Among the reasons given were: (i) 49% felt that supportive data was insufficient, (ii) 32% mentioned the lack of incorporation of hypothermia into advanced cardiovascular life support (ACLS) protocols, and (iii) 28% felt that cooling methods were technically too slow or too difficult (71). Although the controlled studies and several follow-up studies support the use of hypothermia in patients after CA, awareness and education regarding this treatment option must be improved, and hypothermia protocols should be considered for inclusion in future iterations of ACLS.

SECONDARY INJURIES THAT AFFECT NEUROLOGIC OUTCOME

Despite the success of hypothermia, the progression of secondary brain injury is an important consideration in the recovery process of patients. Therefore, preventive strategies to attenuate secondary brain injury are critical. No randomized, controlled trials have been undertaken in relation to secondary brain injuries after CA. The approaches and interventions provided below are from uncontrolled and observational studies in brain injury after CA and other similar ischemic brain injuries.

Cerebral Edema and Intracranial Pressure Elevation

Global cerebral ischemia leads to the development of cytotoxic and vasogenic edema. Up to 47% of patients resuscitated from out-of-hospital arrest have cerebral edema on head CT at day 3 (72). Indirect evidence of ICP elevation, as shown by delayed hyperemia by transcranial-Doppler ultrasound, has been reported (73). However, ICP elevation is not commonly observed, and no conclusive study has been undertaken to show that routine ICP monitoring is needed. In situations where excessive cerebral edema leads to ICP elevation or further neurologic deterioration, short-term acute hyperventilation and bolus mannitol therapy can be used judiciously. These therapies have been used successfully in other pathologies, but their use in edema related to global ischemia has not been well described. Use of steroids does not provide benefit and can lead to adverse outcomes (19).

Cerebrovascular Autoregulation Impairment

A significant number of patients have impaired cerebral autoregulation during the acute phase after resuscitation from CA (74). The abnormality most noted was the absence of, or a right shift in, the cerebral blood flow autoregulatory curve (both of which require higher pressures for adequate perfusion) during the first 24 hours (74). In another study of human CA, survivors with good functional neurologic recovery were independently and positively associated with higher arterial blood pressure during the first two hours after arrest (75). With dysfunction of the auto-regulatory mechanism, improvement of cerebral perfusion might require a higher systemic blood pressure. Although the idea to increase blood pressure to promote cerebral perfusion could theoretically benefit some patients, caution is advised in patients with poor cardiovascular reserve.

Hyperglycemia

In global ischemia from CA, elevated serum glucose has been associated with unfavorable outcome (76,77). Serum glucose elevation is believed to be a marker of the severity of injury. In a series of 145 nondiabetic CA patients, a strong association was found between high median blood glucose levels over 24 hours and poor neurologic outcome (78).

Toward avoidance of potential neurologic injury, American Heart Association guidelines state that during cardiopulmonary resuscitation, drugs should be administered in nonglucose-containing solutions (79). In the absence of controlled human trials that report any benefit of glucose control in stroke and global cerebral ischemia, some insight might be gleaned from the general critical care literature. A randomized, controlled study of general ICU patients with primarily systemic pathology showed that tight control of serum glucose (80 and 110 mg/dL) facilitated reduction of overall mortality by approximately 50% (80). Therefore, glucose monitoring with tight control might prove beneficial to post CA patients.

Hyperthermia

Increasing body temperature after CA has been associated with poor neurologic outcome. In a study of patients presenting in the emergency department with CA, a body temperature higher than 37°C within 48 hours after resuscitation was associated with unfavorable functional neurologic recovery. For every degree higher than 37°C, the study reported an incremental increased association with severe disability, coma, or persistent vegetative state, [odds ratio (OR): 2.26; 95% CI: 1.24–4.12] (81). In another study, body temperature of 39°C or higher after resuscitation from CA was associated with brain death (OR: 37.8; 95% CI: 6.72–212.2) (82).

Fevers due to infection must be controlled, and the cause, properly treated. However, in a significant portion of patients, an infectious source for the fever is not identified. The mechanism by which "noninfectious" hyperthermia occurs after CA is still unclear. Occult infection from intestinal ischemia, the systemic translocation of bacteria or toxins (83), and pulmonary aspiration because of lack of airway protective reflexes in coma (84) are significant causes of hyperthermia in this subset of patients. Hyperthermia might be related to injuries that affect the anterior hypothalamus (85,86). Hyperthermia accentuates the release of neurotransmitters and free radical activity and promotes excitotoxic injury in global ischemia (39,87,88). Therefore, hyperthermia must be avoided during the post-CA period to provide the patient with the best chance of recovery.

Seizures/Myoclonus

Seizures can hinder the recovery of consciousness after CA. Subclinical or nonconvulsive status epilepticus can contribute to poor outcome. EEG should be obtained as soon as possible if seizures are suspected. No controlled studies have been undertaken to address prophylactic antiepileptic therapy. Treatment with anticonvulsants, therefore, must be reserved for those patients with proven seizures and should include a non-sedating, antiepileptic agent.

Postanoxic myoclonus (also known as the Lance-Adams syndrome) has been regarded as a predictor of poor outcome, but a recent report of survivors with postanoxic myoclonus indicates that the myoclonus might improve as neurologic status improves (89). Postanoxic myoclonus tends to occur after respiratory causes of CA and often persists after other signs of neurologic damage have improved. An EEG might be required to differentiate myoclonus from seizures. The treatment of postanoxic myoclonus can be challenging and must be individualized. The following drugs have been reported to reduce clinical myoclonus: valprioc acid, clonazepam, carbamazepine, gabapentin, levodopa, piracetam, methysergide, and leveracetam (90).

Age

Many victims of CA are elderly and have serious underlying comorbidities. Age has been a major concern due to the increasing comorbidities and the perception of increased chance of poor functional outcome following CA. The BRCT clinical trials examined the effect of age (>65 years) on outcome and found that it is associated with decreased overall survival after CA; however, age was not an independent risk factor for poor neurologic outcome (91).

Extracerebral Complications

The cause of death in the majority of patients after resuscitation is mostly extracerebral in nature. In the BRCT 1 study, 63.6% of patients died due to extracerebral causes, whereas 36.4% died from cerebral causes (15). A similar proportion was observed in BRCT 2, with extracerebral causes noted in 72.2% of patients and cerebral causes of death noted in 27.8% (20). In both BRCT 1 and 2, cardiac death accounted for approximately two-thirds of all extracerebral deaths. It is, therefore, noteworthy that the management of extracerebral or systemic complications in these patients, particularly of cardiac injury, is paramount to patient survival. A review of the percentage of mortality in the placebo-treated patients across clinical trials dedicated to brain injury after CA reveals a trend in a reduction in overall mortality over three decades (Fig. 2). With the exception of the 1990 nimodipine study (23), the controlled clinical trials from 1986 to 1993 had a percentage mortality of 80% or greater. The study by Roine selected patients with lesser injury by limiting the duration of CA time and resuscitation time (23). A declining trend in percentage mortality (<80%) is noted in studies from 1997 (27) to 2002 (8,9). Due to the wide variability in trial design, it will be very difficult to precisely determine the factors that lead to the reduction in mortality. However, two key factors might have changed in clinical practice over the time these trials were undertaken: (i) the desire of investigators to include patients with higher chances of survival after CA to allow the assessment of functional outcome, and (ii) the continued improvement in the standard of overall critical care in patients treated with placebo. As we evaluate the therapies to improve neurologic function, we must also consider the need for continued development in the critical care therapies. Only adequate critical care support will allow good functional recovery from brain injury post CA.

CONCLUSIONS

The medical management of brain injury in patients following cardiopulmonary arrest needs a comprehensive approach, starting with the control of the primary hypoxic-ischemic injury from the cessation of blood flow during the arrest and suboptimal perfusion during resuscitation prior to ROSC, to the prevention of secondary insults to the brain (cerebral

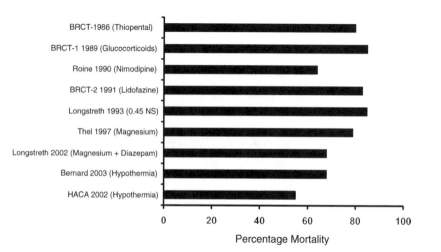

Figure 2   Percentage mortality in the placebo groups of clinical trials for brain injury after cardiac arrest (1986–2002). *Abbreviations*: BRCT, Brain Resuscitation Clinical Trials; HACA, Hypothermia After Cardiac Arrest.

edema, seizures) and reversal of extra-CNS related injuries from such systemic causes as persistent hypoperfusion, hyperthermia and hyperglycemia. Thus far, therapeutic hypothermia (32–34°C) for 12 to 24 hours is the only therapeutic modality that has demonstrated efficacy in improving both survival and functional outcomes following cardiopulmonary arrest. The successful institution of therapeutic hypothermia requires the proper utilization of the methods and devices and timing of cooling and rewarming and prevention of accompanying complications. The extensive preclinical and translational research leading to the favorable results with therapeutic hypothermia proved that brain injury after CA can be ameliorated to yield clinical improvement. Efforts are now on the way to further improve outcomes by enhancing the methods of inducing hypothermia and understanding the optimal period of therapy. Although clinical trials with pharmacological agents have not proven to be beneficial in this paradigm, further studies of agents with novel mechanisms or the use hypothermia in combination with pharmacological neuroprotection hold promise in the future.

REFERENCES

1. Safar P, Escarraga LA, Elam JO. A comparison of the mouth-to-mouth and mouth-to-airway methods of artificial respiration with the chest-pressure arm-lift methods. N Engl J Med 1958; 258:671–677.
2. Kouwenhoven WB, Jude JR, Knickerbocker GG. Closed-chest cardiac massage. JAMA 1960; 173: 1064–1067.
3. Jude JR, Kouwenhoven WB, Knickerbocker GG. An experimental and clinical study of a portable external cardiac defibrillator. Surg Forum 1962; 13:185–187.
4. AHA. Guidelines 2000 for cardiopulmonary resuscitation and emergency cardiovascular care, 2000.
5. Ekstrom L, Herlitz J, Wennerblom B, Axelsson A, Bang A, Holmberg S. Survival after cardiac arrest outside hospital over a 12-year period in gothenburg. Resuscitation 1994; 27:181–187.
6. Stiell IG, Wells GA, Field BJ, et al. Improved out-of-hospital cardiac arrest survival through the inexpensive optimization of an existing defibrillation program: Opals study phase ii. Ontario prehospital advanced life support. JAMA 1999; 281:1175–1181.
7. Grubb NR. Managing out-of-hospital cardiac arrest survivors: 1. Neurological perspective. Heart 2001; 85:6–8.
8. Mild therapeutic hypothermia to improve the neurologic outcome after cardiac arrest. N Engl J Med 2002; 346:549–556.
9. Bernard SA, Gray TW, Buist MD, Jones BM, Silvester W, Gutteridge G, Smith K. Treatment of comatose survivors of out-of-hospital cardiac arrest with induced hypothermia. N Engl J Med 2002; 346: 557–563.
10. Nolan JP, Morley PT, Vanden Hoek TL, et al. Therapeutic hypothermia after cardiac arrest: An advisory statement by the advanced life support task force of the international liaison committee on resuscitation. Circulation 2003; 108:118–121.
11. Kong SE, Blennerhassett LR, Heel KA, McCauley RD, Hall JC. Ischaemia-reperfusion injury to the intestine. Aust NZ J Surg 1998; 68:554–561.
12. Stechmiller JK, Treloar D, Allen N. Gut dysfunction in critically ill patients: A review of the literature. Am J Crit Care 1997; 6:204–209.
13. Carden DL, Granger DN. Pathophysiology of ischaemia-reperfusion injury. J Pathol 2000; 190:255–266.
14. Pittard AJ, Hawkins WJ, Webster NR. The role of the microcirculation in the multi-organ dysfunction syndrome. Clin Intensive Care 1994; 5:186–190.
15. Randomized clinical study of thiopental loading in comatose survivors of cardiac arrest. Brain resuscitation clinical trial i study group. N Engl J Med 1986; 314:397–403.
16. Bleyaert AL, Nemoto EM, Safar P, et al. Thiopental amelioration of brain damage after global ischemia in monkeys. Anesthesiology 1978; 49:390–398.
17. Mullie A, Lust P, Penninckx J, et al. Monitoring of cerebrospinal fluid enzyme levels in postischemic encephalopathy after cardiac arrest. Crit Care Med 1981; 9:399–400.
18. A randomized clinical study of cardiopulmonary-cerebral resuscitation: Design, methods, and patient characteristics. Brain resuscitation clinical trial i study group. Am J Emerg Med 1986; 4:72–86.
19. Jastremski M, Sutton-Tyrrell K, Vaagenes P, Abramson N, Heiselman D, Safar P. Glucocorticoid treatment does not improve neurological recovery following cardiac arrest. Brain resuscitation clinical trial i study group. JAMA 1989; 262:3427–3430.
20. A randomized clinical study of a calcium-entry blocker (lidoflazine) in the treatment of comatose survivors of cardiac arrest. Brain resuscitation clinical trial ii study group [see comments]. N Engl J Med 1991; 324:1225–1231.

21. Cummins RO, Chamberlain DA, Abramson NS, et al. Recommended guidelines for uniform reporting of data from out-of-hospital cardiac arrest: The utstein style. Task force of the American heart association, the european resuscitation council, the heart and stroke foundation of canada, and the australian resuscitation council. Ann Emerg Med 1991; 20:861–874.

22. Cummins RO, Chamberlain D, Hazinski MF, et al. Recommended guidelines for reviewing, reporting, and conducting research on in-hospital resuscitation: The in-hospital "utstein style". American heart association. Ann Emerg Med 1997; 29:650–679.

23. Allen GS, Ahn HS, Preziosi TJ, et al. Cerebral arterial spasm: a controlled trial of nimodipine in patients with subarachnoid hemorrhage. N Engl J Med 1983; 308:619–624.

24. Roine RO, Kaste M, Kinnunen A, Nikki P. Safety and efficacy of nimodipine in resuscitation of patients outside hospital. Br Med J (Clin Res Ed) 1987; 294:20.

25. Roine RO, Kaste M, Kinnunen A, Nikki P, Sarna S, Kajaste S. Nimodipine after resuscitation from out-of-hospital ventricular fibrillation. A placebo-controlled, double-blind, randomized trial. JAMA 1990; 264:3171–3177.

26. Longstreth WT Jr., Diehr P, Cobb LA, Hanson RW, Blair AD. Neurologic outcome and blood glucose levels during out-of-hospital cardiopulmonary resuscitation. Neurology 1986; 36:1186–1191.

27. Thel MC, Armstrong AL, McNulty SE, Califf RM, O'Connor CM. Randomised trial of magnesium in in-hospital cardiac arrest. Duke internal medicine housestaff. Lancet 1997; 350:1272–1276.

28. Longstreth WT Jr., Fahrenbruch CE, Olsufka M, Walsh TR, Copass MK, Cobb LA. Randomized clinical trial of magnesium, diazepam, or both after out-of-hospital cardiac arrest. Neurology 2002; 59:506–514.

29. Voipio V, Kuisma M, Alaspaa A, Manttari M, Rosenberg P. Thrombolytic treatment of acute myocardial infarction after out-of-hospital cardiac arrest. Resuscitation 2001; 49:251–258.

30. Ruiz-Bailen M, Aguayo de Hoyos E, Serrano-Corcoles MC, Diaz-Castellanos MA, Ramos-Cuadra JA, Reina-Toral A. Efficacy of thrombolysis in patients with acute myocardial infarction requiring cardiopulmonary resuscitation. Intensive Care Med 2001; 27:1050–1057.

31. Bottiger BW, Martin E. Thrombolytic therapy during cardiopulmonary resuscitation and the role of coagulation activation after cardiac arrest. Curr Opin Crit Care 2001; 7:176–183.

32. Bottiger BW, Bode C, Kern S, et al. Efficacy and safety of thrombolytic therapy after initially unsuccessful cardiopulmonary resuscitation: a prospective clinical trial. Lancet 2001; 357:1583–1585.

33. Fay T. Observations on generalized refrigeration in cases of severe cerebral trauma. Assoc Res Nerv Ment Dis Proc 1943; 24:611–619.

34. Bigelow WG, Lindsay WK, Greenwood WF. Hypothermia; its possible role in cardiac surgery: an investigation of factors governing survival in dogs at low body temperatures. Ann Surg 1950; 132:849–866.

35. Rosomoff HL. Protective effects of hypothermia against pathological processes of the nervous system. Ann NY Acad Sci 1959; 80:475–486.

36. Safar P, Behringer W, Bottiger BW, Sterz F. Cerebral resuscitation potentials for cardiac arrest. Crit Care Med 2002; 30:S140–S144.

37. Safar P. Cerebral resuscitation after cardiac arrest: a review. Circulation 1986; 74:IV138–IV153.

38. Ginsberg M, Belayev L. The effects of hypothermia and hyperthermia in global cerebral ischemia. In: Maier C, Steinberg G, eds. Hypothermia and Cerebral Ischemia. Totowa, New Jersey: Humana Press, 2004.

39. Ginsberg MD, Sternau LL, Globus MY, Dietrich WD, Busto R. Therapeutic modulation of brain temperature: relevance to ischemic brain injury. Cerebrovasc Brain Metab Rev 1992; 4:189–225.

40. Hicks SD, DeFranco DB, Callaway CW. Hypothermia during reperfusion after asphyxial cardiac arrest improves functional recovery and selectively alters stress-induced protein expression. J Cereb Blood Flow Metab 2000; 20:520–530.

41. Xiao F, Safar P, Radovsky A. Mild protective and resuscitative hypothermia for asphyxial cardiac arrest in rats. Am J Emerg Med 1998; 16:17–25.

42. Sterz F, Safar P, Tisherman S, Radovsky A, Kuboyama K, Oku K. Mild hypothermic cardiopulmonary resuscitation improves outcome after prolonged cardiac arrest in dogs. Crit Care Med 1991; 19:379–389.

43. Safar P. Mild resuscitative hypothermia and outcome after cardiopulmonary resuscitation. J Neurosurg Anesthesiol 1996; 8:88–96.

44. Zeiner A, Holzer M, Sterz F, et al. Mild resuscitative hypothermia to improve neurological outcome after cardiac arrest. A clinical feasibility trial. Hypothermia after cardiac arrest (haca) study group. Stroke 2000; 31:86–94.

45. Bernard SA, Jones BM, Horne MK. Clinical trial of induced hypothermia in comatose survivors of out-of-hospital cardiac arrest. Ann Emerg Med 1997; 30:146–153.

46. Kramer RS, Sanders AP, Lesage AM, Woodhall B, Sealy WC. The effect profound hypothermia on preservation of cerebral ATP content during circulatory arrest. J Thorac Cardiovasc Surg 1968; 56:699–709.

47. Welsh FA, Sims RE, Harris VA. Mild hypothermia prevents ischemic injury in gerbil hippocampus. J Cereb Blood Flow Metab 1990; 10:557–563.

48. Busto R, Globus MY, Dietrich WD, Martinez E, Valdes I, Ginsberg MD. Effect of mild hypothermia on ischemia-induced release of neurotransmitters and free fatty acids in rat brain. Stroke 1989; 20:904–910.

49. Cardell M, Boris-Moller F, Wieloch T. Hypothermia prevents the ischemia-induced translocation and inhibition of protein kinase c in the rat striatum. J Neurochem 1991; 57:1814–1817.

50. Dempsey RJ, Combs DJ, Maley ME, Cowen DE, Roy MW, Donaldson DL. Moderate hypothermia reduces postischemic edema development and leukotriene production. Neurosurgery 1987; 21:177–181.

51. Toyoda T, Suzuki S, Kassell NF, Lee KS. Intraischemic hypothermia attenuates neutrophil infiltration in the rat neocortex after focal ischemia-reperfusion injury. Neurosurgery 1996; 39:1200–1205.

52. Kumar K, Wu X, Evans AT, Marcoux F. The effect of hypothermia on induction of heat shock protein (hsp)-72 in ischemic brain. Metab Brain Dis 1995; 10:283–291.

53. Kumar K, Wu X, Evans AT. Expression of c-fos and fos-b proteins following transient forebrain ischemia: Effect of hypothermia. Brain Res Mol Brain Res 1996; 42:337–343.

54. Colbourne F, Grooms SY, Zukin RS, Buchan AM, Bennett MV. Hypothermia rescues hippocampal ca1 neurons and attenuates down-regulation of the AMPA receptor GluR2 subunit after forebrain ischemia. Proc Natl Acad Sci USA 2003; 100:2906–2910.

55. Nolan JP, Morley PT, Hoek TL, Hickey RW. Therapeutic hypothermia after cardiac arrest. An advisory statement by the advancement life support task force of the international liaison committee on resuscitation. Resuscitation 2003; 57:231–235.

56. Schwab S, Schwarz S, Spranger M, Keller E, Bertram M, Hacke W. Moderate hypothermia in the treatment of patients with severe middle cerebral artery infarction. Stroke 1998; 29:2461–2466.

57. Felberg RA, Krieger DW, Chuang R, et al. Hypothermia after cardiac arrest: Feasibility and safety of an external cooling protocol. Circulation 2001; 104:1799–1804.

58. Diringer MN. Treatment of fever in the neurologic intensive care unit with a catheter-based heat exchange system. Crit Care Med 2004; 32:559–564.

59. Yon S, Magers M, Dobak J, Klos B. A novel system for mild hypothermia. Biomed Instrum Technol 2004; 38:241–246.

60. Mayer SA, Kowalski RG, Presciutti M, et al. Clinical trial of a novel surface cooling system for fever control in neurocritical care patients. Crit Care Med 2004; 32:2508–2515.

61. Zweifler RM, Voorhees ME, Mahmood MA, Parnell M. Rectal temperature reflects tympanic temperature during mild induced hypothermia in nonintubated subjects. J Neurosurg Anesthesiol 2004; 16:232–235.

62. Virkkunen I, Yli-Hankala A, Silfvast T. Induction of therapeutic hypothermia after cardiac arrest in prehospital patients using ice-cold ringer's solution: a pilot study. Resuscitation 2004; 62:299–302.

63. Bernard S, Buist M, Monteiro O, Smith K. Induced hypothermia using large volume, ice-cold intravenous fluid in comatose survivors of out-of-hospital cardiac arrest: a preliminary report. Resuscitation 2003; 56:9–13.

64. Mokhtarani M, Mahgoub AN, Morioka N, et al. Buspirone and meperidine synergistically reduce the shivering threshold. Anesth Analg 2001; 93:1233–1239.

65. Sessler DI. Treatment: meperidine, clonidine, doxapram, ketanserin, or alfentanil abolishes short-term postoperative shivering. Can J Anaesth 2003; 50:635–637.

66. Carhuapoma JR, Gupta K, Coplin WM, Muddassir SM, Meratee MM. Treatment of refractory fever in the neurosciences critical care unit using a novel, water-circulating cooling device. A single-center pilot experience. J Neurosurg Anesthesiol 2003; 15:313–318.

67. Kranke P, Eberhart LH, Roewer N, Tramer MR. Pharmacological treatment of postoperative shivering: A quantitative systematic review of randomized controlled trials. Anesth Analg 2002; 94:453–460 (table of contents).

68. Kliegel A, Losert H, Sterz F, et al. Cold simple intravenous infusions preceding special endovascular cooling for faster induction of mild hypothermia after cardiac arrest—a feasibility study. Resuscitation 2005; 64:347–351.

69. Al-Senani FM, Graffagnino C, Grotta JC, et al. A prospective, multicenter pilot study to evaluate the feasibility and safety of using the coolgard system and icy catheter following cardiac arrest. Resuscitation 2004; 62:143–150.

70. Boelhouwer RU, Bruining HA, Ong GL. Correlations of serum potassium fluctuations with body temperature after major surgery. Crit Care Med 1987; 15:310–312.

71. Abella BS, Rhee JW, Huang KN, Vanden Hoek TL, Becker LB. Induced hypothermia is underused after resuscitation from cardiac arrest: A current practice survey. Resuscitation 2005; 64:181–186.

72. Morimoto Y, Kemmotsu O, Kitami K, Matsubara I, Tedo I. Acute brain swelling afte out of hospital cardiac arrest: Pathogenesis and outcome. Crit Cre Med 1993; 21:104–110.

73. Iida K, Satoh H, Arita K, Nakahara T, Kurisu K, Ohtani M. Delayed hyperemia causing intracranial hypertension after cardiopulmonary resuscitation. Crit Care Med 1997; 25:971–976.

74. Sundgreen C, Larsen FS, Herzog TM, Knudsen GM, Boesgaard S, Aldershvile J. Autoregulation of cerebral blood flow in patients resuscitated from cardiac arrest. Stroke 2001; 32:128–132.

75. Mullner M, Sterz F, Binder M, et al. Arterial blood pressure after human cardiac arrest and neurological recovery. Stroke 1996; 27:59–62.

76. Longstreth WT, Inui TS, Cobb LA, Compass MK. Neurologic recovery after out-of-hospital cardiac arrest. Ann Intern Med 1983; 98:121–132.

77. Longstreth WT Jr., Copass MK, Dennis LK, Rauch-Matthews ME, Stark MS, Cobb LA. Intravenous glucose after out-of-hospital cardiopulmonary arrest: a community-based randomized trial. Neurology 1993; 43:2534–2541.

78. Mullner M, Sterz F, Binder M, Schreiber W, Deimel A, Laggner AN. Blood glucose concentration after cardiopulmonary resuscitation influences functional neurological recovery in human cardiac arrest survivors. J Cereb Blood Flow Metab 1997; 17:430–436.

79. Attitudes of critical care medicine professionals concerning forgoing life-sustaining treatments. The society of critical care medicine ethics committee. Crit Care Med 1992; 20:320–326.

80. van den Berghe G, Wouters P, Weekers F, et al. Intensive insulin therapy in the critically ill patients. N Engl J Med 2001; 345:1359–1367.

81. Zeiner A, Holzer M, Sterz F, et al. Hyperthermia after cardiac arrest is associated with an unfavorable neurologic outcome. Arch Intern Med 2001; 161:2007–2012.

82. Takasu A, Saitoh D, Kaneko N, Sakamoto T, Okada Y. Hyperthermia: is it an ominous sign after cardiac arrest? Resuscitation 2001; 49:273–277.

83. Sterz F, Safar P, Diven W, Leonov Y, Radovsky A, Oku K. Detoxification with hemabsorption after cardiac arrest does not improve neurologic recovery. Review and outcome study in dogs. Resuscitation 1993; 25:137–160.

84. Lawes EG, Baskett PJ. Pulmonary aspiration during unsuccessful cardiopulmonary resuscitation. Intensive Care Med 1987; 13:379–382.

85. Lee-Chiong TL Jr., Stitt JT. Disorders of temperature regulation. Compr Ther 1995; 21:697–704.

86. Powers JH, Scheld WM. Fever in neurologic diseases. Infect Dis Clin North Am 1996; 10:45–66.

87. Madl JE, Allen DL. Hyperthermia depletes adenosine triphosphate and decreases glutamate uptake in rat hippocampal slices. Neuroscience 1995; 69:395–405.

88. Globus MY, Busto R, Lin B, Schnippering H, Ginsberg MD. Detection of free radical activity during transient global ischemia and recirculation: Effects of intraischemic brain temperature modulation. J Neurochem 1995; 65:1250–1256.

89. Werhahn KJ, Brown P, Thompson PD, Marsden CD. The clinical features and prognosis of chronic posthypoxic myoclonus. Mov Disord 1997; 12:216–220.

90. Koenig M, Geocadin R. Global hypoxia-ischemia and critical care seizures. In: Varelas P, ed. Seizures in Critical Care. Totowa, NJ: Humana Press, 2005.

91. Rogove HJ, Safar P, Sutton-Tyrrell K, Abramson NS. Old age does not negate good cerebral outcome after cardiopulmonary resuscitation: Analyses from the brain resuscitation clinical trials. The brain resuscitation clinical trial i and ii study groups. Crit Care Med 1995; 23:18–25.

27 | Prognosis and Neurologic Outcomes Following Cardiopulmonary Arrest

Robert J. Wityk, MD, Director[a], Associate Professor[b]

[a]*Cerebrovascular Division,* [b]*Department of Neurology, Johns Hopkins University School of Medicine, Baltimore, Maryland, USA*

INTRODUCTION

This chapter addresses the following issues concerning cardiopulmonary arrest (CA): (i) prognosis, (ii) clinical syndromes of brain injury, and (iii) clinical and laboratory predictors of outcome. The accurate prognosis and chance for good neurologic recovery is of obvious interest to family members of patients with anoxic coma. In addition, accurate prediction of poor outcome (e.g., mortality or persistent vegetative state) provides important information to intensive care unit teams, so that they are able to provide appropriate support to family members who may be involved in decisions for patients who do not have advanced directives.

The magnitude of out-of-hospital CA is uncertain, with estimates between 200,000 and 500,000 cases annually in the United States (1,2). In one study, the incidence was 7 times higher in subjects with clinically recognized heart disease (5.98/1000 vs. 0.82/1000 subject-years) and was the highest in the subgroup of patients with congestive heart failure (21.9/1000 subject-years) (3). The overall prognosis for anoxic coma is poor, with 85% or more having a poor outcome (death or a vegetative state) within a month of the initial insult (4,5).

Two recent clinical trials of hypothermia in CA-targeted patients who were felt to be at high risk for mortality and severe brain injury. Inclusion criteria were CA due to ventricular fibrillation, with persistent coma after restoration of spontaneous circulation (6,7). Examination of the normothermic control patients provides some idea of the prognosis of anoxic coma in patients receiving optimal resuscitation and intensive care treatment. In one, outcomes measured at hospital discharge among the 34 normothermic patients were as follows: 7 with normal or minimal disability, 2 with moderate disability (discharged to a rehabilitation service), 2 with severe disability (discharged to a long-term nursing facility), and 23 deaths (7). Overall, poor outcome was seen in 74%. In the European study, the outcome assessed at 6 months among 138 normothermic patients was favorable in 39%, but with a 55% mortality rate (6).

CLINICAL SYNDROMES

Neurologic syndromes after an episode of anoxia vary greatly, depending upon the length of anoxia. Patients successfully and promptly resuscitated from out-of-hospital CA are a minority (5–20%), but they generally have good neurologic outcomes and quality of life (8). Brief episodes of anoxia are generally well tolerated, although some patients may develop an amnestic syndrome with severe anterograde amnesia, presumably due to the vulnerability of hippocampal regions involved in memory (9). Longer episodes of anoxia may result in a watershed pattern of cerebral ischemia (10). These patients are typically in a coma for 12 hr or more. Watershed infarctions can cause quadriparesis, with weakness primarily in the proximal arm and leg, typically sparing the hands and feet ("man-in-the-barrel" syndrome). Finally, rare cases of spinal cord stroke occur due to hypotension, in the absence of cerebral injury (11). Plum et al. reported a series of patients who had delayed neurologic deterioration after they awoke from anoxic coma (12). Patients appeared to show good recovery, lasting one to several weeks, but then had recurrent neurologic deterioration, sometimes even to coma and death. Pathologically, the brain shows extensive demyelination, although the pathogenesis remains unclear.

Patients with more prolonged anoxia suffer diffuse cerebral injury, with variable recovery ranging from encephalopathy to persistent coma. Many of these patients develop seizures and/or myoclonus within the first 24 hr of CA. In one report, 17% of patients developed myoclonic status epilepticus, a condition associated with uniformly poor outcome (13).

Selective injury can occur to the large pyramidal cells of layers III and V of the cerebral cortex (laminar necrosis), while the brain stem and spinal cord are preserved (14). The clinical status of patients with this type of injury progresses to a vegetative state, in which the eyes are open but the patient lacks interaction and apparent awareness. Vegetative patients are considered to be in a "persistent" vegetative state if no change in status occurs for 1 month or more, and in a "permanent" vegetative state if no change occurs after 3 months (15). Although laminar necrosis is a common pathologic finding in vegetative patients, it is not the only one that can cause the condition (14,16). The chance of late recovery from a vegetative state is poor. A review of studies found that, after 1 year, 15% of patients in a vegetative state awakened, 32% remained vegetative, and 53% died (4,5). Among the 15% of patients who awakened (*n* = 25), only one had a good neurologic recovery.

Because of this poor prognosis, the ability to predict early on the patients who will die or remain vegetative and to distinguish them from patients who will eventually awaken and possibly have reasonable medical recovery is highly desirable. Such information would be of great value to families of patients trying to decide on continuing life-sustaining treatments.

PROGNOSIS AND CLINICAL PREDICTORS

The neurologic examination is the first step in assessing the prognosis of a comatose patient after CA (17). "Coma" can be defined as a state of unarousable unresponsiveness characterized by the eyes being closed (as in sleep) and the absence of purposeful movements to stimulation (18). "Stupor" refers to a state of deep sleep, with arousal only to vigorous stimulation. In contrast, patients in vegetative states do not appear asleep but open their eyes to stimulation (although diurnal sleep–wake cycles may develop). This state of wakefulness, however, does not include evidence of cognition or awareness. Spontaneous movements might be observed on general observation of the patient, and determination should be made as to whether they are purposeful, semipurposeful (e.g., appropriate withdrawal from a noxious stimulus) or reflex movements. Some very unusual complex reflex movements have been reported even in brain-dead patients and should not be confused with purposeful motor activity (19).

The second step in assessment is determining the degree and duration of arousal (if any) to graded stimulation. One starts with verbal stimuli and then adds increasingly vigorous physical stimulation. Painful stimuli, however, such as sternal rub, pinching, or pinprick, can also elicit reflex responses, which may be difficult to distinguish from purposeful withdrawal. Low-level responses, such as triple flexion or decerebrate posturing are patterned and tend to repeat, regardless of the location or type of stimulus. Semipurposeful withdrawal movements, however, typically display movement of the body part away from the painful stimulus and will change depending upon the location of the stimulus.

A number of studies have attempted to derive rules that predict awakening from postanoxic coma. One of the most widely used studies derives from a series of 210 patients, seen at the Cornell Medical Center, who underwent serial neurologic examinations after being found in a comatose state after CA (20). Noteworthily, two-thirds of the patients in this study had their CA in the hospital. Outcome was determined at 1 year and graded by the following functional scale: (i) coma until death, (ii) vegetative state, (iii) severe disability but conscious, (iv) moderate disability (independent but unable to resume prior level of activity), and (v) good recovery (able to return to prior level of function). By day 3 after CA, 25 (12%) patients awoke from coma. Only 3 more awoke within the next 2 weeks. Of the 28 patients who awoke, 21 (75%) recovered independence. On the other hand, 86 (41%) patients died within the first 3 days, and 134 (64%) died within the first week. The clinical status of the remainder developed into vegetative state. Multivariate analysis with a recursive partitioning algorithm was used to identify portions of the neurologic examination that predicted outcome at 1 year.

The results are presented in (Fig. 1). A series of flow charts shows the actual outcome of patients depending upon key findings on neurologic examination at various time points from initial exam (within 24 hr to 2 weeks). Several important points are evident in the data. First, the certainty of outcome for either worst outcome or best outcome is better at 3 days than at baseline or day 1. Most physicians in clinical practice are uncomfortable with the unacceptably high error rate associated with prognostication prior to day 3. On the other hand, the data is

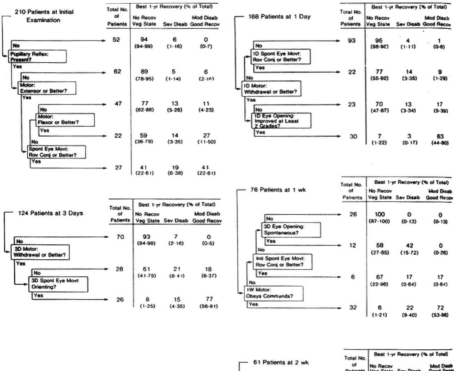

Figure 1 Prediction of best functional outcome at 1 year using neurologic examination at various time points after cardiac arrest. Percentages are given, with 95% confidence interval, in parentheses below the number. The tables also identify the number of patients examined at each time point. *Source*: Adapted from Ref. 20.

limited by a small number of patients in some cells, so that there is still a substantial range to the 95% confidence interval.

A second finding is that a handful of easily obtained clinical findings on examination can carry considerable weight. For example, loss of one of the most basic brain stem reflexes— pupillary response—noted on initial exam was associated with no recovery or a vegetative state in 94% of patients, and no patient had a good or moderate recovery. At day 3, withdrawal to stimuli and spontaneous eye movements was associated with many patients with either good or very poor outcome. An attempt to speak within the first few days, even limited to incomprehensible moaning, has been reported to be a good prognostic sign, although present in only a small number of patients (17,20).

The Glasgow Coma Scale (GCS) (Table 1) utilizes some of the same clinical signs of eye opening and motor response but with an additional feature of verbal response. [Best verbal response was not found to be a useful factor in the Levy study (20).] A Belgian study of 360 patients resuscitated from out-of-hospital CA found good outcome predicted by a GCS of ≥ 10 and poor outcome predicted by a GCS of ≤ 4 (21). In a validation study, they found that these criteria had a sensitivity of 96%, a specificity of 86%, a negative predictive value of 97%, and a positive predictive value of only 77%. A more recent study by the Brain Resuscitation Clinical Trials Study Group supported these findings (22). An analysis of outcome in 262 patients in coma following CA revealed that the most useful predictors were (i) absence of papillary light reaction at baseline predicted poor outcome, (ii) absence of motor response to painful stimuli on day 3 predicted poor outcome, and (iii) use of the Glasgow or Glasgow-Pittsburgh coma scale was no better than use of some of its components.

Table 1 Glasgow Coma Scale

Eyes open
   4—spontaneously
   3—to verbal command
   2—to pain
   1—no response
Best motor response
   6—obeys verbal command
   5—localizes to pain
   4—flexion–withdrawal
   3—decorticate posturing
   2—decerebrate posturing
   1—no response
Best verbal response
   5—oriented and converses
   4—disoriented and converses
   3—inappropriate words
   2—incomprehensible sounds
   1—no response

Neurophysiologic Tests

Among ancillary neurophysiologic tests, electroencephalography (EEG) and somatosensory-evoked potential (SSEP) have been extensively studied in assessing prognosis after brain injury of various etiologies. EEG is particularly useful early in the evaluation of patients by helping to differentiate anoxic coma from psychiatric conditions and from nonconvulsive status epilepticus. Beyond this, the degree of cortical damage roughly correlates with various features of the EEG (23). Several EEG patterns are associated with poor prognosis, including alpha-coma pattern, burst-suppression pattern, and an isoelectric recording. Alpha-coma pattern can be seen with brain stem ischemia after CA and is associated with a mortality rate of about 90% (23). In a systematic review of the literature, Zandbergen found that 5 of 6 studies reported 100% specificity for poor outcome with either an isoelectric or burst-suppression pattern. Using pooled data, the false positive rate for the presence of either pattern was estimated at 0.2% to 5.9%.

Among electrophysiologic tests, median nerve SSEPs have emerged as potentially the most useful. Bilateral absence of cortical SSEP to median nerve stimulation occurs with severe cortical brain injury and is associated with very poor prognosis. Robinson et al. reported an extensive review of the literature of SSEP in predicting prognosis of awaking from coma and extracted data from 41 articles for pooled analysis (24). Among 1136 adults with coma after CA (extracted from 18 articles), 336 had bilateral absence of median nerve SSEP, and none of these patients awoke from coma. The typical follow-up time of these studies was 6 to 12 months after CA. The 95% confidence interval for chance of awakening with bilaterally absent SSEP was 0% to 1%. In contrast, patients with present SSEP of some sort had a 41% chance of awakening, and the chances were better if the SSEP was normal (Fig. 2).

The above analysis was restricted to papers with a sufficient number of patients and data that could be extracted and analyzed. In their literature review, however, Robinson noted two articles reporting a total of 3 patients with absent SSEP who did awaken from postanoxic coma (24). In all cases, however, the SSEP was obtained < 24 hr from CA, and in one of these patients, the SSEP was present when repeated on day 3. Hence, median nerve SSEP may not be useful if obtained within the first 24 hr but should be obtained on day 2 or 3 after CA. Overall, absent median nerve SSEP identified only about half of patients who did not awaken (median sensitivity among studies reviewed, 0.45) but who had a very high specificity (with 95% confidence interval of 0–1% chance of awakening).

Neuroimaging Predictors

MRI has better resolution than CT for subtle brain injury but, overall, has not provided much prognostic value beyond the neurologic examination. In the acute period after CA, MRI is often

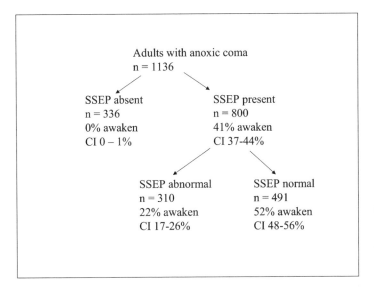

Figure 2 Outcome after anoxic coma, depending upon results of median nerve SSEPs. *Abbreviations*: SSEPs, somatosensory-evoked potentials; CI, Confidence interval. *Source*: Adapted from Ref. 24.

normal, but in the subacute period (<2 weeks), MRI may show abnormal signal in the deep gray matter (GM) nuclei and obscured gray–white matter (WM) distinction (25). Some cases may show cortical laminar necrosis as a strip of high-signal intensity on the T1-weighted images, but this is usually seen in the chronic phase (more than a few weeks after CA) (25,26).

Diffusion-weighted MRI reveals ischemic brain as areas of restricted diffusion in stroke patients within several hours of onset of symptoms. Similar findings have been reported in patients studied within the first few days of CA (25). One study reported restricted diffusion (confirmed by measurements of the mean apparent diffusion coefficient) predominantly in the WM; diffusion weighted imaging (DWI) images showed diffuse, symmetric high signal in the periventricular WM (Fig. 3) (27). Another reported diffuse signal abnormality on DWI in both cortical and WM regions in the majority of patients (28). Widespread abnormality involving cortex, thalamus, and cerebellum on DWI seemed to correlate with poor prognosis, although the number of patients studied was small (*n* = 9) (28).

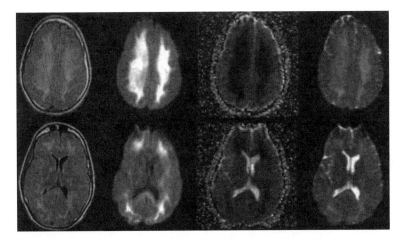

Figure 3 MRI studies of leukoencephalopathy after anoxic brain injury. MRI, for example, of 2 levels of a single patient showing the following sequences (*from left to right*): fluid-attenuated inversion recovery (FLAIR), diffusion-weighted imaging (DWI), apparent diffusion coefficient (ADC) map, T2-weighted image. Note confluent white matter hyperintensity on FLAIR, DWI, and T2, with dark signal on ADC, confirming restricted diffusion. *Source*: Adapted from Ref. 27.

Magnetic resonance spectroscopy after CA demonstrates an elevation in brain lactate and a decrease in the neuronal marker *N*-acetylaspartate (29). The usefulness of this technique over other prognostic methods has not been demonstrated. Given the logistic difficulties of obtaining MRI studies in critically ill patients, the use of MRI for prognosis is not widespread.

Despite its limitations in terms of resolution, CT has the advantage of much greater availability. CT may reveal focal ischemia in some patients after CA but is primarily used to investigate other neurologic causes for coma, such as intracerebral or subarachnoid hemorrhage. Loss of gray–white distinction is a well-known early sign of ischemia on CT. Torbey et al. described a simple method of measuring the CT density in Hounsfield units in the GM of the basal ganglia and in the WM of the internal capsule and calculating a GM/WM ratio (30). In control subjects, this ratio was 1.45, with all controls having a ratio of > 1.30; however, in comatose patients with CA, the median value was 1.18. In this series, all comatose patients who had a ratio of < 1.18 died, whereas the survival rate was 46% among those with a ratio of >1.18. The investigators went on to propose a Brain Arrest Neurological Outcome Scale, which combines scores for duration of CA, a reversed GCS, and scores of the GM/WM index (31). Prognostic cutoffs were derived from a series of 32 comatose patients, but another study should validate these results prospectively.

Laboratory Markers

A number of biochemical markers of brain injury have been studied, including cerebrospinal fluid creatine kinase BB and serum levels of the cytoplasmic enzyme neuron-specific enolase and the astroglial protein S100 (32,33). These proteins are assayed in the blood or cerebrospinal fluid, and high levels at specific times after CA suggest extensive brain injury and correlate with poor outcome. Tirschwell et al. reported the finding that cerebrospinal fluid creatine kinase BB level of 205 U/L had 100% specificity and positive predictive value for predicting poor outcome but a sensitivity of only 48% (32). However, combining median nerve SSEP studies with cerebrospinal fluid creatine kinase BB levels maintained 100% specificity but increased sensitivity to 78% (34). Some concern was noted, however, in performing lumbar puncture after CA in patients who may be developing cerebral edema.

Neuron-specific enolase and S100 have been studied as markers for extent of brain injury in head trauma and after cardiopulmonary bypass (e.g., during cardiac surgery). Levels of enzymes in blood at various time points after CA correlate with outcome, and reduction of neuron-specific enolase levels has been reported in CA patients treated with hypothermia (35,36). Further studies are needed in larger series of patients to determine whether these markers are of added value to the neurologic examination and other laboratory tests.

SUMMARY

To date, no particular test or combination of tests/findings has a sufficiently high sensitivity and specificity to accurately predict outcome after CA. However, if the aim of a prognostic paradigm is to identify the patients who do poorly, then a test with moderate sensitivity would be acceptable, as long as the specificity is high. In a systematic review of predictors of poor outcome after anoxic coma, Zandbergen identified 3 factors with 100% specificity of poor outcome (defined as death or persistent vegetative state): (i) absence of papillary light reflexes on day 3, (ii) absence of motor response to pain on day 3, and (iii) bilateral absence of cortical SSEP within the first week (37). The estimated false-positive rate was lowest with SSEP, leading the authors to conclude that this was the most useful method to predict poor outcome.

Several principles are suggested by the current literature. First, the best time to assess prognosis after CA is approximately 3 days after the event, by which time a number of predictors emerge and carry greater statistical certainty. Second, loss of brain stem function as assessed by pupillary light responses indicates severe brain damage and poor outcome. Third, if brain stem function is relatively intact, prognosis depends on the extent of cortical injury, which might be best assessed by SSEP. Persistent coma after CA suggests significant brain injury, with a poor prognosis for the majority of patients. Much of the current literature focuses on predictors of poor outcome, and little data is available on factors that can identify with certainty patients who will have a good outcome.

REFERENCES

1. Zheng Z-J, Croft JB, Giles WH, et al. Sudden cardiac death in the United States, 1989 to 1998. Circulation 2001; 104:2158–2163.
2. Cobb LA, Fahrenbruch CE, Olsufka M, et al. Changing incidence of out-of-hospital ventricular fibrillation, 1980–2000. JAMA 2002; 288:3008–3013.
3. Rea TD, Pearce RM, Raghunathan TE, et al. Incidence of out-of-hospital cardiac arrest. Am J Cardiol 2004; 93(12):1455–1460.
4. The Multi-Society Task Force on PVS. Medical aspects of the persistent vegetative state. I. N Engl J Med 1994; 330:1499–1508.
5. The Multi-Society Task Force on PVS. Medical aspects of the persistent vegetative state. II. N Engl J Med 1994; 330:1572–1579.
6. The Hypothermia After Cardiac Arrest Study Group. Mild therapeutic hypothermia to improve the neurologic outcome after cardiac arrest. N Engl J Med 2002; 346:549–556.
7. Bernard SA, Gray TW, Buist MD, et al. Treatment of comatose survivors of out-of-hospital cardiac arrest with induced hypothermia. N Engl J Med 2002; 346:557–563.
8. Rea TD, Paredes VL. Quality of life and prognosis among survivors of out-of-hospital cardiac arrest. Curr Opin Crit Care 2004; 10(3):218–223.
9. Finkelstein S, Caronna J. Amnestic syndrome following cardiac arrest. Neurology 1978; 28:280.
10. Caronna JJ. Neurologic syndromes following cardiac arrest and cardiac bypass surgery. In Barnett H, Stein B, Mohr J, Yatsu F, eds. Stroke: Pathophysiology, Diagnosis, and Management. New York: Churchill Livingstone, 1986:747–762.
11. Silver J, Buxton P. Spinal Stroke. Brain 1974; 97:539.
12. Plum F, Posner JB, Hain RF. Delayed neurological deterioration after anoxia. Arch Intern Med 1962; 110:18–25.
13. Krumholz A, Stern BJ, Weiss HD. Outcome from coma after cardiopulmonary resuscitation: Relation to seizures and myoclonus. Neurology 1988; 38:401–405.
14. Dougherty JHJ, Rawlinson DG, Levy DE, et al. Hypoxic-ischemic brain injury and the vegetative state: Clinical and neuropathologic correlation. Neurology 1981; 31:991–997.
15. American Academy of Neurology. Practice Parameters: Assessment and management of patients in the persistent vegetative state. Neurology 1995; 45:1015–1018.
16. Kinney HC, Korein J, Panigrahy A, et al. Neuropathological findings in the brain of Karen Ann Quinlan. The role of the thalamus in the persistent vegetative state. N Engl J Med 1994; 330:1469–1475.
17. Fisher CM. The Neurological Examination of the Comatose Patient. Acta Neurologica Scandinavica 1969; 45(suppl 36):5–56.
18. Plum F, Posner J. The Diagnosis of Stupor and Coma. 3rd ed. Philadelphia: Davis F.A., 1982.
19. Ropper AH. Unusual spontaneous movements in brain-dead patients. Neurology 1984; 34:1089–1092.
20. Levy DE, Coronna JJ, Singer BH, et al. Predicting Outcome from Hypoxic-Ischemic Coma. JAMA 1985; 253(10):1420–1426.
21. Mullie A, Verstringe P, Buylaert W, et al. Predictive value of Glasgow coma score for awakening after out-of-hospital cardiac arrest. Lancet 1988; 1(8578):137–140.
22. Edgren E, Hedstrand U, Kelsey S, et al. Assessment of neurological prognosis in comatose survivors of cardiac arrest. Lancet 1994; 343:1055–1059.
23. Kaplan PW. The EEG in metabolic encephalopathy and coma. J Clin Neurophysiol 2004; 21:307–318.
24. Robinson LR, Micklesen PJ, Tirschwell DL, et al. Predictive value of somatosensory evoked potentials for awakening from coma. Crit Care Med 2003; 31:960–967.
25. Arbelaez A, Castillo M, Mukherji SK. Diffusion-weighted MRI imaging of global cerebral anoxia. AJNR 1999; 20:999–1007.
26. Sawada H, Udaka F, Seriu N, et al. MRI demonstration of cortical laminar necrosis and delayed white matter injury in anoxic encephalopathy. Neuroradiology 1990; 32:319–321.
27. Chalela JA, Wolf RL, Maldjian JA, et al. MRI identification of early white matter injury in anoxic-ischemic encephalopathy. Neurology 2001; 56(4):481–485.
28. Wijdicks EF, Campeau NG, Miller GM. MR imaging in comatose survivors of cardiac resuscitation. AJNR 2001; 22(8):1561–1565.
29. Berek K, Lechleitner P, Luef G, et al. Early determination of neurological outcome after prehospital cardiopulmonary resuscitation. Stroke 1995; 26(4):543–549.
30. Torbey MT, Selim M, Knorr J, et al. Quantitative analysis of the loss of distinction between gray and white matter in comatose patients after cardiac arrest. Stroke 2000; 31(9):2163–2167.
31. Torbey MT, Geocadin R, Bhardwaj A. Brain arrest neurological outcome scale (BrANOS): predicting mortality and severe disability following cardiac arrest. Resuscitation 2004; 63(1):55–63.
32. Tirschwell D, Longstreth WT Jr. Rauch-Matthews M, et al. Cerebrospinal fluid creatine kinase BB isoenzyme activity and neurologic prognosis after cardiac arrest. Neurology 1997; 48:352–357.
33. Madl Ca, Holzer Mb. Brain function after resuscitation from cardiac arrest. Curr Opin Crit Care 2004; 10(3):213–217.

34. Sherman AL, Tirschwell DL, Micklesen PJ, et al. Somatosensory potentials, CSF creatine kinase BB activity, and awakening after cardiac arrest. Neurology 2000; 54(4):889–894.
35. Bottiger BW, Mobes S, Glatzer R, et al. Astroglial protein S-100 is an early and sensitive marker of hypoxic brain damage and outcome after cardiac arrest in humans. Circulation 2001; 103:2694–2698.
36. Tiainen M, Roine RO, Pettila V, et al. Seum neuron-specific enolase and S-100B protein in cardiac arrest patients treated with hypothermia. Stroke 2003; 34:2881–2886.
37. Zandbergen EG, de Haan RJ, Stoutenbeek CP, et al. Systematic review of early prediction of poor outcome in anoxic-ischemic coma. Lancet 1998; 352:1808–1812.

28 | Failure of Neuroprotective Agents to Show Benefit in Clinical Trials

Richard J. Traystman, PhD, FCCM, Professor[a], Associate Vice President[b], and Associate Dean[c]

[a]*Department of Anesthesiology & Perioperative Medicine,* [b]*Research Planning and Development,*
[c]*Research School of Medicine, Oregon Health & Science University, Portland, Oregon, USA*

INTRODUCTION

Stroke and cardiac arrest represent the third leading cause of death and disability in the United States. These diseases strike some 1,400,000 Americans annually, and a high mortality is associated with both. For stroke and cardiac arrest, probably 30% and 50% of individuals, respectively, die immediately, with a large percentage of survivors suffering from severe disability. In fact, stroke itself is the leading cause of disability in the United States and costs the most in terms of health care. Most strokes and cardiac arrests occur in older patients (over 65 years of age); however, a marked increase has been observed in stroke incidence in patients between 45 and 65 years of age (1). Thus, the high incidence and significant morbidity and mortality associated with these diseases and the brain dysfunction in these critically ill patients emphasize the need to identify and test neuroprotective strategies that will be effective in protecting the brain from hemodynamic stressors, such as hypotension and shock states, and in minimizing ischemic damage from stroke and cardiac arrest. The aims of neuroprotection are to optimally match cerebral blood flow with metabolic demand and to stop the complicated pathophysiologic cascades of cellular and molecular events that lead to neuronal, glial, and vascular cell death. Despite ample animal research over the past five decades concerning the pathophysiology of brain injury from ischemia, very little of this work has translated into effective treatment modalities for stroke or cardiac arrest in humans (2). Clinical trials designed to test a variety of neuroprotective agents that have had excellent outcomes in preclinical experimental animal studies have been disappointing. This chapter will discuss some of the potential reasons for the difficulty and lack of success involved in attempting to translate positive experimental results with neuroprotective agents from animals to humans.

MECHANISMS OF INJURY

Cerebral ischemia can produce neuronal death or injury by at least 3 mechanisms: excitotoxicity, oxygen free radicals, and inflammatory mediators (3). Free radicals that are formed following an ischemic event can cause cell membrane destruction (4). Free radical–mediated injury is accompanied by lipid peroxidation, and the involvement of oxygen-derived radicals in cerebral ischemia has been most intensely studied: superoxide anion radical; its protonated form, perhydroxyl radical; hydroxyl radical; the nonradical hydrogen peroxide; and nitric oxide, the endothelium-derived relaxing factor. Ischemia causes the release of a variety of excitotoxic amino acids, such as glutamate and aspartate (5). These affect various receptor sites, including the NMDA site, which mediates calcium flux, and the quisqualate and kainate AMPA receptors, which mediate Na^+K^+ and sodium chloride fluxes, respectively. When these receptors are activated, they cause opening of ionic channels and changes in intracellular ion concentration, eventually leading to cell death. AMPA also binds to metabotropic receptors that stimulate phosphoinositide hydrolysis. Mediators of inflammation, such as leukotrienes and platelet-activating factors, can similarly cause membrane damage and cell death (6). Many inflammatory mechanisms are linked to calcium activation of key cell-signaling enzymes and of proteolytic enzymes, which degrade cytoskeletal proteins (actin and spectrin) and extracellular matrix proteins (laminin). These 3 mechanisms of injury and cell death (excitotoxicity, free radicals, and inflammatory mediators) are probably the best known and studied; however, other mechanisms of injury have also been reported (7).

Each mechanism represents part of a temporal sequence of injury following cerebral ischemia (3). That is to say, each mechanism of injury occurs over a specific time course following ischemic injury. Excitotoxic injury occurs quickly, minutes after the initial injury, and is completed within minutes to a few hours after the onset of ischemia. Inflammation injury and apoptotic injury begin within minutes or the first few hours after injury but may last for days after the initial injury. A temporal sequence of gene expression also follows cerebral ischemia (8). Many genes are expressed following ischemia: the immediate early genes are expressed minutes after ischemia (9), followed quickly by heat-shock proteins, which are expressed hours after the injury (10). Inflammatory mediators (6), apoptotic-related genes (8), and growth factor genes (8,11) are not expressed until hours or even days following the ischemic event. Thus, because of these temporal sequences in mechanisms of injury and gene expression, searching for a neuroprotectant becomes even more complicated. For example, administration of an oxygen radical scavenger or glutamate antagonist long after the release of the oxygen free radical or glutamate may not prove useful for neuroprotection, because the damage may have already been initiated. Similarly, the administration of an antiapoptotic agent, administered long before apoptotic genes begin to be expressed, will likely prove to be unsuccessful. Thus, the search for appropriate neuroprotectants must consider these temporal aspects of the mechanism of injury.

The idea of protecting brain tissue from ischemic injury (neuroprotection) is not a new concept, and over the past five decades, many treatment modalities have been identified and attempted. These include barbiturates, hypothermia, free-radical scavengers, excitatory amino acid antagonists, calcium channel blockers, ionic pump modulators, growth factors, gene and gene-product manipulation, anti-inflammatory agents, antiapoptotic agents, and sex steroids. Unfortunately, although many of these agents have shown great neuroprotective success in a variety of animal models of stroke and cardiac arrest, none have been successful in humans. Barbiturates appeared quite promising in the late 1970s (12), but the initial protective findings could not be reproduced in animals (13,14), and subsequent clinical trials were disappointing (15). However, the idea that both local and general anesthetics may play a role in neuroprotection has been revived and has recently received much attention, although a final opinion has not been rendered (16,17).

Studies concerning hypothermia as a neuroprotectant began 50 years ago (18) but did not receive much attention until the 1990s (19,20). In recent years, interest in hypothermia has greatly increased, and it appears as if this technique has promise in neuroprotection in both focal and global cerebral ischemia (21,22). Much work has been accomplished with oxygen radical scavengers (4) and glutamate antagonists (3), but again, although both classes of drugs have had great success as neuroprotectants in animal models of stroke and cardiac arrest, their use in human disease has been disappointing (23–25). Oxygen radical scavenger type agents continue to be developed and tested. With regard to the use of glutamate antagonists, although these have had great success in ameliorating neuronal damage from cerebral ischemia in preclinical studies, their toxic side effects (hallucinations, neuropsychosis, and seizures) will probably prevent their use in humans. Early preclinical work with such drugs as MK-801, administered both pre- and postischemia, illustrates the research problems that are faced in attempting to correlate animal studies with clinical drug development for stroke victims (26). MK-801 reduces infarct injury by as much as 50% and is effective when administered either prior to or after ischemia is induced in animal models (27), indicating that research with excitatory amino acid antagonists should be pursued, and that attempts should be made to produce a nontoxic glutamate antagonist. Other newer glutamate antagonists, including the MK-801-like agent 2R,4R,5S-[2-amino-4,5- 1,2-cyclohexyl-7-phosphonoheptanoic acid] (NP 17742), also reduce infarction volume by approximately 50% and are effective in several brain areas exposed to ischemic injury (27). Whether these newer glutamate antagonists have toxic effects in humans remains to be determined.

Polyethylene glycol–conjugated superoxide dismutase (PEG–SOD), a potent free-radical scavenger, has been shown to reduce infarct volume by approximately 50% (28). L-NAME, a nitric oxide synthase inhibitor, can also reduce infarct size by 50% when administered either pre- or postischemia (29). Growth factors, such as basic fibroblast growth factor, have also been shown to reduce infarct volume (30), but only at 8 hr following the ischemic event. If infarct size is analyzed at 24 hr, no reduction in infarct size is observed (31). Thus, human fibroblast growth factor may merely delay the injury, but not actually participate as a neuroprotectant. Another consideration with all neuroprotectant drugs is that they may not be equally protective in all brain areas (28,29).

MODELS

Numerous models of focal and global cerebral ischemia have been utilized over the years (32,33); however, it is difficult to compare many of the studies that used different models. Table 1 illustrates the various models of focal stroke (middle cerebral artery occlusion) and global cerebral ischemia. The problems involved in working with many models include differences in measured variables (cerebral blood flow, arterial blood gases, and arterial blood pressure), drug dosages, occlusion duration, and variable measures of outcome, not to mention the plethora of anesthetics used, or the lack thereof. Thus, the experimental conditions utilized by investigators differ from study to study, making comparison difficult, at best. Another confounding factor is that permanent and reversible ischemia are both utilized for stroke or middle cerebral artery occlusion studies in different species and in different strains of animals. Permanent and reversible occlusion models are completely different and probably involve different mechanisms of injury. Some strains of animals are more sensitive to middle cerebral artery occlusion and produce greater injury volumes than do other strains (34,35). Thus, it is important to consider the mouse or rat strain in order to better compare and understand data across laboratories. This holds true for global ischemia models, which also use different techniques to produce ischemia (Table 1) in different species and strains of animals. Producing global ischemia by cephalic vessel occlusion differs from a full cardiac arrest/cardiopulmonary resuscitation (CPR) procedure, and it is likely that the mechanisms of injury during ischemia vary in these models. Finally, regarding animal models and preclinical experimentation, it is critical that experimental protocols be conducted in a blinded and randomized fashion. This has not been the case in many preclinical animal experiments.

DRUG DOSES

Considering the different models of cerebral ischemia and different species used for ischemia studies, it is essential to determine the appropriate concentration of neuroprotective drug to use. Oftentimes, the test drug is administered only at a single dose level, not at high, medium, and low doses, which permits dose–response evaluation of drug-specific putative effects. Dose–response curves for neuroprotection are extremely important to generate but are often neglected in preclinical studies. To be fair, however, one reason that dose–response curves are often not incorporated into preclinical studies is the usually minimal financing available from the pharmaceutical industry for these types of studies. Dose–response development was illustrated by work performed on the 21-aminosteroid agent tirilazad (36). This drug has a vitamin E-like scavenging effect on lipid peroxide radicals, it is a potent scavenger of oxygen radicals (superoxide anion), and it stabilizes membranes. Dose–response characteristics of tirilazad were evaluated in a global ischemia dog model (36). Cerebral perfusion pressure was controlled to a level of ischemia of approximately

Table 1 Global and Focal Models of Cerebral Ischemia

Global		Focal	
Complete	**Incomplete**	**Multifocal**	**Proximal/MCAO**
Cardiac arrest	Hemorrhage	Emboli–patchy CBF	MCAO+carotid
Aortic occlusion	Intracranial hypertension		Photochemical thrombosis
Neck cuff	2 VO		Intraluminal filament
Cephalic artery occlusion	4 VO		Permanent reperfusion
	Permanent reperfusion		

Abbreviations: VO, vessel occlusion; MCAO, middle cerebral artery occlusion; CBF, cerebral blood flow.

10 mmHg. Tirilazad in doses of 0.25, 1.0, or 2.5 mg/kg were compared to placebo in a randomized, blinded study, using nuclear magnetic resonance spectroscopy measurements of brain intracellular pH and bicarbonate as outcome measures. With cerebral ischemia, intracellular brain pH and bicarbonate decreased markedly with all doses of drug or placebo (approximate reductions from 7.2 to 5.7 mM and from 16 to 3 mM, respectively) but returned faster and to higher levels in the drug-treated groups in a dose-dependent fashion. Similarly, somatosensory-evoked potentials were reduced to zero during ischemia but returned in a dose-dependent fashion to approximately 50% of control with tirilazad during reperfusion. Unfortunately, however, not all drugs act in a dose–response fashion, and, in fact, some may have unusual dose–response curves. In addition, the finding that a drug works well in a dose–response fashion in animals does not guarantee that the same dose range will work well in humans. A dose of 10 mg in mice, which is protective, may not be the correct effective dose in humans. Clearly, performing dose–response curves in several animal species is important, if for no other reason than to determine which general range appears to have significant neuroprotective effects. However, even armed with this knowledge, we may not know the best possible dose to use in humans.

WINDOW OF OPPORTUNITY

Once a drug dose is determined, the investigator must then determine the most effective time to administer the drug—the window of opportunity. In many studies, drugs are administered preischemia or at reperfusion; however, although these types of administration may be excellent from the viewpoint of elucidating mechanisms of neuroprotection, they may not have any therapeutic value to the patient with stroke or cardiac arrest ischemia. In the past, few studies have carefully evaluated administration of potential neuroprotective drugs at 5, 15, 30, or 60 min following reperfusion, and even fewer have examined drug administration times of 3, 6, 12, 24 hr, or longer, after the ischemic event. In preclinical animal models, it is precisely known when the ischemia occurs, for the investigators induce it as part of the protocol. Thus, it is easy to choose windows of opportunity for administering a drug; however, ischemia onset is not at all controlled in the clinical situation. Individuals who suffer an ischemic event often require considerable time to obtain treatment; calling the physician, calling 911, waiting for a response, transporting to a hospital, obtaining a brain scan, etc. may require hours, rather than minutes. Thus, to perform expensive clinical trials with proposed neuroprotective drugs administered at 3 hr after the event, when these drugs have never been shown to be efficacious at that time in animal models, seems extremely risky, would not be predictive of success, and might be considered inappropriate. It may well be that the reason clinical trials with NMDA antagonists and other drugs (24,25,37–39) were shown not to be effective in humans was due, in part, to the inability to treat within the window of opportunity demonstrated in animal models. For example, the NMDA antagonists are effective in animal models only in a narrow therapeutic window following ischemia. Another issue is that the best window of opportunity in animal models may be different than that in humans; nevertheless, studies must be performed in animals in order to make an educated guess about which window to use in humans.

ANESTHESIA

Many animal studies of cerebral ischemia are conducted under anesthetic conditions. Two major problems arise in considering the use of anesthesia, and these problems may confound the results obtained. The first concerns the fact that investigators use different anesthetics and analgesics for different species; second, considerable literature supports the idea that anesthetics themselves are neuroprotectant. The theory that anesthesia may have an impact on brain injury following hypoxia or cerebral ischemia is derived from clinical observations that patients under general anesthesia were more tolerant of ischemia than unanesthetized patients (40). Ischemia may be affected by anesthetics via multiple potential mechanisms, including neuroprotection. The mechanisms by which anesthetics produce anesthesia and the pharmacologic characteristics of anesthetics make them likely neuroprotective candidates; these include involvement of NMDA receptors (41), involvement of gamma aminobutyric acid (GABA) A and B receptors (42,43), reduction of oxidative stress (44), inhibition of spontaneous depolarizations in the ischemic penumbra (45), and favorable redistribution of cerebral blood flow (46). Anesthetics have also been demonstrated to increase tolerance of brain to a subsequent ischemic insult (ischemic tolerance) (47). Many investigations of the effects of anesthetics on brain are problematic, because most of these reports have compared various anesthetics to each other, making interpretation of the effect of any one anesthetic difficult or impossible (16). Anesthetics have rarely been compared or evaluated with the unanesthetized state, and only a few studies have evaluated the neuroprotective properties of anesthetics when administered following ischemia onset or at reperfusion. A major problem in those investigations of the effects of neuroprotectants with anesthetized animals is that anesthetics themselves have their own effect on the cerebral vasculature, brain metabolism, brain electrophysiology, temperature, and blood pressure. Generally, patients with stroke or cardiac arrest are not anesthetized at the time of the ischemic event. Thus, whether ischemia in preclinical anesthetized species will mimic ischemic events that occur in awake humans is unlikely.

GENDER DIFFERENCES

The classic comedy statement "women are different from men" apparently holds true for focal and global cerebral ischemia, as well. Postmenopausal women are at high risk for stroke (focal ischemia) and cardiac arrest (global ischemia), but the benefit of hormone replacement therapy (HRT) in stroke prevention is controversial, and HRT in cardiac arrest/CPR is almost completely uninvestigated. Recent clinical trials demonstrated lack of benefit and even potential harm of HRT in stroke, in contrast to earlier epidemiologic studies that demonstrated reduced risk and better outcome from stroke with HRT (48). In experimental models of stroke, estradiol has consistently been shown to reduce lesion size and neuronal death after experimental cerebral ischemia (49) and after cardiac arrest/CPR (50). Adult female mice sustain less histopathologic injury after cardiac arrest/CPR than do age-matched male mice. The sex difference in injury disappears after surgical ovariectomy. It has also been shown that estradiol replacement in ovariectomized animals restores protection from both local stroke (51) and cardiac arrest/CPR (50), suggesting that estradiol is neuroprotective when administered in physiologically relevant concentrations. The apparent disagreement among observational studies, preclinical data, and clinical trials, especially for stroke, emphasizes the complexity of estradiol's actions and indicates the importance of understanding its complex mechanisms of action. It is speculated that testosterone, too, may be an important player in increasing cardiovascular risk (52,53), and although male gender is an acknowledged risk factor for cardiovascular disease, the role of androgens in this pathogenesis is yet unknown. Nevertheless, it seems clear that gender is an important issue concerning focal and global cerebral ischemia, and that clinical trials must have protocols and be appropriately powered, such that male and female groups are evaluated separately for efficacy of neuroprotective agents. It may well be that some neuroprotective drugs are more efficacious in males, some in females, and when gender groups are combined, any significance is masked.

HEALTH CHARACTERISTICS OF ANIMALS

As mentioned above, despite decades of work and literally thousands of manuscripts concerning focal and global models of cerebral ischemia, minimal information has been translated to humans and led to successful clinical trials regarding neuroprotection. Much has been learned from preclinical ischemia studies concerning the complex cellular cascades that underlie mechanisms of ischemic injury and the potential targets for neuroprotection strategies. It must be considered that the animal models of ischemia do not closely mimic human cerebral ischemia. In preclinical animal studies, the animals are usually normal, healthy, young animals, whereas humans who suffer stroke or cardiac arrest /CPR most often have other existing pathologies, such as age, hypertension, diabetes, myocardial infarction, arrhythmia, and/or an assortment of other ongoing disease processes. These other pathologies, however, may alter the way in which stroke or global ischemia presents in humans and may modify the mechanisms involved to produce injury or neuroprotection. Only few studies have been conducted in animals with comorbid diseases and pathologies to evaluate this issue. Thus, the question that must be addressed is whether data accumulated from normal, young, and healthy mice, rats, dogs, and other species can be extrapolated to humans who are aged and possess other comorbid diseases.

COMBINATION DRUG THERAPY

Other mechanisms of neuronal injury exist in addition to the variety that were discussed above. Because there are multiple mechanisms of injury, it is reasonable to consider that there are also multiple mechanisms of neuroprotection. Therefore, although many single agents have been demonstrated to be protective in animal models, a rational approach to therapy is to consider using multiple pharmacologic agents, which affect, or target, more than one potential mechanism or act at several steps in the ischemic cascade (54). It is possible that combined use of an excitatory amino acid antagonist plus a free-radical scavenger may provide greater neuroprotection than either agent alone. The potential synergistic effect of multiple neuroprotective agents has merit. Although some investigators have demonstrated promising results with this technique (55–57), much additional work is required in both small and large animals using various combinations of agents to determine if this approach will be successful. Combination therapy, however, also has its limitations, which may lead to additional problems. With multiple agents, one must consider the potential increase in adverse events due to possible drug interactions that may lead to altered pharmacokinetics. Finally, with combination therapy, arriving at the best combination of drugs for "the combination" requires thinking mechanistically about which targets or receptors involved in the ischemic cascade we are attempting to alter or block in order to ameliorate the effects of ischemic damage.

CLINICAL TRIALS

In past years, clinical trials were always easy to criticize because, inevitably, difficulties were encountered with trial design, poor analysis, inclusion and exclusion criteria, statistical analysis, outcome analysis, lack of blinding and randomization, and heterogeneity of human stroke itself. However, in more recent years, the quality of clinical trials and their criteria in many of these areas has improved. The long-term inability to obtain positive clinical trials may be the result of 3 possible problem areas. The first deals with the preclinical investigator, who oftentimes does not completely evaluate drugs in a manner that can be useful in the clinic, i.e., clarifying dose–response curves, windows of opportunity, and functional and histopathologic outcome measures. The second problem area is that, even when a particular drug is evaluated thoroughly in preclinical animal studies, clinical trial designs are invoked, which do not utilize the important characteristics demonstrated in the preclinical data. Conversely, many times, a clinical trial cannot possibly mimic the animal model and protocol. Third, of course, is that the drug is just not at all neuroprotective in humans. We have learned much from preclinical animal studies concerning basic mechanisms of injury and targets for neuroprotection following ischemia, and, currently, many new technologies are available to evaluate stroke patients and make assessments that were difficult or impossible to make in the past. The technology necessary to image stroke is available at most major health-care facilities and includes early measures of injury, such as diffusion-weighted imaging, magnetic resonance angiography, and perfusion and computed tomography perfusion (58–61). These advanced diagnostic techniques, coupled with better clinical trial designs that include appropriate power analysis, statistical analysis, better inclusion and exclusion criteria, proper blinding and randomization (62,63), should yield clinical trials with few weaknesses. However, even if clinical trial design is perfect, the design and protocol should be based on evidence from preclinical animal studies. In the simplest example, organizing a trial protocol that administers 10 mg of a drug at 3 hr after reperfusion, when those parameters have never been shown to be effective in animal models, would be designing a trial that is unlikely to be successful. Thus, the preclinical evaluation must be stellar and provide critical information in order to plan the most successful of trials. The conditions that should be met before a drug can progress to a clinical trial have been carefully outlined by the Stroke Therapy Academic Industry Roundtable (64) and should be utilized as a guide to preclinical studies that are investigating neuroprotective drugs.

SUMMARY

In this chapter, we have identified the major reasons for failure of neuroprotective agents to show benefit in clinical trials. The discussion has centered on issues of drug dosages, windows of opportunity, multiple mechanisms of injury and neuroprotection, combination therapy, gender differences, and clinical trial design and analysis. Despite the failure of clinical trials to show efficacy with pharmacologic neuroprotection over the years, optimism remains for the future. With newer clinical trial designs and protocols that are based on appropriate preclinical data and utilize the new strategies of stem cell technology, gene therapy, combination therapy, and gender-based differential responses, neuroprotective agents will surely be found in the future.

ACKNOWLEDGMENTS

The author would like to thank Candace Berryman for editorial assistance with this chapter, and the US Public Health Service NIH grants NS20020 and NS46072 for long-term support.

REFERENCES

1. American Heart Association. Heart & Stroke statistical Update. Dallas, TX: American Heart Association, 2000.
2. Kristian T, Siesjo BK. Calcium in ischemic cell death. Stroke 1997; 29:705–718.
3. Iadecola C. Mechanisms of cerebral ischemia. In: Walz W, ed. Cerebral Ischemia: Molecular and Cellular Pathophysiology Study. Totowa, NJ, United States: Humana Press, Inc, 1999:3–32.
4. Traystman RJ, Kirsch JR, Koehler RC. Oxygen radical mechanisms of brain injury following ischemia and reperfusion. J Appl Physiol 1991; 71:1185–1195.
5. Rothman S. Synaptic release of excitatory amino acid neurotransmitter mediates axonic neuronal death. J Neurosci 1996; 4:1884–1891.
6. Kim JS. Cytokines and adhesion molecules in stroke and related disease. J Neurol Sci 1997; 8:i–viii.
7. Fisher M. Characterizing the target of acute stroke therapy. Stroke 1997; 28:866–872.
8. Koisinaho J, Hokfelt T. Altered gene expression in brain ischemia. Neuroreport 1997; 137:69–78.
9. Sharp FR, Sagar SM. Alterations in gene expression as an index of neuronal injury: heat shock and the immediate early gene response. Neurotoxicology 1994; 15:51–59.
10. Uemura Y, Kowall NW, Moskowitz MA. Focal ischemia in rats causes time-dependent expression of c-fos protein immunoreactivity in widespread regions of ipsilateral cortex. Brain Res 1991; 552:99–105.
11. Kovacs Z, Ikezaki K, Samoto K, et al. VEGF and flt expression time kinetics in rat brain infarct. Stroke 1996; 27:1865–1872.
12. Bleyart AL, Nemoto EM, Safar P, et al. Thiopental amelioration of brain damage after global ischemia in monkeys. Anesthesiology 1978; 49:390–398.
13. Gisvold SE, Safar P, Hendrickx HH, et al. Thiopental treatment after global brain ischemia in pigtailed monkeys. Anesthesiology 1984; 60:88–96.
14. Steen PA, Milde JH, Michenfelder JD. No barbiturate protection in a dog model of complete cerebral ischemia. Ann Neurol 1979; 5:343–349.
15. Brain Resuscitation Clinical Trial I Study Group. Randomized clinical study of thiopental loading in comatose survivors of cardiac arrest. N Engl J Med 1986; 314:397–403.
16. Traystman RJ. Anesthetic mediated neuroprotection: established fact or passing fantasy? J Neurosurg Anesthesiol 2004; 16:308–312.
17. Warner DS. Anesthetics provide limited but real protection against acute brain injury. J Neurosurg Anethesiol 2004; 16:303–307.
18. Benson DW, Williams GR Jr., Spencer FC, et al. The use of hypothermia after cardiac arrest. Anesth Analg 1958; 38:423–428.
19. Busto R, Globus MY, Dietrich WD, et al. Effect of mild hypothermia on ischemia-induced release of neurotransmitters and free fatty acids in rat brain. Stroke 1989; 20:904–910.
20. Sterz F, Safar P, Tisherman S, et al. Mild hypothermic cardiopulmonary resuscitation improves outcome after prolonged cardiac arrest in dogs. Crit Care Med 1991; 346:379–389.
21. The Hypothermia After Cardiac Arrest Study Group. Mild hypothermia to improve the neurologic outcome after cardiac arrest. N Engl J Med 2002; 346:549–556.
22. Krieger DW, Yenari MA. Therapeutic hypothermia for acute ischemic stroke: what do laboratory studies teach us? Stroke 2004; 35:1482–1489.
23. Davis SM, Lees KR, Albers GW, et al. Selfotel in acute ischemic stroke: possible neurotoxic effects of an NMDA antagonist. Stroke 2000; 31:347–354.
24. Sacco RL, DeRosa JT, Haley EC Jr., et al. Glycine antagonist in neuroprotection Americas Investigators. Glycine antagonist in neuroprotection for patients with acute stroke: GAIN America. A randomized controlled trial. JAMA 2001; 4:1719–1728.

25. Diener HC, Corten SM, Ford G, et al. Lubeluzole in acute ischemic stroke treatment: a double-blind study with an 8-hour inclusion window comparing a 10-mg daily dose of lubeluzole with placebo. Stroke 2000; 31:2543–2551.

26. Pan Y, Lo EH, Matsumoto K, et al. Quantitative and dynamic MRI of neuroprotection in experimental stroke. J Neurol Sci 1995; 131:128–134.

27. Nishikawa T, Kirsch JR, Koehler RC, et al. Competitive N-methyl-D-aspartate receptor blockade reduces brain injury following transient focal ischemia in cats. Stroke 1994; 25:2258–2264.

28. Matsumiya N, Koehler RC, Kirsch JR, et al. Conjugated superoxide dismutase reduces extent of caudate injury after transient focal ischemia in cats. Stroke 1991; 22:1193–1200.

29. Nishikawa T, Kirsch JR, Koehler RC, et al. Nitric oxide synthase inhibition reduces caudate injury following transient focal ischemia in cats. Stroke 1994; 25:877–885.

30. Bethel A, Kirsch JR, Koehler RC, et al. Intravenous basic fibroblast growth factor decreases brain injury from focal ischemia in cats. Stroke 1997; 28:609–615.

31. Harukuni I, Traystman RJ, Bhardwaj A, et al. Intravenous basic fibroblast growth factor does not ameliorate brain injury resulting from transient focal ischemia in cats. J Neurosurg Anethesiol 1998; 10:160–165.

32. Traystman RJ. Animal models of focal and global cerebral ischemia. Inst Anim Lab Res J 2003; 44:83–93.

33. Kofler J, Traystman RJ. Rodent models of global cerebral ischemia. In: Tatlisumak T, Fisher M, eds. Handbook of Experimental Neurology. Cambridge, MA, United States: Cambridge University Press, 2006; 329–344.

34. Tamura A, Graham DI, McCullough J, et al. Focal cerebral ischemia in the rat: regional cerebral blood flow determined by [14C] iodoantipyrine autoradiography following middle cerebral artery occlusion. J Cereb Blood Flow Metab 1981; 1:61–69.

35. Duverger D, Mackenzie ET. The quantification of cerebral infarction following focal ischemia in the rat: influence of strain, arterial pressure, glucose concentration, and age. J Cereb Blood Flow Metab 1988; 8:449–461.

36. Maruki Y, Koehler RC, Kirsch JR, et al. Tirilazad pretreatment improves early cerebral metabolic and blood flow recovery from hyperglycemic ischemia. J Cereb Blood Flow Metab 1995; 15:88–96.

37. Lyden P, Shuaib A, Ng K, et al. CLASS-1/H/T Investigators. Clomethiazole acute stroke study in ischemic stroke (CLASS-1): final results. Stroke 2002; 33:122–128.

38. Clark WM, Wechsler L, Sabounjian LA, et al. Citicoline Stroke Study Group. A phase III randomized efficacy trial of 200 mg citicoline in acute ischemic stroke patients. Neurology 2001; 57:1595–1602.

39. Albers GW, Goldstein LB, Hall D, et al. Acute Stroke Investigators. Aptigane/hydrochloride in acute ischemic stroke: a randomized controlled trial. JAMA 2001; 286:2673–2682.

40. Wells BA, Keats AC, Cooley DA. Increased tolerance to cerebral ischemia produced by general anesthesia during temporary carotid occlusion. Surgery 1963; 54:216–223.

41. Yang J, Zormski CF. Effects of isoflurane on N-methyl-D-aspartate gated ion channels in cultured rat hippocampal neurons. Ann NY Acad Sci 1991; 625:287–289.

42. Jenkins A, Greenblatt EP, Faulkner HJ, et al. Evidence for a common binding cavity for three general anesthetics within the GABA receptor. J Neurosci 2001; 21:RC136.

43. Harris BD, Moody EJ, Basile AS, et al. Volatile anesthetics bidirectionally and stereospecifically modulate ligand binding to GABA receptors. Eur J Pharmacol 1994; 267:269–274.

44. Wilson JX, Gelb AW. Free radicals, antioxidants, and neurologic injury: possible relationship to cerebral protection by anesthetics. J Neurosurg Anethesiol 2002; 14:66–79.

45. Patel P, Drummond JC, Cole DJ, et al. Isoflurane and pentobarbital reduce the frequency of transient ischemic deep depolarization during focal ischemia in rats. Anesth Analg 1998; 86:773–780.

46. Warner DS, Hansen TD, Vust L, et al. The effects of isoflurane and pentobarbital on the distribution of cerebral blood flow during focal cerebral ischemia. Stroke 1989; 1:219–226.

47. Bhardwaj A, Castro III AF, Alkayed NJ, et al. Anesthetic choice of halothane versus propofol impact on experimental perioperative stroke. Stroke 2001; 32:1920–1925.

48. Hurn PD, Brass LM. Estrogen and stroke: a balanced analysis. Stroke 2003; 34:338–341.

49. Hurn PD, Macrae IM. Estrogen as a neuroprotectant in stroke. J Cereb Blood Flow Metab 2000; 20:631–652.

50. Noppens RR, Kofler J, Hurn PD, et al. Dose-dependent neuroprotection by 17 beta-estradiol after cardiac arrest and cardiopulmonary resuscitation. Crit Care Med 2005; 33:1595–1602.

51. Rusa R, Alkayed NJ, Crain BJ, et al. 17 Beta-estradiol reduces stroke injury in estrogen deficient female animals. Stroke 1999; 30:1665–1670.

52. Fineschi V, Baroldi G, Monociotti F, et al. Anabolic steroid abuse and cardiac sudden death. Arch Pathol Lab Med 2001; 125:253–255.

53. Wigginton JG, Pepe PE, Bedolla JP. Sex-related differences in the presentation and outcome of out-of-hospital cardiopulmonary arrest: a multiyear, prospective population-based study. Crit Care Med 2002; 30:S131–S136.

54. Fisher M, Bogousslavsky J. Evolving toward effective therapy for acute ischemic stroke. JAMA 1993; 270:360–364.

55. Onal MZ, Li F, Tatlisumak T, et al. Synergistic effects of citicoline and MK-801 in temporary experimental focal ischemia in rats. Stroke 1997; 28:1060–1065.
56. Zivin JM, Mazzarella V. Tissue plasminogen activator plus glutamate antagonist improves outcome after embolic stroke. Arch Neurol 1991; 48:1235–1238.
57. Schmid-Elsaesser R, Hungerhuber E, Zausinger S, et al. Combination drug therapy and mild hypothermia: a promising treatment strategy for reversible focal cerebral ischemia. Stroke 1999; 30:1891–1899.
58. Warch S. Stroke neuroimaging. Stroke 2003; 34:345–347.
59. Warch S, Wardlaw J. Advances in imaging 2005. Stroke 2006; 37:297–298.
60. Baron JC, Warch S. Imaging. Stroke 2005; 36:196–199.
61. Kidwell CS, Chalela JA, Saver JL, et al. Comparison of MRI and CT for detection of acute intracerebral hemorrhage. JAMA 2004; 292:1823–1830.
62. Lees KR, Hankey GJ, Hacke W. Design of future acute-stroke treatment trials. Lancet Neurol 2003; 2:51–61.
63. Howard G, Coffey CS, Cutter GR. Is Bayesian analysis ready for use in phase III randomized clinical trials? Beware the sound of sirens. Stroke 2005; 36:1622–1623.
64. Stroke Therapy Academic Industry Roundtable. Recommendations for standards regarding pre-clinical neuroprotective and restorative drug development. Stroke 1999; 30:2752–2758.

29 | Ischemic Preconditioning

Ines P. Koerner, MD, Fellow

Department of Anesthesiology & Perioperative Medicine, Oregon Health & Science University, Portland, Oregon, USA

Nabil J. Alkayed, MD, PhD, Director[a], Associate Professor[b]

[a]*Core Molecular Laboratories and Training,* [b]*Department of Anesthesiology & Perioperative Medicine, Oregon Health & Science University, Portland, Oregon, USA*

INTRODUCTION

The ability to withstand, respond to, and cope with ongoing stress is a fundamental property of all living organisms. At the cellular level, a stress response can be elicited by noxious agents, such as endotoxin and oxygen free radicals, and by disturbances in normal cellular and organ homeostasis, such as those occurring during ischemia and heat stress. When excessive, such stimuli can cause irreversible tissue damage. However, in several organs, including heart and brain, it has been shown that mild stress, including mild ischemic stress, may serve a beneficial role, by rapidly mobilizing existing defense mechanisms to cope with ongoing stress and by inducing a more delayed genomic response to cope with imminent threat. This phenomenon is generally referred to as *preconditioning* or *tolerance*, and rapid and delayed responses define 2 pathophysiologically distinct phases of tolerance, referred to as *early* or *acute* and *delayed* or *late* preconditioning (1). Ischemic preconditioning in brain is of particular importance because brain cells, particularly neurons, are critically dependent on oxygen and nutrients, and the slightest disruption of blood flow can irreversibly damage neurons and lead to permanent functional disability. Unfortunately, despite decades of research, clinically available treatment options for patients who experience cerebral ischemia are still limited. In this chapter, we review the efforts focused on determining endogenous mechanisms of protection that result from ischemic preconditioning and on efforts to translate mechanisms of tolerance into potential stroke therapies.

CLINICAL RELEVANCE

The induction of tolerance to ischemia by preconditioning was first described in the heart 20 years ago (2). It was later observed in brain that brief ischemic insults that did not induce tissue damage, protected the brain against damage caused by subsequent, more severe, and otherwise lethal ischemia (3). It was first observed in gerbils that 2 min of global ischemia protected hippocampal CA1 neurons from lethal 5 min ischemia 24 to 48 hr later. Similar observations were later made in rats (4,5) and mice (6). Whether the human brain can be preconditioned to tolerate ischemia is unknown. A number of recent clinical studies, however, suggest that a transient ischemic attack (TIA) might serve as a preconditioning stimulus, reducing the severity of subsequent strokes (7–10). In contrast, a more recent study failed to detect an association of prior TIA with lesser stroke severity (11). Distinction between the role of TIA as risk factor or protectant is difficult in humans because TIA is a clinical diagnosis of a range of cerebrovascular events that vary in duration, location, severity, and number. TIA frequently precedes severe ischemia, the impact of which might mask any defense mechanisms induced by prior events. Induction of tolerance against ischemia is most beneficial for patients with known elevated risk for developing cerebral ischemic events; for example, patients who have suffered recent TIAs and patients scheduled for surgical procedures that carry increased risk for perioperative ischemia and stroke, such as surgical treatment of cerebral aneurysms, carotid endarterectomy, and cardiac surgery involving cardiopulmonary bypass.

MODELS OF PRECONDITIONING: CROSS-TOLERANCE

Numerous animal models have been described, in which brief episodes of global or focal ischemia are applied, followed by a more severe ischemic stress designed to kill neurons. In the classic experiment, brief global ischemia induced tolerance against subsequent global ischemia (3) in what is referred to as a *global-global* model of ischemic preconditioning. Subsequent studies have demonstrated that tolerance against focal ischemia can also be induced by brief focal ischemia (12), or *focal-focal* preconditioning. Furthermore, brief global ischemia has also been shown to reduce infarct size after focal ischemia induced by middle cerebral artery occlusion (*global-focal*) (13). Finally, transient focal ischemia increases tolerance against subsequent global ischemia. Interestingly, tolerance to ischemia in this *focal-global* paradigm develops in neurons within the region of focal ischemia (14) and in neurons outside the region of primary ischemia (15). Noxious stimuli other than ischemia can also confer tolerance to ischemia. For example, hyperthermia (16,17), as well as hypothermia (18), can protect from subsequent ischemia. Similarly, previous exposure to hypoxia reduces infarct after hypoxic/ischemic injury in neonatal rats (19), and hyperbaric oxygen can induce tolerance against focal ischemia (20). Other conditions and agents shown to induce ischemic tolerance in brain include spreading depression (21–23), status epilepticus (24), hypoglycemia (25), and low doses of the endotoxin lipopolysaccharide (LPS) (26–28). Finally, ischemic tolerance can be induced by chemical preconditioning, using substances that mimic the above-mentioned stimuli. The most extensively studied chemical preconditioning agent is 3-nitropropionic acid (3-NPA), an inhibitor of oxidative phosphorylation that binds to succinate dehydrogenase (SDH) and induces tolerance against *in vitro* ischemia in organotypic hippocampal slices (29), and *in vivo* ischemia in gerbils and rats (30–32).

PHARMACOLOGIC PRECONDITIONING

A more clinically relevant mode of ischemic tolerance induction, known as pharmacologic preconditioning, uses clinically available drugs. For example, promising results have been shown using acetylsalicylic acid (33), as well as the antibiotics kanamycin and erythromycin (34,35). Erythropoietin has also been shown to induce tolerance to ischemia (36). Finally, preischemic exposure to volatile anesthetics, such as halothane and isoflurane, has also been reported to induce ischemic tolerance in the brain (37). In heart, other pharmacologic agents, including nitric oxide (NO) donors, adenosine-receptor agonists, endotoxin derivatives, or opioid-receptor agonists have been shown to mimic the preconditioning effect. Further understanding of the mechanisms underlying the induction and acquisition of tolerance in brain could lead to the development of new clinically useful pharmacologic agents based on their ability to mimic preconditioning and elaborate endogenous mechanisms of ischemic protection. Below, we review mechanisms proposed to mediate ischemic tolerance induction in brain.

MECHANISMS OF ISCHEMIC TOLERANCE

Similar to what has been initially described in heart, ischemic tolerance in brain is biphasic, where tolerance is acquired shortly after the stimulus and at a delayed time point following preconditioning. Early tolerance against subsequent cerebral ischemia starts as early as 30 min after the preconditioning ischemic episode and lasts for approximately 2 hr (rapid preconditioning) (38,39). A second window of tolerance is observed 24 hr later, which lasts for 2 to 7 days (delayed preconditioning) (3,30,31). Early and delayed phases of tolerance represent 2 distinct responses to preconditioning, with different temporal profiles and mechanisms of protection. Acute preconditioning results from rapid changes in activity and posttranslational modifications of existing proteins, whereas delayed tolerance involves gene induction and *de novo* protein synthesis (40). Mechanistically, the early phase of preconditioning is usually attributed to flow-mediated mechanisms or changes in cellular metabolism, whereas delayed tolerance to ischemia represents a long-term, adaptive response to stress and genetic reprogramming in brain toward a more protected phenotype.

ADENOSINE AND K$_{ATP}$ CHANNELS

Studies in heart and brain pointed to an important role for plasmalemmal and, later, mitochondrial ATP-sensitive potassium channels (K$_{ATP}$) in the acquisition of early tolerance. It has been demonstrated that rapid induction of tolerance in brain involves a cascade of events triggered by the liberation of adenosine in response to ischemia, stimulation of adenosine A1 receptors, and opening of plasmalemmal K$_{ATP}$, which leads to membrane hyperpolarization and reduced neuronal excitability (41). Further supporting this finding, ischemic tolerance in hippocampal neurons in gerbils was blocked by adenosine-receptor antagonists (42).

MITOCHONDRIAL K$_{ATP}$ CHANNELS

Opening of mitochondrial K$_{ATP}$ channels (mitoK$_{ATP}$) with diazoxide induces neuronal preconditioning *in vitro* and *in vivo* (43–45), and blockade of mitoK$_{ATP}$ opening with 5-hydroxydecanoate abolishes tolerance induction by ischemic preconditioning (46) and by chemical preconditioning using the mitochondrial enzyme SDH inhibitor 3-NPA (47). Diazoxide also leads to increased free-radical production, possibly by inhibiting SDH, which is part of complex II of the electron transport chain (45). A burst of reactive oxygen species (ROS) might trigger preconditioning mechanisms of protection. For example, tolerance induction by 3-NPA also increases ROS production and induces tolerance to cerebral ischemia (48). SDH has recently been found to be part of a macromolecular complex that forms mitoK$_{ATP}$ (49). Diazoxide and 3-NPA might, therefore, actually act on the same molecule, suggesting that different methods of preconditioning might eventually converge on a common pathway that leads to tolerance induction and neuroprotection.

NMDA RECEPTORS AND CA^{2+}

Influx of calcium ions (Ca^{2+}) following the activation of NMDA-sensitive glutamate receptors has been implicated in tolerance induction. NMDA induces tolerance against oxygen-glucose deprivation (OGD) in neuronal culture and organotypic hippocampal slices (50,51). Furthermore, NMDA-receptor antagonists prevent ischemic preconditioning in gerbils (52). A possible downstream mechanism of protection could be the Ca^{2+}-triggered activation of cAMP-response-element-binding protein (CREB) (53), a transcription factor that induces genes known to protect neuronal cells from ischemic injury and promote neuronal survival (54). CREB phosphorylation is increased in gerbil hippocampal CA1 neurons after global ischemic preconditioning (52) and in surviving penumbral cells in a rat focal ischemic preconditioning model (55). NMDA-receptor activation has also been linked to the activation of nuclear factor-κB (NF-κB), another transcription factor implicated in neuroprotection (56).

NITRIC OXIDE IN PRECONDITIONING

NO is produced in brain by 3 isoforms of nitric oxide synthase (NOS): neuronal (nNOS), endothelial (eNOS), and inducible NOS (iNOS). NO is an important mediator of cell-to-cell communication and regulator of cerebral blood flow and metabolism (57). An increase in NO production, first by nNOS in neurons and later by iNOS in glial cells, has been implicated in cell death after cerebral ischemia (58,59). However, under certain conditions, NO might also induce preconditioning. For example, NOS inhibitors have been shown to abolish tolerance induction by hypoxia (60), transient focal ischemia (61), and LPS (62). Further, iNOS is induced by volatile anesthetics, and its blockage inhibits anesthetic preconditioning (37). NO might contribute to tolerance induction via activation of Ras/ERK and PI3-kinase/Akt neuroprotective signaling pathways (57).

APOPTOSIS INHIBITORS AND BCL-2

Genes that regulate programmed cell death, or apoptosis, are potential downstream mediators of delayed tolerance. Specifically, bcl-2, the prototype of apoptosis-inhibiting genes, has been implicated in the mechanism of protection following preconditioning. Bcl-2 levels are increased after hypoxic preconditioning in cultured neurons (63) and after preconditioning with hyperbaric oxygen *in vivo* (64). Global ischemic preconditioning in gerbils also increases bcl-2 expression (65), and inhibition of bcl-2 expression blocks tolerance induction by focal ischemia in rats (66). Chemical preconditioning with 3-NPA increases bcl-2 expression in ischemia-vulnerable areas of rat brain (48), likely in response to ROS generation (67). During subsequent ischemia, bcl-2 protein can neutralize damaging free radicals (68), inactivate proapoptotic proteins, such as bax (69), stabilize mitochondrial membrane, and prevent the release of cytochrome c and the subsequent caspase activation (70).

REACTIVE OXYGEN SPECIES AND SUPEROXIDE DISMUTASES

Administration of exogenous superoxide dismutase (SOD) during focal ischemic preconditioning abolishes tolerance induction (71), suggesting that induction of ischemic tolerance is triggered by the generation of ROS during preconditioning. However, the role of endogenous antioxidant mechanisms in the induction of tolerance is not clear. Manganese SOD (MnSOD) expression and activity are increased *in vivo* after preconditioning with LPS (72), hyperbaric oxygenation (64) and ischemia (73), and hypoxic preconditioning in cultured neurons (74). In contrast, no differences in expression or activity of either MnSOD or copper-zinc SOD (CuZnSOD) were observed in rats in connection with tolerance induction by spreading depression (75) or focal ischemia (76).

INFLAMMATION IN ISCHEMIC DAMAGE AND ISCHEMIC TOLERANCE

The brain's inflammatory response to ischemia exacerbates ischemic brain damage (77,78). Expression of proinflammatory cytokines, such as tumor necrosis factor α (TNF-α) and interleukin 1 (IL-1), is increased after cerebral ischemia (79), and inhibition of cytokine expression reduces ischemic damage (80). Both cytokines, however, have also been implicated in tolerance induction. Serum IL-1 increases after global ischemic preconditioning in gerbils, and administration of antibody against its receptor blocks tolerance induction (81). Similarly, TNF-α expression in brain is increased after focal ischemic preconditioning in rats, which can be prevented with a neutralizing antibody against TNF-α (82). TNF-α also contributes to *in vitro* tolerance induction by hypoxic preconditioning (83). Because the production of proinflammatory cytokines in brain is probably initiated by signaling through Toll-like receptors (TLRs) that recognize molecules released from ischemia-injured brain tissues, it has been suggested that early preconditioning might be mediated via direct interference with membrane fluidity, disrupting lipid rafts and thereby inhibiting TLR/cytokine signaling pathways (84). Delayed preconditioning, on the other hand, triggers the TLR/cytokine inflammatory pathways, which leads to inflammation and, more importantly, to simultaneous upregulation of feedback inhibitors of inflammation. Activation of the transcription factor NF-κB appears to be a crucial step toward tolerance in these models (85,86). Cyclooxygenase-2 (COX-2), although widely implicated in tolerance induction in the heart (87,88), has not been shown to be relevant to preconditioning in brain.

PRECONDITIONING AND HIBERNATION

The state of increased tolerance to ischemia has been compared to the reduced dependency on oxygen and nutrients that enables hibernation (89). According to this view, preconditioning reprograms brain cells into a hibernation-like state by switching the gene expression profile to one representing a higher state of ischemic tolerance (35,90). Genetic reprogramming into the new protective phenotype involves downregulation of a large number of genes that encode ion channels and enzymes involved in protein turnover, glucose metabolism, and cell cycle regulation (90). Reduced expression of these genes might represent a state of reduced energy consumption and enhanced tolerance to energy deprivation observed in preconditioned and hibernating brains.

HYPOXIA-INDUCIBLE FACTOR 1 AND CYTOCHROME P450

Hypoxia-inducible factor 1 (HIF-1) is a key transcription factor in the brain's response to hypoxic stress (91). Induction of HIF-1α and its downstream targets, such as erythropoietin, have been implicated in hypoxic preconditioning *in vivo* in newborn and adult models (92–94). HIF-1α-mediated induction of cytochrome P450 2C11 expression is an important mechanism of tolerance by hypoxic preconditioning in astrocytes (95). Cytochrome P450 2C11 is an arachidonic acid epoxygenase that is also increased in rats by focal ischemic preconditioning (96). It metabolizes arachidonic acid to epoxyeicosatrienoic acids (EETs), which have been implicated in control of the cerebral circulation (97). EETs have also been shown to protect the heart against ischemia/reperfusion injury (98) and to protect astrocytes from OGD-induced cell death (95). In addition, EETs are antiinflammatory (99), antioxidant (100), and antipyretic (101). Finally, EETs have been shown to stimulate ATP-sensitive potassium channels (102). Therefore, EETs appear to play an important role in mediating ischemic tolerance in brain, and manipulations aimed at increasing their levels, such as increased synthesis or decreased metabolism, constitute a promising therapeutic strategy against ischemic injury.

CONCLUSION AND FUTURE DIRECTIONS

Induced tolerance to ischemia is an attractive strategy for preemptive neuroprotection in patients at high risk for cerebral ischemia in the near future. The mechanisms of preconditioning-acquired ischemic tolerance have not yet been completely characterized. Rapid preconditioning probably involves changes in membrane excitability and mitochondrial function, whereas delayed preconditioning probably involves multiple signaling pathways that activate a set of transcription factors and turn on a set of genes that define a new cellular phenotype that is characterized by increased resilience to ischemic stress. More work is needed to identify relevant molecules and therapeutic targets in the core of this pathway. Mediators of inflammation and pluripotent molecules, such as EETs, are potential targets for such future efforts. Until more specific and efficient inducers of endogenous tolerance are developed, pharmacologic preconditioning might be a feasible alternative for selected patients.

REFERENCES

1. Stein AB, Tang XL, Guo Y, et al. Delayed adaptation of the heart to stress: late preconditioning. Stroke 2004; 35(11 suppl 1):2676–2679.
2. Murry CE, Jennings RB, Reimer KA. Preconditioning with ischemia: a delay of lethal cell injury in ischemic myocardium. Circulation 1986; 74(1124):1136.
3. Kitagawa K, Matsumoto M, Tagaya M. "Ischemic tolerance" phenomenon found in the brain. Brain Res 1990; 528:21–24.
4. Liu Y, Kato H, Nakata N, Kogure K. Protection of rat hippocampus against ischemic neuronal damage by pretreatment with sublethal ischemia. Brain Res 1992; 586(1):121–124.
5. Nishi S, Taki W, Uemura Y, et al. Ischemic tolerance due to the induction of HSP70 in a rat ischemic recirculation model. Brain Res 1993; 615(2):281–288.
6. Wu LY, Ding AS, Ma Q, et al. [Correlation between enhanced anoxic tolerance induced by hypoxic preconditioning and the stability of mitochondrial membrane potential in cultured hypothalamic cells]. Sheng Li Xue Bao 2001; 53(2):93–96.
7. Weih M, Bergk A, Isaev NK, et al. Induction of ischemic tolerance in rat cortical neurons by 3-nitropropionic acid: chemical preconditioning. Neurosci Lett 1999; 272(3):207–210.
8. Moncayo J, de Freitas GR, Bogousslavsky J, et al. Do transient ischemic attacks have a neuroprotective effect? Neurology 2000; 54(11):2089–2094.
9. Sitzer M, Foerch C, Neumann-Haefelin T, et al. Transient ischaemic attack preceding anterior circulation infarction is independently associated with favourable outcome. J Neurol Neurosurg Psychiatry 2004; 75(4):659–660.
10. Wegener S, Gottschalk B, Jovanovic V, et al. Transient ischemic attacks before ischemic stroke: preconditioning the human brain? A multicenter magnetic resonance imaging study. Stroke 2004; 35(3):616–621.
11. Johnston SC. Ischemic preconditioning from transient ischemic attacks? Data from the Northern California TIA Study. Stroke 2004; 35(11 suppl 1):2680–2682.

12. Chen J, Zhu R, Basta K, et al. Inhibition of Bcl-2 protein expression by antisense S-oligodeoxynucleotides treatment exacerbates neuronal death after cerebral ischemia in rats. Neurology 1996; 46:A270.

13. Simon RP, Niiro M, Gwinn R. Prior ischemic stress protects against experimental stroke. Neurosci Lett 1993; 163(2):135–137.

14. Glazier SS, O'Rourke DM, Graham DI, Welsh FA. Induction of ischemic tolerance following brief focal ischemia in rat brain. J Cereb Blood Flow Metab 1994; 14(4):545–553.

15. Miyashita K, Abe H, Nakajima T, et al. Induction of ischaemic tolerance in gerbil hippocampus by pretreatment with focal ischaemia. Neuroreport 1994; 6(1):46–48.

16. Chopp M, Chen H, Ho KL, et al. Transient hyperthermia protects against subsequent forebrain ischemic cell damage in the rat. Neurology 1989; 39(10):1396–1398.

17. Ikeda T, Xia XY, Xia YX, Ikenoue T. Hyperthermic preconditioning prevents blood-brain barrier disruption produced by hypoxia-ischemia in newborn rat. Brain Res Dev Brain Res 1999; 117(1):53–58.

18. Nishio S, Yunoki M, Chen ZF, et al. Ischemic tolerance in the rat neocortex following hypothermic preconditioning. J Neurosurg 2000; 93(5):845–851.

19. Gidday JM, Fitzgibbons JC, Shah AR, Park TS. Neuroprotection from ischemic brain injury by hypoxic preconditioning in the neonatal rat. Neurosci Lett 1994; 168(1–2):221–224.

20. Prass K, Wiegand F, Schumann P, et al. Hyperbaric oxygenation induced tolerance against focal cerebral ischemia in mice is strain dependent. Brain Res 2000; 871(1):146–150.

21. Kawahara N, Ruetzler CA, Klatzo I. Protective effect of spreading depression against neuronal damage following cardiac arrest cerebral ischaemia. Neurol Res 1995; 17(1):9–16.

22. Kobayashi S, Harris VA, Welsh FA. Spreading depression induces tolerance of cortical neurons to ischemia in rat brain. J Cereb Blood Flow Metab 1995; 15(5):721–727.

23. Matsushima K, Hogan MJ, Hakim AM. Cortical spreading depression protects against subsequent focal cerebral ischemia in rats. J Cereb Blood Flow Metab 1996; 16(2):221–226.

24. Lowenstein DH, Simon RP, Sharp FR. The pattern of 72-kDa heat shock protein-like immunoreactivity in the rat brain following flurothyl-induced status epilepticus. Brain Res 1990; 531(1–2):173–182.

25. Bergstedt K, Hu BR, Wieloch T. Initiation of protein synthesis and heat-shock protein-72 expression in the rat brain following severe insulin-induced hypoglycemia. Acta Neuropathol (Berl) 1993; 86(2):145–153.

26. Tasaki K, Ruetzler CA, Ohtsuki T, et al. Lipopolysaccharide pre-treatment induces resistance against subsequent focal cerebral ischemic damage in spontaneously hypertensive rats. Brain Res 1997; 748(1–2):267–270.

27. Dawson DA, Furuya K, Gotoh J, et al. Cerebrovascular hemodynamics and ischemic tolerance: lipopolysaccharide-induced resistance to focal cerebral ischemia is not due to changes in severity of the initial ischemic insult, but is associated with preservation of microvascular perfusion. J Cereb Blood Flow Metab 1999; 19(6):616–623.

28. Deplanque D, Bordet R. Pharmacological preconditioning with lipopolysaccharide in the brain. Stroke 2000; 31(6):1465–1466.

29. Riepe MW, Esclaire F, Kasischke K, et al. Increased hypoxic tolerance by chemical inhibition of oxidative phosphorylation: "chemical preconditioning". J Cereb Blood Flow Metab 1997; 17(3):257–264.

30. Sugino T, Nozaki K, Takagi Y, Hashimoto N. 3-Nitropropionic acid induces ischemic tolerance in gerbil hippocampus in vivo. Neurosci Lett 1999; 259(1):9–12.

31. Wiegand F, Liao W, Busch C, et al. Respiratory chain inhibition induces tolerance to focal cerebral ischemia. J Cereb Blood Flow Metab 1999; 19(11):1229–1237.

32. Nakase H, Heimann A, Uranishi R, et al. Early-onset tolerance in rat global cerebral ischemia induced by a mitochondrial inhibitor. Neuroscience Lett 2000; 290:105–108.

33. Riepe MW, Kasischke K, Raupach A. Acetylsalicylic acid increases tolerance against hypoxic and chemical hypoxia. Stroke 1997; 28:2006–2011.

34. Huber R, Kasischke K, Ludolph AC, Riepe MW. Increase of cellular hypoxic tolerance by erythromycin and other antibiotics. Neuroreport 1999; 10(7):1543–1546.

35. Koerner IP, Brambrink AM. Altered genomic response to ischemia: a means of ischemic tolerance induction in the brain? In: Vincent J-L, ed. Yearbook of Intensive Care and Emergency Medicine 2004. Berlin, Heidelberg: Springer-Verlag, 2004.

36. Dawson TM. Preconditioning-mediated neuroprotection through erythropoietin? Lancet 2002; 359(9301):96–97.

37. Kapinya KJ, Lowl D, Futterer C, et al. Tolerance against ischemic neuronal injury can be induced by volatile anesthetics and is inducible NO synthase dependent. Stroke 2002; 33(7):1889–1898.

38. Pérez-Pinzón MA, Xu G-P, Dietrich WD, et al. Rapid preconditioning protects rats against ischemic neuronal damage after 3 but not 7 days of reperfusion following global cerebral ischemia. J Cerebral Blood Flow Metab 1997; 17:175–182.

39. Stagliano NE, Perez-Pinzon MA, Moskowitz MA, Huang PL. Focal ischemic preconditioning induces rapid tolerance to middle cerebral artery occlusion in mice. J Cereb Blood Flow Metab 1999; 19(7):757–761.

40. Barone FC, White RF, Spera PA, et al. Ischemic preconditioning and brain tolerance: temporal histological and functional outcomes, protein synthesis requirement, and interleukin-1 receptor antagonist and early gene expression. Stroke 1998; 29(9):1937–1950.

41. Heurteaux C, Lauritzen I, Widmann C, Lazdunski M. Essential role of adenosine, adenosine A1 receptors, and ATP-sensitive K+ channels in cerebral ischemic preconditioning. Proc Natl Acad Sci USA 1995; 92(10):4666–4670.

42. Hiraide T, Katsura K, Muramatsu H, et al. Adenosine receptor antagonists cancelled the ischemic tolerance phenomenon in gerbil. Brain Res 2001; 910(1–2):94–98.

43. Domoki F, Perciaccante JV, Veltkamp R, et al. Mitochondrial potassium channel opener diazoxide preserves neuronal-vascular function after cerebral ischemia in newborn pigs. Stroke 1999; 30(12):2713–2718.

44. Shimizu K, Lacza Z, Rajapakse N, et al. MitoK(ATP) opener, diazoxide, reduces neuronal damage after middle cerebral artery occlusion in the rat. Am J Physiol Heart Circ Physiol 2002; 283(3):H1005–H1011.

45. Kis B, Rajapakse NC, Snipes JA et al. Diazoxide induces delayed pre-conditioning in cultured rat cortical neurons. J Neurochem 2003; 87(4):969–980.

46. Yoshida M, Nakakimura K, Cui YJ, et al. Adenosine A(1) receptor antagonist and mitochondrial ATP-sensitive potassium channel blocker attenuate the tolerance to focal cerebral ischemia in rats. J Cereb Blood Flow Metab 2004; 24(7):771–779.

47. Horiguchi T, Kis B, Rajapakse N, et al. Opening of mitochondrial ATP-sensitive potassium channels is a trigger of 3-nitropropionic acid-induced tolerance to transient focal cerebral ischemia in rats. Stroke 2003; 34(4):1015–1020.

48. Brambrink AM, Schneider A, Noga H, et al. Tolerance-inducing dose of 3-nitropropionic acid modulates bcl-2 and bax balance in the rat brain: a potential mechanism of chemical preconditioning. J Cereb Blood Flow Metab 2000; 20(10):1425–1436.

49. Ardehali H, Chen Z, Ko Y, et al. Multiprotein complex containing succinate dehydrogenase confers mitochondrial ATP-sensitive K+ channel activity. Proc Natl Acad Sci USA 2004; 101(32):11880–11885.

50. Raval AP, Dave KR, Mochly-Rosen D, et al. Epsilon PKC is required for the induction of tolerance by ischemic and NMDA-mediated preconditioning in the organotypic hippocampal slice. J Neurosci 2003; 23(2):384–391.

51. Valentim LM, Rodnight R, Geyer AB, et al. Changes in heat shock protein 27 phosphorylation and immunocontent in response to preconditioning to oxygen and glucose deprivation in organotypic hippocampal cultures. Neuroscience 2003; 118(2):379–386.

52. Hara T, Hamada J, Yano S, et al. CREB is required for acquisition of ischemic tolerance in gerbil hippocampal CA1 region. J Neurochem 2003; 86(4):805–814.

53. Tauskela JS, Morley P. On the role of Ca2+ in cerebral ischemic preconditioning. Cell Calcium 2004; 36(3–4):313–322.

54. Walton MR, Dragunow I. Is CREB a key to neuronal survival? Trends Neurosci 2000; 23(2):48–53.

55. Nakajima T, Iwabuchi S, Miyazaki H, et al. Relationship between the activation of cyclic AMP responsive element binding protein and ischemic tolerance in the penumbra region of rat cerebral cortex. Neurosci Lett 2002; 331(1):13–16.

56. Wellmann H, Kaltschmidt B, Kaltschmidt C. Retrograde transport of transcription factor NF-kappa B in living neurons. J Biol Chem 2001; 276(15):11821–11829.

57. Huang PL. Nitric oxide and cerebral ischemic preconditioning. Cell Calcium 2004; 36 (3–4):323–329.

58. Huang Z, Huang PL, Panahian N, et al. Effects of cerebral ischemia in mice deficient in neuronal nitric oxide synthase. Science 1994; 265(5180):1883–1885.

59. Panahian N, Yoshida T, Huang PL, et al. Attenuated hippocampal damage after global cerebral ischemia in mice mutant in neuronal nitric oxide synthase. Neuroscience 1996; 72(2):343–354.

60. Gidday JM, Shah AR, Maceren RG, et al. Nitric oxide mediates cerebral ischemic tolerance in a neonatal rat model of hypoxic preconditioning. J Cereb Blood Flow Metab 1999; 19(3):331–340.

61. Atochin DN, Clark J, Demchenko IT, et al. Rapid cerebral ischemic preconditioning in mice deficient in endothelial and neuronal nitric oxide synthases. Stroke 2003; 34(5):1299–1303.

62. Puisieux F, Deplanque D, Pu Q, et al. Differential role of nitric oxide pathway and heat shock protein in preconditioning and lipopolysaccharide-induced brain ischemic tolerance. Eur J Pharmacol 2000; 389(1):71–78.

63. Bossenmeyer-Pourie C, Koziel V, Daval JL. Effects of hypothermia on hypoxia-induced apoptosis in cultured neurons from developing rat forebrain: comparison with preconditioning. Pediatr Res 2000; 47(3):385–391.

64. Wada K, Miyazawa T, Nomura N, et al. Preferential conditions for and possible mechanisms of induction of ischemic tolerance by repeated hyperbaric oxygenation in gerbil hippocampus. Neurosurgery 2001; 49(1):160–166.

65. Shimazaki K, Ishida A, Kawai N. Increase in bcl-2 oncoprotein and the tolerance to ischemia-induced neuronal death in the gerbil hippocampus. Neurosci Res 1994; 20(1):95–99.

66. Shimizu S, Nagayama T, Jin KL, et al. bcl-2 Antisense treatment prevents induction of tolerance to focal ischemia in the rat brain. J Cereb Blood Flow Metab 2001; 21(3):233–243.

67. Hockenberry DM, Oltvai ZN, Yin XM, et al. Bcl-2 functions in an antioxidant pathway to prevent apoptosis. Cell 1993; 75:241–251.

68. Ellerby HM, Martin SJ, Ellerby LM. Establishment of a cell-free system of neuronal apoptosis: comparison of premitochondrial, mitochondrial, and postmitochondrial phases. J Neurosci 1997; 17:6165–6178.

69. Zamzami N, Brenner C, Marzo I, et al. Subcellular and submitochondrial mode of action of bcl-2 like oncoproteins. Oncogene 1998; 16:2265–2282.

70. Jürgensmeier JM, Xie Z, Deferaux Q. Bax directly induces release of cytochrome c from isolated mitochondria. Proc Natl Acad Sci 1998; 95:4997–5002.

71. Mori T, Muramatsu H, Matsui T, et al. Possible role of the superoxide anion in the development of neuronal tolerance following ischaemic preconditioning in rats. Neuropathol Appl Neurobiol 2000; 26(1):31–40.

72. Bordet R, Deplanque D, Maboudou P, et al. Increase in endogenous brain superoxide dismutase as a potential mechanism of lipopolysaccharide-induced brain ischemic tolerance. J Cereb Blood Flow Metab 2000; 20(8):1190–1196.

73. Kato H, Kogure K, Araki T, et al. Immunohistochemical localization of superoxide dismutase in the hippocampus following ischemia in a gerbil model of ischemic tolerance. J Cereb Blood Flow Metab 1995; 15(1):60–70.

74. Arthur PG, Lim SC, Meloni BP, et al. The protective effect of hypoxic preconditioning on cortical neuronal cultures is associated with increases in the activity of several antioxidant enzymes. Brain Res 2004; 1017(1–2):146–154.

75. Mitchell K, Kariko K, Harris VA, et al. Preconditioning with cortical spreading depression does not upregulate Cu/Zn-SOD or Mn-SOD in the cerebral cortex of rats. Brain Res Mol Brain Res 2001; 96(1–2):50–58.

76. Puisieux F, Deplanque D, Bulckaen H, et al. Brain ischemic preconditioning is abolished by anti-oxidant drugs but does not up-regulate superoxide dismutase and glutathion peroxidase. Brain Res 2004; 1027(1–2):30–37.

77. Barone FC, Feuerstein GZ. Inflammatory mediators and stroke: new opportunities for novel therapeutics. J Cerebral Blood Flow Metab 1999; 19:819–34.

78. Allan SM, Rothwell NJ. Cytokines and acute neurodegeneration. Nat Rev Neurosci 2001; 2(10): 734–744.

79. Berti R, Williams AJ, Moffett JR, et al. Quantitative real-time RT-PCR analysis of inflammatory gene expression associated with ischemia-reperfusion brain injury. J Cereb Blood Flow Metab 2002; 22(9):1068–1079.

80. Barone FC, Arvin B, White RF, et al. Tumor necrosis factor-alpha. A mediator of focal ischemic brain injury. Stroke 1997; 28(6):1233–1244.

81. Ohtsuki T, Ruetzler CA, Tasaki K, Hallenbeck JM. Interleukin-1 mediates induction of tolerance to global ischemia in gerbil hippocampal CA1 neurons. J Cereb Blood Flow Metab 1996; 16(6): 1137–1142.

82. Cardenas A, Moro MA, Leza JC, et al. Upregulation of TACE/ADAM17 after ischemic preconditioning is involved in brain tolerance. J Cereb Blood Flow Metab 2002; 22(11):1297–1302.

83. Liu J, Ginis I, Spatz M, Hallenbeck JM. Hypoxic preconditioning protects cultured neurons against hypoxic stress via TNF-alpha and ceramide. Am J Physiol Cell Physiol 2000; 278(1):C144–C153.

84. Kariko K, Weissman D, Welsh FA. Inhibition of toll-like receptor and cytokine signaling—a unifying theme in ischemic tolerance. J Cereb Blood Flow Metab 2004; 24(11):1288–1304.

85. Ravati A, Ahlemeyer B, Becker A, et al. Preconditioning-induced neuroprotection is mediated by reactive oxygen species and activation of the transcription factor nuclear factor-κB. J Neurochem 2001; 78:909–919.

86. Pradillo JM, Romera C, Hurtado O, et al. TNFR1 upregulation mediates tolerance after brain ischemic preconditioning. J Cereb Blood Flow Metab 2005; 25(2):193–203.

87. Riksen NP, Smits P, Rongen GA. Ischaemic preconditioning: from molecular characterisation to clinical application—part I. Neth J Med 2004; 62(10):353–363.

88. Bolli R, Shinmura K, Tang XL, et al. Discovery of a new function of cyclooxygenase (COX)-2: COX-2 is a cardioprotective protein that alleviates ischemia/reperfusion injury and mediates the late phase of preconditioning. Cardiovasc Res 2002; 55(3):506–519.

89. Bickler PE, Donohoe PH, Buck LT. Molecular adaptations for survival during anoxia: lessons from lower vertebrates. Neuroscientist 2002; 8(3):234–242.

90. Stenzel-Poore MP, Stevens SL, Xiong Z, et al. Effect of ischaemic preconditioning on genomic response to cerebral ischaemia: similarity to neuroprotective strategies in hibernation and hypoxia-tolerant states. Lancet 2003; 362(9389):1028–1037.

91. Sharp FR, Bernaudin M. HIF1 and oxygen sensing in the brain. Nat Rev Neurosci 2004; 5(6):437–448.

92. Jones NM, Bergeron M. Hypoxic preconditioning induces changes in HIF-1 target genes in neonatal rat brain. J Cereb Blood Flow Metab 2001; 21(9):1105–1114.

93. Bernaudin M, Tang Y, Reilly M, et al. Brain genomic response following hypoxia and re-oxygenation in the neonatal rat. Identification of genes that might contribute to hypoxia-induced ischemic tolerance. J Biol Chem 2002; 277(42):39728–39738.

94. Prass K, Scharff A, Ruscher K, et al. Hypoxia-induced stroke tolerance in the mouse is mediated by erythropoietin. Stroke 2003; 34(8):1981–1986.

95. Liu M, Alkayed NJ. Hypoxic preconditioning and tolerance via hypoxia inducible factor (HIF) 1alpha-linked induction of P450 2C11 epoxygenase in astrocytes. J Cereb Blood Flow Metab 2005; 25:939–948.

96. Alkayed NJ, Goyagi T, Joh HD, et al. Neuroprotection and P450 2C11 upregulation after experimental transient ischemic attack. Stroke 2002; 33(6):1677–1684.

97. Alkayed NJ, Birks EK, Hudetz AG, et al. Inhibition of brain P-450 arachidonic acid epoxygenase decreases baseline cerebral blood flow. Am J Physiol 1996; 271(4 Pt 2):H1541–H1546.

98. Wu S, Chen W, Murphy E, et al. Molecular cloning, expression, and functional significance of a cytochrome P450 highly expressed in rat heart myocytes. J Biol Chem 1997; 272(19):12551–12559.

99. Node K, Huo Y, Ruan X, et al. Anti-inflammatory properties of cytochrome P450 epoxygenase-derived eicosanoids. Science 1999; 285(5431):1276–1279.

100. Yang CW, Ahn HJ, Han HJ, et al. Pharmacological preconditioning with low-dose cyclosporine or FK506 reduces subsequent ischemia/reperfusion injury in rat kidney. Transplantation 2001; 72(11):1753–1759.

101. Kozak W, Kluger MJ, Kozak A, et al. Role of cytochrome P-450 in endogenous antipyresis. Am J Physiol Regul Integr Comp Physiol 2000; 279(2):R455–R460.

102. Lu T, VanRollins M, Lee HC. Stereospecific activation of cardiac ATP-sensitive K(+) channels by epoxyeicosatrienoic acids: a structural determinant study. Mol Pharmacol 2002; 62(5):1076–1083.

30 | Therapeutic Potential of Hypothermia in Acute Stroke

Carmelo Graffagnino, MD, FRCPC, Associate Clinical Professor
Department of Medicine/Neurology, Duke University Medical Center, Durham, North Carolina, USA

INTRODUCTION

Although the brain accounts for only 2% of the body's mass, it utilizes 25% of the body's energy and stores and receives 15% to 20% of the total cardiac output. Given these high demands, it makes intuitive sense that even brief periods of anoxia have dire consequences. Cerebral ischemia can be considered either a focal or global process. Focal ischemia is classically exemplified by the syndrome of acute ischemic stroke, whereas global ischemia is most often the consequence of cardiopulmonary arrest (usually due to a malignant cardiac dysrhythmia). The consequences of focal and global ischemia can be profound, ranging from partial to complete disability or death.

The potential lifesaving effects of hypothermia have been evident since early observations that individuals (particularly children) who became immersed in ice-cold water and drowned were able to be resuscitated with no apparent neurologic injury. Although it was understood that the cold water had life-preserving effects, the mechanisms involved remained largely unknown. Certainly, such early physicians as Hippocrates understood that cold water or ice had tissue-preserving and anti-inflammatory effects; however, their beneficial role in preserving brain tissue took several centuries of medical advancement to be realized.

Induced hypothermia as a modern neurologic therapeutic tool dates to the 1940s, when Dr. Temple Fay first reported cooling 124 patients with severe head injury (1). Ten years later, hypothermia was used as a neuroprotective agent during cardiac surgery that required cardiac arrest, which caused global cerebral ischemia (2). Then, in one of the earliest preclinical reports, it was shown that a drop in brain temperature as little as a 2°C to 5°C resulted in marked protection against global ischemia (3). This finding led to the reintroduction of the concept of therapeutic hypothermia for neuroprotection.

BACKGROUND PATHOPHYSIOLOGY OF ISCHEMIA

Cerebral ischemia results in brain injury at the molecular, cellular, and physiologic levels. The mechanisms are many, including energy failure, release of neurotoxins (e.g., excitatory amino acids), and transmembrane electrolyte abnormalities. Secondary injury can occur with reoxygenation and reperfusion. The mechanism of secondary injury appears to involve oxygen radicals and inflammation pathways. A more complete description of proposed mechanisms of brain injury during ischemia and reperfusion can be found in Chapters 17 and 25.

MECHANISMS OF HYPOTHERMIC NEUROPROTECTION

The most attractive feature of induced hypothermia as a neuroprotective strategy is that its neuroprotective action appears to operate via multiple mechanisms. Hypothermia has been shown to alter metabolic rate (4) by decreasing cellular metabolism, thus retarding high-energy phosphate depletion and facilitating postischemic glucose utilization (5). Hypothermia attenuates the cytotoxic cascade by suppressing elevations of intracellular calcium, thereby inhibiting the release of excitotoxic amino acids and reducing intracellular acidosis (6–9).

Hypothermia suppresses the breakdown of the blood–brain barrier (10,11) and reduces free radical formation (9,12). Mild-to-moderate hypothermia might even protect the injured neurovascular tissues against the toxic effects of recombinant tissue plasminogen activator (rtPA), while still allowing the lytic effect to function (13). Hypothermia also prevents cell injury from leading to apoptosis (14), which is believed to be mediated by inhibition of caspase activation (14–16).

PRECLINICAL WORK WITH GLOBAL ISCHEMIA

Exploration of induced hypothermia as a protective strategy for global ischemia injury started with the application of intraischemic hypothermia. Early work demonstrated that intraischemic brain cooling from 33°C to 34°C markedly reduced brain damage following 20 min of forebrain ischemia in rats (3). Similar findings were reproduced in gerbils (17). It was then demonstrated that global ischemic damage could be reduced by selective brain cooling, even following prolonged (30 min) ischemia (18).

Once intraischemic hypothermia was demonstrated to be neuroprotective, experiments that assessed the effectiveness of postischemic induction of hypothermia followed. It was demonstrated that 3 hr of hypothermia (30°C), begun 5 min following a 10-min period of global forebrain ischemia, could reduce ischemic injury by 50% (19). This effect was apparently lost if cooling was delayed by 30 min following the ischemic insult. Subsequent studies demonstrated that the longer the period of postischemic hypothermia was maintained, the more extensive was the degree of the resulting neuroprotection (20–22).

Although studies that utilized intraischemic hypothermia conferred permanent neuroprotection, other studies suggested that postischemic neuroprotection might be transient and that cell death was not prevented, but delayed (23,24). It was later demonstrated that longer periods of ischemia or delays in initiating treatment required prolonged periods of hypothermia in order to demonstrate permanent and effective neuroprotection. In one study, 2 hr of hypothermia at 34°C protected against 8 min of ischemia, but not 12 (25). In another study, 12 hr of hypothermia initiated 1 hr postischemia protected totally against 3 min, and only partially against 5 min, of global ischemia (26). Extending the period of cooling to 24 hr protected completely (26). Subsequently, it was demonstrated that, even if hypothermia was started at as late as 6 hr postischemia, it could be protective as long as it was extended (27). Forty-eight hours of hypothermia started 6 hr after 10 min of global ischemia significantly reduced neuronal loss in a 28-day survival model (27). Not only was this benefit realized in younger animals, but also postischemic hypothermia (32°C for 24 hr) in older animals could be neuroprotective, even when evaluated at 30 days posttreatment (22).

Together, these preclinical experimental results suggest that the longer the period of ischemia and the greater the latency between the ischemic insult and the onset of therapy, the longer the period of hypothermia required to obtain permanent and effective neuroprotection.

PRECLINICAL WORK WITH FOCAL ISCHEMIA

Although transient global ischemia models well resemble the human condition of postcardiac arrest global ischemia, the same cannot be said for focal ischemia. Focal ischemic stroke in humans is a markedly heterogeneous condition, with similar syndromes being produced by quite different pathophysiologic mechanisms. Vascular occlusion in humans can occur from embolic, as well as locally thrombotic, processes. The location and caliber of the occluded vessels vary considerably, as does the collateral flow within a particular vascular distribution. In addition to the anatomical variables listed above, the duration of vascular occlusion also varies from transient events without permanent injury to complete occlusions with irreversible infarction of the supplied territory. Animal studies that attempt to model ischemic stroke are, for the most part, models of either transient or complete large-vessel occlusions. The most commonly used model is the middle cerebral artery occlusion (MCAO) model, which uses either an intraluminal suture or direct ligation or clipping of the vessel (28). Although other models have been developed, including clot embolization and focal cerebral sclerosis, most of the work reviewed here used MCAO models (28,29). Most of these models produce strokes that resemble human large-vessel infarctions [middle cerebral artery (MCA) strokes]. Outcome variables include histopathology, neurotransmitter levels, and functional assessments based on physiologic testing. These outcomes have been measured early (hours to days) in some studies and late (days to weeks) in others.

As variable as the models are in inducing ischemic injury, the treatment paradigms are equally variable. Some investigators initiated hypothermia prior to, or immediately following, onset of ischemia (30–37), whereas others delayed the treatment by minutes to hours postischemia (32,34,35,38). The delay in treatment onset varied from minutes up to 6 hr. It is, therefore, not surprising that the degree of neuroprotection demonstrated ranges from none to as much as 65% reduction in infarct volume (32,34,35,38). Although short periods of hypothermia could result in transient neuroprotection, it became apparent that, if hypothermia (30°C) was prolonged for up to 24 hr, it could result in sustained neuroprotection, even at 3 weeks (48% reduction in infarct volume) (30). No evidence from animal studies shows that hypothermia can be delayed beyond 1 hr after ischemia in permanent focal ischemia and still be protective (32).

The potential benefits of immediate and delayed hypothermia have been evaluated in transient focal ischemia models more extensively and with more consistent results than in permanent occlusion models. In most studies, the duration of ischemia varied from 30 min to 6 hr, with most using 2 hr. Outcomes have been analyzed immediately and at long-term endpoints (1 to 2 months postinfarct).

Nearly all of the studies that utilized intraischemic hypothermia demonstrated neuroprotection (30–92% reduction in infarct volume) when applied for durations as little as 1 hr and up to 24 hr (36,37,39–47). Hypothermia has also been found to be neuroprotective when applied postischemia, although not to the extent observed when instituted intraischemically (37,40,41,43,46,48–54). Delays of greater than 6 hr have not been shown to be effective in focal ischemia, compared to global ischemia, in which prolonged periods of hypothermia might still be beneficial. In general, the longer the delay from the onset of ischemia to hypothermia, the longer hypothermia needs to be applied in order to be beneficial (37,41,43,45,46,50–54). Although moderate hypothermia (32°C) was generally neuroprotective in most models, deeper cooling (27°C) was not shown to be more effective than moderate hypothermia (no protection, versus 46% reduction in infarct volume) (41).

The current evidence overwhelmingly supports moderate hypothermia (32–34°C) as the temperature of choice for neuroprotection. The duration of cooling chosen then depends on the length of the ischemic period and the time delay to onset of therapy.

HUMAN EXPERIENCE WITH HYPOTHERMIA

Measuring Temperature

Although the target organ for hypothermia is the brain, several other sites that require less invasive measures have been evaluated. Direct brain temperature measurements are possible with the use of a thermistor in a ventriculostomy catheter. However, this is not always possible or desirable; therefore, surrogate sites are frequently utilized. Several studies have compared pulmonary artery, bladder, tympanic membrane, and esophageal temperatures with brain temperature and found them to correlate closely (55–57). Although rectal temperature has been shown to correlate with brain temperature in some studies, it is considered less accurate than other sites.

Induction and Maintenance of Hypothermia in Humans

Cranial Cooling

Local brain cooling would be most desirable for hypothermic neuroprotection. However, the effectiveness of surface cooling has been less than desirable. Surface cranial cooling with ice during advanced cardiac life support has been shown to be ineffective in reducing brain temperature (58). One small study demonstrated the effectiveness of a novel cooling helmet in inducing cooling following cardiac arrest (59). The investigators were able to reduce core temperature to 34°C in a median time of 180 min (0.6°C/hr) following return of spontaneous circulation in patients with cardiac arrest with pulseless electrical activity and asystole.

External Surface Cooling

External surface cooling depends on conductive loss of heat from the skin surface. Various methods can be used, including the direct application of ice, cold water, forced cold air, cold water–containing blanket, or cooled gel–containing surface pads. Cold ice packs can reduce core temperature by 0.9°C/hr (60,61); however, this is a labor-intensive method and can result in damage to the skin with prolonged periods of direct ice-to-skin contact. Cold-air cooling is even slower, at a rate of 0.3°C/hr to 0.5°C/hr (62,63). Cold water–containing blankets have been compared to forced cold-air cooling, and no significant advantages have been found with either method (64).

Intravenous Cold Saline

Iced normal saline infusions have been shown to be effective at rapidly reducing core temperatures (65–69). Healthy volunteers were cooled by 2.5°C within an hour of starting a 30-min infusion of 4°C saline (40 mL/kg) after neuromuscular block with vecuronium and general anesthesia (67). Twenty-two patients who were resuscitated from cardiac arrest were cooled by 1.7°C, with 30 mL/kg of 4°C lactated Ringers solution given over 30 min (65). All of these patients received neuromuscular blocking agents. In a similar study, 2 L of 4°C saline was given over 20 to 30 min following return of spontaneous circulation after cardiac arrest (68), resulting in a mean drop of 1.4°C 30 min after initiation of infusion. This drop in temperature did not affect the left ventricular ejection fraction, vital signs, or coagulation parameters.

Recently, a group that studied the feasibility of inducing hypothermia in a prehospital setting, using an infusion of 30 mL/kg of "ice-cold" Ringer's solution given at a rate of 100 mL/min to comatose patients with out-of-hospital cardiac arrest, was able to reduce core temperature from 35.8°C at onset of infusion to 34°C on arrival to hospital (69). Together, these studies demonstrate that the use if intravenous cold saline is a safe, easy-to-use and effective method of inducing systemic hypothermia.

Endovascular Cooling

It has been shown that a closed-loop endovascular system (70) placed in the inferior vena cava can reduce core body temperature by 0.8°C/hr following return of spontaneous circulation in patients with ventricular fibrillation (VF) (71). Similarly, the feasibility of inducing and maintaining moderate hypothermia with the use of endovascular cooling was studied (72). Six patients with severe acute ischemic stroke were treated with moderate hypothermia. Researchers were able to cool patients at a rate of 1.4°C/hr and reached target temperature after 3 hr (range, 2–4.5 hr). None of the patients experienced significant complications in either of these studies.

Extracorporeal Cooling

Extracorporeal cooling is, by far, the most invasive of the methods listed. Rapid core cooling using an extracorporeal heat exchanger has been reported in a small study in which 8 patients were cooled to 32°C within a mean time of 113 min (73).

HUMAN CLINICAL TRIALS WITH HYPOTHERMIA FOR GLOBAL ISCHEMIA (CARDIAC ARREST)

Although initial pilot studies of hypothermia following cardiac arrest showed great promise (61,74–76), two larger, randomized, controlled studies proved the effectiveness of moderate hypothermia for anoxic encephalopathy (60,62). Both of the trials assessed the effectiveness of hypothermia following ventricular tachycardia (VT) or VF. One study randomized 77 patients (43 to hypothermia and 34 to normothermia) (60). The hypothermia group was cooled to 33°C for 12 hr, starting in the ambulance on the way to hospital. At the time of discharge from the hospital, 21 of the 43 (49%) hypothermia-treated patients had a good outcome, compared to 9 of the 34 (26%) in the control group ($p=0.46$). The other study, the Hypothermia After Cardiac Arrest (HACA) study, randomized 273 patients (136 to hypothermia and 137 to normothermia) (62). The hypothermia group was cooled to 33°C for 24 hr. Outcomes were based on 6-month follow-up. Good outcomes were seen in 55% of the hypothermia-treated patients, compared to 39% of the normothermia controls. Although both of these studies limited entry to patients with VT/VF, hypothermia has also been shown to be effective in other cardiac rhythms (asystole) (77).

HUMAN CLINICAL TRIALS WITH HYPOTHERMIA FOR FOCAL ISCHEMIA

Although promising, the experience with hypothermia for the treatment of acute ischemic stroke is less clearly defined than for cardiac arrest. Several small feasibility studies have been published that show that induction and maintenance of hypothermia is possible and might even improve outcome following focal ischemic stroke.

The Copenhagen stroke study (78) was a case control that prospectively included 17 patients who presented with stroke within 12 hr of symptom onset. These patients were cooled with an air-forced cooling blanket for 6 hr. Meperidine was used to suppress shivering. Study patients were compared to 56 historical controls. Core body temperature was decreased from 36.8°C to 35.5°C and was maintained until 4 hr after therapy was discontinued. Although the 6-mo mortality was 12% in cases versus 23% in controls, no significant difference in the Scandinavian stroke scale score was seen at 6 months between groups (78).

Hypothermia has been shown to reduce cerebral edema in the setting of malignant ischemic strokes (79–81). However, hypothermia was not as effective at preventing death as hemicraniectomy (82). Authors randomized 36 patients with severe acute ischemic strokes to either hemicraniectomy ($n=17$) or moderate hypothermia ($n=19$). The hypothermia group had a significantly higher mortality than the hemicraniectomy group (47% vs. 12%, respectively). Although hypothermia has been shown to control intracranial pressure (ICP) in most studies of malignant MCA stroke (79–81), frequently, the result continues to be death, often due to rebound ICP during rewarming. If the rewarming rate is controlled, the rate of rebound ICP can be reduced (83).

The safety of inducing hypothermia following thrombolytic therapy for ischemic stroke was assessed in a small pilot study (84). Ten patients who presented with symptoms of MCA stroke and NIHSS scores of 15 within 6 hr of onset were cooled to 32°C for a period of 12 to 72 hr, depending on vessel patency. Hypothermia was induced using topical cooling blankets. Nine concurrent control patients were chosen for comparison. Three of the hypothermia patients died. The surviving patients had a mean modified Rankin score at 3 months of 3.1±2.3. In this small group of patients, hypothermia was tolerated well and appeared safe in the setting of thrombolysis. Preclinical and small clinical studies have suggested that hypothermia might be protective when added to thrombolytic therapy (84–86).

Intravascular, induced hypothermia for ischemic stroke was first reported in 6 patients with severe acute ischemic stroke who were treated with moderate hypothermia (72). The rate of cooling using this technology was 1.4±0.6°C/hr, and target temperature was reached after 3±1 hr (range, 2–4.5 hr). Singultus was the only device-related complication encountered. Pulmonary infection, arterial hypotension, bradycardia, arrhythmia, and thrombocytopenia were the most common side effects (72).

Controlled Randomized Studies

The largest study to utilize intravascular cooling methods was conducted at the Cleveland Clinic, where 40 patients were randomized to receive either hypothermia at 33°C for 24 hr or best medical care (87). Eighteen patients were cooled. All had MRI scans at 3 to 5 days and 30 to 37 days. At the end of the study, no differences in clinical outcomes between groups were reported. MRI lesion sizes were also similar between groups.

Complications of Hypothermia

Arrhythmias
Although ventricular ectopy can occur in the setting of induced mild to moderate hypothermia, VF is very rare. Even in the setting in which patients present with VT/VF, therapeutic hypothermia is very rare, as seen in the HACA study (62). Bradycardia is the most common arrhythmia seen at temperatures from 32°C to 36.5°C (62).

Electrolyte Abnormalities

The most common ??complication of inducing hypothermia?? is transient hypokalemia. Caution must be noted, as hypokalemia is mostly due to intracellular shift of K and overcorrection might result in life-threatening rebound hyperkalemia during rewarming (88).

Immune System

Hypothermia can suppress the immune system, including T-cell–mediated antibody production (89,90), predisposing patients to infection. It was reported that 7 of 25 stroke patients who underwent hypothermia suffered a septic syndrome (80). In contradistinction to this report, the HACA investigators did not find a significant difference in infections between the control and hypothermia-treated groups (62).

Coagulopathy

Hypothermia can cause coagulation abnormalities, including prolongation of bleeding time and inhibition of the enzymatic reactions of the coagulation cascade (91–93).

CONCLUSIONS AND FUTURE DIRECTIONS

After investment of millions of dollars and treatment of thousands of patients, a neuroprotective pharmaceutical agent has yet to be developed for use in patients with ischemic brain damage, whether it be from a global cause, such as cardiac arrest, or from a focal injury, such as acute vascular occlusion. Most of the agents that have been tested thus far have targeted single mechanisms in the pathophysiologic process that leads to cell death following ischemia. Hypothermia, on the other hand, exerts its influence via multiple mechanisms, and preclinical studies have shown that it is, by far, the most effective neuroprotective strategy currently available. The challenge for clinicians is to translate this strategy into an effective form of therapy for human cerebral ischemia. We have come a long way toward that goal. Randomized, controlled studies have proven that induced moderate hypothermia can reduce cerebral ischemic injury following global ischemia. The next step is to learn how to apply this "old friend" in the management of acute ischemic stroke.

REFERENCES

1. Fay T. Observation on generalized refrigeration in cases of severe cerebral trauma. Assoc Res Nerv Ment Dis Proc 1943; 24:611–619.
2. Bigelow W, Lindsay W, Greenwood W. Hypothermia; its possible role in cardiac surgery: an investigation of factors governing survival in dogs at low body temperatures. Ann Surg 1950; 132:849–866.
3. Busto R, Dietrich W, Globus M-T, Valdes I, Scheingerg P, Ginsberg M. Small differences in intraischemic brain temperature critically determine the extent of ischemic neuronal injury. J Cereb Blood Flow Metab 1987; 7:729–738.
4. Chopp M, Knight R, Tidwell C, Helpern J, Brown E, Welch K. The metabolic effects of mild hypothermia on global cerebral ischemia and recirculation in the cat: comparison to normothermia and hypothermia. J Cereb Blood Flow Metab 1989; 9:141–148.
5. Lanier W. Cerebral metabolic rate and hypothermia: their relationship with ischemic neurologic injury. J Neurosurg Anesthesiol 1995; 7:216–221.
6. Busto R, Globus M, Dietrich D, et al. Effect of mild hypothermia on ischemia induced release of neurotransmitters and free fatty acids in rat brain. Stroke 1989; 20:904–910.
7. Nakashima K, Todd M. Effects of hypothermia on the rate of excitatory amino acid release after ischemic depolarization. Stroke 1996; 27:913–918.
8. Globus M, Busto R, Dietrich W, Martinez E. Intra-ischemic extracellular release of dopamine and glutamate is associated with striatal vulnerability to ischemia. Neurosci Lett 1988; 91:36–40.
9. Globus M, Alonson O, Dietrich D, Busto R, Ginsberg M. Glutamate release and free radical production following brain injury: effects of post-traumatic hypothermia. J Neurochem 1995; 65:1250–1256.
10. Smith S, Hall E. Mild pre- and posttraumatic hypothermia attenuates blood–brain barrier damage following controlled cortical impact injury in the rat. J Neurotrauma 1996; 13(1):1–9.
11. Ishikawa M, Sekizuka E, Sato S, et al. Effects of moderate hypothermia on leukocyte-endothelium interaction in the rat pial microvasculature after transient middle cerebral artery occlusion. Stroke 1999; 30:1679–1686.

12. Globus M, Busto R, Lin B, Schnippering H, Ginsberg M. Detection of free radical activity during transient global ischemia and recirculation: effects of intraischemic brain temperature modulation. J Neurochem 1995; 65:1250–1256.

13. Yenari M, Palmer J, Bracci P, Steinberg G. Thrombolysis with tissue plasminogen activator (tPA) is temperature dependent. Thromb Res 1995; 77:475–481.

14. Xu L, Yenari M, Steinberg G, Giffard R. Mild hypothermia reduces apoptosis of mouse neurons in vitro early in the cascade. J Cereb Blood Flow Metab 2002; 22:21–28.

15. Povlishock J, Buki A, Koiziumi H, Stone J, Okonkwo D. Initiating mechanisms involved in the pathophysiology of traumatically induced axonal injury and interventions targeted at blunting their progression. Acta Neurochir Suppl (Wien) 1999; 73:15–20.

16. Ning X, Chen S, Xu C, et al. Hypothermic protection of the ischemic heart via alterations in apoptotic pathways as assessed by gene array analysis. J Appl Physiol 2002; 92:2200–2207.

17. Clifton G, Taft W, Blair R, Choi S, DeLorenzo R. Conditions for pharmacologic evaluation in the gerbil model of forebrain ischemia. Stroke 1989; 20:1545–1552.

18. Kuluz J, Gregory G, Yu A, Chang Y. Selective brain cooling during and after prolonged global ischemia reduces cortical damage in rats. Stroke 1992; 23:1792–1796.

19. Busto R, Dietrich D, Globus M, Ginsberg M. Postischemic moderate hypothermia inhibits CA1 hippocampal ischemic neuronal injury. Neurosci Lett 1989; 101:299–304.

20. Carroll M, Beek O. Protection against hippocampal CA1 cell loss by post-ischemic hypothermia is dependent on delay of initiation and duration. Metab Brain Dis 1992; 7:45–50.

21. Coimbra C, Wieloch T. Moderate hypothermia mitigates neuronal damage in the rat brain when initiated several hours following transient cerebral ischemia. Acta Neuropathol 1994; 87:325–331.

22. Corbett D, Nurse S, Colbourne F. Hypothermic neuroprotection; a global ischemia study using 18- to 20-month old gerbils. Stroke 1997; 28:2238–2243.

23. Welsh F, Harris V. Postischemic hypothermia fails to reduce ischemic injury in gerbil hippocampus. J Cereb Blood Flow Metab 1991; 11:617–620.

24. Dietrich W, Busto R, Alonso O, Globus M, Ginsberg M. Intraischemic but not postischemic brain hypothermia protects chronically following global forebrain ischemia in rats. J Cereb Blood Flow Metab 1993; 13:541–549.

25. Chopp M, Chen H, Dereski M, Garcia JH. Mild hypothermic intervention after graded ischemic stress in rats. Stroke 1991; 22(1):37–43.

26. Colbourne F, Corbett D. Delayed and prolonged post-ischemic hypothermia is neuroprotective in the gerbil. Brain Res 1994; 654:265–272.

27. Colbourne F, Hui L, Buchan A. Indefatigable CA1 sector neuroprotection with mild hypothermia induced six hours after severe forebrain ischemia in rats. J Cereb Blood Flow Metab 1999; 19:742–749.

28. Ginsberg M, Busto R. Rodent models of cerebral ischemia. Stroke 1989; 20:1627–1642.

29. McAuley M. Rodent models of focal ischemia. Cerebrovasc Brain Metab Rev 1995; 7:153–180.

30. Yanamoto H, Nagata I, Niitsu Y, et al. Prolonged mild hypothermia therapy protects the brain against permanent focal ischemia. Stroke 2001; 32:232–239.

31. Baker C, Onesti S, Barth K, Prestigiacomo C, Solomon R. Hypothermic protection following middle cerebral artery occlusion in the rat. Surg Neurol 1991; 36:175–180.

32. Baker C, Onesti S, Solomon R. Reduction by delayed hypothermia of cerebral infarction following middle cerebral artery occlusion in the rat: a time-course study. J Neurosurgery 1992; 77:438–444.

33. Onesti S, Baker C, Sun P, Solomon R. Transient hypothermia reduces focal ischemic brain injury in the rat. Neurosurgery 1991; 29:369–373.

34. Kader A, Brisman MH, Maraire N, Huh J-T, Solomon RA. The effect of mild hypothermia on permanent focal ischemia in the rat. Neurosurgery 1992; 31(6):1056–1061.

35. Moyer D, Welsh F, Zager E. Spontaneous cerebral hypothermia diminishes focal infarction in rat brain. Stroke 1992; 23:1812–1816.

36. Ridenour T, Warner D, Todd M, McAllister A. Mild hypothermia reduces infarct size resulting from temporary but not permanent focal ischemia in rats. Stroke 1992; 23:733–738.

37. Xue D, Huang Z, Smith K, Buchan A. Immediate or delayed mild hypothermia prevents focal cerebral infarction. Brain Res 1992; 587:66–72.

38. Doerfler A, Schwab S, Hoffmann T, Engelhorn T, Forsting M. Combination of decompressive craniectomy and mild hypothermia ameliorates infarction volume after permanent focal ischemia in rats. Stroke 2001; 32:2675–2681.

39. Chen H, Chopp M, Zhang Z, Garcia J. The effect of hypothermia on transient middle cerebral artery occlusion in the rat. J Cereb Blood Flow Metab 1992; 12:621–628.

40. Karibe H, Chen H, Zarow G, Graham S, Weinstein P. Delayed induction of mild hypothermia to reduce infarct volume after temporary middle cerebral artery occlusion in rats. J Neurosurgery 1994; 80:112–119.

41. Huh P, Belayev L, Zhao W, Koch S, Busto R, Ginsberg M. Comparative neuroprotective efficacy of prolonged intraischemic and postischemic hypothermia in focal cerebral ischemia. J Neurosurgery 2000; 92:91–99.

42. Maier C, Ahern K, Cheng M, Lee J, Yenari M, Steinberg G. Optimal depth and duration of mild hypothermia in a focal model of transient cerebral ischemia: effects on neurologic outcome, infarct size, apoptosis, and inflammation. Stroke 1998; 29:2171–2180.

43. Maier C, Sun G, Kunis D, Yenari M, Steinberg G. Delayed induction and long-term effects of mild hypothermia in focal model of transient cerebral ischemia: neurological outcome and infarct size. J Neurosurgery 2001; 94:90–96.

44. Morikawa E, Ginsberg M, Dietrich W, et al. The significance of brain temperature in focal cerebral ischemia: histopathological consequences of middle cerebral artery occlusion in the rat. J Cereb Blood Flow Metab 1992; 12:380–389.

45. Schmid-Elsaesser R, Hungerhuber E, Zausinger S, Baethmann A, Reulen HJ. Combination drug therapy and mild hypothermia: a promising treatment strategy for reversible, focal cerebral ischemia. Stroke 1999; 30:1891–1899.

46. Yanamoto H, Nagata I, Nakahara I, Tohnai N, Zhang Z, Kikuchi H. Combination of intraischemic and postischemic hypothermia provides potent and persistent neuroprotection against temporary focal ischemia in rats. Stroke 1999; 30(12):2720–2726.

47. Zausinger S, Hungerbuber E, Baethmann A, Reulen H, Schmid-Elsaesser R. Neurological impairment in rats after transient middle cerebral artery occlusion: a comparative study under various treatment paradigms. Brain Res 2000; 863:94–105.

48. Kawai N, Okauchi M, Morisaki K, Nagao S. Effects of delayed intraischemic and postischemic hypothermia on a focal model of transient cerebral ischemia in rats. Stroke 2000; 31:1982–1989.

49. Kollmar R, Schabitz W, Heiland S, et al. Neuroprotective effect of delayed moderate hypothermia after focal cerebral ischemia: an MRI study. Stroke 2002; 33:1891–1904.

50. Colbourne F, Corbett D, Zhao Z, Yang J, Buchan A. Prolonged but delayed postischemic hypothermia: a long-term outcome study in the rat middle cerebral artery occlusion model. J Cereb Blood Flow Metab 2000; 20:1702–1708.

51. Corbett D, Hamilton M, Colbourne F. Persistent neuroprotection with prolonged postischemic hypothermia in adult rats subjected to transient middle cerebral artery occlusion. Exp Neurol 2000; 163:200–206.

52. Yanamoto H, Hong S, Soleau S, Kassell N, Lee K. Mild postischemic hypothermia limits cerebral injury following transient focal ischemia in rat neocortex. Brain Res 1996; 718(1–2):207–211.

53. Zhang R-L, Chopp M, Chen H, Garcia JH, Zhang ZG. Postischemic (1 hour) hypothermia significantly reduces ischemic cell damage in rats subjected to 2 hours of middle cerebral artery occlusion. Stroke 1993; 24:1235–1240.

54. Zhang Z, Chopp M, Chen H. Duration dependent post-ischemic hypothermia alleviates cortical damage after middle cerebral artery occlusion in the rat. J Neurol Sci 1993; 117:240–244.

55. Veerloy J, Heytens L, Veeckmans G, et al. Intracerebral temperature monitoring in severely head injured patients. Acta Neurochir (Wien) 1995; 134:76–78.

56. Henker R, Brown D, Marion M. Comparison of brain temperature with core (rectal and bladder) temperatures in head injured adults. Crit Care Med 1997; 25:A73.

57. Stone J, Goodman R, Baker K, Baker C, Solomon R. Direct intraoperative measurement of human brain temperature. Neurosurgery 1977; 41:20–24.

58. Callaway C, Tadler S, Katz L, Lipinski C, Brader E. Feasibility of external cranial cooling during out-of-hospital cardiac arrest. Resuscitation 2002; 52:159–165.

59. Hachimi-Idrissi S, Corne L, Ebinger G, Michotte Y, Huyghens L. Mild hypothermia induced by a helmet device: a clinical feasibility study. Resuscitation 2001; 51:275–281.

60. Bernard S, Gray T, Buist M, et al. Treatment of comatose survivors of out-of-hospital cardiac arrest with induced hypothermia. N Engl J Med 2002; 346:557–563.

61. Bernard S, Jones B, Horne M. Clinical trial of induced hypothermia in comatose survivors of out-of-hospital cardiac arrest. Ann Emerg Med 1997; 30:146–153.

62. The Hypothermia After Cardiac Arrest Study Group. Mild therapeutic hypothermia to improve the neurologic outcome after cardiac arrest. N Engl J Med 2002; 346:549–556.

63. Felberg R, Krieger D, Chuang R, et al. Hypothermia after cardiac arrest: feasibility and safety of an external cooling protocol. Circulation 2001; 104:1799–1804.

64. Theard M, Temelhoff R, et al. Convection versus conduction cooling for induction of mild hypothermia during neurovascular procedures in adults. J Neurosurg Anesthesiol 1997; 9:250–255.

65. Bernard S, Buist M, Monteiro O, Smith K. Induced hypothermia using large volume, ice-cold intravenous fluid in comatose survivors of out-of-hospital cardiac arrest: a preliminary report. Resuscitation 2003; 56:9–13.

65. Rijnsburger E, Girbes A, Spijkstra J, et al. Induction of hypothermia using large volumes of ice-cold intravenous fluid: A feasibility study [abstr]. Intensive Care Med 2004; 30 (suppl 1):S143.

67. Rajek A, Greif R, Sessler D, et al. Core cooling by central venous infusion of ice-cold (4 degrees and 20 degrees C) fluid: Isolation of core and peripheral thermal compartments. Anesthesiology 2000; 93:629–637.

High-Risk Group for Herniation

Gaze deviation, hemiplegia, and neglect (NIHSS >15 right hemisphere)

OR

Hemiplegia and global aphasia (NIHSS >20 left hemisphere) consistent with a total anterior circulation syndrome

AND

one of the following:

1. Nausea or vomiting

   OR

2. Early CT > 50% MCA territory hypodensity ± ACA or PCA territory hypodensity

   OR

3. DWI evidence of > 82 mL infarction

   OR

4. Carotid "T" occlusion by MRA, CTA, or conventional angiography

Consider the following algorithm with early repeat CT or MRI imaging.

Proposed Hemicraniectomy Management Algorithm

1. If high-risk group, repeat CT scan within 6–12 hr of initial evaluation.

   If follow-up CT evidence of complete MCA or MCA+ACA/PCA infarction or DWI > 145 mL, consider hemicraniectomy with durotomy/duroplasty.

2. If not, repeat CT scan again in 6–12 hr; if new anisocoria or any decreasing level of consciousness (LOC), repeat CT scan.

   If CT scan reveals midline shift (anteroseptal shift ≥ 5 mm), consider hemicraniectomy with durotomy/duroplasty.

Figure 1 Algorithm for management of high-risk patients with large hemispheric infarctions.

Hemicraniectomy involves removal of bone on one side of the skull and simultaneously performing a generous dural opening. The minimal adequate decompression is defined by the following bony boundaries (Fig. 2):

1) anterior, frontal to midpupillary line
2) posterior, approximately 4 cm to the external auditory canal
3) superior, to the superior sagittal sinus
4) inferior, to the floor of the middle cranial fossa

Bone removed during a hemicraniectomy can be saved in the peritoneum or in a bone bank in antibiotic solution at −80°C. Bone is replaced after the swelling has subsided in one to three months. Cruciate or circumferential durotomy must be performed over the entire region of bony decompression to insure that nothing resists the expanding brain from being able to herniate outward. Dural grafting is recommended. No brain amputation or ventriculostomy is required or necessary. This complete procedure achieves a new pathway of least resistance for the swelling brain ipsilateral to the lesion and causes less compression of the vital brain structures not otherwise involved in the primary disease process (such as the brain stem). The brain acts as a sphere rather than a cylinder when herniating through the decompression opening (Fig. 3). The size of the bone flap determines the magnitude of decompression achieved and significantly increases when the diameter exceeds 12 cm. Small bone flaps do not achieve the desired decompression needed.

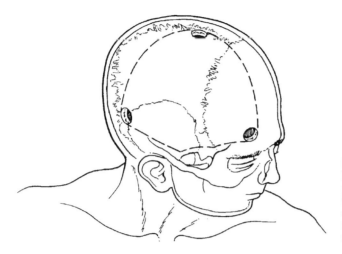

Figure 2 Surgical sketch of the bony boundaries recommended in an ongoing prospective, randomized, controlled trial for hemicraniectomy in massive hemispheric stroke. *Source*: Courtesy of Douglas Chyette, MD, Cleveland Clinic Foundation, Cleveland, Ohio.

KEY ISSUES TO ADDRESS PRIOR TO HEMICRANIECTOMY

Evidence that hemicraniectomy reduces mortality is largely derived from uncontrolled case series and retrospective studies. Early animal studies revealed that trephination surgery, a form of hemicraniectomy in rats, reduces the seven-day mortality from 35% in the nonsurgical group to almost 0% in the surgical group (15,16). Neurologic behavior and infarct volume were favorable in those treated with ultra-early surgery within four hours of occlusion, confirming the importance of early intervention. Compared to control groups, hemicraniectomy in rats increases perfusion in the cortex and reduces the infarct volume, as shown by MRI (17).

Hemicraniectomy can also be combined with other techniques that can synergistically help to reduce brain edema. Comparison of moderate hypothermia to hemicraniectomy in massive cerebral infarctions reveals that hemicraniectomy is, in fact, better, with no difference in intensive medical treatment or duration of stay in the neurologic intensive care unit. In one retrospective study, the mortality rate was 47% for the hypothermia group versus 12% for the hemicraniectomy group (18). In a case series that combined hemicraniectomy with resection of infarcted tissue, 10 of 12 patients who underwent the procedure survived, 5 had independent or moderate disability, and 5 were left with severe disability. The mortality rate was 16%, but the disability rate was high at 41%, compared to other published case reports (19). Table 1 contains a review of all of the current hemicraniectomy trials.

A number of issues arise when one considers hemicraniectomy for massive cerebral infarctions, as discussed below.

Hemicraniectomy Following Large Hemispheric Infarctions

Hemicraniectomy is usually considered when unequivocal clinical and radiological signs suggest impending brain edema and when all other medical measures have failed. Common predictors of brain edema following large hemispheric infarction include young age, nausea and vomiting in the first 24 hours of admission, NIHSS of ≥15 for right hemisphere MCA infarction and ≥20 for left hemisphere MCA infarction, early hypodensity on CT scan, midline shift of more than 10 mm at the septum pellucidum level, and early hypodensity that involves more than 50% of the MCA territory (6). Some authors advocate repeating CT scan within 6 to 12 hours for those at high risk for brain edema (4). Evidence of anteroseptal shift ≥5 mm on follow-up CT is strongly associated with fatal outcome and might act as an important warning sign of further shift to come (8). Early hemicraniectomy should be considered before brain herniation and irreparable brain damage occurs. Women with malignant MCA infarction had worse outcomes than men in one retrospective study (20). The presence of vascular territory involvement beyond the MCA territory also serves as a marker of progression (8). Anterior choroidal artery infarction involving the uncus and hippocampal head can predispose to a greater degree of herniation and secondary brain stem compression. MRI offers advantages in detecting malignant MCA

(A)   **(B)**

(C)   **(D)**

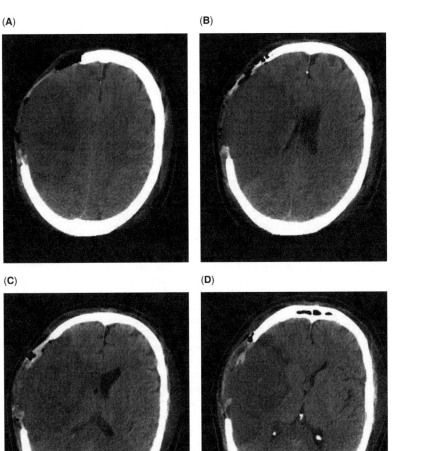

Figure 3 Decompressive hemicraniectomy and duraplasty in a 44-year-old male following carotid dissection from motor vehicle accident. The ischemic/infarcted brain tissue in the right hemisphere has room for herniation outward and prevents downward displacement of vital structure.

infarction by allowing assessment of volumes of diffusion-weighted and perfusion-weighted abnormality. A diffusion-weighted imaging abnormality of median volume >145 mL 14 hours from onset was associated with a malignant course, with 100% sensitivity and 94% specificity (21). An apparent diffusion coefficient <80%, involving greater than 82 mL of brain tissue less than 6 hours from onset had similar high sensitivity and specificity for malignant course (22). Serum markers, such as S100B, have also been shown to predict a malignant course of MCA infarction (23). Unfortunately, no single parameter can signal that malignant MCA infarction will definitely occur. A combination of clinical and imaging prognostic factors should be present before hemicraniectomy is contemplated.

The Impact of Age on Hemicraniectomy Outcome
The impact of age on outcome has been poorly studied in patients with large hemispheric infarctions. Case reports have clearly shown that older patients who undergo hemicraniectomy have poor functional outcomes and increased mortality (24–27), perhaps because older patients have other comorbid conditions. In one recent study, age >60, severe neurologic deficit on admission, longer duration of intensive care treatment, and mechanical ventilation were significantly associated with more severe disability (Barthel Index <50) (28). Health-related quality of life was considerably impaired in the subscales of mobility, household management, and

Table 1 Clinical Trials of Hemicraniectomy in Stroke

Trial	Status	Design	Results
DESTINY (Decompressive Surgery for Treatment of Malignant Infarction of the Middle Cerebral Artery)	Ongoing	68 patients, 9 centers. Prospective, randomized, open, controlled, multicentered study: To compare the efficacy of conservative treatment alone to decompressive surgery+conservative treatment after malignant hemispheric ischemic cerebral infarction. Patients randomized between 12 and 36 hr of onset of deterioration symptoms; treatment/surgery within 6 hr of randomization	Not available
HAMLET (Hemicraniectomy After MCA Infarction with Life-Threatening Edema Trial)	Ongoing	112 patients, 7 centers. Open, randomized, multicentered clinical trial: Patients randomized to either decompressive surgery (consisting of large hemicraniectomy and duroplasty, followed by intensive care treatment) or conservative treatment (consisting of either intensive care treatment or "standard" therapy on a stroke unit). Randomization stratified according to the intended mode of conservative treatment	Not available
HeaDDFIRST (Hemicraniectomy and Durotomy for Deterioration from Infarction-Related Swelling Trial)	Completed	Multicentered pilot clinical trial with a planned enrollment of 75 patients: All patients receive standardized medical therapy (SMT). Patients who develop severe brain swelling within 96 hr of stroke onset are randomized to receive SMT alone or SMT+standardized hemicraniectomy and durotomy	Not available
Hemicraniectomy and moderate hypothermia in patients with severe ischemic stroke	Completed	Retrospective study comparing moderate hypothermia to hemicraniectomy ($n=36$)	Mortality was 12% for hemicraniectomy group versus 47% for hypothermia group
HeMMI (Hemicraniectomy for Malignant Middle Cerebral Artery Infarctions)	Ongoing	56 patients. Open, randomized clinical trial: Patients randomized to receive either standard medical treatment or hemicraniectomy with duroplasty within 72 hr from symptom onset	Not available

body care. Some authors strongly recommend hemicraniectomy for younger patients (age <45) on the assumption that, given fewer comorbid conditions, they are better able to tolerate brain edema and have better functional outcomes. However, some critics argue that this could be a result of selection bias. A study of the natural history of 42 patients found the mortality rate to be 28% in patients <45 years of age, compared to 90% in those >45 years of age (29). Analysis of pooled data from case reports and retrospective studies supports this observation (30); 14% of patients <50 years of age died following surgery, compared to 32% of those >50 years of age. At the same time, younger patients have less room for expansion due to absence of age-related atrophy, and this could increase the risk of herniation and death. Thus, age might be a crucial factor in determining which patients should undergo hemicraniectomy.

Timing of Hemicraniectomy

Animal and clinical studies have provided evidence for benefit from early surgery. In animal MCA occlusion models, early hemicraniectomy at one hour versus 24 hours reduced infarct volume significantly (15). A 1998 analysis of the influence on functional outcome and mortality of early hemicraniectomy (<24 hours after symptom onset) versus late surgery (>24 hours after first reversible signs of herniation), based on clinical status at admission and initial CT findings showed that, out of 31 patients who underwent early hemicraniectomy, mortality was 16%, and 84% had a Barthel index >60 at 3-month follow-up (31). Early hemicraniectomy led to a significant reduction in ICU admission (7.4 vs. 13.3 days, $p < 0.05$). On the other hand, late intervention has been shown to affect neither outcome nor recovery. Early decompressive surgery should be performed to prevent irreversible damage to adjacent brain tissues. Several other case reports and retrospective studies have revealed the same results (24,26). Analysis of pooled published reports suggests that signs of herniation have no impact on the timing of surgery and outcomes (30). Randomized, controlled trials are necessary to determine the optimal timing for hemicraniectomy. Current ongoing clinical trials randomize patients who present between 12 and 96 hours from symptom onset (Table 1).

Hemicraniectomy and Large Dominant-Hemisphere Infarctions

Performing hemicraniectomy in patients who have suffered large dominant-hemisphere infarctions is highly controversial. The benefit of hemicraniectomy in dominant-hemisphere infarctions appears less convincing due to the mistaken perception that the procedure might leave patients with severe aphasia and poor quality of life. Functional MRI studies have demonstrated that most functional recovery from aphasia is due to cortical reorganization of the unaffected (right) hemisphere. A significant shift of activation areas into homologous areas of the right hemisphere is seen (32,33). However, conflicting evidence suggests that functionally important cortical reorganization occurs in adjacent areas of normal brain tissue that surrounds language areas (32,34), which might explain the somewhat surprising degree of clinical recovery reported in subsets of patients with dominant-hemisphere infarctions who undergo hemicraniectomy. One study reported mild-to-moderate aphasia outcomes in dominant-hemisphere hemicraniectomy if performed early (31). Another group retrospectively studied 14 patients who were admitted with dominant-hemisphere infarction and were subsequently treated with hemicraniectomy; 13 had significant improvement in communication ability. Younger age group and early decompressive hemicraniectomy were identified as main predictors for recovery from aphasia (35). Thus, it can be argued that younger patients with dominant-hemisphere infarction might be offered early hemicraniectomy, as their natural history favors a trend toward improved mortality and better recovery. We should not underestimate the extent of functional recovery possible via cortical reorganization to the unaffected nondominant hemisphere.

CONCLUSION

Hemicraniectomy is a life-saving procedure in patients with massive cerebral infarctions. At this time, it is not very clear which age group of patients have a better functional outcome. Younger patients with massive cerebral infarctions should be monitored carefully for brain edema and strongly considered for hemicraniectomy. We require a better understanding of the pathophysiology of massive cerebral infarctions in this group of patients.

No therapy has been proven optimal for massive cerebral infarctions. It is difficult to form a coherent inference from case series and retrospective studies because selection bias prevents valid conclusions. The key pathophysiologic concept is that focal increases in ICP are different from global increases. Although surgical decompressive craniectomy can save lives and appears more promising than moderate hypothermia, it remains unclear whether these management strategies are appropriate, given the expected severe disability. Quality-of-life and social-disability measures might be the most important outcomes for future randomized clinical trials. Finally, randomized trials are difficult to execute for both strategies because massive cerebral infarction occurs relatively rarely and expertise in its treatment, with either hypothermia or surgical management, is in the development stage.

REFERENCES

1. Hacke W, Schwab S, Horn M, et al. "Malignant" middle cerebral artery territory infarction: clinical course and prognostic signs. Arch Neurol 1996; 53(4):309–315.
2. Rothwell PM, Coull AJ, Giles MF, et al. Change in stroke incidence, mortality, case-fatality, severity, and risk factors in Oxfordshire, U.K. from 1981 to 2004 (Oxford Vascular Study). Lancet 2004; 363(9425):1925–1933.

3. Frank JI. Large hemispheric infarction, deterioration, and intracranial pressure. Neurology 1995; 45(7):1286–1290.

4. Demchuk AM, Krieger DW. Mass effect with cerebral infarction. Curr Treat Options Neurol 1999; 1(3):189–199.

5. Kasner SE, Demchuk AM, Berrouschot J, et al. Predictors of fatal brain edema in massive hemispheric ischemic stroke. Stroke 2001; 32(9):2117–2123.

6. Krieger DW, Demchuk AM, Kasner SE, et al. Early clinical and radiological predictors of fatal brain swelling in ischemic stroke. Stroke 1999; 30(2):287–292.

7. von Kummer R, Meyding-Lamade U, Forsting M, et al. Sensitivity and prognostic value of early CT in occlusion of the middle cerebral artery trunk. AJNR Am J Neuroradiol 1994; 15(1):9–15; discussion 16–18.

8. Barber PA, Demchuk AM, Zhang J, et al. Computed tomographic parameters predicting fatal outcome in large middle cerebral artery infarction. Cerebrovasc Dis 2003; 16(3):230–235.

9. Ropper AH. Lateral displacement of the brain and level of consciousness in patients with an acute hemispheral mass. N Engl J Med 1986; 314(15):953–958.

10. von Kummer R, Allen KL, Holle R, et al. Acute stroke: usefulness of early CT findings before thrombolytic therapy. Radiology 1997; 205(2):327–333.

11. Berrouschot J, Barthel H, von Kummer R, et al. 99m technetium-ethyl-cysteinate-dimer single-photon emission CT can predict fatal ischemic brain edema. Stroke 1998; 29(12):2556–2562.

12. Firlik AD, Kaufmann AM, Wechsler LR, et al. Quantitative cerebral blood flow determinations in acute ischemic stroke. Relationship to computed tomography and angiography. Stroke 1997; 28(11):2208–2213.

13. Kucinski T, Koch C, Grzyska U, et al. The predictive value of early CT and angiography for fatal hemispheric swelling in acute stroke. AJNR Am J Neuroradiol 1998; 19(5):839–846.

14. Ransohoff J, Benjamin V. Hemicraniectomy in the treatment of acute subdural haematoma. J Neurol Neurosurg Psychiatry 1971; 34(1):106.

15. Forsting M, Reith W, Schabitz WR, et al. Decompressive craniectomy for cerebral infarction. An experimental study in rats. Stroke 1995; 26(2):259–264.

16. Doerfler A, Forsting M, Reith W, et al. Decompressive craniectomy in a rat model of "malignant" cerebral hemispheric stroke: experimental support for an aggressive therapeutic approach. J Neurosurg 1996; 85(5):853–859.

17. Engelhorn T, von Kummer R, Reith W, et al. What is effective in malignant middle cerebral artery infarction: reperfusion, craniectomy, or both? An experimental study in rats. Stroke 2002; 33(2):617–622.

18. Georgiadis D, Schwarz S, Aschoff A, et al. Hemicraniectomy and moderate hypothermia in patients with severe ischemic stroke. Stroke 2002; 33(6):1584–1588.

19. Robertson SC, Lennarson P, Hasan DM, et al. Clinical course and surgical management of massive cerebral infarction. Neurosurgery 2004, 55(1):55–61; (discussion 61–52).

20. Maramattom BV, Bahn MM, Wijdicks EF. Which patient fares worse after early deterioration due to swelling from hemispheric stroke? Neurology 2004; 63(11):2142–2145.

21. Oppenheim C, Samson Y, Manai R, et al. Prediction of malignant middle cerebral artery infarction by diffusion-weighted imaging. Stroke 2000; 31(9):2175–2181.

22. Thomalla GJ, Kucinski T, Schoder V, et al. Prediction of malignant middle cerebral artery infarction by early perfusion- and diffusion-weighted magnetic resonance imaging. Stroke 2003; 34(8):1892–1899.

23. Foerch C, Otto B, Singer OC, et al. Serum S100B predicts a malignant course of infarction in patients with acute middle cerebral artery occlusion. Stroke 2004; 35(9):2160–2164.

24. Carter BS, Ogilvy CS, Candia GJ, et al. One-year outcome after decompressive surgery for massive nondominant hemispheric infarction. Neurosurgery 1997; 40(6):1168–1175; (discussion 1175–1166).

25. Koh MS, Goh KY, Tung MY, et al. Is decompressive craniectomy for acute cerebral infarction of any benefit? Surg Neurol 2000; 53(3):225–230.

26. Walz B, Zimmermann C, Bottger S, et al. Prognosis of patients after hemicraniectomy in malignant middle cerebral artery infarction. J Neurol 2002; 249(9):1183–1190.

27. Curry WT Jr., Sethi MK, Ogilvy CS, et al. Factors associated with outcome after hemicraniectomy for large middle cerebral artery territory infarction. Neurosurgery 2005; 56(4):681–692; (discussion 681–692).

28. Foerch C, Lang JM, Krause J, et al. Functional impairment, disability, and quality of life outcome after decompressive hemicraniectomy in malignant middle cerebral artery infarction. J Neurosurg. 2004; 101(2):48–254.

29. Wijdicks EF, Diringer MN. Middle cerebral artery territory infarction and early brain swelling: progression and effect of age on outcome. Mayo Clin Proc 1998; 73(9):829–836.

30. Gupta R, Connolly ES, Mayer S, et al. Hemicraniectomy for massive middle cerebral artery territory infarction: a systematic review. Stroke 2004; 35(2):539–543.

31. Schwab S, Steiner T, Aschoff A, et al. Early hemicraniectomy in patients with complete middle cerebral artery infarction. Stroke 1998; 29(9):1888–1893.

32. Heiss WD, Karbe H, Weber-Luxenburger G, et al. Speech-induced cerebral metabolic activation reflects recovery from aphasia. J Neurol Sci 1997; 145(2):213–217.
33. Abo M, Senoo A, Watanabe S, et al. Language-related brain function during word repetition in post-stroke aphasics. Neuroreport 2004; 15(12):1891–1894.
34. Cao Y, Vikingstad EM, George KP, et al. Cortical language activation in stroke patients recovering from aphasia with functional MRI. Stroke 1999; 30(11):2331–2340.
35. Kastrau F, Wolter M, Huber W, et al. Recovery from aphasia after hemicraniectomy for infarction of the speech-dominant hemisphere. Stroke 2005.

32 | Blood-Pressure Management in Subarachnoid Hemorrhage, Acute Ischemic Stroke, and Intracerebral Hemorrhage

Wendy C. Ziai, MD, Assistant Professor

Departments of Neurology, Neurosurgery, and Anesthesia/Critical Care Medicine, Johns Hopkins University School of Medicine, Baltimore, Maryland, USA

INTRODUCTION

The brain and cerebral circulation are highly vulnerable to the effects of blood pressure (BP) instability. Untreated hypertension is an important risk factor for cerebral infarction, intracerebral hemorrhage (ICH), and, to a lesser extent, subarachnoid hemorrhage (SAH) (1–4). The deleterious effects of acutely elevated BP in the presence of these and other cerebral insults, however, must be balanced against the physiologic regulation of cerebral perfusion pressure (CPP) and risks of reduced cerebral blood flow (CBF). After a surge in intracranial pressure (ICP), such as following subarachnoid or other intracranial hemorrhage, ICP may temporarily surpass mean arterial BP (MABP), such that CPP falls to zero, with resultant loss of consciousness. The elevated systemic BP after such events is presumably an autoregulatory phenomenon and may represent a component of the Cushing response, along with bradycardia and irregular respiratory effort, if ICP continues to be elevated. Rapid treatment of such hypertension is thought to be detrimental because decreased CPP may worsen brain injury by aggravating ischemia (5–7). Systemic hypertension has been shown to be protective in several brain injury paradigms, including mass lesions, infarction, and traumatic brain injury (7–10). The rationale for lowering BP in these same conditions is to decrease the risk for new or ongoing hemorrhage, depending on the mechanism of injury. The optimal BP might depend on several factors, including presence of chronic hypertension, suspected intracranial hypertension, age, etiology of injury, and time since onset (5). Guidelines for acute BP control are often controversial, vague, or nonexistent. It is therefore important to review the relevant pathophysiology in order to make rational decisions under a variety of clinical conditions.

This chapter focuses on the causes of acute hypertension in SAH, acute ischemic stroke, and ICH; the effects of hypertension on the cerebral vasculature; and the optimization of BP management in these neurologic diseases.

CEREBROVASCULAR PHYSIOLOGY

CBF is controlled by the following relationship between CPP and cerebrovascular resistance (CVR), such that CBF=CPP/CVR. CPP is the difference between the MABP and the backpressure produced by the intracranial contents (venous blood, cerebrospinal fluid, and brain tissue, i.e., the ICP), such that CPP=MABP–ICP.

Under normal conditions, ICP is negligible, and arterial BP determines CPP. Because of the ability of cerebral blood vessels to autoregulate, CBF in normal patients stays relatively constant over a wide range of CPP (Fig. 1). Both pial and small parenchymal arterioles are thought to take part in the mechanism of autoregulation (11). As MABP decreases below the lower limit (60 mmHg in adults), vasodilatation occurs, but eventually CPP becomes insufficient, causing CBF and cerebral blood volume (CBV) to decrease with resultant cerebral ischemia (12). With increasing MABP, vasoconstriction occurs in response to increasing CBF and CBV. As the upper limit of the autoregulatory curve is exceeded, however, increasing intraluminal pressure forcefully dilates segments of arterioles, causing damage to the blood–brain barrier, with resultant cerebral edema and hypertensive encephalopathy (13–15).

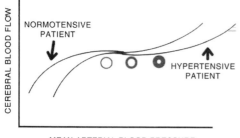

Figure 1 Autoregulation curves in normotensive and hypertensive patients.

MEAN ARTERIAL BLOOD PRESSURE

In chronic hypertension, both the lower and the upper ends of the autoregulation curve are shifted to the right, toward higher pressures (12,16–18). Anatomically, the smaller resistance blood vessels undergo degenerative changes that include thickening and fibrosis of the media (in muscular arteries) and intima and patchy degeneration of smooth muscle cells, producing luminal narrowing and increased vascular resistance (19). Although the resting CBF is the same in normotensive and hypertensive individuals, these structural changes limit the capacity of the resistance vessels for maximal vasodilatation and impair tolerance of lower BPs, while improving tolerance to hypertension through vasoconstriction of these same vessels. Long-term antihypertensive treatment can reverse these adaptive changes and shift the autoregulation curve back to its normal range, although only limited reversibility occurs in elderly hypertensive patients (20,21).

Myogenic and metabolic mechanisms have been proposed to explain autoregulation. The myogenic hypothesis by which vessels change caliber in response to changes in the transmural pressure gradient is supported by observations of a purely myogenic response *in vitro* and would be consistent with the rapidity of the response on the order of seconds (22). The metabolic hypothesis suggests that changing periarteriolar concentrations of metabolites, such as adenosine, might mediate autoregulatory vasodilatation; however, the vasoconstriction response is not well explained by metabolic mechanisms (23).

Although hypertension is frequently associated with acute neurologic insult as a physiologic response to inadequate CBF or ICP elevation, clinical evaluation of hypertension should consider all possible etiologies that require unique treatment, including pain (headache), anxiety, withdrawal of medications, and certain illicit drugs.

SUBARACHNOID HEMORRHAGE

SAH typically results from a ruptured intracranial aneurysm, trauma, or arteriovenous malformation. At the time of rupture, acute arterial hypertension occurs, reflecting a compensatory response to transient elevation of ICP. If ICP remains elevated, such as may occur with development of hydrocephalus, systemic BP may remain high, as a manifestation of the Cushing reflex. Often, however, hypertension is present without overt signs of increased ICP, reflecting a hyperadrenergic state secondary to excess release of catecholamines and/or response to headache and neck pain. The management of hypertension in patients with SAH may therefore involve therapies other than antihypertensive agents. Early hydrocephalus may be managed with placement of an intraventricular catheter, with care not to acutely increase transmural pressure and cause aneurysm rerupture. Pain is optimally treated with a short-acting reversible agent, such as intermittent fentanyl. These agents have no direct effect on ICP and CBF but may lead to respiratory depression, elevation in carbon dioxide, and resultant increase in CBF and ICP. In poor-grade patients, hypertension, along with tachycardia and restlessness, might be the only manifestations of pain (24). Later in the course of SAH, the effects of vasospasm on CBF should be taken into consideration, as permissive and induced hypertension is often the goal of therapy.

Acute Subarachnoid Hemorrhage (Preclipping/Prevasospasm)
Prior to the development of vasospasm, autoregulation is often intact, unless complicating factors exist, such as hydrocephalus or ICH (25). Brain perfusion might be dependent on arterial

BP because the range between the upper and lower limits of autoregulation narrows (26). If autoregulation is compromised in certain areas, aggressive reduction of MABP might cause ischemia. The risk of not treating BP spikes prior to aneurysm clipping is thought to be an increase in the rate of rebleeding. Although no controlled trial has demonstrated this association, in the Cooperative Aneurysm Study conducted between 1963 and 1970, two of the treatment arms (affecting 1005 patients with ruptured aneurysms) were pharmacologic lowering of BP and bed rest alone (27). Antihypertensive therapy did not reduce the mortality rate or rate of rebleeding in the intention-to-treat analysis but did decrease rebleeding in the treatment analysis. The rebleeding rate was 16% if systolic BP (SBP) was between 170 and 240 mmHg, compared to 9% if SBP was in the range of 94 to 169 mmHg. This study was performed in the pre-CT era and was therefore likely inaccurate for the diagnosis of rebleeding. A subsequent study in the 1980s compared patients who were previously hypertensive with SAH [to maintain diastolic BP (DBP) at less than 100 mmHg] to normotensive controls. A lower rate of rebleeding was reported for treated patients (15% vs. 33%; $p=0.012$), but a higher rate of cerebral infarction was also reported (43% vs. 22%; $p=0.03$), although the average BPs were still higher than in the controls (28). In the International Cooperative Study on the Timing of Aneurysm Surgery (1980–1983), BP on admission was an independent predictor of death and disability in the multivariate analysis (4). Higher BP was also associated with altered level of consciousness and older age, both independent predictors of poor outcome. The presence of hypertension, therefore, most likely reflects the severity of the SAH (4).

Recommendations for management of BP in the SAH population range considerably. One group suggests avoiding antihypertensive therapy, with the exception of "extreme" BP elevation or evidence of end-organ damage, such as clinical signs of encephalopathy, retinopathy, and cardiac failure, or laboratory findings of proteinuria, elevated creatinine, and oliguria, and chest X-ray findings of left ventricular failure (29). A more conservative guideline is to treat SBP greater than 150 mmHg, or greater than 10% of the premorbid level if that is known (30). Patients who fail to respond to pain control or reversal of other systemic abnormalities need antihypertensive medication, preferably a rapid-acting intravenous agent, such as labetalol, nicardipine infusion, or hydralazine. We do not use nitroglycerin due to the potential for increasing ICP from venous dilation, although some authors recommend it for patients with cardiac dysfunction (24). If ICP is elevated, CPP must be maintained above 70 mmHg, which in some patients may require BP augmentation.

Late Subarachnoid Hemorrhage (Postclipping/Vasospasm)

Once the aneurysm has been secured by clipping or coiling, BP management is directed to optimizing CBF in the setting of vasospasm. In the presence of large artery vasospasm, autoregulation is impaired in the majority of patients (31,32). Yundt et al. (25) used positron-emission tomography to study CBV in response to global or regional reductions in CPP and found that in patients with aneurysmal SAH without vasospasm, CBF, cerebral metabolic rate of oxygen (CMRO$_2$), and CBV were reduced with normal oxygen extraction fraction. In patients with arteriographic vasospasm, CBF and CBV were decreased, with minimal change in CMRO$_2$ and with increased oxygen extraction fraction. This pattern is consistent with misery perfusion and suggests that parenchymal vessels distal to arteries with vasospasm are not capable of normal autoregulatory vasodilation (25). More practically, cerebral autoregulation can be assessed clinically with tests, such as the cuff deflation test (33) and transient hyperemic response test (34), or by continuously using transcranial Doppler methods (35).

BP management in the presence of clinical vasospasm has largely been incorporated as part of triple-H therapy, which also includes hypervolemia and permissive hemodilution. The evidence for resolution of ischemic deficits that result from this therapy is based on uncontrolled, nonrandomized studies (4,36). In one series of 58 patients with progressive neurologic deterioration from angiographically confirmed cerebral vasospasm, induced arterial hypertension reversed neurologic deficits transiently in 47 patients, with permanent improvement in 43 cases (36). Reversal of ischemia by increasing CBF is the main goal of triple-H therapy. In another study, increases in cortical CBF of 34% (mean CBF increased 21%) were recorded in 43 SAH patients over the first 24 hr of triple-H therapy (37). However, values for CBF were within the normal range, and a control group was not evaluated in this study. Still unknown are the optimal levels of BP and volume status, as well as which component of triple-H therapy is the most important. Pharmacologically induced hypertension has been shown to improve

CBF in ischemic regions in patients with symptomatic vasospasm (31,38). Raising MABP from $90 + 11$ mmHg to $111 + 13$ mmHg with dopamine infusion in 13 SAH patients with suspected clinical vasospasm increased CBF to above the ischemic range (defined as $25 \, mL/100 \, gm/min$) in more than 90% of uninfarcted ischemic territories (identified by using xenon-enhanced CT) and decreased local CBF in one-third of the nonischemic territories (31). The increase may be explained by passive perfusion-dependent flow in areas with impaired autoregulation, by mechanical vasodilation, by increased collateral flow, or by direct vasodilatory response to dopamine, mediated by dopaminergic receptors at low doses (31).

The case against prophylactic use of triple-H therapy to prevent vasospasm was made by another randomized, controlled study in 32 patients who presented within 72 hr of SAH. Half of the patients were treated with triple-H therapy, and half with normovolemic fluid therapy (39). No statistical differences were found between groups regarding the frequency or severity of clinical or transcranial Doppler-defined vasospasm, regional CBF evaluated by Single Photon Emission CT (SPECT), or 1-year outcome assessed by Glasgow coma scale (GCS) and neuropsychologic tests (39). In addition, additional costs and more complications were involved in the hyperdynamically treated group. The results of this study are consistent with findings that only a proportion of patients with vasospasm respond to triple-H therapy, which may also reflect the realization that the causes of delayed ischemic neurologic deficits in the SAH population are probably multifactorial, including vasospasm, as well as embolization, thrombosis, reperfusion injury, and cerebral edema.

Kim et al. demonstrated in humans with vasospasm after SAH that raising cardiac output ($4.1–6.0 \, L/min/m^2$) with dobutamine was equally as efficacious as raising MABP ($102–132$ mmHg) with phenylephrine in producing significant elevation of CBF, measured by xenon CT (40). Studies comparing clinical benefits of a cardiac output strategy versus a MABP strategy for clinical vasospasm are not available. However, patients with unsecured aneurysms or neurogenic-stunned myocardium and clinical vasospasm may be more safely managed with CO rather than MABP optimization. In the setting of an unsecured aneurysm, the risk of rerupture must be carefully weighed against the risk of cerebral ischemia secondary to vasospasm. In one series, 3 out of 16 patients with unclipped ruptured aneurysms rebled, all with arterial pressures greater than 160 mmHg (36). Although it cannot be proven that hypertension was the cause of rebleeding, the potential stress of increased arterial pressure in this setting suggests that BP should be carefully controlled and that alternative treatments for vasospasm should be considered.

ISCHEMIC STROKE

Transient hypertension is observed frequently following acute ischemic stroke and might be the result of a combination of factors, including anxiety, pain, neuroendocrine factors, stroke location, or a compensatory response to increased ICP (41–44). Acutely elevated BP is associated with increased early mortality after stroke, although whether this represents the consequence of stroke severity or its cause is presently unknown (1,2,45). Interestingly, low SBP and DBP, as well as elevated SBP, DBP, and MABP have been associated with poor stroke outcome, producing a U-shaped relationship between SBP and outcome (46–50). Analysis of a single SBP measurement prior to randomization in the International Stroke Trial in 17,398 patients with confirmed ischemic stroke also found a U-shaped relationship between baseline SBP and both early death and late death or dependency (50). In addition, patients with admission SBP greater than 200 mmHg had more than a 50% greater risk of recurrent stroke, compared to those with SBP of 130 mmHg. The relationship of low BP with poor outcome was associated with an excess of early deaths from coronary events and possible cerebral reinfarctions. It was not clear whether these associations were causal.

From a retrospective analysis of 1455 ischemic strokes from the Glycine Antagonist in Neuroprotection (GAIN) international trial, elevated pulse pressure during acute ischemic stroke was found to be independently associated with poor stroke outcome at three months, after correcting for baseline NIHSS, age, gender, treatment group (Gavestinel vs. placebo), heart rate, stroke risk factors, and stroke, type (51). Another issue is the potential compounding effect of BP on overall cardiovascular risk. A meta-analysis of approximately 1 million subjects by The Prospective Studies Collaboration found that stroke and other types of cardiovascular mortality increase exponentially with BP (52). A follow-up report stated a doubling of mortality for every 20/10 mmHg increase in BP, starting as low as 115/75 mmHg (53). However, BP reduction in the acute stages of stroke might not be beneficial and might be potentially harmful.

The Nimodipine West European Stroke Trial randomized 295 patients within 24 hr of stroke to placebo, low-dose nimodipine (1 mg/hr), or high-dose nimodipine (2 mg/hr) (54). For patients who had less than total anterior circulation strokes, lowering of DBP worsened neurologic outcome and high-dose nimodipine worsened both neurologic and functional outcome, compared to placebo-treated patients. However, nimodipine treatment and lowering of BP had no significant effect on outcome for patients with total anterior circulation infarcts (50).

Early BP elevations often decline spontaneously during the first minutes to hours of monitoring and may not require pharmacologic treatment (55). SBP and DBP decrease spontaneously by 12 and 7 mmHg within the first 24 hr after stroke, and by 22 and 12 mmHg within the first week (46). Because cerebral autoregulation is impaired in ischemic brain regions, CBF is pressure dependent, and further reduction may irreversibly injure the ischemic penumbra and increase stroke volume. A prospective study of 115 patients with acute ischemia, whose serial SBP was recorded for 24 hr, found on multivariate analysis, that poor outcome at 3 months was independently significantly associated with only initial NIHSS and the degree of reduction in SBP (56). An odds ratio (OR) of 1.89 for each 10% decrease in SBP was reported. Antihypertensive medication use was unrelated to initial BP levels and was not significantly associated with outcomes, suggesting that even spontaneous reductions in SBP may be detrimental in acute ischemia (57).

Further evidence for the effect of reduction in BP comes from a prospective study of 372 patients with acute ischemic stroke that evaluated the relationship between changes in SBP and DBP from hospital admission to 24 hr after admission with dichotomized Rankin Scale outcome (score ≤ 2). Outcome assessment was performed at day 5 after admission (58). Multivariate logistic regression analysis showed that a DBP reduction of more than 25% from admission to 24 hr after admission was associated with a 3.8-fold increase in adjusted odds for poor neurologic outcome on day 5. This result was independent of whether the reduction was spontaneous or induced by antihypertensive treatment. No significant association was found for SBP reduction and outcome.

It is probably safe to conclude that optimal BP management has not been established in ischemic stroke. The Stroke Council of the American Stroke Association has produced consensus guidelines that state that antihypertensive agents should be withheld unless DBP is greater than 120 mmHg or SBP is greater than 220 mmHg (59). This recommendation, however, is based on level V, or anecdotal evidence. Labetalol is a preferred drug, but intravenous infusion of nicardipine may be warranted when BP is difficult to control. Oral nicardipine and captopril are also suggested. Avoiding sublingual use of calcium antagonists, such as nifedipine, is recommended due to anecdotal evidence of rapid absorption, causing precipitous BP reduction (60).

In patients who present with hypotension, the differential diagnosis includes aortic dissection, volume depletion, and decreased cardiac output secondary to myocardial ischemia or cardiac arrhythmias (59). Treatment should begin with volume replacement with normal saline and correction of underlying causes, such as arrhythmia, followed by vasopressor agents if initial management is unsuccessful.

Acute treatment of elevated BP should be considered for patients undergoing thrombolysis and patients with severe hypertension, hemorrhagic transformation of the infarct, acute myocardial infarction, aortic dissection, acute pulmonary edema, hypertensive encephalopathy, or severe left ventricular failure (61). For patients receiving thrombolysis with recombinant tissue plasminogen activator (rtPA), the National Institute of Neurological Disorders and Stroke (NINDS) rtPA Stroke Study Group Guidelines recommend maintaining BP at less than 185/110 mmHg prior to thrombolysis and less than 180/105 mmHg during and after administration of rtPA (62). Intravenous labetalol is the agent of choice. The rate of BP control is also important, because rapid decreases in systemic pressure can worsen neurologic condition and responses to antihypertensives may be exaggerated in these patients (43,63,64)

Increasing BP in patients with small infarcts on diffusion-weighted imaging (DWI) and a large area of hypoperfusion on MRI perfusion-weighted imaging or CT perfusion scan might improve neurologic outcomes (65). Patients with completed stroke without a large diffusion–perfusion mismatch might alternatively have worse outcomes with elevated BP due to exacerbation of edema or hemorrhage.

A few animal and patient studies have even provided preliminary data that suggest that raising BP with intravenous vasopressors might be effective in improving neurologic function in acute/subacute stroke, especially in patients with large diffusion–perfusion mismatch on MRI (10,66). For example, in patients with more than 20% diffusion–perfusion mismatch up to 7 days post onset of symptoms, 9 patients with induced hypertension showed significant improvement from day 1 to day 3 and at 3-month follow-up in NIHSS (3-day mean, 5.6 vs. 9.7; $p < 0.02$; 3-month NIHSS: $p < 0.04$) and cognitive scores (mean 28% errors vs. 67% errors; $p = 0.03$) compared to "untreated" patients (64). Only treated patients demonstrated a significant reduction in the volume of hypoperfused tissue on perfusion weighted imaging (mean of 132–58 ml; $p < 0.02$). BP elevation involved increasing the MABP in 10% increments over 12 hr (achieved with a combination of intravenous saline and phenylephrine infusion) until motor/cognitive function improved or a MABP of 130 to 140 was reached. At 24 hr, patients were started on midodrine (up to 10 mg orally t.i.d.), fludrocortisone (up to 0.2 mg t.i.d.), and NaCl tablets, while weaning the phenylephrine to keep MABP in the goal range. Oral medications were tapered off at 4 weeks, as long as no clinical deterioration was observed. Two patients resumed oral medication for up to 3 months. No adverse effects of pharmacologic BP elevation with phenylephrine occurred. The authors concluded that patients in this study were highly selected, because all had severe stenosis or complete occlusion of the proximal middle cerebral artery (M1 segment) and/or internal carotid artery. These characteristics had shown the best response to BP elevation in earlier studies (67). Improvement in neurologic function, therefore, could be ascribed to recanalization of middle cerebral arterial branches, development of collateral blood supply, or reduction of edema. The risks of this treatment strategy have not been fully evaluated and include hemorrhagic conversion of infarct, cardiac ischemia, bradycardia, and congestive heart failure (68). Ideally, an ongoing NIH-sponsored clinical trial will assess this issue and fully evaluate efficacy of induced BP elevation in acute and subacute strokes.

In another study to evaluate the effect of dexamphetamine in acute ischemic stroke, 45 patients were randomized within 72 hr of symptom onset to 1 of 3 dose levels (2.5, 5, or 10 mg) orally b.i.d. or placebo for 5 days (69). At 7 days, dexamphetamine was associated with significant increases in SBP (mean increase 14 mmHg; $p < 0.004$) and DBP (mean increase 8 mmHg; $p = 0.01$) and significant improvement in Scandinavian Stroke Scale and functional outcome (based on motor function and Barthel index). The 1- and 3-month outcomes, however, were not different from those of placebo patients. The improvement in function may have been related to BP elevation or to other effects of amphetamine reported in experimental models (70).

Finally, evidence has been reported that lowering SBP at some point after stroke reduces the risk of recurrent stroke, both ischemic and hemorrhagic, as well as other vascular complications. The PROGRESS trial (perindopril protection against recurrent stroke) randomized 6105 patients who had had transient ischemic attack (TIA) or stroke in the previous five years to placebo or antihypertensive treatment with perindopril and, if no contraindication, to a diuretic, indapamide (71,72). A relative risk reduction of 43% (95% confidence interval (CI): 30–54) was realized in patients who received the combination regiment but not perindopril alone. The BP reduction in the combination therapy group was 12/5 mmHg, compared to 5/3 mmHg in the monotherapy group. The risk reduction was greatest in patients with baseline intracranial hemorrhage (49%; 95% CI: 18–68) and was significant in patients with baseline ischemic stroke (26%; 95% CI: 12–38) but not in patients with baseline TIA (23%; 95% CI: 23–52). Subgroup analysis showed no significant reduction for the stroke subtypes of lacunar stroke or cardio-embolic stroke (73).

BP reduction probably should not be the goal, however, in patients with bilateral carotid stenosis of 70% or greater or with unilateral carotid occlusion (57). This recommendation is based on a meta-analysis of data from the United Kingdom TIA (UK-TIA) trial, the European Carotid Surgery Trial, and the North American Symptomatic Carotid Surgery Trial, which showed a significant negative relationship between SBP reduction and stroke risk in patients, with greater than 70% stenosis in both carotid arteries, who did not receive endarterectomy, as well as a trend toward higher stroke risk in patients with carotid occlusion and lower diastolic pressure (74). The 5-year stroke risk was significantly higher in patients with SBP below the median compared to those with SBP above the median (64% vs. 24%; $p < 0.002$). If endarterectomy was performed, the stroke risk was reversed to 13.5% in the high-SBP group and 18.3% in the low SBP group but was not significantly different ($p = 0.6$). In the UK-TIA trial, patients with TIA had significantly reduced stroke risk with lower SBP.

In conclusion, based on the ASA consensus guidelines and studies evaluating outcomes in relation to BP, it is recommended that BP not be lowered in the first week after ischemic stroke, except for SBP greater than 220 mmHg, DBP greater than 120 mmHg, or medical conditions requiring urgent BP lowering (59,61). From the International Stroke Trial, patients with admission SBP between 140 and 179 mmHg had the most favorable outcomes. Early death occurred in patients with SBP both above and below this range (50). Induced hypertension may benefit certain patients, notably those with severe intracranial stenosis and a large diffusion–perfusion mismatch on MRI (67). Considering the PROGRESS trial data, SBP should eventually be lowered in almost all stroke patients by 1 to 6 months after stroke onset by approximately 12/5 mmHg. Caveats include lesions that may reduce cerebral perfusion (intracranial large vessel stenosis, bilateral carotid stenosis, and carotid occlusion), which may require initial management prior to BP lowering (57).

INTRACEREBRAL HEMORRHAGE

The most important risk factors associated with acute ICH are advancing age and hypertension (3). The pathophysiology of ICH most commonly involves hypertension-induced changes in the small arteries and arterioles, with formation of microaneurysms at juncture points of major feeding and small penetrating arteries (75,76). Systemic hypertension is common after ICH, occurs in up to 90% of patients, is usually higher than after ischemic stroke, and often lasts for several days (41,77,78). By the tenth day after ICH, a third of patients remain hypertensive (41). High BP on admission and during the first 24 hr has been associated with increased mortality in some series but not in others (79–81). The major reason to aggressively treat hypertension is that elevated BP might result in early rebleeding from ruptured small arteries and arterioles, which causes hematoma enlargement and occurs in approximately 38% of patients within the first 24 hr after presentation (82). The converse risk is whether reducing arterial pressure reduces CBF with resulting cerebral ischemia (2,5).

Although ICH is caused by many conditions, such as cerebral amyloid angiopathy, vascular malformations, aneurysms, anticoagulant use and coagulation disorders, tumors, hemorrhagic transformation of infarcts, and drug abuse, the prevalence of chronic hypertension in the ICH population implies that most patients will have a shifted autoregulatory curve at onset (19,26). Another reason for abnormal autoregulation is increased ICP, which causes reduced CPP (2,83). Both animal and human studies have reported CBF values close to the threshold of ischemia in the perihematoma region, where autoregulation is impaired (84,85). One study measured changes in regional CBF using SPECT following drug-induced BP reduction in 68 patients with hypertensive ICH in the thalamus and putamen (86). In the acute period (3 days after onset on average), mean CBF decreased only if MABP was lowered by more than 20% (86). In the chronic period, greater reductions in MABP were required to cause CBF reduction. Other studies have found no difference in CBF with lowering of BP, one in a dog model of ICH and the other a human study (83,87). Although a follow-up study in humans did report significant reductions in periclot CBF and $CMRO_2$, compared with contralateral values in 19 patients with acute ICH at 5 to 22 hr after onset (88), $CMRO_2$ was reduced to a greater degree than CBF, arguing against the idea that the tissue was ischemic. MRI studies have also failed to show evidence of hypoperfusion surrounding hematomas (89,90); therefore, aggressive treatment of hypertension may not be detrimental to periclot cerebral perfusion (91). For very large ICH, no data are available regarding the effect of lowering BP. The effect of increased ICP on BP and cerebral perfusion may be significant in these patients.

The rationale for treating BP is to prevent hematoma growth, increase in ICP, and possible edema formation. The risk of ongoing hemorrhage in the setting of uncontrolled hypertension is difficult to attribute to BP alone. One retrospective and one prospective observational study did not find baseline BP to be associated with hematoma enlargement, although early use of antihypertensive agents may have obscured this relationship (Table 1) (82,93). A retrospective analysis of 186 patients with spontaneous ICH did report SBP greater than 200 mmHg as an independent factor predisposing to ICH growth in the acute phase (94). Another retrospective study of 87 patients found that cases in which initial MABP was less than or equal to 145 mmHg

Table 1 Antihypertensive Agents for Acute Blood Pressure Control

Drug	Mechanism of action	Onset of action	Duration of action	Dosage	Drug-specific adverse effects
Diazoxide	Activates adenosine triphosphate-sensitive potassium channels	1–5 min	1–12 hr	IV bolus: 50–100 mg q 10 min; continuous infusion: 15–30 mg/min	Severe hyperglycemia, salt and water retention
Hydralazine	Nitric oxide interferes with calcium mobilization in smooth muscle	15–30 min	3–4 hr	2.5–10 mg IV bolus (up to 40 mg)	Drug-induced lupus syndrome, serum-sickness-like illness
Sodium nitroprusside	Nitric oxide	Immediate	2–3 min	0.25–10 µg/kg/min IV	Cyanide toxicity
Labetalol	α-1, β-1, β-2 receptor antagonist	5–10 min	2–12 hr	10–80 mg IV q 10 min up to 300 mg/d IV infusion: 0.5–2 mg/min	Congestive heart failure, bronchospasm, hypoglycemia, bradycardia
Esmolol	Selective β-1 antagonist	Immediate	<15 min	0.25–0.5 mg/kg IV bolus, then 50–200 µg/kg/min	Bradycardia, congestive heart failure
Nicardipine	Calcium channel antagonist	1–5 min	3–6 hr	5 mg/hr IV, increase by 1–2.5 mg/hr q 15 min, up to 15 mg/hr	Hypotension, reflex tachycardia
Enalaprilat	Angiotensin converting enzyme inhibitor	5–15 min	6 hr	0.625–1.25 mg IV over 15 min	Renal dysfunction
Clonidine	α-2 receptor agonist	Hours	8–12 hr	0.1 mg orally q 12 h; up to 2.4 mg/day	Sedation, bradycardia, rebound hypertension
Phentolamine	α-1, α-2 receptor antagonist	2 min	10–15 min	5–20 mg IV	Tachycardia, arrhythmias
Thiopental	Activation of Gamma amino butytic acid receptor	2 min	5–10 min	30–60 mg IV	Myocardial depression
Fenoldopam	Dopamine-1, α-2 receptor agonist	15 min	10–20 min	0.01–1.6 µg/kg/min IV; no bolus	Tachycardia–bradycardia, hypokalemia
Trimethaphan	Ganglionic blockade	Immediate	5–10 min	1–5 mg/min IV	Cycloplegia, mydriasis, urinary retention, bronchospasm
Adenosine	Adenosine receptor agonist	<1 min	1–2 min	Up to 220 mg/kg/min	None
Nitroglycerin	Nitric oxide	1–2 min	3–5 min	5–100 µg/kg/min	Methemoglobin production

Abbreviations: IV, intravenous; GABA, Gamma-aminobutyric acid; DA, Dopamine.
Source: From Ref. 92.

and MABP was maintained at below 125 mmHg in the first 2 to 6 hr of presentation were associated with better outcomes in both mortality and severe morbidity (admission MABP: $p < 0.005$; 2–6 hr MABP: $p < 0.005$) (95). This study, however, did not adjust for variables, such as hematoma volume, ventricular blood, and initial GCS, which may have confounded the results. A different study reported an opposing result using serial MABP recordings over the first 24 hr after presentation in 105 patients with spontaneous ICH (96). Each patient's MABP was calculated as a slope, and the effect of MABP slope on mortality and functional outcome was determined, with adjustment for other predictive factors. The MABP slope (faster rate of decline) was significantly associated with increased mortality ($p = 0.04$), independent of initial GCS and hematoma volume (96). The MABP slope, however, did not predict functional outcome among the survivors. The main explanation for this finding was thought to be a reduction in CPP, which worsened ischemic injury in the perihematoma zone, resulting in increased edema and mass effect by compensatory vasodilation in regions with intact autoregulation that exacerbated preexisting intracranial hypertension (95). Ohwaki et al. retrospectively studied associations of serial BP from admission to the second CT scan, with change in hematoma size in 76 patients with hypertensive ICH (97). Medical management attempted to lower SBP below targets of 140 to 170 mmHg. Hematoma enlargement (increase in volume ≥140% or 12.5 cm³) occurred in 16 patients (21%) and was significantly and independently associated with maximum SBP (OR, per mmHg: 1.04; 95% CI: 1.01–1.07) after adjusting for hematoma volume and GCS at admission. A target SBP of greater than or equal to 160 mmHg was significantly associated with hematoma enlargement, compared to patients with a target SBP of less than or equal to 150 mmHg (97). Although this retrospective study cannot conclude that increased BP caused hematoma enlargement, the authors conclude that efforts to lower SBP to below 150 mmHg may prevent hematoma enlargement.

The only randomized study that evaluated BP management reported better outcomes with BP control, although the lack of CT data in this early study compromises its validity (98). Qureshi et al. assessed the feasibility and safety of aggressive antihypertensive treatment in a multicenter prospective study of 27 patients with ICH and acute hypertension (99). The target was SBP less than 160 mmHg and DBP less than 90 mmHg within 24 hr of symptom onset. Hematoma expansion was documented in 9% of patients, and patients treated within 6 hr of symptom onset were more likely to be functionally independent, according to modified Rankin scale, compared to patients treated at between 6 and 24 hr ($p = 0.03$) (99).

Considering the combined risks of inadequate CPP as a consequence of aggressive control of elevated BP and rebleeding, which may be related to very high SBP, the American Heart Association guidelines recommend maintaining MABP to less than 130 mmHg in patients with a history of hypertension and CPP greater than 70 mmHg in patients with an ICP monitor (5,100). Finally, SBP less than 90 mmHg should be treated with vasopressor agents.

In the chronic phase, hypertension has been identified as a major risk factor for development of primary and recurrent ICH with an association that is stronger than that observed for ischemic stroke (71,101). In the Systolic Hypertension in the Elderly Program study (102), the relative risk reduction with antihypertensive treatment for hemorrhagic stroke was 0.46 (95% CI: 0.21–1.02), compared to 0.63 (95% CI: 0.48–0.82) for ischemic stroke. The treatment effect was observed within the first year of treatment for hemorrhagic stroke but not until the second year for ischemic stroke. In the case of recurrent ICH, 74 patients with hypertensive ICH studied prospectively for a mean of 2.8 years were found to have significantly higher DBP in the recurrence group, compared to the nonrecurrence group (88 ± 8 vs. 82 ± 7 mmHg; $p = 0.04$). Recurrence rates were 10.0% per patient year in patients with DBP more than 90 mmHg, compared with less than 1.5% per patient year in patients with lower DBP ($p < 0.001$) (103).

In conclusion, BP is often significantly elevated during the acute period after ICH and returns spontaneously to baseline values after the first week. The best current guidelines for managing BP in ICH are those provided by the AHA Stroke Council and are based on nonrandomized retrospective and anecdotal studies. Although many physicians believe in a conservative approach to BP management in these patients due to concern for decreasing CPP and belief that hematomas stop active bleeding within minutes, it is likely that careful lowering of arterial pressure to at least below 180 mmHg will have therapeutic benefit in reducing hematoma expansion. Moreover, the data supporting exacerbation of secondary neuronal injury in perihematoma regions with lowering of BP are not well supported, at least for small- to moderate-sized hemorrhages. Instead, it has been postulated that regions of increased DWI are due to "metabolic suppression" rather than ischemia, the clinical effects of which remain unknown at this time (89,90). A large randomized, controlled study of lowering of acute BP in ICH would be needed to resolve much of the controversy surrounding this topic.

Although hypertension is a primary cause of SAH and ischemic and hemorrhagic stroke, BP management in these conditions remains a controversial subject. The optimal strategy likely differs across individual patients, depending on mechanism of injury and determinants of cerebral perfusion. The challenge remains to identify these factors in an efficient way to produce rational approaches to BP control.

REFERENCES

1. Britton M, Carlsson A. Very high blood pressure in acute stroke. J Intern Med 1990; 228:611–615.
2. Powers WJ. Acute hypertension after stroke: the scientific basis for treatment decisions. Neurology 1993; 43:461–467.
3. Broderick J. Intracerebral hemorrhage. In: Gorelick PBAM, ed. Handbook of Neuroepidemiology. New York: Marcel Dekker, Inc.; 1994:141–167.
4. Kassell NF, Torner JC, Haley EC Jr., Jane JA, Adams HP, Kongable GL. The international coopera-tive study on the timing of aneurysm surgery. Part 1: overall management results. J Neurosurg 1990; 73:18–36.
5. Broderick JP, Adams HP Jr., Barsan W, et al. Guidelines for the management of spontaneous intra-cerebral hemorrhage: a statement for healthcare professionals from a special writing group of the stroke council, American Heart Association. Stroke 1999; 30:905–915.
6. Lisk DR, Grotta JC, Lamki LM, et al. Should hypertension be treated after acute stroke? A ran-domized controlled trial using single photon emission computed tomography. Arch Neurol 1993; 50:855–862.
7. Rosner MJ, Daughton S. Cerebral perfusion pressure management in head injury. J Trauma 1990; 30:933–40; discussion 940–941.
8. Schrader H, Zwetnow NN, Morkrid L. Regional cerebral blood flow and CSF pressures during Cush-ing response induced by a supratentorial expanding mass. Acta Neurol Scand 1985; 71:453–463.
9. Schrader H, Lofgren J, Zwetnow NN. Influence of blood pressure on tolerance to an intracranial expanding mass. Acta Neurol Scand 1985; 71:114–126.
10. Drummond JC, Oh YS, Cole DJ, Shapiro HM. Phenylephrine-induced hypertension reduces ischemia following middle cerebral artery occlusion in rats. Stroke 1989; 20:1538–1544.
11. Kontos HA, Wei EP, Navari RM, Levasseur JE, Rosenblum WI, Patterson JL. Responses of cerebral arteries and arterioles to acute hypotension and hypertension. Am J Physiol 1978; 234:H371–H383.
12. Strandgaard S. Autoregulation of cerebral blood flow in hypertensive patients. The modifying influ-ence of prolonged antihypertensive treatment on the tolerance to acute, drug-induced hypotension. Circulation 1976; 53:720–727.
13. Westergaard E, van Deurs B, Brondsted HE. Increased vesicular transfer of horseradish peroxi-dase across cerebral endothelium, evoked by acute hypertension. Acta Neuropathol (Berl) 1977; 37: 141–152.
14. Sokrab TE, Johansson BB, Kalimo H, Olsson Y. A transient hypertensive opening of the blood-brain barrier can lead to brain damage. Extravasation of serum proteins and cellular changes in rats sub-jected to aortic compression. Acta Neuropathol 1988; 75:557–565.
15. Johansson B. Hypertension and the blood brain barrier. In: Neuvelt E, ed. Implications of the blood-brain barrier and its manipulation. Vol. 2. New York: Plenum Press; 1988:557–565.
16. Jones JV, Fitch W, MacKenzie ET, Strandgaard S, Harper AM. Lower limit of cerebral blood flow autoregulation in experimental renovascular hypertension in the baboon. Circ Res 1976; 39:555–557.
17. Barry DI, Strandgaard S, Graham DI, et al. Cerebral blood flow in rats with renal and spontane-ous hypertension: resetting of the lower limit of autoregulation. J Cereb Blood Flow Metab 1982; 2:347–353.
18. Strandgaard S, Jones JV, MacKenzie ET, Harper AM. Upper limit of cerebral blood flow autoregula-tion in experimental renovascular hypertension in the baboon. Circ Res 1975; 37:164–167.
19. Paulson OB, Waldemar G, Schmidt JF, Strandgaard S. Cerebral circulation under normal and patho-logic conditions. Am J Cardiol 1989; 63:2C–5C.
20. Strandgaard S, Paulson OB. Cerebral autoregulation. Stroke 1984; 15:413–416.
21. Vorstrup S, Barry DI, Jarden JO, et al. Chronic antihypertensive treatment in the rat reverses hypertension-induced changes in cerebral blood flow autoregulation. Stroke 1984; 15:312–318.
22. Osol G, Halpern W. Myogenic properties of cerebral blood vessels from normotensive and hyperten-sive rats. Am J Physiol 1985; 249:H914–H921.
23. Phillis JW, Walter GA, O'Regan MH, Stair RE. Increases in cerebral cortical perfusate adenosine and inosine concentrations during hypoxia and ischemia. J Cereb Blood Flow Metab 1987; 7:679–686.
24. Le Roux PD, Winn HR. Management of the ruptured aneurysm. In: Mayberg MR, Winn HR, eds. Neurosurgery Clinics of North America. Philadelphia: WB Saunders Company, 1998:(3):525–540.
25. Yundt KD, Grubb RL, Diringer MN, Powers WJ. Autoregulatory vasodilation of parenchymal vessels is impaired during cerebral vasospasm. J Cereb Blood Flow Metab 1998; 18:419–424.
26. Kaneko T, Sawanda T, Niimi T, et al. Lower limit of blood pressure in treatment of acute hyperten-sive intracranial hemorrhage. J Cereb Blood Flow Metab 1983; 3:S51–S52.

27. Torner JC, Kassell NF, Wallace RB, Adams HP Jr. Preoperative prognostic factors for rebleeding and survival in aneurysm patients receiving antifibrinolytic therapy: report of the Cooperative Aneurysm Study. Neurosurgery 1981; 9:506–513.

28. Wijdicks EF, Vermeulen M, Murray GD, Hijdra A, van Gijn J. The effects of treating hypertension following aneurysmal subarachnoid hemorrhage. Clin Neurol Neurosurg 1990; 92:111–117.

29. van Gijn J, Rinkel GJ. Subarachnoid haemorrhage: diagnosis, causes and management. Brain 2001; 124:249–278.

30. Bernardini G, Mayer SA, Solomon RA. Subarachnoid hemorrhage. In: Miller DH RE, ed. Critical Care Neurology. Boston: Butterworth-Heinemann; 1999:233.

31. Darby JM, Yonas H, Marks EC, Durham S, Snyder RW, Nemoto EM. Acute cerebral blood flow response to dopamine-induced hypertension after subarachnoid hemorrhage. J Neurosurg 1994; 80:857–864.

32. Voldby B, Enevoldsen EM, Jensen FT. Cerebrovascular reactivity in patients with ruptured intracranial aneurysms. J Neurosurg 1985; 62:59–67.

33. Aaslid R, Lindegaard KF, Sorteberg W, Nornes H. Cerebral autoregulation dynamics in humans. Stroke 1989; 20:45–52.

34. Giller CA. A bedside test for cerebral autoregulation using transcranial Doppler ultrasound. Acta Neurochir (Wien) 1991; 108:7–14.

35. Soehle M, Czosnyka M, Pickard JD, Kirkpatrick PJ. Continuous assessment of cerebral autoregulation in subarachnoid hemorrhage. Anesth Analg 2004; 98:1133–1139.

36. Kassell NF, Peerless SJ, Durward QJ, Beck DW, Drake CG, Adams HP. Treatment of ischemic deficits from vasospasm with intravascular volume expansion and induced arterial hypertension. Neurosurgery 1982; 11:337–343.

37. Origitano TC, Wascher TM, Reichman OH, et al. Sustained increased cerebral blood flow with prophylactic hypertensive hypervolemic hemodilution ("triple-H therapy") after subarachnoid hemorrhage. Neurosurgery 1990; 27:729–739.

38. Muizelaar JP, Becker DP. Induced hypertension for the treatment of cerebral ischemia after subarachnoid hemorrhage: direct effect on cerebral blood flow. Surg Neurol 1986; 25:317–325.

39. Egge A, Waterloo K, Sjoholm H, Solberg T, Ingebrigtsen T, Romner B. Prophylactic hyperdynamic postoperative fluid therapy after aneurysmal subarachnoid hemorrhage: a clinical prospective, randomized, controlled study. Neurosurgery 2001; 49:593–606.

40. Kim DH, Joseph M, Ziadi S, Nates J, Dannenbaum M, Malkoff M. Increases in cardiac output can reverse flow deficits from vasospasm independent of blood pressure: a study using xenon computed tomographic measurement of cerebral blood flow. Neurosurgery 2003; 53:1044–1052.

41. Wallace JD, Levy LL. Blood pressure after stroke. JAMA 1981; 246:2177–2180.

42. Chamorro A, Vila N, Ascaso C, Elices E, Schonewille W, Blanc R. Blood pressure and functional recovery in acute ischemic stroke. Stroke 1998; 29:1850–1853.

43. Carlberg B, Asplund K, Hagg E. Factors influencing admission blood pressure levels in patients with acute stroke. Stroke 1991; 22:527–530.

44. Jansen PA, Schulte BP, Poels EF, Gribnau FW. Course of blood pressure after cerebral infarction and transient ischemic attack. Clin Neurol Neurosurg 1987; 89:243–246.

45. Torner J, Nibbelink DW, LF B. Statistical comparison of end results of a randomized treatment study. In: Sahs AL, Nibbelink DW, Tonner JC, eds. Aneurysmal subarachnoid hemorrhage. Baltimore: Urban & Schwarzenberg, 1981:249–275.

46. Jorgensen H, Nakayama H, Raaschou H, Olsen T. Effect of blood pressure and diabetes on stroke progression. Lancet 1994; 344:156–159.

47. Linsberg PJ, Soinne L, Roine RO, et al. Community-based thrombolytic therapy of acute ischemic stroke in Helsinki. Stroke 2003; 34:1443–1449.

48. Ahmed N, Näsman P, Wahlgren NG. Effect of intravenous nimodipine on blood pressure and outcome after acute stroke. Stroke 2000; 31:1250–1255.

49. Dawson SL, Mankletow BN, Robinson TG, Panerai RB, Potter JF. Which parameters of beat to beat blood pressure and variability best predict early outcome after acute ischemic stroke? Stroke 2001; 31:463–468.

50. Leonardi-Bee Jo, Bath PMW, Phlilips SJ, Sandercock PAG, for IST Collaborative Group. Blood pressure and clinical outcome in the international stroke trial. Stroke 2002; 33:1315–1320.

51. Aslanyan S, Weir CJ, Lees KR. Elevated pulse pressure during the acute period of ischemic stroke is associated with poor stroke outcome. Stroke 2004; 35:3153–3155.

52. Lewington S, Clarke R, Qizilbash N, Peto R, Collins R. Prospective studies collaboration. Age-specific relevance of usual blood pressure to vascular mortality: a meta-analysis of individual data for one million adults in 62 prospective studies. Lancet 2002; 360:1903–1913.

53. Chobanian AV, Bakris GL, Black HR, et al. National high blood pressure education program coordinating committee. Seventh report of the joint national committee on prevention, detection, evaluation, and treatment of high blood pressure. Hypertension 2003; 42:1206–1252.

54. Ahmed N, Wahlgren NG. Effects of blood pressure lowering in the acute phase of anterior circulation infarcts and other stroke subtypes. Cerebrovasc Dis 2003; 15:235–243.

55. Broderick J, Brott T, Barsan W, et al. Blood pressure during the first minutes of focal cerebral ischemia. Ann Emerg Med 1993; 22:1438–1443.

56. Oliveira-Filho J, Silva SC, Trabuco CC, Pedreira BB, Sousa EU, Bacellar A. MD. Detrimental effect of blood pressure reduction in the first 24 hr of acute stroke onset. Neurology 2003; 61:1047–1051.

57. Hillis AE. Systemic blood pressure and stroke outcome and recurrence. Curr Atheroscler Rep 2004; 6:274–280.

58. Vlcek M, Schillinger M, Lang W, Lalouschek W, Bur A, Hirschl MM. Association between course of blood pressure within the first 24 hr and functional recovery after acute ischemic stroke. Ann Emerg Med 2003; 42:619–626.

59. Adams, HP, Adams,RJ, et al. ASA guidelines for the early management of patients with ischemic stroke: a scientific statement from the stroke council of the American Stroke Association. Stroke 2003; 34:1056–1083.

60. Grossman E, Messerli FH, Grodzicki T, Kowey P. Should a moratorium be placed on sublingual nifedipine capsules given for hypertensive emergencies and pseudoemergencies? JAMA 1996; 276:1328–1331.

61. Adams HP Jr., Brott TG, Crowell RM, et al. Guidelines for the management of patients with acute ischemic stroke. A statement for healthcare professionals from a special writing group of the stroke council, American Heart Association. Stroke 1994; 25:1901–1914.

62. Adams H, Brott TG, AJ F. Guidelines for thrombolytic therapy for acute stroke: a supplement to the guidelines for the management of patients with acute ischemic stroke. A statement for healthcare professionals from a special writing group of the stroke council, American Heart Association. Circulation 1996; 94:1167–1174.

63. Guidelines for cardiopulmonary resuscitation and emergency cardiac care. Emergency cardiac care committee and subcommittees, American Heart Association. Part IV. Special resuscitation situations. Jama 1992; 268:2242–2250.

64. Britton M, de Faire U, Helmers C. Hazards of therapy for excessive hypertension in acute stroke. Acta Med Scand 1980; 207:253–257.

65. Hillis AE, Ulatowski JA, Barker PB, et al. A pilot randomized trial of induced blood pressure elevation: effects on function and focal perfusion in acute and subacute stroke. Cerebrovasc Dis 2003; 16:236–246.

66. Rordorf G, Cramer SC, Efird JT, et al. Pharmacological elevation of blood pressure in acute stroke. Clinical effects and safety. Stroke 1997; 28:2133–2138.

67. Rordorf G, Koroshetz W, Ezzeddine MA, Segal AZ, Buonanno FS. A pilot study of drug-induced hypertension for treatment of acute stroke. Neurology 2001; 56:1210–1213.

68. Fagan SC, Bowes MP, Lyden PD, Zivin JA. Acute hypertension promotes hemorrhagic transformation in a rabbit embolic stroke model: effect of labetalol. Exp Neurol 1998; 150:153–158.

69. Martinsson L, Gunnar N, Wahlgren G. Safety of dexamphetamine in acute ischemic stroke. A randomized, double blind, controlled dose-escalation trial. Stroke 2003; 34:475–481.

70. Stoemer RP, Kent TA, Hulsebosch CE. Enhanced neocortical neural sprouting, synaptogenesis, and behavioral recovery with d-amphetamine therapy after neocortical infarction in rats. Stroke 1998; 29:2381–2395.

71. Progress Collaborative Group. Randomized trial of a perindopril-based blood pressure-lowering regimen among 6105 individuals with previous stroke or transient ischemic attack. Lancet 2001; 358:1033–1041.

72. Messerli FH, Hanley DF, Gorelick PB. Blood pressure control in stroke patients: what should the consulting neurologist advise? Neurology 2002; 1:23–25.

73. Chapman N, Huxley R, Anderson C, et al. Effects of perindopril-based blood pressure lowering regimen on the risk of recurrent stroke according to stroke subtype and medical history: the PROGRESS trial. Stroke 2004; 35:116–121.

74. Rothwell PM, Howard SC, Spence JD. Relationship between blood pressure and stroke risk in patients with symptomatic carotid occlusive disease. Stroke 2003; 34:2583–2590.

75. Cole F, Yates PO. Pseudo-aneurysms in relationship to massive cerebral hemorrhage. J Neurol Neurosurg Psychiatry 1967; 30:61–66.

76. Fisher CM. Pathological observations in hypertensive cerebral hemorrhage. J Neuropathol Exp Neurol 1971; 30:536–550.

77. Britton M, Carlsson A, de Faire U. Blood pressure course in patients with acute stroke and matched controls. Stroke 1986; 17:861–864.

78. Harper G, Castleden CM, Potter JF. Factors affecting changes in blood pressure after acute stroke. Stroke 1994; 25:1726–1729.

79. Fogelholm R, Avikainen S, Murros K. Prognostic value and determinants of first-day mean arterial pressure in spontaneous supratentorial intracerebral hemorrhage. Stroke 1997; 28:1396–1400.

80. Terayama Y, Tanahashi N, Fukuuchi Y, Gotoh F. Prognostic value of admission blood pressure in patients with intracerebral hemorrhage. Keio Cooperative Stroke Study. Stroke 1997; 28:1185–1188.

81. Qureshi AI, Safdar K, Weil J, et al. Predictors of early deterioration and mortality in black Americans with spontaneous intracerebral hemorrhage. Stroke 1995; 26:1764–1767.

82. Brott T, Broderick J, Kothari R, et al. Early hemorrhage growth in patients with intracerebral hemorrhage. Stroke 1997; 28:1–5.

83. Powers W, Adams RE, KD Y. Acute pharmacological hypotension after intracerebral hemorrhage does not change cerebral blood flow. The American Heart Association Conference, Nashville, TN, 1999.

84. Mayer SA, Lignelli A, Fink ME, et al. Perilesional blood flow and edema formation in acute intracerebral hemorrhage: a SPECT study. Stroke 1998; 29:1791–1798.

85. Sills C, Villar-Cordova C, WP. Demonstration of hypoperfusion surrounding intracerebral hematomas in humans. J Stroke Cerebrovasc Dis 1996; 6:17–24.

86. Kuwata N, Kuroda K, Funayama M, Sato N, Kubo N, Ogawa A. Dysautoregulation in patients with hypertensive intracerebral hemorrhage. A SPECT study. Neurosurg Rev 1995; 18(4):237–245.

87. Qureshi AI, Wilson DA, Hanley DF, Traystman RJ. Pharmacologic reduction of mean arterial pressure does not adversely affect regional cerebral blood flow and intracranial pressure in experimental intracerebral hemorrhage. Crit Care Med 1999; 27:965–971.

88. Zazulia AR, Diringer MN, Videen TO, Adams RE, Yundt K, Aiyagari V, Grubb RL, Powers WJ. Hypoperfusion without ischemia surrounding acute intracerebral hemorrhage. J Cerebral Blood Flow Metab 2001; 21:804–810.

89. Kidwell RW, Saver JL, Mattiello J, et al. Diffusion-perfusion MR evaluation of perihematomal injury in hyperacute intracerebral hemorrhage. Neurology 2001; 57:1611–1617.

90. Schellinger PD, Fiebach JB, Hoffmann K, et al. Stroke MRI in intracerebral hemorrhage: is there a perihemorrhagic penumbra? Stroke 2003; 34:1674–1679.

91. NINDS ICH Workshop Participants. Priorities for Clinical Research in Intracerebral Hemorrhage. Report From a national institute of neurological disorders and stroke workshop. Stroke 2005; 36:e23–e41.

92. Tietjen CS, Hurn PD, Ulatowski JA, Kirsch JR. Treatment modalities for hypertensive patients with intracranial pathology: options and risks. Crit Care Med 1996; 24:311–322.

93. Fujii Y, Takeuchi S, Sasaki O, Minakawa T, Tanaka R. Multivariate analysis of predictors of hematoma enlargement in spontaneous intracerebral hemorrhage. Stroke 1998; 29:1160–1106.

94. Kazui S, Minematsu K, Yamamoto H, Sawada T, Yamaguchi T. Predisposing factors to enlargement of spontaneous intracerebral hematoma. Stroke 1997; 28:2370–2375.

95. Dandapani BK, Suzuki S, Kelley RE, Reyes-Iglesias Y, Duncan RC. Relation between blood pressure and outcome in intracerebral hemorrhage. Stroke 1995; 26:21–24.

96. Qureshi AI, Bliwise DL, Bliwise NG, Akbar MS, Uzen G, Frankel MR. Rate of 24-hour blood pressure decline and mortality after spontaneous intracerebral hemorrhage: A retrospective analysis with a random effects regression model. Critical Care Med 1999; 27(3):480–485.

97. Ohwaki K, Yano, E, Nagashima H, Hirata M, Nakagomi T, Tamura A. Blood pressure management in acute intracerebral hemorrhage. Stroke 2004; 35:1364–1367.

98. McKissock W, Richardson A, Taylor J. Primary intracerebral hemorrhage: a controlled trial of surgical and conservative treatment in 180 unselected cases. Lancet 1961; 2:222–226.

99. Qureshi AI, Mohammad YM, Yahia AM, et al. A prospective multicenter study to evaluate the feasibility and safety of aggressive antihypertensive treatment in patients with acute intracerebral hemorrhage. J Intesive Care Med 2005; 20(1):34–42.

100. Diringer MN. Intracerebral hemorrhage: pathophysiology and management. Crit Care Med 1993; 21:1591–1603.

101. Tanaka H et al. Risk factors for cerebral hemorrhage and cerebral infarction in a Japanese rural community. Stroke 1982; 13:62–73.

102. Perry H et al. Effects of treating isolated systolic hypertension on the risk of developing various types and subtypes of stroke: the systolic hypertension in the elderly program (SHEP). J Am Med Assoc 2000; 284:465–471.

103. Arakawa S et al. Blood pressure control and recurrence of hypertensive brain hemorrhage. Stroke 1998; 29:1806–1809.

33 | Diagnosis and Treatment of Cerebral Arteriovenous Malformations

Abhishek Srinivas, MD
Stephen Chang, MD, Resident
Philippe Gailloud, MD, Associate Professor
Division of Interventional Neuroradiology, The Johns Hopkins Hospital, Baltimore, Maryland, USA

INTRODUCTION

The term "cerebral vascular malformations" covers a range of vascular anomalies that involve the brain and its surrounding tissue. Due to their slow-flow state, capillary telangiectasias and cavernous angiomas, both abnormalities of the capillary network, are not documented by cerebral angiography and are, therefore, defined as "angiographically occult" cerebrovascular malformations. Developmental venous anomalies (also known as venous angiomas) are aberrant venous drainage pathways that most commonly remain asymptomatic. Dural arteriovenous fistulas (AVFs) are high-flow vascular malformations that primarily involve the dural venous sinuses. Finally, arteriovenous malformations (AVMs) consist of tumorlike aggregations of abnormal blood vessels with high-flow arteriovenous shunting. This chapter focuses on the diagnosis and treatment of cerebral AVMs.

Cerebral AVMs occur in 0.14% to 0.50% of the population, with a mean diagnosis age of 31.2 years (1). The distribution is nearly equal between sexes, approximately 55% of the lesions being found in men. Ninety percent of cerebral AVMs are supratentorial, with only 10% located within the posterior fossa. Cerebral AVMs account for 1% to 2% of all strokes, 3% of strokes in young adults, and 9% of subarachnoid hemorrhages (1). Usually, they are single lesions, unless associated with hereditary hemorrhagic telangiectasia (2).

Nearly 53% of AVMs present with hemorrhage (3). On average, the annual risk of hemorrhage from a cerebral AVM has been estimated to range between 2% and 4% (4,5). However, patients who initially present with a hemorrhage have a high risk of recurrent bleed—between 6% and 17% in the first year after the event, decreasing to a baseline level after three years (6–8). After a second hemorrhage, the risk of further hemorrhage is even higher, reaching up to 25% within the first year (8). A prior bleed is, therefore, a strong predictor of the risk of hemorrhage (9). Other less prognostic, but nevertheless associated, predictors of hemorrhage include deep or impaired venous drainage, and presence of aneurysms on the feeding arteries of intranidal aneurysms or of multiple aneurysms (9). The mortality rate associated with the hemorrhagic presentation of an AVM ranges between 10% and 15%, with an overall morbidity rate of approximately 50% (10). Other common presentations include focal seizures in 30% of patients (11), persistent or progressive neurologic deficit in 12%, and headache in approximately 4% (12).

The basic pathophysiologic element of a cerebral AVM is an abnormal connection (or shunt) between a "feeding" artery and a "draining" vein. A cortical AVF is a vascular malformation limited to a single or a few arteriovenous shunts, whereas an AVM contains a large number of shunts, entangled in a central tumorlike component called the AVM nidus (1). The capillary bed, which is usually located between the arteries and the veins, is congenitally absent in AVMs. As a consequence, the arterial blood pressure is directly transmitted to the venous side of the lesion, contributing to the venous sinuosity and dilation typical of the disease. In addition, the high-flow nature of AVMs contributes to the development of flow-related phenomena, such as arterial and venous aneurysms, high-flow arteriopathy, and vascular steal phenomenon.

IMAGING OF AVMs

Despite the recent progress in noninvasive neurovascular imaging, digital subtraction angiography (DSA) remains the most accurate technique for the diagnosis of cerebrovascular disorders; however,

CT and MR imaging play a significant role in the diagnosis and management of cerebral AVMs. Fast and widely available, CT is the first-line imaging technique for patients presenting to the emergency department with a suspicion of acute intracranial hemorrhage. As such, CT is often the first imaging study obtained in patients with AVM (Fig. 1A). Although contrast-enhanced CT can confirm the presence of abnormal blood vessels in or around the hematomas, the role of CT angiography in the characterization of cerebral AVMs remains unknown. Nonruptured AVMs might be apparent on nonenhanced CT, in particular, when associated with large draining veins. Compression of the nidus by a hematoma can lead to underestimation of the actual size of an AVM by any imaging technique, and sometimes might completely prevent its detection (Fig. 1B and C). Such mass effect represents a pitfall, both for accurate diagnosis and for treatment planning of AVMs (1,13). MR imaging is a sensitive modality for the detection and localization of the nidus and its draining veins (Fig. 2A) and plays an important role in the planning of radiosurgical therapy, as well as in the follow-up of treated AVMs, as the nidus volume can be measured and followed temporally (1). MR angiography provides limited information on the nature of the feeding arteries and draining veins, the dynamic characteristics of the arteriovenous shunts, and the presence of associated vascular lesions such as extranidal and intranidal aneurysms (9). MR angiography is also poor at evaluating high-flow vascular malformations.

DSA remains the gold-standard imaging technique for evaluation of cerebral AVMs. Modern DSA is associated with extremely low complication risks (2). It offers precise information about the nidus configuration, the number, size, location, and characteristics of arterial feeders and draining veins. DSA also documents associated vascular anomalies with significant management implications, such as arterial and/or venous stenoses or occlusions, extranidal and intranidal aneurysms, or the presence of surrounding moya-moya-like vasculature that can

(A)   **(B)**

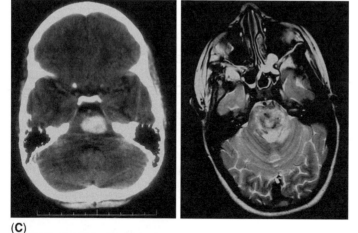

(C)

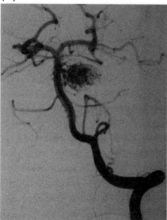

Figure 1 A 12-year-old girl with sudden headache and drowsiness. (**A**) Axial nonenhanced computed tomography showing a spontaneously hyperdense lesion within the pons consistent with acute hemorrhage. (**B**) Axial T2-weighted magnetic resonance imaging showing inhomogeneous signal in the pons corresponding to the hematomas, as well as several "flow-void" images that indicate the presence of fast-flowing vessels and suggest the presence of an arteriovenous malformation (AVM). (**C**) Digital subtraction angiography, left vertebral injection, showing a left paramedian pontine AVM nidus.

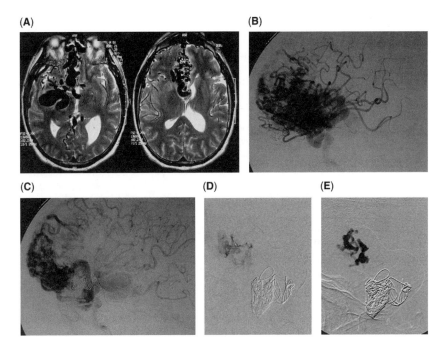

Figure 2 A 50-year-old man with new onset of seizures. (**A**) Axial T2-weighted magnetic resonance images showing a right paramedian frontal arteriovenous malformation (AVM) nidus and a large draining vein (*right image*), as well as an associated arteriovenous fistula (AVF) with prominent venous aneurysms (*left image*). The exact nature of the AVF was defined by subsequent digital subtraction angiography (DSA). (**B**) DSA, right internal carotid injection, showing the combination of the AVM nidus and large AVF. (**C**) digital subtraction angiography (DSA), right internal carotid injection, after treatment of the AVF by a combination of coiling and N-butyl-2-cyanoacrylate (NBCA) glue injection. The remaining part of the lesion consists of a now-typical AVM nidus that can be treated by staged NBCA embolization. (**D**) DSA, superselective injection of one of the AVM feeders through a flow-guided 1.2-French microcatheter (1 French = 0.33 mm). The fast-flowing arteriovenous connections dilute the contrast agent, resulting in a faint outline of the targeted nidus portion. (**E**) DSA, NBCA injection showing good casting of the targeted portion of the nidus without extension into the venous system.

simulate an AVM. Critical hemodynamic characteristics of the AVM, including the presence of very high-flow arteriovenous shunts within the nidus, are also better analyzed by angiography (Fig. 2A and B). Intraoperative DSA, i.e., angiography performed in the operating room to assist surgical treatment, is used both to help localize the AVM as the surgery progresses and to confirm the absence of residual AVM at the end of the resection (14).

AVM GRADING SYSTEM

The Spetzler–Martin scale is the most commonly used AVM gradation system in clinical practice. However, it is important to understand that the Spetzler–Martin scale is a surgical scale that categorizes AVMs by predicting the likelihood of satisfactory surgical outcome and, therefore, has little practical value for alternate therapeutic options, such as embolization and radiosurgery. The Spetzler–Martin grade of an AVM is determined by summing three individual scores. For the first score, based on size (as determined by measuring the largest diameter of the nidus on angiography), 1 is given for an AVM<3cm, 2 for an AVM between 3 and 6cm, and 3 for an AVM>6cm. For the second score, based on the eloquence (i.e., the functional importance of the adjacent brain tissue), 1 is given if the AVM is adjacent to eloquent tissue, 0 is attributed if it is not. Eloquent areas of brain tissue include sensorimotor, visual, and language areas, as well as thalamus, hypothalamus, internal capsule, brain stem, cerebellar peduncles, and deep cerebellar nuclei. The third score depends on whether the venous drainage of the AVM is superficial (score of 0) or has a deep component (score of 1). The sum of the three partial scores ranges between 1 and 5, the highest grades being associated with increased difficulty in surgical resection and poor surgical outcome (15).

MANAGEMENT OF CEREBRAL AVMs

Comprehensive management of cerebral AVMs requires a balanced, multidisciplinary, team approach that covers every treatment option offered by a specialized, tertiary care setting, including the service of vascular neurosurgeons, interventional neuroradiologists, radiation therapy specialists, neurointensivists, neuroanesthesiologists, and neurorehabilitation specialists. The choice of a treatment modality must take into account multiple factors that include the patient's clinical status and personal inclinations, initial presentation of the AVM, and its angioarchitecture and location. The available treatment options include radiosurgery, resection surgery, and endovascular embolization, as well as conservative management and observation.

AVM Surgery

Surgery has long been the gold standard for the treatment of intracranial AVMs. The most significant development to occur in this field has been the introduction and generalization of microsurgical techniques. In a series of more than 1200 patients treated over a 50-year period, a fivefold decrease in the mortality rate and a twofold decrease in the morbidity rate were documented for patients who underwent microsurgery as opposed to conventional surgery (16). Microsurgical resection of a small AVM located in the superficial or noneloquent brain achieves high-cure rates with low morbidity and remains the treatment of choice for such lesions (17). Besides microsurgery, such new technologies as functional MR imaging, intraoperative electrophysiologic cortical mapping, and neurosurgical navigation systems have also helped to decrease surgical morbidity and mortality. Functional MR imaging is a sensitive planning tool when used to detect critical cortical areas in patients with AVMs located near the language centers (18). Intraoperative stimulation mapping and corticography play a similar role during resection of AVMs located within eloquent tissue. Stimulation mapping can be used to delineate motor, sensory, and language areas, thus decreasing the risk of neurologic deficits during excision of critically located AVMs (19). Intraoperative DSA also plays an important role in the efficacy and safety of AVM resection by allowing precise localization of the nidus and its different feeders as the resection progresses and confirming the completeness of the treatment before skull closure (14). The latter is particularly important, as subtotal resection of cerebral AVMs alone does not reduce the risk of bleeding from the lesion (20). Embolization of an AVM as a preparation to the surgical resection also helps to decrease the surgical risk and will be discussed later in this chapter.

The reported efficacy of surgery in obtaining an angiographic cure ranges between 94% and 100%. The likelihood of angiographic cure varies slightly with the AVM location: Complete obliteration has been reported in 100% of patients with AVMs located in the Sylvian fissure or in the lateral ventricles and in 89% of patients with brain stem lesion (11). The efficacy of surgery also varies with the Spetzler–Martin grade of AVM (21). Larger AVMs and those with deep-draining veins are understandably associated with an increased operative risk. In general, AVMs<4cm located in noneloquent cortex can be resected with a 5% risk of complication, whereas the surgical risk of larger AVMs located adjacent to or within functional areas can be 10% to 20% (9). The risk of permanent major neurologic morbidity has been reported to be 0% in patients with Spetzler–Martin grade I, II, and III AVMs, whereas patients with grade IV and V AVMs had permanent, major, neurologic deficit rates of 22% and 17%, respectively (22). A retrospective assessment of the determinants of neurologic outcome in 124 patients who underwent surgical resection of their AVMs, at a mean follow-up duration of 12 months, revealed that the rates of disabling and nondisabling neurologic deficits were 6% and 32%, respectively (11,23). The clinical presentation obviously influences the functional outcome. One series showed that patients who presented with ruptured AVM and underwent microsurgical resection tended to improve clinically after therapy, whereas patients treated for unruptured AVMs were more susceptible to worsening of their neurologic function. The mean change in Modified Rankin Scale was +0.89 for patients with a ruptured AVM and –0.38 for patients with unruptured AVM (24).

AVM Radiosurgery

Stereotactic radiosurgery is a form of radiation therapy in which the radiation beam is precisely aimed at a focal spatial point localized by CT, MR imaging, and/or DSA (Fig. 3A–C). Stereotactic radiosurgery techniques include gamma knife, heavy-charged particles generated

(A)

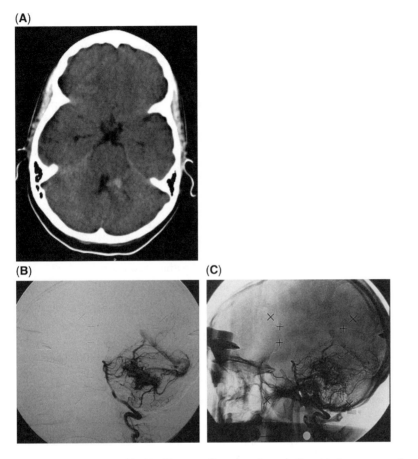

(B)   **(C)**

Figure 3 A 11-year-old girl with a small, ruptured cerebellar arteriovenous malformations (AVM). (**A**) Axial nonenhanced computed tomography showing a small hemorrhage near the left middle cerebellar pedicle. (**B**) Digital subtraction angiography (DSA), left vertebral artery injection (lateral view), showing the AVM nidus, fed by multiple small cerebral branches and draining into the straight sinus via the precentral vein. (**C**) DSA, same view as in (**B**), nonsubtracted image showing the stereotactic frame used for radiosurgery planning.

in a cyclotron, and linear accelerator (Linac). Gamma knife, which focuses a large number of cobalt-gamma radiation beams on the targeted nidus, is currently the most commonly used radiosurgical modality for AVM treatment. The principle of AVM radiation therapy is to create a radio-induced vascular injury that leads to nidus obliteration by endothelial cell proliferation (9). Complete obliteration occurs in approximately 80% of cases over a 1 to 3 year period of latency after radiosurgery. Radiosurgery has proven to be particularly useful in the treatment of cerebral AVMs that were previously considered inoperable due to their size, critical location, and/or deep venous drainage (high Spetzler–Martin grades) (25). Other advantages of radiosurgery include its fairly noninvasive nature (painless and short recovery time) and the lack of visible posttreatment markings (no skin incision); however, the risk of hemorrhage persists until the lesion has been totally eradicated (26). A series review of patients treated with gamma knife showed that lesions between 79.2% and 84.1% were obliterated at 2 year follow-up (27,28). Another study reported a total obliteration rate of 78.9% for a follow-up period of 2 years or more (29). The importance of documenting long-term clinical follow-up was evidenced in a study that showed that 4 of 48 (8%) patients with previously documented angiographic cures presented with new hemorrhages and recanalization of the AVM (30). Concerns have been raised that the hemorrhagic risk might increase during the latency period. It has been shown, however, that the annual risk of hemorrhage during the 1 to 3 year period of latency after radiosurgery remains comparable to the natural risk of hemorrhage of an untreated AVM (26,31). In fact, in a study of more than 500 patients, it was found that radiosurgery might actually decrease the risk of hemorrhage even before angiographic evidence of obliteration is seen (32).

Factors that contribute to potential treatment failures include changes in the nidus morphology after radiosurgery, because of resolution of a hematoma, poor technical planning, recanalization of a previously embolized portion of the AVM, and large AVM volume (>10 cc). Decreasing the radiation dose, because of the proximity of adjacent eloquent brain tissue, is also associated with treatment failure (11). Radiosurgery is most effective for AVMs with a volume <10 mL or a maximum diameter of <3 cm (27,33,34). Some view the ideal treatment volume for stereotactic radiosurgery to be between 1 and 10 mL, which correlates to grades I through III on the Spetzler–Martin Scale (35). However, a review of a series of 838 patients with radiosurgery-treated AVMs suggested that nidus obliteration was directly related to the radiation dose at the periphery of the AVM only and was independent of the AVM volume itself (36). Larger AVMs can be treated with staged-volume radiosurgery (37). By allowing a higher radiation dose to be delivered to the entire AVM volume, this staged approach increases the probability of total AVM obliteration, while considering the dose–volume relationship. In addition to nidus obliteration, radiosurgery has been shown to relieve AVM-related symptoms. In another series, 75% of patients with headache and 51% of patients with seizures reported improvement in their symptoms, whereas only 2% of patients experienced worsening (33). In a third series, 92% of patients with AVMs treated by radiosurgery could return to their previous employment, 72% were able to resume normal activities, 63% had decreased headache severity, and 52% had improved seizure control (38).

Reported complication rates for AVM radiosurgery range from 3.2% to 12.5%. A correlation has been noted between the incidence of radiation-related complications, the volume of tissue treated with > 12 Gy, and AVMs of deeper location (39). Delayed complications of radiosurgery include radiation necrosis, the development of tumefactive cysts (40), radio-induced Vasculitis, and chronic ischemia. A long-term follow-up of 53 patients treated with gamma-knife radiosurgery noted a 9.4% rate of radiation-related morbidities, including hemi–Parkinson syndrome, hemiparesis, and visual field disturbances (41). The risk of late stochastic effects of radiation, such as the occurrence of cerebral malignancy, has been raised more recently. Secondary malignancies have been reported to occur as early as 6 years after radiosurgery, and benign tumors have been reported to occur as late as 16 to 19 years postsurgery. Three of the 4 radio-induced malignancies reviewed in a study reported in 2003 (42) were glioblastoma multiforme; however, the authors considered the risk of secondary malignancy to be low.

AVM Embolization

The principles behind the endovascular approach to cerebral AVMs are (i) superselective access of the AVM feeders and nidus using minimally invasive, image-guided techniques and (ii) obliteration of the nidus and/or its feeders with an embolic agent (hence the name embolization) (Fig. 2D and E). Transarterial AVM embolization is safe and efficient in trained hands and with the support of adequate angiographic equipment. Although embolization can be curative in selected cases, with cure rates reaching 22% in certain series (43), its main role is currently the preparation of the AVM for either surgery or radiosurgery. By reducing the AVM volume and removing its highest flow components (frequently including large-caliber arteriovenous shunts "hidden" within the AVM nidus), embolization helps to minimize blood loss, to make surgical resections safer and shorter, and to increase the likelihood of successful radiosurgery.

Transarterial embolization of cerebral AVMs principally involves the use of liquid embolic agents such as N-butyl-2-cyanoacrylate (NBCA) and ethanol. Other less commonly used agents include calibrated microparticles, silk threads, and detachable microcoils. The efficacy of embolization depends on nidus penetration by the embolic agent. Therefore, microcoils should only be used to assist embolization with a penetrating agent, such as NBCA. Occasionally, microcoils are used in conjunction with glue to treat a fast-flow AVF located close to or within a more typical AVM nidus (Fig. 2B and C). Lower complication rates have been reported with NBCA than with other materials in the endovascular treatment of brain AVMs (44). Further, NBCA has been found to be better able to penetrate AVMs than polyvinyl alcohol (PVA) particles and is more biocompatible than other acrylate agents, and, because it can be used at a lower concentration than other acrylates, NBCA carries almost no risk of permanent microcatheter gluing (44). Preoperative AVM embolization with NBCA decreases the difficulty of surgery for AVMs of larger size and higher grade by reducing the operative time and intraoperative blood loss (45). NBCA is currently the embolic agent of choice for preoperative embolization of AVMs.

Although NBCA embolization is widely performed prior to radiosurgery or used as the sole AVM treatment modality, these indications presently constitute off-label use of the device.

Although acrylate agents have been routinely used in Europe for more than 20 years, PVA particles were the main embolic agent for preoperative embolization of AVMs in the United States prior to the approval of NBCA by the Food and Drug Administration. Because embolization with PVA particles does not penetrate the nidus of the AVM efficiently, the degree of devascularization of the lesion tends to be overestimated, and the chance of recanalization increases (46,47). Ethanol represents another alternative agent for AVM embolization. One series found no evidence of recanalization in patients after a mean follow-up time of 13 months (48). Although complications occurred in 8 of 17 patients (47%) (including short-term memory loss in one patient and subarachnoid hemorrhage and death in two patients), it was concluded that ethanol has a permanence not observed in most other embolic agents (48). A new biocompatible liquid ethylene vinyl alcohol copolymer preparation is the most recently developed agent for AVM embolization. Several advantages of this new agent over NBCA have been suggested, including better penetration of the nidus and easier use, while disadvantages include a relative inability to treat high-flow shunts due to slow polymerization and relatively high microcatheter retention rates. At the time of writing of this chapter, this new agent has not been approved for AVM embolization in the United States.

CONCLUSION

Cerebral AVMs are complex congenital vascular malformations with significant clinical implications, including the risks of intracranial hemorrhage, seizure, stroke, and death. Although cerebral AVMs are most often detected by CT and/or MR imaging, DSA remains the optimal technique for precise characterization of the AVM nidus, its feeders, and its draining veins, as well as for the detection of associated significant anomalies, such as intranidal and extranidal aneurysms and high-flow AVFs. Optimal therapeutic planning requires a multidisciplinary approach, including expertise in vascular neurosurgery, radiation therapy, and interventional neuroradiology. The best treatment option is a case-by-case decision and might involve one or a combination of the following techniques: conventional surgical resection, stereotactic radiosurgery, and endovascular embolization.

REFERENCES

1. Al-Shahi R, Warlow C. A systematic review of frequency and prognosis of arteriovenous malformations of the brain in adults. Brain 2001; 124:1900.
2. Jessurum GA, Kamphuis DJ, van der Zande FH, Nossent JC. Cerebral arteriovenous malformations in the Netherlands Antilles: high prevalence of hereditary hemorrhagic telangiectasia-related single and multiple cerebral arteriovenous malformations. Clin Neurol Neurosurg 1993 Sep; 95(3):193-198.
3. Hofmeister C, Stapf C, Hartmann A, et al. Demographic, morphological, and clinical characteristics of 1289 patients with brain arteriovenous malformation. Stroke 2000; 31:1307–1310.
4. Kondziolka D, McLaughlin MR, Kestle JR. Simple risk predictions for arteriovenous malformation hemorrhage. Neurosurgery 1995; 37:851–855.
5. Brown RD Jr. Simple risk predictions for arteriovenous malformation hemorrhage (letter). Neurosurgery 2000; 46:1024.
6. Graf CJ, Perret GE, Torner JC. Bleeding from cerebral arteriovenous malformation as part of their natural history. J Neurosurg 1983; 58:331–337.
7. Mast H, Young WL, Koennecke HC, et al. Risk of spontaneous haemorrhage after diagnosis of cerebral arteriovenous malformation. Lancet 1997; 350:1065–1068.
8. Forster DM, Steiner L, Hakanson S. Arteriovenous malformations of the brain: a long-term clinical study. J Neurosurg 1972; 37:562–570.
9. Brown RD, Flemming KD, Meyer FB, Cloft HJ, Pollock BE, Link ML. Natural history, evaluation, and management of intracranial vascular malformations. Mayo Clin Proc. 2005; 80(2):269–281.
10. Samson DS, Batjer HH. Preoperative evaluation of the risk/benefit ratio for arteriovenous malformations of the brain: a 24-year follow-up assessment. J Neurosurg 1990; 73:387–391.
11. Fleetwood IG, Steinberg GK. Arteriovenous malformations. Lancet 2002; 359:863–873.
12. Brown RDJ, Wiebers DO, Torner JC, O'Fallon WM. Frequency of intracranial hemorrhage as a presenting symptom and subtype analysis: a population-based case study of intracranial vascular malformations in Olmsted Country, Minnesota. J Neurosurg 1996; 85:29–32.

13. The Arteriovenous Malformation Study Group. Arteriovenous malformations of the brain in adults. N Engl J Med 1999; 340(23):1812–1818.

14. Hashimoto H, Iida J, Hironaka Y, Sakaki T. Surgical management of cerebral arteriovenous malformations with intraoperative digital subtraction angiography. J Clin Neuroscience 2000; 7 (Suppl 1):33–35.

15. Spetzler RF, Martin NA. A proposed grading system for arteriovenous malformations. J Neurosurg 1986; 65:476–483.

16. Zhao J, Wang S, Jingsheng L, Wei Q, Sui D, Zhao Y. Clinical characteristics and surgical results of patients with cerebral arteriovenous malformations. Surg Neurol 2005; 63:156–161.

17. Schaller C, Schramm J, Haun D. Significance of factors contributing to surgical complications and to late outcome after surgery of cerebral arteriovenous malformations. J Neurol Neurosurg Psychiatry 1998; 65:547–554.

18. Pouratian N, Bookheimer SY, Rex DE, Martin NA, Toga AW. Utility of preoperative functional magnetic resonance imaging for identifying language cortices in patients with vascular malformations. Neurosurg Focus 2002; 15:13–14.

19. Burchiel KJ, Clarke H, Ojemann GA, Dacey RG, Winn. Use of stimulation mapping corticography in the excision of arteriovenous malformations in sensorimotor and language-related neocortex. Neurosurgery 1989; 24:322–327.

20. Drake CG. Cerebral arteriovenous malformation: considerations for and experience with surgical treatment in 166 cases. Clin Neurosurg 1979; 26:145–208.

21. Lawton MT. UCSF Brain Arteriovenous Malformation Study Project. Spetzler-Martin Grade III arteriovenous malformations: surgical results and a modification of the grading scale. Neurosurgery 2003; 52(4):740–748.

22. Hamilton MG, Spetzler RF. The prospective application of a grading system for arteriovenous malformations. Neurosurgery 1994; 34:2–7.

23. Hartmann A, Stapf C, Hofmeister C, et al. Determinants of neurological outcome after surgery for brain arteriovenous malformation. Stroke 2000; 31:2361–2364.

24. Lawton MT, Du R, Tran MN, Achrol AS, McCulloch CE, et al. Effect of presenting hemorrhage on outcome after microsurgical resection of brain arteriovenous malformations. Neurosurgery 2005; 56:485–493.

25. Jawahar A, Jawahar LL, Nanda A, et al. Stereotactic radiosurgery using leksell gamma knife: current trends and future directives. Frontiers Biosci 9:932–938.

26. Friedman WA, Blatt DL, Bova FJ, Buatti JM, Mendenhall WM, Kubilis PS. The risk of hemorrhage after radiosurgery for arteriovenous malformations. J Neurosurg 1996; 84:912–919.

27. Ogilvy CS. Radiation therapy for arteriovenous malformations: a review. Neurosurgery 1990; 26:725–735.

28. Levy RP, Fabrikant JI, Frankel KA, et al. Stereotactic heavy-charged-particle Bragg peak radiosurgery for the treatment of intracranial arteriovenous malformations in childhood and adolescence. Neurosurgery 1989; 24:841–852.

29. Chang JH, Chang JW, Park YG, et al. Factors related to complete occlusion of arterio-venous malformations after gamma knife radiosurgery. J Neurosurg 2000; 3:96–101.

30. Lindqvist M, Karlsson B, Guo WY, Kihlostrom L, Lippitz B, Yamamoto M. Angiographic long-term follow-up data for arteriovenous malformations previously proven to be obliterated after gamma knife radiosurgery. Neurosurgery 2000; 46:803–810.

31. Pollock BE, Flickinger JC, Lundsford LD, Bissonette DJ, Kondziolkalnm D. Hemorrhage risk after stereotactic radiosurgery of cerebral arteriovenous malformations. Neurosurgery 1996; 38:652–659.

32. Maruyama K, Kawahara N, Masahiro S, et al. The risk of hemorrhage after radiosurgery for cerebral arteriovenous malformations. New Engl J Med. 2005; 25:146–153.

33. Lunsford LD, Kondziolka D, Flickinger JC, et al. Stereotactic radiosurgery for arteriovenous malformations of the brain. J Neurosurg 1991; 75:512–524.

34. Steiner L, Lindquist C, Adler JR, et al. Clinical outcome of radiosurgery for cerebral arteriovenous malformations. J Neurosurg 1992; 77:1–8.

35. Lawton MT, Hamilton MG, Spetzler RF. Multimodality treatment of deep arteriovenous malformation: thalamus, basal ganglia, and brainstem. Neurosurgery 1995; 37:29–36.

36. Karlsson B, Lax I, Soderman M. Can the probability for obliteration after radiosurgery for arteriovenous malformations be accurately predicted? Int J Radiat Oncol Biol Phys 1999; 43:313–319.

37. Pollock BE, Kline RW, Stafford SL, Foote RL, Schomber PJ. The rationale and technique of staged-volume arteriovenous malformation radiosurgery. Int J Radiat Oncol Biol Phys 2000; 48:817–824.

38. Pollock BE, Lunsford LD, Kondziolka D, et al. Patient outcomes after stereotactic radiosurgery for operable arteriovenous malformations. Neurosurgery 1994; 35:1–8.

39. Flinkinger JC, Kondziolka D, Lunsford LD, et al. Arteriovenous malformation radiosurgery study group. Development of a model to predict permanent symptomatic postradiosurgery injury for arteriovenous malformation patients. Int J Radiat Oncol Biol Phys 2000; 46:1143–1148.

40. Edmister WB, Lane JI, Gilbertson JR, Brown RD, Pollock BE. Tumefactive cysts: a delayed complication following radiosurgery for cerebral arterial venous malformations. AJNR Am J Neuroradiol 2005; 26(5):1152–1157.
41. Yamamoto M, Hara M, Ide M, Ono Y, Jimbo M, Saito I. Radiation-related adverse effects observed on neuro-imaging several years after radiosurgery for cerebral arteriovenous malformations. Surg Neurol 1998; 49:385–398.
42. Loeffler JS, Niemierko A, Chapman PH. Second tumors after radiosurgery: tip of the iceberg or a bump in the road? Neurosurgery 2003; 52(6):1436–1440; discussion 1440–1442.
43. Yu SC, Chan MS, Lam JM, Tam PH, Poon WS. Complete obliteration of intracranial arteriovenous malformation with endovascular cyanoacrylate embolization: initial success and rate of permanent cure. AJNR Am J Neuroradiol 2004; 25(7):1139–1143.
44. Liu HM, Huang YC, Wang YH. Embolization of cerebral arteriovenous malformations with n-butyl-2-cyanoacrylate. J Formos Med Assoc 2000; 99(12):906–913.
45. Jafar JJ, Davis AJ, Berenstein A, Choi IS, Kupersmith MJ. The effect of embolization with N-butyl cyanoacrylate prior to surgical resection of cerebral arteriovenous malformations. J Neurosurg 1993; 78(1):60–69.
46. Sorimachi T, Koike T, Takeuchi S, et al. Embolization of cerebral arteriovenous malformations achieved with PVA particles: angiographic reappearance and complications. AJNR Am J Neuroradiol 1999; 20(7):1323–1328.
47. Germano IM, Davis RL, Wilson CB, Hieshima GB. Histopathological follow-up study of 66 cerebral arteriovenous malformations after therapeutic embolization with polyvinyl alcohol. J Neurosurg 1992; 76(4):607–614.
48. Yakes WF, Krauth L, Ecklund J, et al. Ethanol endovascular management of brain arteriovenous malformations: initial results. Neurosurgery 1997; 40(6):1145–1152; discussion 1152–1154.

34 | Endovascular Therapy for Carotid Stenosis

Alison J. Nohara, MD, Medical Director
Interventional Neuroradiology, Eden Medical Center,
Castro Valley, California, USA

INTRODUCTION

As the population ages, the number of reported age-associated diseases increases. One of these diseases is atherosclerosis. Although atherosclerosis can occur in any arterial location, one critical location is at the carotid bifurcation, as it restricts blood flow to the internal carotid artery and, hence, the brain. Stroke is the third leading cause of death, and the leading cause of adult disability in the United States. More than 80% of these strokes are ischemic in nature, and 35% to 40% of ischemic strokes are direct results of large-vessel atherosclerosis (1). Carotid endarterectomy (CEA), surgical removal of plaque, was pioneered in the 1950s and has become established as the preferred intervention for treating carotid artery stenosis.

In the late 1990s, the first carotid angioplasty/stenting procedures were conducted (2–5), whereby, via a catheter and under fluoroscopic observation, a balloon (with or without a balloon-expandable stent) was placed at the level of the stenosis and used to expand the narrowing. This procedure represented a potential alternative to CEA and a significant development in the field of endovascular intervention. However, the rates of risk associated with those early procedures—approximately 10% (3,6,7)—did not compare favorably with complication rates for CEA. The 1991 North American Symptomatic Carotid Endarterectomy Trial (NASCET) documented significant benefits of CEA for symptomatic patients who had stenosis of >70% and reported an overall rate of 6.5% for perioperative stroke or death and a rate of 2% for permanent disability or death (8). It is important to recognize, however, that these results were achieved with specific sets of patient and surgeon selection criteria that limit the validity of comparisons to the few existing studies of carotid stenting. For example, centers were excluded from the NASCET if their rates of complication were >6%. Complication rates <6% for CEA might be found among experienced surgeons who perform the procedure frequently but are not as common in the wider community; hence, this biased selectivity became the major criticism of the collaborative work. The 1995 Asymptomatic Carotid Atherosclerosis Study (ACAS) (9), which reported benefit from surgery in patients with stenosis >60%, used an even more selective surgical complication rate of 3%. Even so, data from both of these studies is frequently utilized to make patient management decisions.

The Carotid Revascularization Endarterectomy versus Stent Trial was initiated to develop comparable data for the 2 procedures but has been slow to achieve patient enrollment and is still underway. Given the improvements in technology in carotid stenting, including the development of distal protection devices, carotid stenting might well be proven to be a viable alternative to CEA. However, until that time, its use is likely to remain limited to 2 patient populations: those who are poor surgical candidates for CEA and those who suffer restenosis.

In part, because the NASCET excluded high-risk surgical candidates, resistance to the use of carotid stenting for such patients has been considerably less. The benefit of carotid stenting in these patients was given further support by the Stenting and Angioplasty with Protection in Patients at High Risk for Endarterectomy (SAPPHIRE) study (10,11), which showed slightly improved outcomes and shorter hospitalizations in patients with endovascular treatment, compared to those with surgical treatment. In 2005, the Centers for Medicare and Medicaid Services approved Medicare coverage for carotid stenting for high-risk CEA patients with symptomatic stenosis >70% and for high-risk CEA patients who are enrolled in Category B investigational device exemption clinical trials and have symptomatic stenosis between 50% and 70% or asymptomatic stenosis >80% (12).

Restenosis, or *recurrent stenosis*, is a condition that is present in approximately 20% of patients who receive CEA (13–16). Its etiology has a biphasic distribution. In the first 24 months post CEA, restenosis usually represents intimal hyperplasia from the surgical manipulation. After 2 years, it is more commonly due to recurrent atherosclerotic disease. Intimal hyperplasia is smooth and easily expanded by balloon angioplasty. Embolic phenomena are rare, as the lesion is not as friable as atheromatous plaque. The risk of repeat surgery is approximately 12%, and increases in these patients (6,17) due to risk of nerve injury at the prior operative site. Therefore, carotid angioplasty, with or without stents, is commonly performed in this patient population.

When making the recommendation for carotid angioplasty/stenting, it is important to consider the marginal improvements of outcome. From a procedural viewpoint, it has become easier to perform these interventions. Hence, now the more difficult question must be addressed: which patients truly benefit from the revascularization? For the surgical opening of the carotid artery, NASCET has made it clear that patients who have 69% or greater stenosis with symptoms referable to the distribution should be treated (8). ACAS additionally provided proof that patients with 80% or greater stenosis would benefit, even if asymptomatic (9). The SAPPHIRE study demonstrated that patients with high degrees of stenosis who are poor candidates for CEA can still benefit from revascularization in the form of carotid stenting. The length of time that a patient needs to live after the procedure to reap the benefits of the risks involved, and the therapy that current medical management can provide for patients without intervention remain unclear factors. For example, with the introduction of Statin medications, a 20% to 35% reduction in stroke has been documented in patients with atherosclerotic disease (18–20). The NASCET study did not take these newer drugs into account; therefore, the marginal improvement of risk from surgical or endovascular repair might now be reduced.

PREPARATION FOR CAROTID STENTING

As mentioned above, patient selection is critical. Using the standards established in NASCET for measuring the degree of stenosis, patients should have symptomatic disease >69% or asymptomatic disease >80%. They should be poor surgical candidates but have a life expectancy >5 years. Although noninvasive methods can document stenosis, assessment of the degree of stenosis is fairly inaccurate. In NASCET, as well as ACAS, official cervical angiograms were used to assess the degree of stenosis.

The patient should be placed on an antiplatelet regimen, either clopidogrel or ticlopidine hydrochloride, as well as aspirin. Clopidogrel loading takes at least 4 days at a dose of 75 mg/day. Some prefer to load with 300 mg on the day before the procedure. However, a subset of patients will be resistant to this load and require more days to obtain therapeutic levels of clopidogrel. Presently, no laboratory level exists for testing the efficacy of this dosing regimen. The literature does not establish an exact level of aspirin, but 81 mg is the minimal dose. Tests should be performed to assess renal function through the blood urea nitrogen (BUN)/creatinine levels and ratio. Iodinated contrast is excreted by the kidneys, and if the renal creatinine is >2.0, it predisposes the patient to acute renal toxicity and failure. In patients with marginally elevated renal creatinines (1.6–2.0), protocols to maximize renal excretion and protect the working nephrons can be used. The major emphasis of these regimens is aggressive hydration. Prothrombin time and partial thromboplastin time should be obtained to evaluate bleeding risk, both at the access point as well as to the poorly perfused brain. Some patients in the stenting group might require warfarin sulfate, and they will require placement on heparin sodium periprocedurally. The heparin sodium can be continued until the time of the procedure, as heparin sodium is routinely used for cerebral angiograms. Hematocrit and white count can be performed as a general assessment to ensure reasonable cardiac reserve and no active bacterial infection. Standards vary by institution, but if anesthesia is used for these cases, preoperative evaluation with the anesthesia service is recommended.

Patients should be nothing by mouth (NPO) from midnight, the night before the procedure. Careful consideration should be given to which medications are taken prior to the procedure. Withholding antihypertensives could lead to uncontrolled hypertension, which could cause hemorrhagic stroke during reperfusion. Oral hyperglycemic medications are potentially associated with postprocedure lactic acidosis. On the other hand, hyperglycemia is detrimental to the ischemic brain. Therefore, preprocedural hyperglycemia should be treated with insulin. (The patient does need to continue aspirin and antiplatelet regimens.) Examination should be performed prior to the procedure by the procedural team to establish the patient's baseline. The patient will need to be consented and consulted by the anesthesiology team, if that is the norm. It is helpful to place a urinary catheter, as the patient will be supine for at least 2 hr. If the patient has never had a CEA or previous manipulation of the carotid bulb, it is recommended that an external pacemaker be placed on the patient or available in the room to treat possible bradycardia, resulting from parasympathetic excitation during dilation of the bulb. This response is exaggerated occasionally, requiring emergent pharmacotherapy.

PROCEDURE

A thorough diagnostic angiogram should be performed to observe both the lesion and the collateral flow to the brain. Although the carotid artery is the immediate target for repairing flow, the overall goal is to improve cerebral perfusion; thus, the true target of the intervention is the brain. Knowing the level of diminished flow to the brain and the potential conduits for collateral flow facilitates establishment of the necessity for the procedure and the potential risks to the patient during the procedure. The Circle of Willis is not complete in all patients and may exhibit many variations with only 20% to 25% of the population having complete collateral pathways (21).

Ideally, carotid stenting should be performed under moderate sedation, allowing the team members to quickly evaluate the neurologic consequences of intervention. However, some patients will not be able to stay motionless at critical points in the procedure, which could lead to a devastating outcome. These patients would benefit from a general anesthetic technique that will allow for rapid emergence following completion of the procedure and immediate postprocedure neurologic evaluation.

The procedure is initiated with catheterization of the common carotid artery on the side of stenosis. Via an exchange over a guidewire or via direct catheterization, the equivalent of an 8-French guiding catheter is stably placed into the common carotid artery. Angiograms are performed, measurements are taken, and careful determination of the appropriate diameter is made. Then length of the balloon (stent) is selected based on the length of the stenosis and the diameter of the native vessel. After the balloon/stent system is chosen, the common carotid artery is accessed. Distal protection, usually a wire-mounted basket, can be placed over a micro-guidewire, and the balloon (stent) is placed through the lesion. Distal protection devices should be placed below the skull base in a straight segment of the carotid. The device is inflated, and deployment of the stent is performed. Angiograms are performed until the operator is satisfied with the diameter restoration. Additional balloon inflations with the same or larger balloons might be required for optimal dilation. Final angiograms are performed intracranially to document normalization of flow and transit time from the arteries to the veins, thereby ensuring no significant emboli. The system can then be removed, and the patient can emerge from anesthesia.

ROUTINE POSTPROCEDURAL CARE

It is recommended that the patient remain heparinized overnight, with international normalised ratios of approximately 2.0 to 2.5 to protect against clot formation along the stent. To ensure that the patient does not bleed from the access site, either the sheath should be secured into place or a closure device should be used. If it is decided that the sheath stay in place overnight, the patient must remain supine and the sheath must be monitored and kept open throughout the period of risk. Patients who still have a sheath in place can be placed in a reverse Trendelenburg position, so that they have some ability to eat and socialize while in the unit.

Patients should remain on aspirin and clopidogrel for 4 to 8 weeks to prevent the development of in-stent thrombosis. Dose variation is usually determined by the level of medical risk to the patient. Usually, patients who develop carotid disease also have vascular disease in other territories; therefore, aspirin is usually recommended indefinitely, unless it is contraindicated by some other factor.

Post procedure, the patient should recover in an intensive care unit setting, preferably a unit dedicated to neurosciences, as frequent neurologic checks are recommended no less than once every 2 hr. Groin checks are frequent (every 15 min for the first hour, and once per hour thereafter).

COMPLICATIONS

Although carotid stenting patients are generally older with many medical comorbidities, due to the lower invasiveness of the endovascular approach, these patients now emerge from the procedure with relatively low complications—hence, its Medicare approval. Following are the more common complications and the associated postprocedural concerns.

Cardiovascular

As stated earlier, in patients who have not already undergone carotid surgery, the barorecep-tors are present in the carotid bulb. During stretching of the stenosis, the baroreceptors can be activated, causing bradycardia. In some patients, this response is overly exaggerated, caus-ing asystole. Usually, when the stimulus is removed, the heart rate responds, but not always. Again, these patients have many comorbidities, including cardiac disease. Patients who have prolonged bradycardia or asystole will require close monitoring to observe and treat any fur-ther stress on the heart.

Additionally, during the procedure, all of the lines infuse heparinized saline. Depending on the length of the procedure and the rate of administration, patients could receive >3 L of fluids. In younger patients, this might be identified as only a slight dilution of the hematocrit (hematocrit reduction of 3–6% is commonly seen in this scenario). However, in older patients, excess fluid can critically raise the cardiac filling pressures, resulting in pulmonary edema and frank cardiac failure.

Neurologic

Patients who have critically low perfusion to a hemisphere can have what is termed as "shock brain," in which, in spite of good reperfusion of a hemisphere, the patient has a globally dimin-ished neurologic examination for approximately 24 hr. This condition is usually limited in time, and with time, the brain function responds to the new perfusion.

Recent stroke in a patient is a relative contraindication to stent placement, because, if the stroke is large enough, reperfusion hemorrhage will occur if the territory is reperfused when the blood–brain barrier is still considered regulated to a lower perfusion pressure. The larger the territory of stroke, the more profound the repercussions of bleeding into the site and the stronger the contraindication for doing the procedure in the first place. Obviously, patient selection is performed on a case-by-case basis, with knowledge of other perfusion that the patient may or may not have had. Small lacunar infarcts can be treated in the acute setting, depending on the patient's symptoms and vascular reserve. These cases harbor more hazards, as the team performing the procedure and the team receiving the patient must be aware of the increased risks of hemorrhage. If any patient has a focal neurologic change during examination, noncontrast head computed tomography is the first study that should be performed to assess hemorrhage and/or stroke. Although the goal of neurointerventional procedures (carotid stenting or angioplasty) is to prevent stroke, stroke is the most common and most devastating complication of these procedures.

Renal

As mentioned above, the iodinated contrast that is used in angiography, although safer than in previous years, still is a significant cause of renal toxicity. The higher the dose, the more common is renal failure. A longer, more complicated procedure usually is indicative of a larger contrast dose. The patient's creatinine level should be checked before discharge to ensure nor-mal or baseline function. Additional risk of renal toxicity exists for patients who take oral hyperglycemic medications. Therefore, their medications should be held for 48 hr, and their renal function should be checked more frequently after discharge.

Groin

A small but real risk of groin complications exists for patients who undergo an angiogram. The risk increases slightly with prolonged sheath placement, use of closure devices, and anti-coagulation, with the main risk being hemorrhage and vessel damage. Significant hematocrit shifts might indicate a retroperitoneal hemorrhage, and significant compartmentalization into the muscles of the thigh might occur, without external detection. Contained hematomas in the groin are uncomfortable for the patient but not life threatening. Pseudoaneurysm in the groin vessels can occur as a late complication secondary to large local hematoma.

SUMMARY AND CONCLUSIONS

Since the advent of carotid angioplasty and stenting, practitioners have become more proficient, and the tools available to them have become smaller and more sophisticated. The procedures are used routinely for patients who are poor candidates for CEA and in cases of restenosis. Complications include surgical comorbidities common among older patients, those associated with insertion of catheters and the use of contrast, stroke (the risk of which is slightly increased over other cerebral angiographic procedures due to the presence of atherosclerotic disease), and bradycardia and assytoli resulting from the stretching of the baroreceptors in the carotid bifurcation. The use of carotid stenting is likely to increase, as it has recently been approved for coverage under Medicare to treat carotid stenosis >80% in patients with high-surgical risk. Given that the most recent improvements in all types of treatment—CEA, stenting, and nonsurgical—have not yet been fully evaluated and compared, it remains important for the field to continue to try to understand the natural history of atherosclerotic disease and to better understand what and when a plaque becomes unstable. For individual practitioners, the decisions of if, when, and how to intervene must be weighed carefully in each case.

REFERENCES

1. Marks M, Do HM. Endovascular and Percutaneous Therapy of the Brain and Spine. Philadelphia, Pennsylvania: Lippincott Williams and Wilkins, 2002.
2. Roubin GS, Yadav S, Iyer SS, et al. Carotid stent-supported angioplasty: a neurovascular intervention to prevent stroke. Am J Cardiol 1996; 78:8–12.
3. Diethrick EB, Ndiaya M, Reid DB. Stenting in the carotid artery: initial experience in 110 patients. J Endovasc Surg 1997; 3:42–62.
4. Criado FJ, Wellons E, Clark NS. Evolving indications for and early results of carotid artery stenting. Am J Surg 1997; 174:111–114.
5. Vozzi CR, Rodriguez AO, Paolantionio D, et al. Extracranial carotid angioplasty and stenting: initial results and short-term follow-up. Tex Heart Inst J 1997; 24:167–172.
6. Kasiragan K. Regarding "Preprocedural risk stratification: identifying an appropriate population for carotid stenting." J Vasc Surg 2002; 35(2):407–408.
7. Brooks WH, McClure RR, Jones MR, et al. Carotid angioplasty and stenting versus carotid endarterectomy: randomized trial in a community hospital. J Am Coll Cardiol 2001; 38(6):1589–1595.
8. North American Symptomatic Carotid Endarterectomy Trial Collaborators. Beneficial effect of carotid endarterectomy in symptomatic patients with high-grade carotid stenosis. N Engl J Med 1991; 325(7): 445–453.
9. Executive Committee for the Asymptomatic Carotid Atherosclerosis Study. Endarterectomy for asymptomatic carotid artery stenosis. JAMA 1995; 273(18):1421–1427.
10. Yadav JS. Carotid stenting in high-risk patients: design and rationale of the SAPPHIRE trial. Cleveland Clin J Med 2004; 71(suppl):S45–S46.
11. Yadav JS, Wholey MH, Kuntz RE, et al. Protected carotid-artery stenting versus endarterectomy in high-risk patients. N Engl J Med. 2004; 351(15):1493–1501.
12. Phurrough S, Salive M, Hogarth R, et al. Coverage Decision Memorandum for Carotid Artery Stenting; Centers for Medicare and Medicaid Services: Washington, D.C., March 17, 2005.
13. Archie J. Reoperations for carotid artery stenosis: role of primary and secondary reconstructions. J Vasc Surg 2001; 33(3):495–503.
14. Dillavou ED, Kahn MB, Carabasi RA, et al. Long-term follow-up of reoperative carotid surgery. Am J Surg 1999; 178:197–200.
15. Ricotta J, O'Brian-Irr M. Conservative management of residual and recurrent lesions after carotid endarterectomy: long-term results. J Vasc Surg 1997; 26(6):963–969.
16. Samson RH, Showalter DP, Yunis JP, et al. Hemodynamically significant early recurrent carotid stenosis: an often self-limiting and self-reversing condition. J Vasc Surg 1999; 30(3):446–452.
17. AbuRahma AF, Jennings TG, Wulu JT, et al. Redo carotid endarterectomy versus primary carotid endarterectomy. Stroke 2001; 32:2787–2792.

18. Blauw GJ, Lagaay AM, Smelt AH, et al. Stroke, statina and cholesterol. A meta-analysis of randomized, placebo-controlled, double-blind trials with HMG-CoA reductase inhibitors. Stroke 1997; 28:946–950.

19. Warshafsky S, Packard D, Marks SJ, et al. Efficacy of 3-hydroxy-3-methylglutaryl coenzyme A reductase inhibitors for prevention of stroke. J Gen Intern Med 1999; 14:763–774.

20. Di Mascio R, Marchioli R, Tognoni G. Cholesterol reduction and stroke occurrence: an overview of randomized clinical trials. Cerebrovasc Dis 2000; 10:85–92.

21. Osborn, AG. Diagnostic Neuroradiology. Mosby: St. Louis, 1994.

35 | Acute Stroke Care Units: A Critical Appraisal

Paul A. Nyquist, MD, MPH, Assistant Professor of Neurology

Neurosciences Critical Care Division, Departments of Neurology, Neurological Surgery, Anesthesiology, and Critical Care Medicine, Johns Hopkins University School of Medicine, Baltimore, Maryland, USA

Anish Bhardwaj, MD, FAHA, FCCM, Professor[a] and Director[b]

[a] Departments of Neurology, Neurological Surgery, and Anesthesiology & Perioperative Medicine,
[b] Neurosciences Critical Care Program, Oregon Health & Science University, Portland, Oregon, USA

INTRODUCTION

The effect of an acute stroke unit (ASU) on the care of stroke patients in the United States has never been adequately tested. Consequently, many critical questions remain. Do ASUs represent an improvement in health-care delivery in the U.S. health-care system? Can ASUs in the United States improve functional independence if most rehabilitation is provided at a separate facility from the ASU? Is the emphasis in the United States on reduction of acute care costs, morbidity, and mortality enough to justify the development of ASUs? Despite these unanswered critical questions, the ASU will soon emerge as a growing presence in the U.S. hospital system. ASUs are growing in number as the need for certified primary stroke centers increases. Their presence will offer new opportunities for stroke professionals to expand and improve the treatment options available to patients with acute stroke.

The most common portal of entry for patients with acute stroke in the U.S. medical system is through the emergency department, where they are triaged and rendered acute treatment. A limited number of therapeutic interventions is available in the emergency setting for patients with ischemic stroke and involve two primary modalities: intravenous (IV) recombinant tissue plasminogen activator (rtPA) and intra-arterial thrombolysis (1,2). In the coming years, newer technology will be widely utilized for efficacious treatment of acute stroke, even when administered in a delayed fashion after the onset of stroke symptoms. Clinicians will be using technologies, such as diffusion-weighted and perfusion-weighted MRI and CT studies, to identify patients with perfusion/diffusion mismatch (3,4), who will be potential candidates for a host of new treatments, including new types of thrombolytics and intra-arterial recannalization, with new mechanical clot removing devices (5). These new technologies will require training and equipping a group of dedicated health-care providers with the proper resources.

Strategies for interventions focused on improved outcomes in specific disease states require highly trained medical personnel with an array of therapeutic options that allow for flexibility in the care of patients with complex pathology. The specialty concept has led to the development of specialty units, such as cardiac care units, ICU, and neurocritical care units. The increased treatment and observational vigilance implemented in these units work synergistically with increased resource density to improve outcomes and reduce costs (6,7). Neurologic units that specialize in critically ill neurologic patients are associated with decreased lengths of stay, increased organ donation, and improved outcomes (8–10). Endpoints that have been utilized to determine benefits of such units include care of patients with craniotomies, decreased use of unnecessary neuroimaging studies, and rapid identification of patients with deteriorating neurologic conditions by specially trained nurses.

HISTORIC PERSPECTIVE

Conceived in the 1960s, ASUs originally were developed with the goals of cost containment and improved outcomes (11,12). The first ASUs were simply wards in which patients were placed for the purpose of observation (13,14). The goal was to establish a single, designated location for patients with a set of diagnoses for the purposes of cost reduction, administrative simplification, and standardization of care. Soon, the ASU became a place for the implementation of early rehabilitation, and it was observed that this specialized care resulted in improved outcomes (15,16). In these units, complications, such as deep vein thrombosis, urinary tract infections, and aspiration pneumonia, were more easily identified and treated (17,18). However, many hospitals were forced to combine these units with general neurology wards, as the number of neurology inpatients declined. Economic forces that required increased efficiency and cost containment presented incentives to reduce beds (19,20). At the same time, in Europe, literature emphasizing the care of patients in an ASU had been growing since the 1960s (15,20).

ASU IN THE UNITED STATES VS. EUROPE

In most European health systems, the ASU is the primary modality for the care of stroke patients. The European model emphasizes rehabilitation, secondary prevention, and the treatment of side effects of stroke. With the exception of Germany, ASUs in Europe are not critical care units, and the acute treatment of stroke is de-emphasized. The benefits of ASU in the European system are now supported by multiple studies that demonstrate reduced cost and improved outcomes. However, these cost and mortality reductions are observed in a system with highly centralized planning, in which cost containment is less dependent on the length of hospital stay, and more focused on the issues of resource restraint (21,22). In the U.S. system, cost savings are often realized through acute treatment modalities that reduce the long-term cost of patient care. However, in this system, patients who have suffered stroke receive more fragmented care over the long term. The cost savings associated with high-intensity acute treatment have not been demonstrated in the literature.

A number of studies have examined the impact of ASUs on functional independence, morbidity, and mortality. Most of the sentinel work has been completed in the Northern European countries of the United Kingdom, Sweden, and Denmark. These studies were strongly influenced by the various organizational structures in the regions where the studies were completed and resulted in a concept of the stroke unit that can be classified into two types: long-term and short-term acute care units. The long-term care approach is best exemplified by the United Kingdom and Scandinavian systems (23), which de-emphasize the acute care of patients with stroke and emphasize the role of patients as stroke survivors. Treatment is oriented toward long-term rehabilitation, earlier community placement, and cost-effective secondary stroke prevention. Stroke patients stay for extended periods, receiving acute care and rehabilitation in the same ward. The short-term care model emphasizes aggressive interventionalism and is considered more resource intensive. The German system is also based on this concept. In this system, a highly centralized organization of ASUs rapidly identifies, refers, and transports patients to specialized stroke centers in which aggressive interventional strategies are employed. The goal of these units is to aggressively intervene to minimize brain injury from acute stroke. However, they have not proven to improve outcomes or survival (24).

The European systems discussed above have many commonalities, even though their therapeutic philosophies are different. They have established standards of care and an organization that extends to the regional and national levels. Conversely, some European countries do not have organized stroke care on a national level or incorporated ASUs. The French and Italian medical systems utilize medical wards as the primary location of stroke care. General neurologic wards act as secondary organizational units (25). In these countries, the care of stroke patients is often supplemented by stroke teams.

The U.S. system is quite different. Acute care occurs in a local or regional hospital over a period of days to weeks (26,27). Once stabilized, the patient is transported to a rehabilitation hospital that is in a different location, often in a different region. Cost curtailment in this system is almost always realized through reduced length of stay in the acute care setting (28,29). The intensity of medical resource utilization in this system is almost always higher than in the traditional European model. Additionally, follow-up care for patients might be fragmented and incomplete, and the system does not have centralized organization (30–35).

EUROPEAN LITERATURE AND DATABASES

Studies that demonstrate the efficacy of ASUs in ameliorating mortality date back to the 1960s. A 1993 summary article of these studies demonstrated that the odds of improved outcome were greater in a specialized unit than in a general medical ward (36). Reduction in mortality was 28%. This reduction persisted up to 12 months (odds ratio, OR: 0.79; 95% CI: 0.63–0.99, $p < 0.05$), with improved survival in patients treated in the specialized ASU. The most recent large analysis of morbidity and mortality in ASUs versus general medical wards was published as a meta-analysis in the Cochrane review based on the Stroke Unit Trialist Collaboration in the United Kingdom. The conclusions of the study were that patients treated in an ASU were more likely to be alive, independent, and living at home one year after stroke. The OR of death at one year was 0.83. The odds of institutionalization or death were lower (0.76), as were those of death and dependency (0.75) (23,37). These findings were not restricted to any one subgroup of stroke patients.

A number of trials have evaluated the cost-effectiveness of ASUs and how outcomes are influenced by interventions in the ASU. Most deaths in an ASU are prevented within the first 4 weeks after stroke onset (38,39). Other data have suggested that patients in ASUs are discharged earlier. A substantial amount of the benefit derived by care in this setting might be the avoidance of complications associated with prolonged hospitalization (23).

Literature that emphasizes the success of ASUs in changing stroke outcomes is expanding, and many databases and investigator collaborations have evolved over the past two decades. Examples of such databases include: The Riks-Stroke Collaboration, a Swedish national quality register for stroke care (40–44); the Stroke Trialist Collaboration in the United Kingdom (23); the Japanese Standard Stroke Registry Database (45); the Besancon Stroke Registry in France (46); Parma Stroke Data Bank: atherothrombotic and lacunar stroke in Italy (47); the German Stroke Study Collaboration (48); the Austrian Stroke Registry (49); and the National Audit of Stroke in the United Kingdom (50). These databases have allowed for critical observation of the efficacy of ASUs in different populations. Some studies have attempted to contrast national experiences with the stroke unit model to compare differences in efficacy and cost-effectiveness in different locations (14). These comparisons are always hindered by a lack of consistency in study design and data gathering, which is reflected in differences in quantity and type of data gathered. As these collaborations continue, undoubtedly the quality of the studies and the validity of the conclusions will improve.

NEED FOR ASU IN THE UNITED STATES

The cerebrovascular center is a stroke center, with an increased ability to care for all cerebrovascular disease, including ischemic stroke, subarachnoid hemorrhage, and intracranial hemorrhage. The need for development of cerebrovascular centers is increasing, and certification of these centers by the Joint Commission for Hospital Accreditation (JCAHO) is eminent (51). One of the by-products of standardization and certification of these units might be the development of a state triage system that encourages the diversion of specific disease entities to cerebrovascular centers.

In June 2000, guidelines for the establishment of primary stroke centers in the United States were published (52) (i) that recognized the need for a core of stroke professionals, with emphasis on the development of a "stroke team," and that the ideal location for the delivery of stroke care is in a stroke center, and (ii) that recommended that institutions that provide care beyond the emergency department should provide care in an ASU setting. The guidelines recognized a 17% reduction in death, a 7% increase in patients returning to independence, and an 8% reduction in the length of stay in patients who were managed in an ASU. As the JCAHO has taken the lead in certifying centers as primary stroke centers, the implementation of the guidelines will become integral to certification. Below is a limited list of issues that provide a clear rationale for the existence and development of ASUs.

- Acute stroke patients are at a risk for neurologic, cardiopulmonary, and other medical complications.
- Stroke management involves great variability, which sometimes leads to increased morbidity and mortality.
- Coordinated care in the ASU decreases morbidity and mortality, and improves functional outcome.

- An ASU provides the optimal setting for follow-up of stroke patients who are at risk for neurologic deterioration.
- Twenty-four-hour monitoring is mandatory for patients after thrombolytic therapy or for patients enrolled in investigative trials.
- Use of stroke critical care pathways improves efficiency of care, reduces length of hospital stay, and lowers the cost of stroke care.

As new technologies for ischemic stroke are developed and implemented, the ASU will become a place where they will be utilized to manage patients in a manner that improves outcome. The ASU promises to be a more complex environment, where more critically ill patients will be sustained with more technologically complex life support systems.

ACUs: DEFINITION AND COMPOSITION

Although the ASU employs specialized technologies in one location, it is at the same time a nonphysical construct in which specialists engage in dedicated stroke care that is primarily behaviorally dependent, as opposed to technologically driven. ASUs should be staffed by those who have an interest and specialized training in the care of patients who have suffered from stroke. This training requires a significant amount of dedicated continuing medical education, as well as additional clinical training, such as clinical fellowships. Stroke units should employ computerized databases, have written care protocols, and have the capability to monitor patients frequently. An ASU can acquire the characteristics of an ICU, with invasive and complex monitoring equipment; however, it is more likely that the ASU will employ minimal specialized clinical monitoring and focus on basic cardiac monitoring. Physicians in the ASU can be intensivists or general internists, even though most physicians who direct or run the ASU are neurologists. All physicians responsible for specialized care in these units should have special education and advanced training in the management of the sequelae of stroke. In the future, those physicians designated as medical directors of ASUs should have additional training and certification in neurovascular neurology.

Any physician managing an ASU should be familiar with guidelines pertaining to standard care of patients who have suffered a stroke. Information regarding the performance and management of the ASU should be immediately available, such as written admission and discharge protocols, patient census, outcome data, educational, and continuing medical education records for all members of the unit staff. The configuration and size of an ASU can vary. However, the unifying principle is organized care of patients who have suffered a stroke, delivered by trained professionals who specialize in the care of these patients.

Many studies within and outside the United States have examined the issue of how an ASU affects outcomes. Still, the consensus about what constitutes an ASU is often unclear. This lack of standardization is important when attempting to abstract data on ASU efficacy and to identify and describe specific practices and skills that result in measurable improvements in outcome.

In the literature, the following are considered essential elements of an ASU (36,37):

- Staffed with a special interest in stroke or rehabilitation;
- Routine involvement of caregivers in the rehabilitation process;
- Coordinated multidisciplinary team care that incorporates meetings at least weekly;
- Information provided to patients and caregivers; and
- Regular programs of education and training.

In our opinion, the following elements are also essential components of an ASU:

- Accessible geographical location;
- Capability to continuously monitor cardiac function, blood pressure, and oxygen saturation;
- Specialized nursing staff;
- Small patient-to-nurse ratio;
- Multidisciplinary stroke team headed by a physician, with expertise in cerebrovascular disease;
- Dedicated beds;

Table 1 Number of Beds and Staffing Ratios for 175 Stroke Units, United Kingdom National Audit, 2001–2002

	Average	Range
Total number of stroke beds	20	14–27
Ratio of stroke patients/stroke beds	1.45	1.04–2.13
Ratio of stroke beds/qualified nurses at 10 hr on a normal weekday	7.70	5.6–9.5
Ratio of stroke beds/qualified nurses plus care assistants at 10 hr on a normal weekday	3.20	2.4–3.8
WTE establishment		
WTE clinical psychologist per 10 stroke beds	0.16	0.08–0.32
WTE dietitians per 10 stroke beds	0.16	0.09–0.33
WTE occupational therapists per 10 stroke beds	0.83	0.56–1.17
WTE physiotherapists per 10 stroke beds	1.18	0.82–1.67
WTE speech and language therapists per 10 stroke beds	0.36	0.18–0.56

Abbreviation: WTE, whole-time equivalent.
Source: Adapted from Ref. 50.

- Stroke critical pathway, with a case manager overseeing its execution;
- Preprinted orders;
- Ready access to and active role of rehabilitation services;
- Regular stroke team rounds to facilitate a coordinated plan of care;
- Participation in stroke clinical research trials;
- Specialized nursing protocols to identify neurologic deterioration and limit medical complications (deep venous thromboses, aspiration, etc.); and
- Protocols for early bedside swallowing evaluation and proper limb positioning.

However, it is not clear which of the characteristics listed above directly affect outcome.
Often, an ASU offers services not included in the above listings. These resources are valuable and can contribute to improved care for patients. Examples of these resources were seen in the national audit of stroke care in the United Kingdom, which included 240 hospitals in England, Wales, and Northern Ireland and reported data on the number of ancillary services provided besides those characterized as essential for ASU classification. This data was extracted from the 175 hospitals, with identified ASUs. Table 1 includes the staffing ratios at the 175 stroke units audited in the UK national audit, and Table 2 represents the composition in full-time equivalents of the Queen Elizabeth II Health Sciences Center Acute Stroke Team in Halifax, Canada.

Table 2 Subspecialties that Compose the Acute Stroke Team at the Queen Elizabeth II Health Sciences Center, Halifax, Canada (20 Beds)

Specialists	FTE
Neuroscience nurses	28.3
Neurologist/physicians	0.5
Neuropsychologist	0.2
Occupational therapist	1.7
Pharmacist	0.8
Physiotherapist	1.2
Rehabilitation medicine	0.1
Social work	0.8
Speech-language pathologist	1.1
Spiritual care	0.8
Team coordinators	0.5
Food and nutrition	1.3

Full-time equivalents, which reflect resources at the Queen Elizabeth II and do not necessarily represent recommended staffing levels.
Abbreviation: FTE, full-time equivalents.
Source: Adapted from Ref. 53.

HUMAN RESOURCES IN THE ASU

The ASU is an interdisciplinary environment that utilizes expertise from a wide range of clinical specialties. Neurologists, as well as intensivists and internists, practice in the unit, and nurses with specialized neuroscience training fuel its clinical engine. It is important that the nurses have adequate training to detect early neurologic decline in patients following stroke. Physical and occupational therapists facilitate the progression of patients from a bed-bound state to functional independence. During multidisciplinary rounds that occur every day in most ASUs, the care of each patient is organized; plans for acute care, rehabilitation, and secondary prevention of stroke are addressed; and decisions are made concerning the distribution of human resources within the unit. Economic and social issues confronting patients are resolved, and discharge plans are made.

CAPABILITIES OF AN ASU

The goal of the ASU is to provide optimal care for patients following acute stroke and transient ischemic attack (TIA), including prevention of deep venous thromboses, avoidance of aspiration pneumonia, treatment of urinary tract infections, and cardiac monitoring to identify arrhythmias that might be associated with stroke. The rapid evaluation of patients with TIA within a 24-hour period results in increased safety and reduced cost, and requires "critical" pathways and arrangements for ultrasound and neuroimaging to ensure adequate and immediate care of these patients to reduce their length of stay and avoid their discomfort and alienation typically associated with long hospitalization. The rapid treatment with IV rtPA of patients who progress to a stroke following a TIA is a function that can most easily be accomplished in an ASU.

Patients who are eligible to receive interventional treatment following acute stroke, such as rtPA or other intravascular therapies, are cared for in the ASU 24 hours after receiving rtPA, when their ICU observational stay is complete. All patients who suffer acute stroke and come to the ASU are rapidly assessed and treated. The unit optimizes the treatment of risk factors associated with secondary stroke (elevated blood pressure, hyperlipidemia, smoking cessation, and treatment of atrial fibrillation). The diagnostic methods by which to define the sources of cerebral ischemia include carotid ultrasonography, echocardiography, MRI, magnetic resonance angiography (MRA), Computed tomography angiography (CTA), and digital duplex angiography. Patients who undergo procedures performed by interventional radiologists or vascular surgeons can complete their postoperative course in a monitored environment. Patients who receive elective surgical procedures, such as carotid endarterectomy, can also be cared for in this environment.

CONFIGURATION OF ASU

The physical configuration of the ASU has implications for patient care. In the setting of such units as the medical, surgical, or coronary care ICU, the patient is placed in proximity to devices necessary for revival and treatment. The overall goal of the ASU is to observe the patient with monitoring devices that result in the early detection of clinical decline. In the ASU, there is no electronic apparatus that accurately detects the onset of a stroke. Thus, architectural design that emphasizes visibility and easy access to the patient is essential for optimal care, e.g., configurations, in which one nurse can easily observe four patients, who are always in his/her line of sight and can be reached with relatively few steps. In a closed ward configuration, in which each patient is housed in a single room, frequent neurologic evaluations are required in the acute phase of illness to appropriately monitor the patient. The most important element in any ward situation is the matching of an appropriately trained nurse to the afflicted patient. In many hospitals today, the ability to house like patients together is limited, which we believe creates a less-than-optimal care environment.

SPECIFIC ISSUES SURROUNDING CARE IN ASUs

Studies have clearly determined that ASUs are associated with a decrease in patient morbidity and mortality and an increase in functional independence following stroke. The influence of individual traits of ASUs on outcomes is not clear from most of the large, randomized studies. Studies that evaluate key aspects of care received in ASUs are now being conducted.

A single question that confronts advocates of accredited ASUs is whether patient care following stroke is better in an ASU than in a general medical ward. A number of studies have compared stroke teams to ASUs or stroke wards. The most recent study, completed in the United Kingdom, prospectively followed 267 patients after moderately severe ischemic stroke. They were randomized to stroke teams that functioned as a general medical ward and an ASU. Outcomes that evaluated mortality, institutionalization, neurologic function, quality of life, and resource utilization were obtained at three months and one year after stroke onset. An intention-to-treat design was used, with a multifactorial logistic regression analysis. Institutionalization and mortality were significantly higher at three months and one year (OR: 2.8; 95% CI: 1.3–6.2) for patients with large-vessel infarcts treated in general medical wards. Those patients with small-vessel infarcts faired equally well with care from a stroke team in a general medical ward (23). Based on this study, the application of the limited resources associated with an ASU might best be reserved for those patients with large-vessel or embolic stroke.

The transition of the patient from an acute setting to the home setting involves other issues of cost containment and improved outcome. Most patients report that their primary goal after a stroke is to return to their home environment. Strategies that promote early progression to the home environment result in both improved patient satisfaction and decreased costs. Ultimately, it must be determined whether the outcomes in a home setting and in a modified hospital setting are comparable. Is the decreased cost that is associated with home care associated with greater patient well being? In the United Kingdom, a study compared the efficacy of three treatment settings in outcome, their acceptability to patients, and their acceptability to caregivers. The three settings were (i) a specialized ASU, (ii) general medical wards with a stroke team in attendance, and (iii) home care with a visiting stroke care therapist, and a general practitioner who had special interest in stroke. The primary outcome was death or institutionalization at 1 year. Secondary measures included functional abilities, mood, quality of life, resource use, length of stay, and patient and caregiver satisfaction; 457 patients were randomized, with equal numbers in each group. The groups were well matched for baseline characteristics. The mortality and institutionalization at 1 year were lower for the ASU group. Significantly fewer patients in the ASU group died, and those alive without disability were significantly associated with the ASU. ASU patients had shorter and more complete rehabilitation. The greatest dissatisfaction was associated with care on the general medical ward. The greatest satisfaction was associated with care at home. This study did not support a role for care of stroke patients in a general ward or at home. The ASU was also more cost-effective per day of life than either of the other modalities. These data suggest that the benefits of stroke care in an ASU in the United Kingdom clearly outweigh the costs and that the trend toward early discharge seen in the United States might have negative consequences for those patients who are discharged without complete rehabilitation (54). Studies that have evaluated the effectiveness of home care have had contradictory results. Another post hoc analysis of the cost-effectiveness data from the above study suggests that, when early-cost considerations were included and long-term costs were excluded, the short-term costs of ASU care were much greater (55).

Why do ASUs work? The specific traits of ASUs that result in improvements in morbidity and mortality have not been identified. Resource availability does not seem to be the limiting factor influencing improved outcomes. Research that emphasizes the paradigms of stroke care that include access to rehabilitation, stroke specialist care, and attentive nursing do not adequately explain the benefits associated with improved outcomes. A recent study that examined the differences in management of patients in various settings might provide an explanation for the improved outcomes associated with care received in stroke units (56). In a randomized prospective study, 304 patients with similar characteristics were randomized to ASUs or general medical wards. ASU patients were monitored more frequently and received more treatments (e.g., oxygen and antipyretics) that were thought to improve stroke outcomes. Patients received increased interventions that decreased aspiration rates and resulted in early return to enteral feeding, and those who were treated in ASUs experienced fewer complications and attenuated progression of symptoms, including fewer secondary strokes and less chest pain. The conclusion of the study was that differences in functional independence and reduced mortality were attributable to differences in medical management (56).

SUMMARY AND CONCLUSIONS

ASUs have been proven by prospective, randomized trials to reduce morbidity, mortality, and costs and to increase functional independence. Improved outcomes for patients who suffer from stroke are influenced as much by available resources as they are by the management decisions made by the dedicated professionals who operate ASUs. As new treatments for acute stroke are developed and proven technologic interventions become available for the care of stroke patients, the ASU will be the place where these new techniques are applied, consequently transitioning these units into critical care units. In the near future, the need for certification of primary stroke centers will increase. As a result of these powerful trends in medicine, stroke centers will be a growing presence in the U.S. hospital system. They will undoubtedly have a positive impact on the care and recovery of patients who suffer from stroke.

ACKNOWLEDGMENTS

This work is supported in part by the U.S. Public Health Service National Institutes of Health grant NS 046379.

REFERENCES

1. Adams H, Adams R, Del Zoppo G, Goldstein LB. Guidelines for the early management of patients with ischemic stroke: 2005 guidelines update: a scientific statement from the stroke council of the American Heart Association/American Stroke Association. Stroke 2005; 36:916.
2. Wardlaw JM, Zoppo G, Yamaguchi T, Berge E. Thrombolysis for acute ischaemic stroke. Cochrane Database Syst Rev 2003; 3.
3. Latchaw RE, Yonas H, Hunter GJ, et al. Guidelines and recommendations for perfusion imaging in cerebral ischemia a scientific statement for healthcare professionals by the writing group on perfusion imaging, from the council on cardiovascular radiology of the American Heart Association. Stroke 2003; 34:1084.
4. Butcher K, Parsons M, Baird T, et al. Perfusion Thresholds in Acute Stroke Thrombolysis. Stroke 2003; 34:2159–2164.
5. Smith WS, Sung G, Starkman S, et al. Safety and efficacy of mechanical embolectomy in acute ischemic stroke. Results of the MERCI trial. Stroke 2005; 36:1432–1438.
6. Pronovost PJ, Angus DC, Dorman T, Robinson KA, Dremsizov TT, Young TL. Physician staffing patterns and clinical outcomes in critically ill patients. JAMA 2002; 288:2151–2162.
7. Pronovost PJ, Jencks M, Dorman T, et al. Organizational characteristics of intensive care units related to outcomes of abdominal aortic surgery. JAMA 1999; 281:1310–1312.
8. Suarez JI, Zaidat OO, Suri MF, et al. Length of stay and mortality in neurocritically ill patients: impact of a specialized neurocritical care team. Crit Care Med 2004; 32:2311–2317.
9. Helms AK, Torbey MT, Hacein-Bey L, Chyba C, Varelas PN. Standardized protocols increase organ and tissue donation rates in the neurocritical care unit. Neurology 2004; 23(63):1955–1957.
10. Mirski MA, Chang CW, Cowan R. Impact of a neuroscience intensive care unit on neurosurgical patient outcomes and cost of care: evidence-based support for intensivist-directed specialty ICU model of care. J Neurosur Anesthesiol 2001; 13:83–92.
11. Isaacs B. Stroke units. Br Med J 1971; 4:492.
12. Hewer RL. Stroke units. Br Med J 1972; 1(791):52.
13. Large H, Tuthill JE, Kennedy FB, Pozen TF. In the first stroke intensive care unit. Am J Nurs 1969; 69:76–80.
14. Grieve R, Porsdal V, Hutton J, Wolfe C. A comparison of the cost-effectiveness of stroke care provided in London and Copenhagen. Int J Technol Assess Health Care 2000; 16:684–695.
15. Stevens RS, Ambler NR, Warren MD. A randomized controlled trial of a stroke rehabilitation ward. Age Ageing 1984; 13:65–75.
16. Stevens RS, Isaacs B. Stroke rehabilitation units in the United Kingdom. Health Trends 1984; 16:61–63.
17. Norris JW, Hachinski VC. Intensive care management of stroke patients. Stroke 1976; 7:573–577.
18. Drake WE Jr., Hamilton MJ, Carlsson M, Blumenkrantz J. Acute stroke management and patient outcome: the value of Neurovascular Care Units (NCU). Stroke 1973; 4:933–945.
19. Garraway WM, Walton MS, Akhtar AJ, Prescott RJ. The use of health and social services in the management of stroke in the community: results from a controlled trial. Age Ageing 1981; 10:95–104.
20. Schmidt SM, Guo L, Scheer SJ. Changes in the status of hospitalized stroke patients since inception of the prospective payment system in 1983. Arch Phys Med Rehabil 2002; 83:894–898.

21. Czlonkowska A, Milewska D, Ryglewicz D. The polish experience in early stroke care. Cerebrovasc Dis 2003; 15:14–15.
22. Indredavik B. Stroke units—the Norwegian experience. Cerebrovasc Dis 2003; 15:19–20.
23. How do stroke units improve patient outcomes? A collaborative systematic review of the randomized trials. Stroke Unit Trialists Collaboration [Review]. Stroke 1997; 28:2139–2144.
24. Busse O. Stroke units and stroke services in Germany. Cerebrovasc Dis 2003; 15.
25. Hommel M, Deblasi A, Garambois K, Jaillard A. The French stroke program. Cerebrovasc Dis 2003; 15:11–13.
26. Centers for Disease Control. Hospitalizations for stroke among adults aged over 65 years—United States, 2000. JAMA 2003; 290:1023–1024.
27. Fang J, Alderman MH. Trend of stroke hospitalization, United States, 1988–1997. Stroke 2001; 32:2221–2226.
28. Dobrez DG, Lo Sasso AT, Heinemann AW. The effect of prospective payment on rehabilitative care. Arch Phys Med Rehabil 2004; 85:1909–1914.
29. Stuart M, Ryser C, Levitt A, et al. Stroke rehabilitation in Switzerland versus the United States: a preliminary comparison. Neurorehabil Neural Repair 2005; 19(2):139–147.
30. Stroke Stineman MG, Ross RN, Hamilton BB, et al. Inpatient rehabilitation after stroke: a comparison of lengths of stay and outcomes in the veterans affairs and non-veterans affairs health care system. Med Care 2001; 39:123–137.
31. Kelly PJ, Furie KL, Shafqat S, Rallis N, Chang Y, Stein J. Functional recovery following rehabilitation after hemorrhagic and ischemic stroke. Arch Phys Med Rehabil 2003; 84:968–972.
32. Rodgers H, Mackintosh J, Price C, et al. Does an early increased-intensity interdisciplinary upper limb therapy programme following acute stroke improve outcome? Clin Rehabil 2003; 17:579–589.
33. Hoenig H, Sloane R, Horner RD, Zolkewitz M, Reker D. Differences in rehabilitation services and outcomes among stroke patients cared for in veterans hospitals. Health Serv Res 2001; 35:1293–1318.
34. Horner RD, Swanson JW, Bosworth HB, Matchar DB. VA acute stroke (VAST) study team. Effects of race and poverty on the process and outcome of inpatient rehabilitation services among stroke patients. Stroke 2003; 34:1027–1031.
35. Lai SM, Alter M, Friday G, Lai SL, Sobel E. Disposition after acute stroke: who is not sent home from hospital? Neuroepidemiology 1998; 17:21–29.
36. Langhorne P, Dennis MS. Stroke units: the next 10 years. Lancet 2004; 363:834–835.
37. Organized inpatient (stroke unit) care for stroke. Stroke Unit Trialists' Collaboration. Cochrane Database Syst Rev 2000; 2:CD000197. Review. Update in: Cochrane Database Syst Rev 2002; 1:CD000197.
38. Millikan CH. Stroke intensive care units; objectives and results. Stroke 1979; 10:235–237.
39. Bamford J, Sandercock P, Dennis M, Burn J, Warlow C. Classification and natural history of clinically identifiable subtypes of cerebral infarction. Lancet 1991; 337:1521–1526.
40. Asplund K, Hulter Asberg K, Norrving B, Stegmayr B, Terent A, Wester PO. Riks-Stroke collaboration Riks-Stroke—a Swedish national quality register for stroke care. Cerebrovasc Dis 2003; 15:5–7.
41. Glader EL, Stegmayr B, Johansson L, Hulter-Asberg K, Wester PO. Differences in long-term outcome between patients treated in stroke units and in general wards: a 2-year follow-up of stroke patients in Sweden. Stroke 2001; 32:2124–2130.
42. Bokemark L, Blomstrand C, Fagerberg B. Considerable differences in the management of stroke. A study of structured vs. conventional care. Lakartidningen 1996; 21(93):681–685 (in Swedish).
43. Glader EL, Stegmayr B, Norrving B, et al. Riks-Stroke collaboration. Sex differences in management and outcome after stroke: a Swedish national perspective. Stroke 2003; 34:1970–1975.
44. Stegmayr B, Asplund K, Danielsson BP, et al. Stroke unit care saves lives. The Swedish national quality assessment registry of stroke care is the first of its kind in the world. Lakartidningen 1999; 96:2719–2724.
45. Shiotsuki H, Ogushi Y, Fushimi K, Kobayashi S. Japanese Standard Stroke Registry Study (JSSRS) Group. Evaluation of applied cases of thrombolytic therapy against ultra-acute ischemic stroke. Using the Japanese Standard Stroke Registry Database. Tokai J Exp Clin Med 2005; 30:49–62.
46. Moulin T, Tatu L, Vuillier F, Berger E, Chavot D, Rumbach L. Role of a stroke data bank in evaluating cerebral infarction subtypes: patterns and outcome of 1776 consecutive patients from the Besancon stroke registry. Cerebrovasc Dis 2000; 10:261–271.
47. Finzi G, Catamo A, Mombelloni A, et al. Parma stroke data bank: atherothrombotic and lacunar stroke. Minerva Med 1994; 85:579–588.
48. German Stroke Study Collaboration. Predicting outcome after acute ischemic stroke: an external validation of prognostic models. Neurology 2004; 62:581–585.
49. Steiner MM, Brainin M. Austrian Stroke Registry for acute stroke units. The quality of acute stroke units on a nation-wide level: the Austrian Stroke Registry for acute stroke units [Review]. Eur J Neurol 2003; 10:353–360.
50. Rudd AG, Hoffman A, Irwin P, Pearson M, Lowe D. Intercollegiate working party for stroke. Stroke units: research and reality. Results from the national sentinel audit of stroke. Qual Saf Health Care 2005; 14:7–12.

51. Alberts MJ, Latchaw RE, Selman WR, et al. Recommendations for comprehensive stroke centers. A consensus statement from the brain attack coalition. Stroke 2005; 36:1597–1616.

52. Alberts MJ, Hademenos G, Latchaw RE, et al. Recommendations for the establishment of primary stroke centers. Brain Attack Coalition. JAMA 2000; 283:3102–3109.

53. Phillips SJ, Eskes GA, Gubitz GJ. On behalf of the Queen Elizabeth II health sciences centre acute stroke team. Description and evaluation of an acute stroke units. CMAJ 2002; 167(6).

54. Kalra L, Evans A, Perez I, Knapp M, Swift C, Donaldson N. A randomised controlled comparison of alternative strategies in stroke care. Health Technol Assess 2005; 9:1–94.

55. Patel A, Knapp M, Perez I, Evans A, Kalra L. Alternative strategies for stroke care: cost-effectiveness and cost-utility analyses from a prospective randomized controlled trial. Stroke 2004; 35:196–203.

56. Evans A, Perez I, Harraf F, et al. Can differences in management processes explain different outcomes between stroke unit and stroke-team care? Lancet 2001; 358:1586–1592.

36 | Telemedicine Applied to Stroke Care

Marian P. LaMonte, MD, MSN, Associate Professor
Departments of Neurology and Emergency Medicine, University of Maryland School of Medicine, University of Maryland Medical Center, Baltimore, Maryland, USA

Mona N. Bahouth, MSN, CRNP, Director
Department of Neurology, University of Maryland School of Medicine, University of Maryland Medical Center, Baltimore, Maryland, USA

Yan Xiao, PhD, Associate Professor
Peter Hu, MS, CNE, Instructor
Colin Mackenzie, MBChB, Professor and Director
Department of Anesthesiology, University of Maryland School of Medicine, University of Maryland Medical Center, Baltimore, Maryland, USA

INTRODUCTION

Many nations face public health crises related to services required by aging populations. Stroke, a disease most prevalent in the aging population, is one of the leading causes of death and disability worldwide and is among the costliest. In the United States, recommendations for improving stroke services can be found through various vascular associations and, more recently, through the Joint Commission on Accreditation of Hospitals (1,2). However, health-care providers face significant challenges in enacting recommendations for stroke specialty services, and telemedicine has been explored as a means to surmount some of them. This chapter focuses on key research that involves telemedicine for stroke services, particularly those studies that provide the foundation for the future growth of the technology. We also summarize issues that impede more widespread use of this new technology and offer possible solutions.

CURRENT CHALLENGES IN PROVIDING EMERGENCY ACCESS TO STROKE SPECIALTY CARE

The major factors that hinder seamless emergency care for patients who suffer from stroke can be sorted into 4 categories: lack of on-site stroke specialty resources, geographic distance to specialty services, need for rapid access to multimodal services, and difficulty in obtaining reimbursement for services. Most recommendations for quality stroke services stress that providers have special training in stroke evaluation, diagnosis, and treatment. Currently, personnel qualified to administer acute stroke care and who are available 24 hr per day, 7 days per week can be found in only a small number of health-care facilities in the United States. However, most stroke care is rendered distant from these resource-rich locations. Ensuring patients a timely emergency evaluation for ischemic stroke treatment with intravenous thrombolysis places additional stress on sparse specialty resources. Finally, although guidelines for improved stroke care are based on outcome measures, reimbursement for these services is often lacking.

TELEMEDICINE AS A BRIDGE FROM ON-SITE EMERGENCY PROVIDERS TO SPECIALISTS

From the early 1990s, audiovisual data transmission has been used to provide specialty support for emergency services (3,4). The common theme of this early research was the recognition that telemedicine links between specialty and field providers could collapse the barrier of geographic distance and time for patient evaluation and treatment. In an evaluation of the appropriateness of incorporating telemedicine systems in emergency departments, it was concluded that the emergency department is a suitable place for establishing a telemedicine center, because telemedicine linkage may decrease unnecessary transfer of patients from their local hospitals (3). In addition, the Telemedicine Emergency Neurosurgical Network (TENN) confirmed the clinical efficacy and cost effectiveness of neurosurgical consultation in a population of 329 at risk, underserved patients (4). In the TENN review, no transport risks or radiologic review discrepancies were identified within the evaluated data collected over 35 months.

FUNDAMENTAL RESEARCH ADVANCING TELEMEDICINE FOR STROKE CARE

Several groups have reported that National Institute of Health Stroke Scale (NIHSS) scores acquired by telemedicine transmission were comparable to those obtained in face-to-face clinical examinations (5–7). Reported inter-rater evaluations between teletransmitted and bedside evaluators in these studies were similar or exceeded kappa values reported for the original validation study of the NIHSS (8). The earliest of these, in 1998, also tested reliability of NIHSS scoring by 2 stroke specialists while viewing patient examinations via wireless teletransmission (5). Scores among specialists were reliable; assuring that the technology posed no limit to deficit ascertainment.

The first successful telemedicine systems for acute stroke consultation and treatment were reported at the University of Maryland Medical Center (9–14). Researchers created a test-bed to pilot projects that involved the technology's application (12). This group tested the advantages of real time, 2-way transmission of audio–video recording of a remotely located patient to stroke clinicians at the medical center, versus telephonic transmission of data alone. They found that 2-way audiovisual linkage added diagnostic and management certainty, provided prearrival time to prepare for treatment, and increased the number of patients with ischemic stroke treated with intravenous recombinant tissue plasminogen activator (Fig. 1) (10,11). Other important information gleaned from early study of this technology included clinician acceptance of the technology, patient and family satisfaction with remote specialty consultant care, and improved ability to diagnose and appropriately treat other neurologic disorders, including subarachnoid hemorrhage, intracerebral hemorrhage, seizure, hypoglycemia, transient ischemic attack, and pseudostroke (11). Provisos for the further growth of these services were enunciated, including the need for ongoing funding and a future optimal system that would allow wireless transmission from the community hospital to a specialist at any location (11).

The University of Maryland test bed advanced the capability of the technology, enabling stroke specialists to examine patients while they were en route by ambulance to the hospital (5). The study found that earlier knowledge and assurance of the patient's stroke diagnosis and deficits improved

Patient is asked to raise his arms (Note 12 seconds interval)

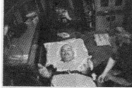
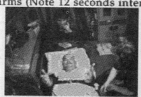
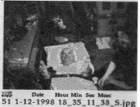

51 1-12-1998 18_34_59_79_S.jpg   51 1-12-1998 18_35_05_89_S.jpg   51 1-12-1998 18_35_11_38_S.jpg

Toward the end of the transport, note the patient's left arm drops from his lap indicating possible weakness.

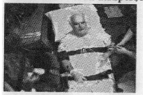
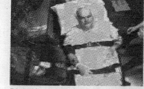
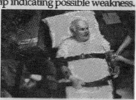

51 1-12-1998 18_42_11_89_S.jpg   51 1-12-1998 18_42_31_01_S.jpg   51 1-12-1998 18_42_42_32_S.jpg

Paramedic recognizes decline in status and repeats exam, but patient's left arm is paretic.

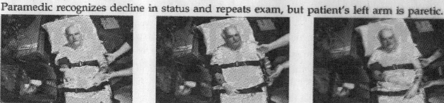
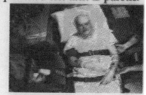

51 1-12-1998 18_42_51_67_S.jpg   51 1-12-1998 18_43_03_58_S.jpg   51 1-12-1998 18_43_09_24_S.jpg

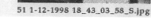

Figure 1   Teletransmission of patient experiencing stroke during transport.

upon the standard 911 medic audio description. Visual confirmation of patient status prior to arrival enhanced the team's preparedness and ultimately shortened the time to treatment. Mean door-to-needle times were 17 min in the telemedicine group and 33 min in the control group ($p = 0.003$).

In 1999, researchers documented the importance of developing telemedicine networks as a potential solution for barriers to acute stroke treatment (13). Descriptions of several stroke telemedicine networks and outcomes from their implementation have been published (10,13–19). Systems in Maryland, New York, Ontario, and, more recently, Georgia, Massachusetts, and Germany have reported their findings. Still others are forming. Outcomes from each suggest that acute stroke consultation rendered via telemedicine can provide safe administration of thrombolytic therapy with low complication rates to ischemic stroke patients in remote locations, who otherwise would not have access to specialty care.

Telemedicine networks are generally organized between a stroke specialty center that has personnel and capital resources available and one or more facilities that lack clinical resources for specialized stroke care. Aside from the obvious fixed locality of the patient in an emergency department, most current networks also have a fixed physical location from which the on-call specialist operates. The advancement of the technology toward cellular wireless communication should allow for mobility of the stroke specialist and more rapid connection between the referring provider and consultant. Telemedicine networks provide an advantage in keeping the operating costs lower due to less potential duplication of equipment, less maintenance cost due to use of compatible equipment, and less redundancy in on-call effort by a stroke specialist. An important disadvantage is that stroke specialists who are on call for larger networks can become overwhelmed with simultaneous consult requests. Except for those networks that are delineated in the Rural Health Act, equitable reimbursement for services rendered by the specialists is lacking (20).

Table 1 provides a summary of supporting literature that relates to key activities in telemedicine for stroke. We believe that further research of these activities is necessary and will validate their importance in advancing the field of telemedicine for stroke care.

Table 1 Status of Supporting Literature for Key Stroke Telemedicine Activities[a]

Activity performed via telemedicine	Supporting literature			
	>1 study	1 study	Emerging data	Data needed
Architecture review	X			
Validity of remote neurologic exam	X			
Reliability of remote neurologic exam	X			
Neurologist delivers tPA remotely	X			
Nurse practitioner delivers tPA remotely	X			
Field emergency physician delivers tPA with consultant	X			
Field nurse practitioner delivers tPA with consultant		X		
Telemedicine network services demonstrate increased stroke services to remote site	X			
Long-term outcomes of patients receiving telemedicine delivered care				X
Economic factors research				X
Wireless data transmission	X			
End-to-end cellular wireless transmission			X	
Legal encumbrances				X
Risk management issues				X
Privacy concerns				X
Privatization				X
Reimbursement strategies/mechanisms			X	
Rehabilitation services				

[a] This summary is not intended to be a complete list of activities nor a comprehensive compilation of the literature for each activity. Instead, activities and publications specific to stroke telemedicine have been categorized in order to visually depict opportunities for further research.
Abbreviation: tPA, tissue plasminogen activator.

Table 2 Funding Sources for University of Maryland
Telemedicine Stroke Test Bed Projects

Federal/state/foundation
  Department of Defense
  National Library of Medicine
  National Medical Technology Test Bed
  National Emergency Medicine Association
  State of Maryland, Cigarette Restitution Funds
Medical center/industry
  The University of Maryland Medical Center
  St. Mary's Hospital
  TRW, Inc.
  Bell Atlantic/Verizon
  Vtel Products Corporation
  American Personal Communication (Sprint)
  Genentech, Inc.
Contractual
  The University of Maryland–St. Mary's Hospital
  The University of Maryland–Doctor's Hospital

REIMBURSEMENT CHALLENGES AND ALTERNATIVES FOR RENEWABLE FUNDING FOR TELEMEDICINE PROGRAMS

Third-party payers seldom recognize services that are rendered by means other than face-to-face patient care. The Rural Telehealth Act does not recognize service needs based on lack of specialty care providers for each region. Most telemedicine programs started as funded research or with unrestricted sponsored grants; few have attracted ongoing payment for these services (Table 2).

The practice of contractually based services is a solution that is gaining acceptance. Our medical center group, in conjunction with a member of our telemedicine network, agreed to develop a contract for services (21). Legal, financial, administrative, clinical, technical support, and medical practice compliance representatives from each institution comprised our contract development team. Critical components of the contract were defined, by committee consensus of the issues related to this care model, as follows: relationship of the parties, professional and hospital services, patient consent and confidentiality, insurance and definitions of liabilities, and billing and compensation. Professional fees were based on current medicare consultation reimbursement.

The contract defined terms and duties specific to the referring hospital and consultant's hospital. Duties of the referring hospital included accessing the specialty stroke service, obtaining consent from the patient to transmit audio–video recording for their care, providing staff responsibilities during the remote stroke consultation, making available medication and clinical services, and planning for emergency department after care. Duties specific to the consultants included details about appropriate times for response to a referring provider, hours of coverage, protocol development, and educational services provided.

A separate contract was developed for the technology portion of the service, and terms for equipment costs, linkage line fees, technology expertise, maintenance, and hours of technology support were defined.

CONCLUSIONS AND FUTURE DIRECTIONS

Facilities that provide emergency services, including radiologic studies, have the basic components to identify stroke and differentiate ischemic from hemorrhagic stroke type. However, recommended standards now extend stroke expertise beyond these basic capabilities to include professionals who can evaluate best therapeutic strategies and determine the benefit and risk of acute stroke therapy (1). Given that approximately 61 million people are considered underserved for specialty medical care (22), the use of this technology supports a more efficient and equitable distribution of stroke care to neurologically underserved and resource-scarce populations. Moreover, telemedicine has garnered governmental sanction as a tool for providing emergency stroke specialty consultation and treatment (23).

Further prospective study of patient outcomes and effect on health-care costs should be undertaken. Funding and reimbursement mechanisms must be established in order to promote widespread use of telemedicine. Exploring and developing less-expensive and portable wireless communication methods will be helpful to move care to the prehospital arena and allow for greater mobility of the consultant on call. Finally, third-party payers must address reimbursement for technology and professional services.

Technology is advancing at a rapid pace, and merging this technology with clinician expertise holds promise for national improvement in stroke care. Establishing novel technology-based services may be the key to providing health care to our growing aging populations.

REFERENCES

1. Alberts MJ, Hademenos G, Latchaw RE, et al. Recommendations for the establishment of primary stroke centers. JAMA 2000; 283:3102–3109.
2. http://www.jcaho.org/dscc/dsc/certification+information/stroke_brochure.pdf.
3. Chi CH, Chang I, Wu WP. Emergency department-based telemedicine. Am J Emerg Med 1999; 17(4):408–411.
4. Chodroff PH. A three-year review of telemedicine at the community level—clinical and fiscal results. J Telemed Telecare 1999; 5(1):28–30.
5. LaMonte MP, Xiao Y, Hu P, et al. Shortening time to stroke treatment using ambulance telemedicine: TeleBAT. J Stroke Cerebrovasc Dis 2004; 13(4):148–154.
6. Wang S, Lee SB, Pardue C, et al. Remote evaluation of acute ischemic stroke: reliability of the National Institutes of Health Stroke Scale via telestroke. Stroke 2003; 34:e188–191.
7. Handschu R, Littman R, Reulbach U, et al. Telemedicine in emergency evaluation of acute stroke: interrater agreement in remote stroke video examination with a novel multimedia system. Stroke 2003; 34:2842–2846.
8. Lyden P, Brott T, Tilley B, et al. Improved reliability of the NIH stroke scale using video training. Stroke 1994; 25(11):2220–2226.
9. LaMonte MP, Xiao Y, Hu P, Gaasch W, Gunawardane R, Mackenzie CF. Design and evaluation of a real-time mobile telemedicine system for ambulance transport. Proc Am Med Informatics Assoc 1998; 1:1102.
10. LaMonte MP, Xiao Y, Mackenzie C, et al. Tele-BAT: mobile telemedicine for the brain attack team. J Stroke Cerebrovasc Dis 2000; 9(3):128–135.
11. LaMonte MP, Bahouth MN, Hu P, et al. Telemedicine for acute stroke: triumphs and pitfalls. Stroke 2003; 34:725–728.
12. Cullen JS, Gagliano D, Gaasch W, et al. Mobile medicine testbed. TRW Syst Inform J Rev 1999; 7(1):1–16.
13. LaMonte MP, Hu P, Xiao Y, Page CW, Mackenzie CF. Telemedicine networks: a potential solution for emergency department barriers to stroke treatment. 24th American Heart Association International Conference on Stroke and Cerebral Circulation. Stroke 1999; 1:66.
14. LaMonte MP, Bates V, Bahouth MN, et al. Administration for ischemic stroke during telemedicine consultation. Stroke 2001; 32(1):374.
15. Merino JG, Silver B, Wong E, et al. Extending tissue plasminogen activator use to community and rural stroke patients. Stroke 2002; 33:141–146.
16. Wiborg A, Widder B. Teleneurology to improve stroke care in rural areas: the Telemedicine in Stroke in Swabia (TESS) Project. Stroke 2003; 34:1763–1768.
17. Audebert HJ, Kukla C, Clarmann von Claraau S, et al. Telemedicine for safe and extended use of thrombolysis in stroke: the Telemedic Pilot Project for Integrative Stroke Care (TEMPiS) in Bavaria. Stroke 2005; 36:287–291.
18. Wang S, Gross H, Lee SB, et al. Remote evaluation of acute ischemic stroke in rural community hospitals in Georgia. Stroke 2004; 35:1763–1768.
19. Schwamm LH, Rosenthal ES, Hirshberg A, et al. Virtual Telestroke support for the emergency department evaluation of acute stroke. Acad Emerg Med 2004; 11:1193–1197.
20. http://telehealth.hrsa.gov/pubs/legis.htm (Rural Telehealth Act, 1999).
21. LaMonte MP, Bahouth MN. Developing a telemedicine contract for acute stroke consultation. Telemed J E Health 2005; 11:2.
22. Laff W. Rural medicine programs aimed to reverse physician shortage in outlying regions. AAMC Reporter Nov 2004. http://www.aamc.org/newsroom/reporter/nov04/rural.htm.
23. Provider Support Systems. National Institute of Neurological Disorders and Stroke. Improving the chain of recovery for acute stroke in your community. Task Force Reports 2003; 87–89.

37 | Multimodality Neuromonitoring in Acute Stroke

Wolf-Dieter Heiss, MD, Professor, Christian Dohmen, MD
Rudolf Graf, PhD, Assistant Professor
Department of Neurology, Max-Planck Institute for Neurological Research,
University of Cologne, Cologne, Germany

INTRODUCTION

Based on extensive experience in experimental models (1–4), invasive multimodal monitoring was introduced into neurointensive care of patients with severe disorders of the brain, especially in those with severe head injury (5,6). In these patients, repetitive or continuous recordings of brain tissue oxygenation, substrate delivery and concentration (e.g., glucose, lactate, pyruvate, and amino acids), and alterations of the ionic homeostasis supplement the established monitoring of intracranial pressure (ICP) and cerebral perfusion pressure (CPP) (5,7–11). Because progressive interruption of substrate delivery, which affects patients after severe head injury, is also the main factor for tissue damage in subarachnoid hemorrhage (SAH), multimodal neuroimaging was also utilized to predict the development of brain damage, such as infarction or brain swelling (12–14). Recently, multimodal neuromonitoring was also introduced into the management of patients with acute ischemic stroke (15), especially aiming at an early prediction of development of space-occupying edema (malignant infarction) (16) and at an online assessment of treatment effects. This application of neuromonitoring represents a valid example of translational research, as variables determined in experimental models of focal ischemia can be compared to those obtained in patients with acute ischemic stroke.

STUDIES IN EXPERIMENTAL STROKE MODELS

The various neuromonitoring tools, including invasive recording of ICP and CPP, neurochemical recording with microdialysis, high-performance liquid chromatography (HPLC) or tissue-oxygen sensors, and electrophysiologic recording, that are now used in stroke patients in intensive care units, have been tested for many years in experimental studies, and it still seems as if many of the benefits of these tools are best obtained in the experimental situation. For example, the ability to accomplish almost continuous recordings immediately following insult is one of the major benefits of invasive monitoring tools. However, this immediacy can only be achieved in experimental conditions, in the acute phase of ischemia, and, typically, even in the preischemic control stage; whereas, under clinical conditions, the start of monitoring is often delayed by many hours following stroke onset. Similarly, simultaneous measurement with multiple sensors in differently affected tissue compartments seems essential for effective monitoring—a protocol easily achieved in experimental settings if the brain size of the experimental animal allows such multiple approaches. In the clinic, by contrast, the site of sensor implantation is often predetermined by surgical needs for a craniotomy or other surgical procedure, such as catheter implantation for ventricular drainage. Optimal positioning of sensors is not possible because application of additional burr holes is unethical. Another problem is the small volume of tissue that is analyzed by most of the invasive techniques in a laboratory. In view of the large human brain, results might be easily misinterpreted because of inadequate sensor positioning, compared to assessments with the same tools in smaller animal brains. It is, therefore, not surprising that invasive neuromonitoring has been performed only in stroke patients in whom extended secondary, damage-like, space-occupying edema or bleeding is to be expected.

The decision to use invasive monitoring in an individual patient is usually based on neuroimaging results. A malignant course is characterized by edema formation and delayed, secondary deterioration due to rise in ICP and allows more time for indication for such treatments as hemicraniectomy than is available in the first hours after stroke onset, when the decision whether to use thrombolysis must be made. In this somewhat longer timeframe, advantages of neuromonitoring can be realized, particularly if introduced to supplement noninvasive neuroimaging modalities, such as MRI or positron-emission tomography (PET). In this chapter, we will mainly focus on experimental results obtained in a focal ischemia model that is prone to malignant stroke in a certain percentage of animals. In this context, one should consider that single modalities, such as electrophysiologic tools or micro-dialysis, have often been experimentally applied but that invasive multimodality monitoring, including ICP/CPP recording, has rarely been performed in other than so-called malignant models.

We investigated, in various series of experiments, a model of focal ischemia in cats that has been shown to be prone to secondary deterioration in a percentage of cats during permanent occlusion (17) and, particularly, during reperfusion if the duration of a transient ischemic episode is prolonged (18). To investigate mechanisms of primary and secondary glutamate accumulation in relation to a malignant course of edema formation and global cerebral blood flow (CBF) reduction, the studies, using a multiparametric approach, focused on time-course relationships between ICP and CPP, CBF, extracellular alterations of neuro-chemical substances (19,20), and changes in electrophysiologic parameters, such as peri-infarct depolarization (21).

The studies were performed in halothane- or α–chloralose-anesthetized adult cats. With an occlusion device implanted at the proximal portion of the middle cerebral artery (MCA), we occluded and reperfused the left MCA for desired periods. A pressure transducer mea-sured mean arterial blood pressure (MABP), a strain-gauge MicroSensor measured ICP, and a thermocouple measured regional brain temperature. Microdialysis probes were inserted into cortical core (ectosylvian gyrus, $n = 10$) and perifocal regions (marginal gyrus, $n = 9$) within the MCA territory. Concentrations of amino acids, such as glutamate, and of purine catabolites, such as adenosine, inosine, and hypoxanthine in dialysate, were analyzed by HPLC. Adjacent to microdialysis probes, laser-Doppler flow (LDF) probes measured regional CBF (rCBF). In all experiments, the skull was sealed after preparation.

MCA occlusion (MCAO) (Fig. 1) reduced CBF in all animals below 25% and below 35% of control in respective core and perifocal regions. In experiments with transient 3-hour MCAO, almost 50% of cats showed pupil dilation in the course of reperfusion and were, there-fore, defined as "malignant MCA infarction." MABP did not change throughout MCAO but increased slightly in nonmalignant cases and decreased in malignant cases following reper-fusion. Similar to MABP, ICP did not change during MCAO but started to increase in both malignant and nonmalignant cases almost immediately after reopening of the MCA, an effect that was noted from the beginning to be more pronounced in malignant cases. Furthermore, in these animals, ICP continued to increase throughout the reperfusion period; in a final stage of steep rise, values well above 70 mmHg were reached. As a result, CPP was dramatically altered, with a decrease below 30 mmHg at the time of the steep ICP increase. Maximum values of ICP during reperfusion were significantly higher in malignant than in nonmalignant cases; consequently, minimum values of CPP during reperfusion were significantly lower in malig-nant than in nonmalignant cases. Furthermore, the volume of neuronal necrosis, evaluated in paraffin-embedded brain sections stained with hematoxylin-eosin and Luxol fast blue, was significantly larger in malignant than in nonmalignant cases.

Extracellular glutamate evaluated by microdialysis/HPLC (Fig. 1) increased approxi-mately 20-fold during MCAO in the ischemic core of malignant animals, and this rise was significantly higher than in benign cases. In the perifocal zone, such a rise was not observed in either malignant or in benign cases. Thus, microdialysis determinations in the core region seemed most predictive regarding the fatal course. Upon reperfusion, LDF–CBF and gluta-mate primarily recovered. In malignant cats, however, a secondary elevation of glutamate was apparent during the reperfusion period. In this "secondary elevation group," glutamate started to rise when CPP decreased below ~60 mmHg. Almost simultaneously, symptoms of transtentorial herniation were recognized. Minimal CPP values in the animals of this group were below 50 mmHg, and brains showed midline-shift and neuronal necrosis even in the contralateral hemisphere. Surprisingly, extracellular adenosine (a marker of Adenosine tri-phosphate depletion) rose transiently during MCAO but not during secondary ischemia that

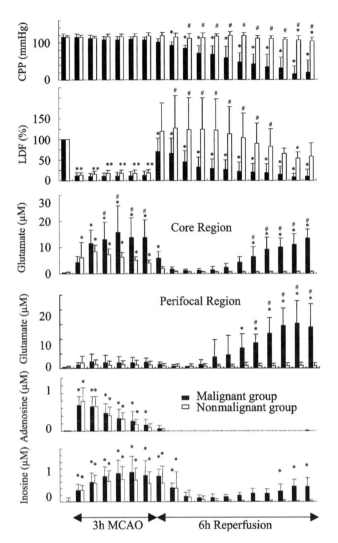

Figure 1 Changes in CPP, LDF, glutamate (measured independently in core and perifocal regions), and the purine catabolites, adenosine and inosine, in the two groups exhibiting a nonmalignant course (*white bars*; n = 5) and a malignant course (*black bars*; n = 5) of infarction, as a function of time. Mean ± SD is plotted every half hour. *p < 0.05: significantly different from preischemic control. #p < 0.05: significantly different from group exhibiting a malignant course. Note significant elevation of glutamate during MCAO in core but not in perifocal, region. Note also secondary elevation of glutamate and inosine, but not adenosine, in the "malignant" group in the course of reperfusion, documenting metabolic derangement in these animals. *Abbreviations*: CPP, cerebral perfusion pressure; LDF, laser-Doppler flow; MCAO, middle cerebral artery occlusion.

resulted from decreased CPP in the late reperfusion period, where as other purins (inosine and hypoxanthine) increased in both phases. We hypothesize that, after reperfusion, salvage pathways are able to resynthesize inosine monophosphate (IMP), but not adenosine monophosphate (AMP), because inosine and hypoxanthine, as precursors for IMP synthesis, have been formed in excess during MCAO, but adenosine, as the precursor of AMP synthesis, is only transiently elevated during MCAO.

The role of elevated glutamate as an endogenous excitotoxin (22) has been challenged (23). For example, glutamate concentration in neuropil, where receptors are activated, is not detectable by microdialysis. In addition, inhibitory substances, such as Gama-amino butyric acid and adenosine, increase when glutamate is elevated (24,25). Therefore, glutamate has been hypothesized to have another detrimental role as an induction factor for the generation of transient, spreading, depression-like depolarizations in peri-infarct regions (26). These depolarizations are generated at multiple sites, including cortex and striatum (21), and might be suppressed by glutamate antagonists (27,28). The depolarizations propagate into surrounding, metabolically stressed, at-risk tissue. Because repolarization is an energy-consuming process, these repetitive depolarizations are associated with progressive deterioration. Evidence shows that they might cause expansion of infarction, including the transformation into malignant infarction (17,21,29). To observe these phenomena, experimental multimodal monitoring has predominantly used direct current potential recordings and assessment of extracellular ion activities with ion selective electrodes (17,21), techniques that are not readily available for use in human patients. In a recent study in human trauma patients, however, it was shown that spreading, depression-like events can be detected by subdural electroencephalogram recordings using multiple strip electrodes (30), and an attempt is currently being undertaken to measure depolarizations in hemispheric stroke patients.

Although more multimodality neuromonitoring techniques are available in experimental than in clinical settings, many have found their way into clinical research. For example, the introduction of microdialysis has opened a rather wide analytic spectrum, because, with the use of a single "sensor," various classes of markers for glucose metabolism (glucose, lactate/pyruvate ratio), ATP depletion (purine catabolites), membrane degradation (glycerol), excitotoxicity (glutamate), and nitric oxide formation (nitrate, nitrite) can be analyzed in the same dialysate sample. Obviously, the clinical relevance of these methods can best be shown in models that closely mimic clinical conditions. It must be recognized, however, that besides ICP, none of the techniques can be introduced into routine clinical management due to limitations associated with the site of sensor implantation in relation to injury, problems with quantification, and the small volume of tissue that can be analyzed.

APPLICATION OF MULTIMODAL MONITORING IN THE NEUROLOGIC INTENSIVE CARE UNIT

Until recently, the only widely accepted parameters, by which, to continuously monitor the cerebral status of patients in the neurologic intensive care unit have been ICP and CPP. Both measures can be helpful to guide further treatment in patients with traumatic brain injury and poor-grade SAH (31). However, their use in monitoring secondary deleterious events in SAH and occlusive stroke is doubtful, and their influence on overall outcome has never been proven in controlled trials (32,33). As ischemia and hypoxia are the common pathophysiologic mechanisms of cerebral tissue damage in traumatic brain injury, SAH, and ischemic stroke, monitoring focuses on oxygenation, metabolism, and CBF in brain tissue. Current monitoring devices are small, fiber-like microprobes that are implanted into the tissue of interest.

Oxygen tension in brain tissue (P_tO_2) can be measured by either a polarographic technique or optical luminescence using a microcatheter that is fixed in the skull by a special bolt, and resulting data can be combined with determination of tissue carbon dioxide and pH. For measurement of rCBF, probes that estimate CBF by the thermal diffusion principle are now available. In contrast to the single variables obtained with these probes, microdialysis is able to monitor a broad spectrum of substances. Glucose, lactate, pyruvate, urea, glutamate, and glycerol can be measured and displayed at bedside. As each of the monitoring devices yields important information about the injured brain, monitoring can be maximized when devices are combined for multimodal neuromonitoring, which can be achieved by implantation of several probes via a single burr hole using a multichannel bolt kit that reduces risk of bleeding or infection. First introduced in traumatic brain injury, the new monitoring techniques are now used in patients with SAH and ischemic stroke.

In patients with SAH, multimodal neuromonitoring is used to detect clinical events that lead to secondary ischemia (e.g., hematoma, edema, or secondary ischemia due to vasospasm). For this purpose, probes are implanted (mainly intraoperatively during aneurysmal clipping) into the tissue territory supplied by the aneurysmatic artery. Several studies showed that ischemic events correlate with distinct patterns of changes in monitoring parameters, which led to identification of markers for ischemia: increased levels of brain tissue lactate, lactate/pyruvate ratio, glutamate, glycerol, aspartate, and hypoxanthine, as well as a drop in glucose and P_tO_2 (12,14,34–42). Consistent with the finding of markers of secondary brain damage, a correlation between ischemia markers and clinical outcome after SAH was found. Poor outcome after SAH correlated with high lactate, high lactate/pyruvate, and high lactate/glucose ratios, and high values of glycerol and glutamate, a decrease in glucose and pyruvate, and a decrease in P_tO_2 below 10 mmHg (11–14,36–38,42–49). In addition to these bedside parameters, post hoc analysis of microdialysate by HPLC revealed further characteristics of patients with poor outcome—high average concentrations of hypoxanthine, taurine, and serine (13) and increased GABA concentrations (50). A 2003 study demonstrated the particular importance of P_tO_2 measurements in detection and prediction of cerebral edema in SAH patients (51). Other groups demonstrated that a delayed ischemic neurologic deficit (DIND) after SAH that manifested as secondary paresis, deterioration of mental status, and aphasia, was associated with an increase in brain lactate and glutamate and a decrease in glucose (39,40). Yet another group reported in 2001 that in 83% of patients who developed DIND, excessive increases of lactate, lactate/pyruvate ratio, and glutamate preceded clinical onset of DIND by several hours (5–42 hr) (52). Early decreases of P_tO_2 were found to indicate vasospasm that was confirmed in angiography and, in another study, pCO_2 increases to 60 mmHg and pH decreases to 6.7 were indicative of vasospasm (53,54). Measurement of rCBF by thermal diffusion seems to be a reliable tool for prediction of vasospasm and might be superior to transcranial-Doppler ultrasonography (55).

Multimodal neuromonitoring can also be used to guide therapies aimed at restoring blood supply to the tissue. Lactate/pyruvate ratio was increased and P_tO_2 and glucose were decreased due to vasospasm and were normalized after transluminal balloon angioplasty (53). P_tO_2 values were monitored for verification of the effect of hypervolemic hypertension or nimodipine therapy (49,56). Aside from detecting secondary damage, multimodal monitoring can be used as a control tool during aneurysmal clipping to prevent perioperative primary ischemic transition (35).

Multimodal neuromonitoring has recently been introduced in patients with large hemispheric infarction who are in danger of developing a space-occupying brain edema with subsequent transtentorial herniation, so-called malignant MCA infarction (16). In these patients, multimodal neuromonitoring is applied to detect secondary ischemia and malignant clinical course. Accurate prediction of clinical course is of particular importance for the timely implementation of such invasive therapies as hemicraniectomy, by which mortality rates can be reduced with conservative treatment from ~80% to 20–30% (57). The potential of microdialysis to detect secondary ischemic events and predict a malignant clinical course was first demonstrated in 1999 (58). All monitoring parameters increased when a massive, space-occupying edema developed, indicating secondary ischemia of the primary healthy hemisphere. Interestingly, changes of glutamate and glycerol occurred several hours earlier than ICP changes or clinical deterioration. In further studies involving a greater number of patients with large MCA infarction, in whom probes were placed in the ipsilateral peri-infarct region, markers for secondary ischemia were consistent with the observations in SAH; namely, increased levels of lactate, lactate/pyruvate ratio, glutamate, glycerol, aspartate, GABA, and hypoxanthine, and a reduction of P_tO_2 below 10 mmHg (59,60) (Fig. 2). Furthermore, these parameters correlated strongly with clinical outcome (using modified Rankin scale), and with the extent of space-occupying brain edema. Neuromonitoring markers for ischemia showed excellent sensitivity, specificity, and predictive values for malignant course; however, peak values were reached only at time points at which deterioration had progressed beyond the point of efficacy for hemicraniectomy (60). Concentrations of nontransmitter amino acids, such as arginine, asparagine, isoleucine, leucine, methionine, phenylalanine, serine, and valine, have been shown to correlate closely with clinical course (61). Low concentrations of nontransmitter amino acids were able to predict malignant brain edema early, at a time point when hemicraniectomy could be effective (Fig. 2). The lower concentrations of nontransmitter amino acids in patients later developing mass edema were attributed to dilution of substances due to an early expansion of vasogenic edema into the peri-infarct tissue.

As in SAH, multimodal neuromonitoring can be used to evaluate the effect of therapeutic interventions and thereby guide treatment in patients with large hemispheric infarcts. Effects of different antiedema drugs were evaluated by means of multimodal neuromonitoring in patients with malignant MCA infarction (62,63). Based on their results, researchers concluded that the value of ICP measurement as a surrogate marker for therapeutic efficacy was inferior to that of P_tO_2 (62). Effects of hypothermia on brain metabolism measured by microdialysis

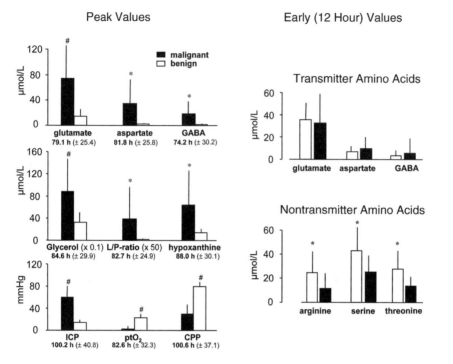

Figure 2 Multimodal monitoring in peri-infarct tissue of patients with large middle cerebral artery infarction. *Left column*: Peak values (mean ± SD) of interstitial metabolites and ICP and minimal values of CPP and P_tO_2 for patients with malignant and benign clinical course after infarction, respectively (significant differences between groups: *$p < 0.05$, #$p < 0.01$). In patients with malignant course, significantly higher values were observed for all microdialysis parameters and ICP; significantly lower values were seen for P_tO_2 and CPP. Time point of mean peak value of patients with malignant course is indicated below name of the parameter (hours after stroke). *Right column*: Extracellular concentrations of nontransmitter amino acids and transmitter amino acids, expressed as mean ± SD of the first 12 hr of microdialysis measurement. Concentrations of transmitter amino acids were not significantly different at this early time point, whereas nontransmitter amino acids showed marked differences between malignant and benign clinical course. *Abbreviations*: CPP, cerebral perfusion pressure; ICP, intracranial pressure.

have also been investigated and found to be neuroprotective on tissue at risk for secondary ischemia, a finding that was evidenced by reduction of glutamate, lactate, and lactate/pyruvate ratio, and by a rise in pyruvate (64).

Several methodologic limitations must be considered before applying multimodal neuromonitoring. First, invasive monitoring of metabolism with microdialysis probes and of tissue oxygen with sensors are regional measurements in a small tissue volume. Therefore, only focal and selective information can be obtained from tissue compartments already lesioned or in danger of becoming damaged. This drawback can be overcome by integrating monitoring techniques that yield global information about the cerebral status, such as measurements of ICP, CPP, or jugular bulb oximetry. With microdialysis, quantification of parameters is difficult to achieve, and, so far, relative changes in concentrations must be interpreted over time. Implantation of probes into brain tissue is invasive and associated with risk of bleeding and infection. The risk of invasive measurement with implantable microdialysis, oxygen, or CBF probes is comparable to the risks of ICP measurement in the parenchyma. Fixation of probes with a multichannel bolt kit might reduce the risk of bleeding and infection and help to control placement of probes in the white matter. Innovations in microdialysis technique make monitoring of larger peptides possible, which might include measurements of several peptides relevant in the pathophysiology of stroke, such as interleukins or matrix-metalloproteinases. Furthermore, microdialysis can be used to monitor drug delivery to the brain, which might become part of multimodal monitoring in the future.

COMPARISON TO FUNCTIONAL IMAGING

Multimodal neuromonitoring permits the clinician to continuously or repeatedly follow alterations in several variables responsible for pathophysiologic conditions in the brain over prolonged periods of time, but it is restricted to small volumes of brain tissue (2). Therefore, the site of monitoring probes must be carefully selected to reflect the brain regions in which reliable pathophysiologic changes occur in the course of the disease. To select the appropriate location of the monitoring probe, imaging techniques [computed tomography (CT) or MRI] are used, and the border zone in which progression of damage can be expected is defined. However, applying functional imaging for assessment of perfusional and metabolic disturbances can yield independent markers of the condition of various tissue compartments in whole brain. Therefore, a combination of both approaches—repeated, continuous determination of physiologic variables in related small brain volumes and assessment of perfusion and metabolism of the whole brain at a defined time point after the attack—might improve the insight into pathophysiology and the prediction of course and prognosis of the disorder.

To evaluate the potential of microdialysis as an instrument for chemical brain monitoring, the changes in extracellular concentrations of various substrates were related directly to the metabolic states as assessed by PET in MCAO and reperfusion in primates (65). Measurements of the cerebral metabolic rate of oxygen (CMRO$_2$), CBF, and the oxygen extraction fraction (OEF) by ^{15}O-PET and H$_2$^{15}O-PET were used to identify regions of severe ischemia (CMRO$_2$ less than 60% of contralateral area) and penumbra (increased OEF), and to detect reperfusion. Regions with severe ischemia during MCAO displayed high increases in lactate/pyruvate ratio, hypoxanthine, and glutamate; and irrespective of the extent of reperfusion, those levels never decreased to baseline. Regions classified as penumbra (increased OEF) displayed only slight transient increases in those substrates, which returned to baseline during reperfusion. The study proved that extracellular changes of energy-related metabolites and glutamate differed according to the ischemic state of tissue during MCAO and a successful reperfusion. However, this early study also indicated the necessity to observe relative changes over time. In a further study, the value of glycerol as a marker of lipid degradation and irreversible tissue damage was tested (66,67). In this primate stroke model, a marked and sustained increase in interstitial glycerol indicated severe ischemia, and a transient and slight increase of this substrate reflected the penumbra condition. These dialysate compounds might be useful in following the sequence of secondary pathophysiologic changes.

In a complex experimental set-up, several variables were followed before, during, and up to 6 hr after 3-hour MCAO in 11 cats (68). MABP and ICP were measured simultaneously, and CPP was calculated. The extracellular concentration of glutamate was determined by microdialysis and HPLC and was followed for the entire experiment (Fig. 3). Regional changes in CBF and cerebral metabolic rate for glucose (CMRGlc) were determined by PET after 15O-water or 18F-fluorodeoxyglucose injection. Extent of ischemia in core and border zones was determined during MCAO, and flow and substrates were followed in these defined regions. In 3 animals, a malignant course was observed with excessive rise in ICP, drop in CPP, secondary deterioration of CBF (Fig. 3), and symptoms of herniation, including dilatation of pupils. Severe ischemia extended over 55% to 75%, and moderate ischemia extended over 5% to 10% of the hemisphere. Extracellular concentration of glutamate increased significantly in the core of ischemia during MCAO and spread to border zones during the reperfusion. In the other eight cats, severe ischemia covered 10% to 45%, and moderate ischemia, 15% to 30%, of the hemisphere. Perfusional and metabolic deficits were confined to the ischemic regions for the duration of follow-up, and ICP was only transiently increased after reopening of the MCA, without leading to persisting changes in ICP, CPP, CBF, or glutamate concentrations. In this study, functional imaging identified the large region of damage at the end of the occlusion period and predicted the malignant course, which was reflected in the sequential changes of ICP, CPP, and metabolic substrates.

The validity of monitoring physiologic variables in small focal volumes was established by comparing these results to measurements of flow and energy metabolism of the whole brain that were obtained by PET in patients with head injury (69) and with SAH (34,70). In patients with head injury, the lactate/pyruvate ratio correlated with OEF, but a significant relationship between dialysate substrates (glucose, lactate, lactate/pyruvate, and glutamate) and CBF was not found. In SAH, alterations in dialysate levels of energy-related metabolites and excitatory

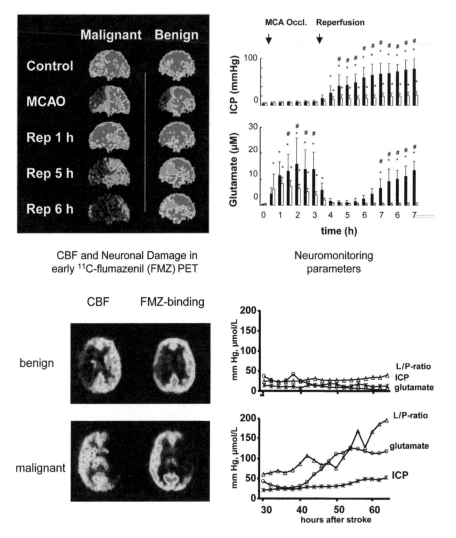

Figure 3 Comparison of multimodal monitoring and functional imaging in an experimental stroke model and in patients with large MCA infarction. (*Upper panel, left*) Sequential PET CBF images in two cats with malignant (*left*) and benign courses after transient MCAO. Note hyperperfusion immediately following recirculation and subsequent deterioration, extending into the contralateral hemisphere in the malignant animal. (*Upper panel, right*) ICP and glutamate (mean ± SD, plotted every half hour) in two groups of cats exhibiting malignant (*black bars*) or nonmalignant (*white bars*) infarction. Note significantly higher glutamate rise in the core of infarction in the malignant group already during ischemia. (*Lower panel, left*) CBF and FMZ binding determined by PET before implementation of monitoring devices in benign and malignant infarction. In benign infarcts, volumes of severe hypoperfusion and neuronal damage (i.e., reduced FMZ binding) were smaller than in patients with malignant course. (*Lower panel, right*) Sequential recordings of lactate/pyruvate ratio and glutamate concentration in benign versus malignant MCA infarction starting 30 hr after onset of symptoms. In the benign course, no changes in the variables were observed, whereas in malignant infarct, substrate concentrations and ICP increased progressively. *Abbreviations*: ICP, intracranial pressure; MCA, middle cerebral artery; CBF, cerebral blood flow; PET, positron-emission tomography; MCAO, middle cerebral artery occlusion; FMZ, flumazenil.

amino acids directly correlated to the energy state, as defined by PET (34), and glutamate, glycerol, and lactate/pyruvate ratio correlated to the CBF in the respective region (70). Therefore, these compounds can be used as extracellular markers of ischemia, especially when probes for continuous chemical monitoring can be inserted into at-risk tissue, as defined by PET studies.

The concept of a combination of early PET imaging (for identifying ischemic damage and tissue at risk) with prolonged multimodal monitoring (for tracing the course of pathophysiologic changes) was realized in a study of 34 patients with infarcts expanding over more than 50% of the MCA territory, demonstrated in early cerebral CT (60). In these cases, PET of

11C-flumazenil (FMZ), a ligand of central benzodiazepine receptors that is established as a marker of neuronal integrity, was used to assess CBF and irreversible neuronal damage within 24 hr after stroke. After the PET study, probes for microdialysis and for measurement of ICP and P_tO_2 were placed into the ipsilateral frontal lobe in the vicinity of the infarct on CT (Fig. 3). The clinical course of these patients was followed and regarded as malignant when signs of uncal herniation developed with a unilaterally dilated pupil and when the follow-up CT showed space-occupying brain edema with midline shift.

The volume of critically hypoperfused tissue as determined by the distribution of FMZ (CBF less than 50% of contralateral mean) 3 to 38 hr (mean, 17 hr) after symptom onset was larger in patients with malignant course ($n=17$, $144.5 \pm 27.6 \, cm^3$) than in the benign group ($n=17$, $62.2 \pm 37.2 \, cm^3$), as was the volume of irreversible damage (malignant, $157.9 \pm 37.9 \, cm^3$; benign, $47.0 \pm 46.9 \, cm^3$) (Fig. 3). Mean CBF values within the ischemic core were significantly lower ($21.5 \pm 3.7\%$ vs. $34.7 \pm 6.6\%$), and the volume of the ischemic penumbra was significantly smaller (42.6 ± 14.4 vs. $58.0 \pm 14.4 \, cm^3$) in the malignant group, as compared to the benign group. The volume of irreversible damage and the volume of severe ischemia correlated significantly with patient outcome (expressed by modified Rankin scale score after 3 months).

In patients with malignant course, CPP dropped to less than 50 to 60 mmHg at 22 to 72 hr (mean 52.0 hr) after onset of symptoms. Subsequently, P_tO_2 dropped and glutamate increased, indicating secondary ischemia (Fig. 3). Maximal changes in the monitored variables reached significant levels for glutamate, aspartate, GABA, glycerol, lactate/pyruvate ratio, hypoxanthine, ICP, CPP, and P_tO_2. The mean peak values for glutamate, aspartate, and GABA were significantly lower for patients with benign course than for patients with a malignant course. Similarly, lactate, lactate/pyruvate ratio, hypoxanthine, and ICP increased significantly in the malignant group, and CPP and P_tO_2 were significantly lower in these cases.

CONCLUSIONS AND FUTURE DIRECTIONS

In conclusion, PET allowed prediction of malignant MCA infarction at an early state and long before determinations of ICP and P_tO_2 or microdialysis recorded the ongoing progression and detrimental pathophysiologic changes that accompany the critical stage of clinical deterioration. The combination of these methods helps to identify patients at risk for formation of space-occupying edema and could be useful for the selection of patients who might benefit from invasive interventional therapeutic strategies.

REFERENCES

1. Benveniste H, Hansen AJ, Ottosen NS. Determination of brain interstitial concentrations by microdialysis. J Neurochem 1989; 52(6):1741–1750.
2. Ungerstedt U. Microdialysis–principles and applications for studies in animals and man. J Intern Med 1991; 230(4):365–373.
3. Kehr J. A survey on quantitative microdialysis: theoretical models and practical implications. J Neurosci Methods 1993; 48(3):251–261.
4. Robinson TE, Justice JB. Microdialysis in the Neurosciences. Amsterdam: Elsevier, 1991.
5. De Georgia MA, Deogaonkar A. Multimodal monitoring in the neurological intensive care unit. Neurologist 2005; 11(1):45–54.
6. Hillered L, Vespa PM, Hovda DA. Translational neurochemical research in acute human brain injury: the current status and potential future for cerebral microdialysis. J Neurotrauma 2005; 22(1):3–41.
7. Bullock R, Chesnut RM, Clifton G, et al. Guidelines for the management of severe head injury. The American Association of Neurological Surgeons & the Brain Trauma Foundation, 1995.
8. Tsubokawa T, Marmarou A, Robertson C, et al. Neurochemical Monitoring in the Intensive Care Unit. New York: Springer, 1995.
9. Meixensberger J, Kunze E, Barcsay E, et al. Clinical cerebral microdialysis: brain metabolism and brain tissue oxygenation after acute brain injury. Neurol Res 2001; 23(8):801–806.
10. Bellander BM, Cantais E, Enblad P, et al. Consensus meeting on microdialysis in neurointensive care. Intensive Care Med 2004; 30(12):2166–2169.
11. Sarrafzadeh A, Haux D, Sakowitz O, et al. Acute focal neurological deficits in aneurysmal subarachnoid hemorrhage: relation of clinical course, CT findings, and metabolite abnormalities monitored with bedside microdialysis. Stroke 2003; 34(6):1382–1388.

12. Nilsson OG, Brandt L, Ungerstedt U, et al. Bedside detection of brain ischemia using intracerebral microdialysis: subarachnoid hemorrhage and delayed ischemic deterioration. Neurosurgery 1999; 45(5):1176–1184.

13. Staub F, Graf R, Gabel P, et al. Multiple interstitial substances measured by microdialysis in patients with subarachnoid hemorrhage. Neurosurgery 2000; 47(5):1106–1116.

14. Persson L, Valtysson J, Enblad P, et al. Neurochemical monitoring using intracerebral microdialysis in patients with subarachnoid hemorrhage. J Neurosurg 1996; 84(4):606–616.

15. Hillered L, Persson L, Pontén U, et al. Neurometabolic monitoring of the ischaemic human brain using microdialysis. Acta Neurochir 1990; 102:91–97.

16. Hacke W, Schwab S, Horn M, et al. 'Malignant' middle cerebral artery territory infarction: clinical course and prognostic signs. Arch Neurol 1996; 53(4):309–315.

17. Ohta K, Graf R, Rosner G, et al. Calcium ion transients in peri-infarct depolarizations may deteriorate ion homeostasis and expand infarction in focal cerebral ischemia in cats. Stroke 2001; 32(2): 535–543.

18. Taguchi J, Graf R, Rosner G, et al. Prolonged transient ischemia results in impaired CBF recovery and secondary glutamate accumulation in cats. J Cereb Blood Flow Metab 1996; 16(2):271–279.

19. Toyota S, Graf R, Valentino M, et al. Malignant infarction in cats after prolonged middle cerebral artery occlusion. Glutamate elevation related to decrease of cerebral perfusion pressure. Stroke 2002; 33(5):1383–1391.

20. Toyota S, Graf R, Valentino M, et al. Prediction of malignant infarction: perifocal neurochemical monitoring following prolonged MCA occlusion in cats. Acta Neurochir Suppl 2003; 86:153–157.

21. Umegaki M, Sanada Y, Waerzeggers Y, et al. Peri-infarct depolarizations reveal penumbra-like conditions in striatum. J Neurosci 2005; 25(6):1387–1394.

22. Olney JW. Excitatory neurotoxins as food additives: an evaluation of risk. Neurotoxicology 1981; 2(1):163–192.

23. Obrenovitch TP. High extracellular glutamate and neuronal death in neurological disorders. Cause, contribution or consequence? Ann NY Acad Sci 1999; 890:273–286.

24. Hagberg H, Andersson P, Lacarewicz J, et al. Extracellular adenosine, inosine, hypoxanthine, and xanthine in relation to tissue nucleotides and purines in rat striatum during transient ischemia. J Neurochem 1987; 49(1):227–231.

25. Matsumoto K, Graf R, Rosner G, et al. Flow thresholds for extracellular purine catabolite elevation in cat focal ischemia. Brain Res 1992; 579(2):309–314.

26. Hossmann KA. Periinfarct depolarizations. Cerebrovasc Brain Metab Rev 1996; 8(3):195–208.

27. Gill R, Andine P, Hillered L, et al. The effect of MK-801 on cortical spreading depression in the penumbral zone following focal ischaemia in the rat. J Cereb Blood Flow Metab 1992; 12(3):371–379.

28. Iijima T, Mies G, Hossmann KA. Repeated negative DC deflections in rat cortex following middle cerebral artery occlusion are abolished by MK-801: effect on volume of ischemic injury. J Cereb Blood Flow Metab 1992; 12(5):727–733.

29. Back T, Kohno K, Hossmann KA. Cortical negative DC deflections following middle cerebral artery occlusion and KCl-induced spreading depression: effect on blood flow, tissue oxygenation, and electroencephalogram. J Cereb Blood Flow Metab 1994; 14(1):12–19.

30. Strong AJ, Fabricius M, Boutelle MG, et al. Spreading and synchronous depressions of cortical activity in acutely injured human brain. Stroke 2002; 33(12):2738–2743.

31. Czosnyka M, Pickard JD. Monitoring and interpretation of intracranial pressure. J Neurol Neurosurg Psychiatry 2004; 75(6):813–821.

32. Frank JI. Large hemispheric infarction, deterioration, and intracranial pressure. Neurology 1995; 45(7):1286–1290.

33. Schwab S, Aschoff A, Spranger M, et al. The value of intracranial pressure monitoring in acute hemispheric stroke. Neurology 1996; 47(2):393–398.

34. Enblad P, Valtysson J, Andersson J, et al. Simultaneous intracerebral microdialysis and positron emission tomography in the detection of ischemia in patients with subarachnoid hemorrhage. J Cereb Blood Flow Metab 1996; 16(4):637–644.

35. Hutchinson PJ, Al-Rawi PG, O'Connell MT, et al. Monitoring of brain metabolism during aneurysm surgery using microdialysis and brain multiparameter sensors. Neurol Res 1999; 21(4):352–358.

36. Kett-White R, Hutchinson PJ, Al-Rawi PG, et al. Cerebral oxygen and microdialysis monitoring during aneurysm surgery: effects of blood pressure, cerebrospinal fluid drainage, and temporary clipping on infarction. J Neurosurg 2002; 96(6):1013–1019.

37. Persson L, Hillered L. Chemical monitoring of neurosurgical intensive care patients using intracerebral microdialysis. J Neurosurg 1992; 76(1):72–80.

38. Schulz MK, Wang LP, Tange M, et al. Cerebral microdialysis monitoring: determination of normal and ischemic cerebral metabolisms in patients with aneurysmal subarachnoid hemorrhage. J Neurosurg 2000; 93(5):808–814.

39. Sakowitz OW, Sarrafzadeh AS, Benndorf G, et al. On-line microdialysis following aneurysmal subarachnoid hemorrhage. Acta Neurochir Suppl 2001; 77:141–144.
40. Unterberg AW, Sakowitz OW, Sarrafzadeh AS, et al. Role of bedside microdialysis in the diagnosis of cerebral vasospasm following aneurysmal subarachnoid hemorrhage. J Neurosurg 2001; 94(5):740–749.
41. Hillered L, Valtysson J, Enblad P, et al. Interstitial glycerol as a marker for membrane phospholipid degradation in the acutely injured human brain. J Neurol Neurosurg Psychiatry 1998; 64(4):486–491.
42. Meixensberger J, Vath A, Jaeger M, et al. Monitoring of brain tissue oxygenation following severe subarachnoid hemorrhage. Neurol Res 2003; 25(5):445–450.
43. Sarrafzadeh A, Haux D, Kuchler I, et al. Poor-grade aneurysmal subarachnoid hemorrhage: relationship of cerebral metabolism to outcome. J Neurosurg 2004; 100(3):400–406.
44. Cesarini KG, Enblad P, Ronne-Engstrom E, et al. Early cerebral hyperglycolysis after subarachnoid haemorrhage correlates with favourable outcome. Acta Neurochir (Wien) 2002; 144(11):1121–1131.
45. Kanthan R, Goplen G, Griebel R, et al. Clinical evaluation of vasospasm in subarachnoid haemorrhage by in vivo microdialysis. J Neurol Neurosurg Psychiatry 1995; 59(6):646–647.
46. Nilsson OG, Saveland H, Boris-Moller F, et al. Increased levels of glutamate in patients with subarachnoid haemorrhage as measured by intracerebral microdialysis. Acta Neurochir Suppl 1996; 67:45–47.
47. Saveland H, Nilsson OG, Boris-Moller F, et al. Intracerebral microdialysis of glutamate and aspartate in two vascular territories after aneurysmal subarachnoid hemorrhage. Neurosurgery 1996; 38(1):12–19.
48. Runnerstam M, von EC, Nystrom B, et al. Extracellular glial fibrillary acidic protein and amino acids in brain regions of patients with subarachnoid hemorrhage–correlation with level of consciousness and site of bleeding. Neurol Res 1997; 19(4):361–368.
49. Vath A, Kunze E, Roosen K, et al. Therapeutic aspects of brain tissue pO2 monitoring after subarachnoid hemorrhage. Acta Neurochir Suppl 2002; 81:307–309.
50. Hutchinson PJ, O'Connell MT, Al-Rawi PG, et al. Increases in GABA concentrations during cerebral ischaemia: a microdialysis study of extracellular amino acids. J Neurol Neurosurg Psychiatry 2002; 72(1):99–105.
51. Strege RJ, Lang EW, Stark AM, et al. Cerebral edema leading to decompressive craniectomy: an assessment of the preceding clinical and neuromonitoring trends. Neurol Res 2003; 25(5):510–515.
52. Sarrafzadeh AS, Sakowitz OW, Lanksch WR, et al. Time course of various interstitial metabolites following subarachnoid hemorrhage studied by on-line microdialysis. Acta Neurochir Suppl 2001; 77:145–147.
53. Hoelper BM, Hofmann E, Sporleder R, et al. Transluminal balloon angioplasty improves brain tissue oxygenation and metabolism in severe vasospasm after aneurysmal subarachnoid hemorrhage: case report. Neurosurgery 2003; 52(4):970–974.
54. Charbel FT, Du X, Hoffman WE, et al. Brain tissue PO(2), PCO(2), and pH during cerebral vasospasm. Surg Neurol 2000; 54(6):432–437.
55. Vajkoczy P, Horn P, Thome C, et al. Regional cerebral blood flow monitoring in the diagnosis of delayed ischemia following aneurysmal subarachnoid hemorrhage. J Neurosurg 2003; 98(6):1227–1234.
56. Stiefel MF, Heuer GG, Abrahams JM, et al. The effect of nimodipine on cerebral oxygenation in patients with poor-grade subarachnoid hemorrhage. J Neurosurg 2004; 101(4):594–599.
57. Schwab S, Steiner T, Aschoff A, et al. Early hemicraniectomy in patients with complete middle cerebral artery infarction. Stroke 1998; 29(9):1888–1893.
58. Berger C, Annecke A, Aschoff A, et al. Neurochemical monitoring of fatal middle cerebral artery infarction. Stroke 1999; 30(2):460–463.
59. Schneweis S, Grond M, Staub F, et al. Predictive value of neurochemical monitoring in large middle cerebral artery infarction. Stroke 2001; 32(8):1863–1867.
60. Dohmen C, Bosche B, Graf R, et al. Prediction of malignant course in MCA infarction by PET and microdialysis. Stroke 2003; 34(9):2152–2158.
61. Bosche B, Dohmen C, Graf R, et al. Extracellular concentrations of non-transmitter amino acids in peri-infarct tissue of patients predict malignant middle cerebral artery infarction. Stroke 2003; 34(12):2908–2913.
62. Steiner T, Pilz J, Schellinger P, et al. Multimodal online monitoring in middle cerebral artery territory stroke. Stroke 2001; 32(11):2500–2506.
63. Berger C, Sakowitz OW, Kiening KL, et al. Neurochemical monitoring of glycerol therapy in patients with ischemic brain edema. Stroke 2005; 36(2):e4–e6.
64. Berger C, Schabitz WR, Georgiadis D, et al. Effects of hypothermia on excitatory amino acids and metabolism in stroke patients: a microdialysis study. Stroke 2002; 33(2):519–524.
65. Enblad P, Frykholm P, Valtysson J, et al. Middle cerebral artery occlusion and reperfusion in primates monitored by microdialysis and sequential positron emission tomography. Stroke 2001; 32(7):1574–1580.

66. Frykholm P, Hillered L, Langström B, et al. Increase of interstitial glycerol reflects the degree of ischaemic brain damage: a PET and microdialysis study in a middle cerebral artery occlusion-reperfusion primate model. J Neurol Neurosurg Psychiatry 2001; 71(4):455–461.

67. Paschen W, van den KW, Hossmann KA. Glycerol as an indicator of lipid degradation in bicuculline-induced seizures and experimental cerebral ischemia. Metab Brain Dis 1986; 1(1):37–44.

68. Heiss WD, Dohmen C, Sobesky J, et al. Identification of malignant brain edema after hemispheric stroke by PET-imaging and microdialysis. Acta Neurochir Suppl 2003; 86:237–240.

69. Hutchinson PJ, Gupta AK, Fryer TF, et al. Correlation between cerebral blood flow, substrate delivery, and metabolism in head injury: a combined microdialysis and triple oxygen positron emission tomography study. J Cereb Blood Flow Metab 2002; 22(6):735–745.

70. Sarrafzadeh AS, Haux D, Ludemann L, et al. Cerebral ischemia in aneurysmal subarachnoid hemorrhage: a correlative microdialysis-PET study. Stroke 2004; 35(3):638–643.

38 | Gender Differences in Stroke Pathobiology: Therapeutic Implications

Louise D. McCullough, MD, PhD, Assistant Professor and Director of Stroke Research
Department of Neurology, University of Connecticut Health Center,
Farmington, Connecticut, USA

Julia Kofler, MD, Resident
Department of Neuropathology, University of Pittsburgh School of Medicine,
Pittsburgh, Pennsylvania, USA

Patricia D. Hurn, PhD, Professor and Vice Chairman of Research
Department of Anesthesiology & Perioperative Medicine, Oregon Health &
Science University, Portland, Oregon, USA

INTRODUCTION

Biologic sex is an important genetic factor in the incidence and outcome of cerebral ischemia and clinical stroke. Emerging experimental data suggest that gender and background reproductive steroids shape ischemic cell death in the brain. The principal mammalian estrogen (17β-estradiol) is neuroprotective in many types of brain injury, whereas androgens appear to exacerbate ischemic damage. These hormones clearly contribute to, but do not fully account for, sex-specific responses to cerebral ischemia. The purpose of this chapter is (i) to review the importance of biologic sex to clinical and experimental stroke outcome and injury mechanisms, (ii) to summarize the controversy behind estradiol's neuroprotective properties, and (iii) to introduce the novel concept that androgens contribute to ischemic sensitivity in the male brain.

ROLE OF BIOLOGIC SEX

Clinical Observations

Ischemic stroke occurs with greater frequency in men than in women across diverse ethnic backgrounds and nationalities (1). This sexually dimorphic epidemiology is present until late in life, well beyond the menopausal years. For example, in the Northern Manhattan Stroke Study, stroke rates in women do not equalize to those of men until beyond 75 years of age (2). However, women's strokes occur later in life, perhaps explaining the alarming statistic that more than 60% of stroke fatalities occur in women (3). Although mortality from cardiovascular disease appears to be declining in men, this advance has not been evident in women (470,000 deaths per year in 1970 vs. 500,000 per year in 2001) (3). Knowledge of the mechanisms of ischemic cell death and neuroprotective therapies in both sexes is clearly important; however these factors might not be identical in men and women.

Experimental Models

When female and male animals are evaluated side by side, a male phenotype of "ischemic sensitivity" can be uncovered. A remarkable rodent study of more than 2000 genetically hypertensive and stroke-prone animals showed that life expectancy is longer in the female than in the male. Evidence of cerebral hemorrhage and vascular lesions was absent in females until an advanced age (4). These early observations mimic human epidemiology. Furthermore, outcome from brain injury is clearly sex linked in standard animal models. Female rats and mice of many different inbred and outbred strains sustain smaller tissue damage and improved functional outcome from focal or global cerebral ischemia than do males for an equivalent insult. Similarly, male animals sustain greater injury than do age-matched females after traumatic brain injury or cardiac arrest (5). We have explored complicated rodent strains that have been engineered for the expression of diseases that are important risk factors in clinical stroke, including insulin-dependent diabetes, noninsulin-dependent diabetes, and hypertension. In each genetic strain and despite deleterious systemic complications, females appear less sensitive to a controlled ischemic insult than males.

Similar sex specificity can be modeled in cell culture when background sex steroids are removed from the media. For example, female neurons tolerate toxic dopamine exposure and survive twofold, relative to male cells (6). Further, female neurons obtained from the cortex or the periventricular zone live longer in culture than do male cells, potentially due to their ability to better utilize protective phosphorylation mechanisms (7). Neuronal sensitivity to pharmacologic insults that are used to simulate brain injury (e.g., glutamate, peroxynitrite, hydrogen peroxide, and staurosporine) is also sex specific. Male neurons are more susceptible to excitotoxic challenges than are female neurons. In contrast, response to oxidants, such as hydrogen peroxide, is gender neutral (8). These observations do not appear to be limited to neurons. Cell death after oxygen–glucose deprivation is decreased in female versus male astrocytes at postnatal day 3 (9) and in female-derived hippocampal slices (10), suggesting that sex-specific sensitivity to cerebral ischemia is due in part to differences in the utilization of molecular cell-death pathways.

Sex-Specific Molecular Mechanisms and Targets

New studies confirm sex-specific outcomes in mice deficient in genes known to be important to cell-death pathways, e.g., inducible and neuronal nitric oxide synthase (nNOS) and the DNA repair enzyme poly(ADP-ribose) polymerase (PARP-1). Based on data in male animals and mixed-sex cultures, these molecules have been postulated to play an important role in neurodegeneration and stroke. For example, nitric oxide generated during ischemia has been well documented to kill neurons, in part from a rapid reaction with superoxide anion, which leads to peroxynitrite formation, protein nitration, and DNA damage. New studies show that female nNOS knockout mice, or wild-type female mice treated with NOS inhibitors, sustain *paradoxically increased, not decreased*, damage after experimental stroke (Fig. 1) (11). Another well-established cell-death mechanism involves PARP-1 activation after DNA damage consequent to prooxidant mechanisms in ischemia and reperfusion. Data obtained from male models or mixed-sex neuronal cultures emphasize that halting PARP-1 activation improves cell recovery. However, loss of PARP-1 activity in female knockouts, or in wild-type females treated with novel and specific PARP inhibitors, enormously *exacerbates* ischemic damage (Fig. 2) (11). Sex also influences the benefit of PARP-1 deletion in postnatal female and male mice that are subjected to hypoxia–ischemia. Whereas male PARP-1–deficient newborns enjoy an approximate 50% reduction in histologic damage, damage in female knockouts is unchanged (12). The point of divergence for the male vs. female is not well established; however, it might be related to ability of PARP-1 to squander energy in the form of NAD^+ during ischemia/reperfusion. In the face of extensive DNA damage, PARP-1 activation rapidly depletes NAD^+ as the enzyme ribosylates defective DNA for processing. A 2004 study demonstrated that NAD^+ utilization was more pronounced in tissue homogenates from male pups, suggesting that energy depletion might be more profound during hypoxia–ischemia in the male (12).

Although it is not clear how the nitric oxide and PARP-1 death pathways diverge in males and females, these data suggest that sex can alter the molecular context of brain injury. A logical extension of this concept is that preclinical data should be obtained in both sexes to avoid erroneous conclusions, just as clinical trials of new therapies and drugs require representation of both sexes. An excellent example arises in a recent publication in which the efficacy of a selective κ-opioid-receptor agonist, BRL 52537 hydrochloride, in reducing damage in a standardized rat focal stroke model was evident only in males, not in females (13). The agent acts, in part, by attenuating nitric oxide toxicity and could be promising because of its long therapeutic window and low toxicity. Accordingly, further testing in human stroke is warranted, but stratification by sex will be required.

Although the gender differences in *experimental* stroke are provocative, the relevance of these findings to clinicians who see stroke patients is unclear at present. However, as we increase our understanding of pharmacologic and physiologic differences in preclinical studies, clinical investigators are discovering clear sex differences in therapies that are used in the treatment of stroke patients. A very recent example comes from data derived from the Women's Health Study in which 39,876 healthy women were studied to evaluate the efficacy of aspirin in the primary

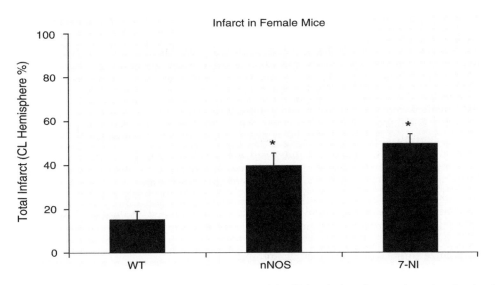

Figure 1 Total infarction expressed as a percentage of the CL hemisphere in ovary-intact female mice. Genetic deletion of nNOS or enzyme inhibition by pharmacologic means is well known to ameliorate ischemic damage after middle cerebral artery occlusion in male mice. In contrast, these manipulations dramatically increase damage in females. As shown here, WT female mice sustain significantly smaller infarcts than do female nNOS knockouts or WT females treated with the selective nNOS inhibitor 7-NI (25 mg/kg IP given prior to stroke onset, compared to oil-treated WT mice; data not shown). *p<0.01 compared to WT females. *Abbreviations*: WT, wild-type; nNOS, neuronal nitric oxide synthase; 7-NI, 7-nitroindazole; CL, contralateral. *Source*: From Ref. 11.

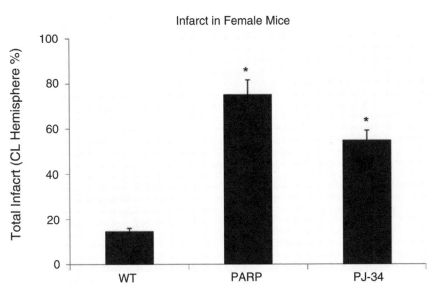

Figure 2 Total infarction expressed as a percentage of the CL hemisphere in ovary-intact female mice. Observations that genetic deletion of PARP-1 or enzyme inhibition by pharmacologic means improves ischemic outcome in male rodents provide the evidence for the concept that PARP is a deleterious player in stroke damage. In contrast, similar maneuvers in female mice fail to protect and exacerbate ischemic damage, suggesting that PARP-1 plays a different role in the female. As shown here, WT female mice demonstrate smaller infarcts after middle cerebral artery occlusion than do PARP-deficient females or WT females treated with the specific PARP inhibitor PJ-34 (10 mg/kg given at stroke onset, as compared to vehicle-treated females, data not shown). *p<0.01 compared to WT females. *Abbreviations*: CL, contralateral; WT, wild-type; PARP-1, poly-ADP ribose polymerase. *Source*: From Ref. 11.

prevention of cardiovascular events, including stroke, and in the reduction of mortality from cardiovascular causes (14). Subjects were randomized to receive 100 mg of aspirin or placebo every other day and were followed for 10 years. Aspirin lowered the risk of ischemic stroke in these women by 24% but did not alter the risk of myocardial infarction or death. This finding is in direct contrast to the findings of the Physicians Health study, which examined a similar, but male-only, cohort in which aspirin had *no effect* on stroke (15). Interestingly, women were more likely to have a stroke than a myocardial infarction in the Women's Health study—a finding in contrast with male disease patterns in which risk for myocardial infarction is greater than that of stroke. These striking differences in disease epidemiology appear to be accounted for solely by gender. Similar sex-specific responses to standard *acute* stroke therapeutics are also emerging. In a recent pooled analysis of randomized clinical trials, women responded more favorably than did men when treated with recombinant tissue plasminogen activator within 6 hours of stroke (16). In part, this result might be explained by the poor outcomes observed in placebo-treated women. These initial observations do not suggest a biologic mechanism; however, they do emphasize that biologic sex could be an important variable in acute response to stroke therapy. Future studies of gender as an independent-response variable are needed if we are to optimize stroke therapy in women and in men.

ESTROGEN: MULTIPLE ACTIONS, CURRENT CONTROVERSIES

The previous discussion of sex differences does not imply that female or male sex steroids are unimportant to ischemic pathobiology. Without doubt, estrogen is an important endogenous neuroprotectant and might play a large role in women's early protection from stroke. By the year 2015, approximately 50% of women in the United States will be over 45 years of age and facing increasing stroke risk in the context of a postmenopausal physiology, where native estrogens are lost. Accordingly, potential benefits and hazards of hormone replacement therapy (HRT) are currently a subject of much controversy and concern for women. Exogenous estrogens, particularly 17β-estradiol, have been well studied in translational models of brain injury, with positive results, i.e., reduced cell death, reduced infarction size, and improved functional recovery. Nevertheless, these favorable data for acute stroke treatment are frequently submerged by reports from prospective, randomized, clinical trials that show that estrogen is not favorable for primary or secondary stroke prevention.

Estradiol as an Acute Neuroprotectant

Endogenous estrogens strongly influence outcome to an ongoing ischemic event in the female. In rodents, ischemic outcome varies with the stage of the estrous cycle, with lesser infarct volumes in proestrus (period of high estradiol) as compared to metestrus (period of low estradiol) (17). Male–female differences in stroke sensitivity can be blunted by ovariectomy or by natural declination of estrogen levels with aging (18,19). Exogenous estradiol treatment before or after focal cerebral ischemia at physiologic levels reduces ischemic tissue death. Almost universally, the steroid reduces brain injury after an ischemic, glutamatergic, pro-oxidant, or proapoptotic insult (20,21). Accordingly, it is potentially important as an acute neuroprotectant.

However, several points should be critically evaluated in the plethora of animal and cell injury studies. In both permanent and transient focal cerebral ischemia models, estrogen is effective in estrogen-deficient rodents (males, ovariectomized females, and reproductively senescent females). However, the therapeutic range of "neuroprotective" steroid doses is not large; best results are obtained in most studies with low, physiologic levels of the steroid. No studies of long-term estrogen exposure have been conducted; therefore, the effect of treatment duration is unclear. Almost all of our understanding of estrogen's neuroprotection arises from rodent data. Few data are available in higher-order, gyroencephalic animals, such as cat or nonhuman primates. Most studies have evaluated 17β-estradiol, not the potent estrogen conjugates that are utilized in HRT. Few laboratories have demonstrated deleterious effects of estrogen, although a large variety of animal and cell models have been evaluated. In two studies of severe cerebral ischemia induced by permanent focal cerebral ischemia (22) or global cerebral ischemia from four-vessel occlusion (23), estradiol enhanced tissue damage. Accordingly, we have few data that define and distinguish the neuroprotectant estrogen from the proinjury estrogen.

Lastly, it must be emphasized that estrogen's actions in the brain and in the cerebral vasculature are quite complex. Most estrogens are vasoactive and have potent effects on endothelium and vascular smooth muscle cells of brain blood vessels. For example, 17β-estradiol can increase cerebral blood flow during and after vascular occlusion, but high doses are prothrombotic. The steroid likely utilizes multiple cellular signaling mechanisms; likely mechanisms include gene transcription of neuroprotective genes, as well as rapid receptor-mediated and receptor-independent effects. These latter actions involve phosphorylation cascades and intracellular signaling that activate ion channels, neurotransmitter receptors, and enzymes, such as endothelial nitric oxide synthase. Many estrogens have potent, concentration-dependent lipid antioxidant activity, although typically at supraphysiologic concentrations. In total, estrogen's very breadth of actions as a multifunctional molecule makes it an ideal prototype for developing future neuroprotectants.

Role in Prevention and Clinical Trials

Over the past 30 years, observational studies have found lower risks of coronary heart disease (CHD) and stroke in women who take postmenopausal estrogens, suggesting that estrogen is vasoprotective (24). Observational reports were not as clearly positive for stroke, but most describe no increased risk or some benefit in prevention of fatal strokes (25). The Heart and Estrogen-Progestin Replacement Study (HERS) was the first randomized, blinded trial to use combined estrogen and progestin [medroxyprogesterone acetate (MPA)]. After four years of hormone replacement therapy (HRT), the HERS found no reduction in the risk for CHD, stroke, or transient ischemic attack, with a threefold increase in venous thromboembolism (26). An important observation in the HERS was that patients who received HRT sustained an early increased risk of cardiovascular events that was offset by a lower event rate in subsequent years. It was presumed that this was due to an early prothrombotic risk, followed by a later protective effect, and that prolonged follow-up would demonstrate an overall beneficial effect for HRT. However, the release of the 6.8-year follow-up on the HERS cohort (HERS II) in 2002 showed prolonged HRT to have no benefit on cerebrovascular end points (27), demonstrating that HRT was ineffective for the secondary prevention of cardiovascular events.

The HERS study was designed to investigate the effects of HRT on coronary disease progression, with stroke and transient ischemic attack as secondary endpoints. In contrast, the Women's Estrogen for Stroke Trial (WEST) was the first randomized trial designed to examine stroke recurrence as the primary endpoint and to use estrogen without progestin as the replacement therapy (28). WEST found no benefit on total stroke incidence and a surprising increase in fatal stroke among women who were assigned to estradiol therapy. However, this trial, like HERS, examined women with *known* vascular disease, some of whom were postmenopausal for many years. One explanation for the lack of effect of estrogen is that it is ineffective in preventing vascular disease once the disease is already established and cannot reverse atherosclerotic damage accumulated over time. In addition, the dose of estrogen evaluated in these studies was higher than in current HRT formulations.

The National Institutes of Health (NIH)-sponsored Women's Health Initiative (WHI) was the first large, randomized trial of *primary prevention* of stroke and vascular disease (as well as numerous other endpoints) among healthy hormone users (29). Two parallel trials were originally designed. In one arm, women with a prior hysterectomy were randomized to receive either conjugated equine estrogen (0.625 mg/day; ERT) treatment or placebo. A second arm examined women with intact uteri, who were randomized to either combined estrogen plus progestin (HRT) or placebo, in acknowledgment of the increased risk of endometrial cancer with unopposed estrogen therapy. The primary outcome measure was the incidence of CHD, and the primary adverse outcome was invasive breast cancer. Secondary endpoints included the effect of HRT on stroke, pulmonary embolism, endometrial cancer, colorectal cancer, hip fracture, and death.

The HRT arm of the trial, which was to have continued until 2005, was terminated in July 2002 on the basis of recommendations by the WHI Data and Safety Monitoring Board, which found that overall risks from the use of combined HRT outweighed the benefits. In addition to an increased risk of breast cancer, other adverse effects included an increased stroke risk, with 8 more strokes per year for every 10,000 women in the HRT group. Other outcomes also suggested an overall negative effect on health, including increases in cardiovascular events and pulmonary embolism. In April 2004, the results of the estrogen-alone arm (ERT) of the WHI were reported (total subjects, 10,739). Similar to HRT, estrogen replacement (ERT) did not reduce the risk of stroke. After an average follow-up of 6.8 years, they reported an absolute excess risk of 12 additional strokes per 10,000 person-years, with no effect on CHD incidence (30). The numerous position statements that have been produced since the publishing of the WHI trial results are still considered to be quite controversial. Issues involving the appropriateness of dose, timing of administration after menopause, and "real-risk" to women have been strongly debated. It is important to note that the women enrolled in this trial were otherwise healthy, so that *any* adverse effect on their health could represent a real increase in risk. Current recommendations from the American Heart Association and the Food and Drug Administration state "hormone replacement therapy, either with combined therapy or with estrogen alone should neither be initiated nor continued for prevention or treatment of heart disease or stroke." If replacement therapy is prescribed for postmenopausal symptoms, the lowest effective dose should be used for the shortest possible time to alleviate symptoms.

In a further analysis of the HRT trial arm, classification of strokes into specific stroke subtypes has now been completed (31). After 5.6 years of follow-up, 151 strokes were reported in the HRT group (1.8%) versus 107 strokes (1.3%) in the placebo group; most were classified as ischemic strokes. Women who received HRT sustained a 31% increased risk of stroke, as compared to placebo-treated woman. The risk appears to be unrelated to interactions with other risk factors, such as hypertension, diabetes, or age. Risk was largely evident after year 1 reinforcing the concept that short-term HRT for relief of postmenopausal symptoms of vasomotor instability remains low risk. This observation is somewhat different from the WEST and HERS secondary prevention studies, in which the increased risk was seen in the first year of therapy. Again, a possible related issue is that women in these secondary prevention trials were at much greater risk for vascular events. The severity of stroke was equivalent in both groups, suggesting that treatment with HRT also does not reduce stroke damage when stroke occurs.

Surprisingly, younger women had a similar, if not greater, risk of stroke (46% increase in the 50- to 59-year-old cohort) when randomized to HRT, compared with older woman, suggesting that early initiation of HRT does not reduce stroke risk nor prevent progression of vascular disease. In terms of stroke outcome, based on the secondary analysis of the WHI HRT cohort (utilizing inflammatory biomarkers), it is unlikely that any subgroup of women will benefit from HRT as it is currently prescribed. Although combined estrogen/progestin compounds comprise the most commonly prescribed hormone regimen in the United States, it is not known if progestins interact with estrogen and diminish its neuroprotective effects. Experimental data suggest that progesterone increases subcortical damage after vascular occlusion in animals (32) and can reverse the beneficial effect seen on atherosclerotic plaque formation in nonhuman primates (33). However, recent clinical data argue against this hypothesis. The Estrogen Replacement and Atherosclerosis trial utilized estrogen with or without a progestin and found no benefit in coronary disease progression, as measured angiographically in either treatment group (34). Results from the Estrogen in the Prevention of Re-infarction Trial (35) demonstrate that estradiol valerate also did not reduce risk of recurrent myocardial infarction. Furthermore, the WEST did not demonstrate a beneficial effect of estradiol for secondary prevention of stroke and ischemic injury, nor did the WHI demonstrate benefit with estrogen replacement therapy (ERT).

In summary, results from recent randomized clinical studies conflict with earlier epidemiologic and observational data on hormone use for prevention of stroke. The total evidence for the clinical benefit of HRT or ERT in reduction of fatal stroke is arguably quite small (36). The data emphasize that unanticipated and paradoxic effects accompany estrogen as it is currently administered in women. In light of the WHI, estrogen's neuroprotective properties and potential benefit in human cerebral ischemic injury must be re-assessed. Lastly, recent evidence of gender-specific responses to standard stroke therapies should be integrated into this framework, because estrogen might interact with underlying biologic sex differences in stroke pathobiology.

Hormones, Contraceptives, and Stroke

Stroke in the premenopausal woman is a rare event. However, many women in this age group are treated with sex steroids through estrogen-progestin oral contraceptives (OCs). Currently, OCs are used by more than 10 million women in the United States and more than 78.5 million women worldwide. The potential for enhancement of stroke risk in OC users has been extensively investigated. Early studies of first-generation high-dose estrogen OCs (e.g., 250 µg) showed a significant association with increased risk of stroke (37,38). More recent case–control studies indicate that risk is clearly dependent on the estrogen dose (39,40). With the low-dose preparations most commonly used today (30–35 µg), the majority of studies report very low or no increased risk of stroke (41). Based on background incidence rates, absolute risk for stroke has been estimated to be 6.7 per 100,000 women per year in users of low-dose OCs and 12.9 in users of high-dose OCs. The consensus is that the contraceptive and noncontraceptive benefits of OCs use far outweigh the risk. However, subpopulations of women are susceptible to ischemic complications of OCs and require special attention. These subgroups include women who smoke and those with migraine headaches, with or without aura manifestation (39). Again, risk is dependent on the estrogen dose, and the addition of smoking leads to a dramatic increase in relative risk (42).

TESTOSTERONE: ROLE IN MALE SENSITIVITY TO ISCHEMIA

Despite the fact that male sex is a well-acknowledged risk factor for human stroke, most research aimed at understanding gender differences in stroke has focused exclusively on female sex steroids. Available epidemiologic studies suggest that testosterone, the major mammalian androgen, has a neutral or favorable effect on cardiovascular disease (43). This possibility is likely related, in part, to beneficial effects on vascular endothelial function and the vasodilatory properties of testosterone at physiologic concentrations. In the clinical setting, testosterone declines in men after stroke, presumably as a stress response (44). However, testosterone has recently emerged as another sex steroid that has the potential to alter ischemic cell death. For example, surgical castration and subsequent low testosterone decrease histologic damage after focal cerebral ischemia in the young adult male rat (45,46) and negatively affect outcome from experimental spinal cord injury (47). When administered in supraphysiologic doses, testosterone increases brain damage after cardiac arrest and cardiopulmonary resuscitation (48). These new studies suggest that gender differences in stroke outcome are not solely due to female sex and/or sex steroids and that androgens might adversely shape experimental stroke outcome. However, many questions remain to be addressed. We do not know how "andropause," the natural decline of androgen levels in aging men, affects cerebrovascular function and sensitivity to cerebral ischemia. Current observations suggest that when testosterone is replaced in aging male animals to levels similar to that of young males, the steroid protects the brain from ischemic injury (49). Thus, it seems that testosterone acts in an age-specific manner during ischemia. Testosterone can act either directly on the androgen receptor or indirectly via conversion to dihydrotestosterone by 5-reductase. Alternatively, testosterone can exert its effects via metabolism to estrogen by the cytochrome P450 enzyme aromatase. Both aromatase and the androgen receptor pathway are important for the effects of testosterone on brain function, but it is not yet clear which mechanism is the major mediator of the deleterious effects of testosterone in cerebral ischemia.

CONCLUSIONS

In summary, biologic sex and sex steroids are important factors in the incidence and outcome from cerebral ischemia and clinical stroke. Physiologic estradiol replacement has uniformly been shown to ameliorate a variety of experimental injuries to the central nervous system. However, results from recent randomized clinical studies of standard HRT conflict with these data and with earlier epidemiologic and observational data on hormone use for the prevention of stroke. In light of the WHI, estrogen's neuroprotective properties and potential benefits in human cerebral ischemic injury must be reassessed. Lastly, the roles of sex and androgens as contributors to male stroke risk and the apparent inherent sensitivity to cerebral ischemia present a new and novel area for bench and clinical research.

ACKNOWLEDGMENTS

This work was supported by U.S. Public Health Service NIH grants NS33668, NR03521, NS20020, the American Heart Association, and the Hazel K. Goddess Fund for Stroke Research in Women.

REFERENCES

1. Sudlow CL, Warlow CP. Comparable studies of the incidence of stroke and its pathological types: results from an international collaboration. International Stroke Incidence Collaboration. Stroke 1997; 28:491–499.
2. Sacco RL, Boden-Albala B, Gan R, et al. Stroke incidence among white, black and Hispanic residents of an urban community. Am J Epidemiol 1998; 147:259–2683.
3. American Heart Association Website; Statistics for 2005. www.AHA.org
4. Yamori Y, Horie R, Handa H, et al. Pathogenetic similarity of strokes in stroke-prone spontaneously hypertensive rats and humans. Stroke 1976; 7:46–53.
5. Hurn PD, Vannucci SJ, Hagberg H. Adult or perinatal brain injury: Does sex matter? Stroke 2005; 36:193–195.
6. Lieb K, Andrae J, Reisert I, et al. Neurotoxicity of dopamine and protective effects of the NMDA receptor antagonist AP-5 differ between male and female dopaminergic neurons. Exp Neurol 1995; 134:222–229.
7. Zhang L, Li PP, Feng X, et al. Sex-related differences in neuronal cell survival and signaling in rats. Neurosci Lett 2003; 337:65–68.
8. Du L, Bayir H, Lai Y, et al. Innate gender-based proclivity in response to cytotoxicity and programmed cell death pathway. J Biol Chem 2004; 279:38563–38570.
9. Liu M, Hurn PD, Roselli CE, et al. Role of P450 aromatase in sex-specific astrocyte cell death. J Cereb Blood Flow Metab 2006; May 17th epub.
10. Li H, Pin S, Zeng Z, et al. Gender differences in neuronal cell death. Ann Neurology 2005; 58(2):317–321.
11. McCullough LD, Blizzard KK, Zeng Z, et al. Ischemic NO and PARP activation in brain: male toxicity, female protection. J Cereb Blood Flow Metab 2005; 25(4):502–512.
12. Hagberg H, Wilson MA, Matsushita H, et al. Parp-1 gene disruption in mice preferentially protects males from perinatal brain injury. J Neurochem 2004; 90:1068–1075.
13. Zeynalov E, Massaki N, Hurn PD, et al. Neuroprotective effect of selective kappa opioid receptor agonist is gender specific and linked to reduced neuronal nitric oxide. J Cereb Blood Flow Metab 2006; 26(3):414–420.
14. Ridker PM, Cook NR, Lee IM, et al. A randomized trial of low-dose aspirin in the primary prevention of cardiovascular disease in women. N Engl J Med 2005; 352(13):1293–1304.
15. Final report on the aspirin component of the ongoing Physicians' Health Study. Steering Committee of the Physicians' Health Study Research Group. N Engl J Med 1989; 321(3):129–135.
16. Kent DM, Price LL, Ringleb P, et al. Sex-based differences in response to recombinant tissue plasminogen activator in acute ischemic stroke: a pooled analysis of randomized clinical trials. Stroke 2005; 36(1):62–65.
17. Carswell HVO, Dominiczak AF, Macrae IM. Am J Physiol Heart Circ Physiol 2000; 278:H290–H294.
18. Alkayed NJ, Harukuni I, Kimes AS, et al. Gender-linked brain injury in experimental stroke. Stroke 1998; 29:159–166.
19. Alkayed NJ, Murphy SJ, Traystman RJ, et al. Neuroprotective effects of female gonadal steroids in reproductively senescent female rats. Stroke 2000; 31:161–168.
20. Hurn PD, Brass LM. Estrogen and stroke: a balanced analysis. Stroke 2003; 34:338–341
21. McCullough LD, Hurn PD. Estrogen and ischemic neuroprotection: an integrated review. Trends Endrocrinol Metab 2003; 14:228–235.
22. Gordon KB, Macrae IM, Carswell HV. Effects of 17 beta oestradiol on cerebral ischemic damage and lipid peroxidation. Brain Res 2005; 1036:155–162.
23. Harukuni I, Hurn PD, Crain BJ. Deleterious effect of beta-estradiol in a rat model of transient forebrain ischemia. Brain Res 2001; 900:137–142.
24. Langer RD. Hormone replacement and the prevention of cardiovascular disease. Am J Cardiol 2002; 89:36E–46E; discussion 46E.
25. Paganini-Hill A. Hormone replacement therapy and stroke: risk, protection or no effect? Maturitas 2001; 38:243–261.
26. Hulley S, Grady D, Bush T, et al. Randomized trial of estrogen plus progestin for secondary prevention of coronary heart disease in postmenopausal women. Heart and Estrogen/progestin Replacement Study (HERS) Research Group. JAMA 1998; 280:605–613.
27. Hulley S, Furberg C, Barrett-Connor E, et al. Noncardiovascular disease outcomes during 6.8 years of hormone therapy: Heart and Estrogen/progestin Replacement Study follow-up (HERS II). JAMA 2002; 288:58–66.
28. Viscoli CM, Brass LM, Kernan WN, et al. A clinical trial of estrogen-replacement therapy after ischemic stroke. N Engl J Med 2001; 345:1243–1249.
29. Writing Group for the Women's Health Initiative Investigators (2002). Risks and benefits of estrogen plus progestin in healthy postmenopausal women. JAMA 288(3), 321–333.
30. Anderson GL, Limacher M, Assaf AR, et al. Effects of conjugated equine estrogen in postmenopausal women with hysterectomy: the Women's Health Initiative randomized controlled trial. JAMA 2004; 291:1701–1712.

31. Wassertheil-Smoller S, Hendrix SL, Limacher M, et al. Effect of estrogen plus progestin on stroke in postmenopausal women: the Women's Health Initiative: a randomized trial. JAMA 2003; 289: 2673–2684.
32. Murphy SJ, Traystman RJ, Hurn PD, Duckles SP. Progesterone exacerbates striatal stroke injury in progesterone-deficient female animals. Stroke 2000; 31:1173–1178.
33. Williams JK, Honore EK, Washburn SA, Clarkson TB. Effects of hormone replacement therapy on reactivity of atherosclerotic coronary arteries in cynomolgus monkeys. J Am Coll Cardiol 1994; 24:1757–1761.
34. Herrington DM, Reboussin DM, Brosnihan KB, et al. Effects of estrogen replacement on the progression of coronary-artery atherosclerosis. N Engl J Med 2000; 343:522–529.
35. Cherry N, Gilmour K, Hannaford P, et al. Oestrogen therapy for prevention of reinfarction in postmenopausal women: a randomised placebo controlled trial. Lancet 2002; 360:2001–2008.
36. Nelson HD, Humphrey LL, Nygren P, et al. Postmenopausal hormone replacement therapy: scientific review. JAMA 2002; 288:872–881.
37. Gillum LA, et al. Ischemic Stroke Risk with Oral Contraceptives: A meta-analysis. JAMA 2000; 284(1): 72–78.
38. Leys D et al. Stroke prevention: management of modifiable vascular risk factors. J Neurol 2002; 249: 507–517.
39. Bousser MG, Kittner SJ. Oral Contraceptives and stroke. Cephalalgia 2000; 20:183–189.
40. Kemmeren JM, et al. Risk of arterial thrombosis in relation to oral contraceptives (RATIO) study: oral contraceptives and the risk of ischemic stroke. Stroke 2002; 33:1202–1208.
41. Schwartz SM, et al. Stroke and use of low-dose oral contraceptives in young women: a pooled analsis of two US studies. Stroke 1998; 29:2277–2284.
42. Tietjen GE. The relationship of migraine and stroke. Neuroepidemiology 2000; 1913–1919.
43. Alexandersen P, Haarbo J, Christiansen C. Relationship of natural androgens to coronary heart disease in males: a review. Atherosclerosis 1996; 125:1–13.
44. Jeppesen LL, Jorgensen HS, Nakayama H, et al. Decreased serum testosterone in men with acute ischemic stroke. Arterioscler Thromb Vasc Biol 1996; 16:749–754.
45. Hawk T, Zhang YQ, Rajakumar G, et al. Testosterone increases and estradiol decreases middle cerebral artery occlusion lesion size in male rats. Brain Res 1998; 796:296–298.
46. Yang SH, Perez E, Cutright J, et al. Testosterone increases neurotoxicity of glutamate in vitro and ischemia-reperfusion injury in an animal model. J Appl Physiol 2002; 92:195–201.
47. Hauben E, Mizrahi T, Agranov E, et al. Sexual dimorphism in the spontaneous recovery from spinal cord injury: a gender gap in beneficial autoimmunity? Eur J Neurosci 2002; 16:1731–1740.
48. Kofler J, Noppens R, Roselli CE, et al. Testosterone increases neuronal injury after cardiac arrest/ cardiopulmonary resuscitation (CA/CPR) in middle-aged male mice. Anesthesiology 2004; 101:A872.
49. Hurn PD, Ardelt AA, Alkayed NJ, et al. Estrogen and testosterone as neuroprotectants in stroke. In: Pharmacology of Cerebral Ischemia. Krieglstein J, ed. Stuttgart, Germany: Medpharm Scientific Publishers, 457–464.

39 | Ultrasonography in the Management of Acute Stroke

Andrei V. Alexandrov, MD, Director
Stroke Research and Neurosonology Program, Barrow Neurological Institute, Phoenix, Arizona, USA

Marc Ribo, MD, Stroke Neurologist
Unitat Neurovascular Hospital Vall d'Hebron, Universitat Autónoma de Barcelona, Barcelona, Spain

INTRODUCTION

Stroke is a major social and health-care burden, with more than 700,000 people suffering from it annually in the United States. It is the leading cause of permanent disability, and its annual cost to patients, hospitals, and society is estimated at $51 billion (1). Cerebrovascular ultrasound has established applications in the detection of stroke risk factors and mechanisms; in screening for therapeutic, surgical, and catheter-based interventions; and in monitoring of arterial lesions that are responsible for stroke symptoms. Ultrasound provides a fast, portable, non-invasive, repeatable, and inexpensive technique for vascular diagnosis. Ultrasound in stroke care directly affects clinical decision-making in the following situations (2):

- Early detection, quantification, and characterization of extracranial atherosclerosis and occlusive disease, especially at the carotid bifurcation
- Consequences of proximal arterial occlusive disease on the distal cerebral vasculature
- Detection of microemboli associated with cardiac and aortic pathology and carotid artery surgical manipulation (and perhaps gauging response to antiplatelet therapy)
- Selection of children with sickle cell disease for blood transfusion as an effective tool in primary stroke prevention
- Natural history and response to treatment of acute arterial occlusion that causes hyperacute stroke
- Augmentation of the fibrinolytic effect of thrombolytic drugs in the treatment of acute ischemic stroke
- Time course and reversibility of cerebral vasospasm after subarachnoid hemorrhage

This chapter describes the use of cerebrovascular ultrasound tests at bedside for patients with acute stroke symptoms. Vascular ultrasound assessment has evolved as an extension of the neurologic examination that helps to define vascular origin of patient symptoms and location of arterial obstruction to flow.

TRANSIENT ISCHEMIC ATTACK VS. STROKE

Transient ischemic attack (TIA) and acute ischemic stroke are often difficult to differentiate in the emergency room if patients are seen acutely within minutes or hours of symptom onset. In fact, TIA and stroke may represent a spectrum of ischemic stroke. Recent evidence suggests that TIA is a medical emergency. When focal cerebral ischemic symptoms completely resolve within 24 hours, the event has been considered a TIA, not a stroke. However, the majority of TIAs resolve within minutes, and advanced neuroimaging studies demonstrate that events with longer-lasting symptoms are likely to be strokes (3). TIAs have a more serious prognostic implication than previously appreciated. After a TIA occurs, approximately 10% of patients will have a stroke in the next three months, and almost half of these strokes will develop within the first two days of the initial symptoms (4). Simple symptom duration/risk factor scales (4,5) can be used with imaging to identify patients at high risk for TIA. Patients with TIAs that have persistent arterial occlusion on ultrasound or brain lesion(s) on diffusion-weighted MRI are at particularly high risk of early stroke recurrence (6,7). Because TIA is a serious risk factor that is highly predictive of stroke, patients suspected of having TIA must be evaluated in a timely and comprehensive manner. Clinical history, knowledge of neurologic symptoms, and timely performance of brain imaging tests are essential in the workup of these patients.

Data from the National Institutes of Neurological Disorders and Stroke (NINDS) recombinant tissue plasminogen activator (rtPA) study demonstrate that, in most cases, symptoms of ischemia, which persist for at least one hour, progress to permanent deficits. In this pivotal trial of thrombolytic therapy for ischemic stroke, half of the patients with ischemic symptoms persistent at 1 hour received placebo. Unfortunately, at 24 hours after symptom onset, only 2.6% of patients who received placebo had complete recovery of neurologic function (8). Therefore, from a clinical perspective, patients who have symptoms that last for at least 1 hour have a 97% chance of having a stroke and should be evaluated emergently. The current time window for the only approved therapy with systemic rtPA is 3 hours after symptom onset. However, the majority of patients who suffer stroke arrive at the hospital outside this strict time window. Despite this, diagnostic testing of patients with symptoms that last longer than 3 hours should still be prioritized and accomplished in a timely manner, as effective measures to prevent stroke recurrence exist and depend on a stroke pathogenic mechanism (9).

TARGETS OF CEREBROVASCULAR ULTRASOUND TESTING

One of the most established reasons for carotid duplex testing is to screen for significant carotid artery disease. Stroke neurologists often use the Trial of Org 10172 in Acute Stroke classification (10) to delineate plausible etiologies of ischemic stroke:

- Large-vessel atherothrombotic stroke
- Cardioembolic stroke
- Lacunar stroke
- Other (dissection, coagulopathy, paradoxical embolism, etc.)
- Undetermined

Patients with "large-vessel atherothrombotic stroke" have imaging evidence of reduction of more than 50% of the diameter of the vessel by plaque or thrombus. These patients suffer stroke due to hypoperfusion with severe proximal internal carotid artery (ICA) stenosis and poor collateralization or due to artery-to-artery embolization, commonly from a thrombogenic plaque surface with variable degrees of carotid stenosis. Up to 90% of ischemic strokes occur in the carotid artery territories. These patients represent the target group for screening carotid arteries with ultrasound of the neck.

Patients with "cardiogenic strokes" suffer from embolism that originates in heart chambers. For example, patients with atrial fibrillation are at high risk of forming an atrial thrombus and of subsequent brain vessel embolization. This risk is reduced by anticoagulation (11). Carotid plaques and stenoses may also be found in these patients, adding complexity to the choice of medications for secondary stroke prevention.

In patients who suffer from so-called "lacunar strokes," occlusive lesions are developing in the small perforating vessels of the brain, which are currently below the resolution of ultrasound imaging systems. Nevertheless, strokes in the small-vessel territory still require diagnostic workup to exclude concomitant large-vessel atherosclerosis as a risk factor that may have caused artery-to-artery embolization with an acute lacunar syndrome at presentation.

Large-vessel atherothrombotic, cardiogenic, and lacunar strokes account for approximately 30%, 35%, and 10% of all strokes, respectively, whereas other types usually represent 10% of cases. In approximately 15% of stroke patients, clinical, radiologic, and other diagnostic studies reveal no identifiable risk factor, and stroke mechanism in these patients remains undetermined.

Overall, indications for the carotid duplex ultrasound examination include (i) symptoms of stroke or TIA attributable to carotid artery distribution, (ii) carotid bruit, (iii) suspicion of carotid stenosis from other imaging tests, such as magnetic resonance angiography (MRA), (iv) suspicion of carotid or aortic dissection, and (v) preoperative screening for carotid stenosis (12–14).

Major carotid endarterectomy trials were pivotal in finding effective stroke prevention measures in patients with carotid atherosclerosis (12–14). These trials established the levels

Table 1 The Society of Radiologists in Ultrasound Consensus Criteria for Grading Carotid Stenosis

Stenosis range N method	ICA PSV	ICA/CCA PSV ratio	ICA EDV	Plaque
Normal	<125 cm/sec	<2.0	<40 cm/sec	None
<50%	<125 cm/sec	<2.0	<40 cm/sec	<50% diameter reduction
50–69%	125–230 cm/sec	2.0–4.0	40–100 cm/sec	≥50% diameter reduction
70%–near occlusion	>230 cm/sec	>4.0	>100 cm/sec	≥50% diameter reduction
Near occlusion	May be low or undetectable	Variable	Variable	Significant, detectable lumen
Occlusion	Undetectable	Not applicable	Not applicable	Significant, no detectable lumen

Abbreviations: ICA, internal carotid artery; PSV, peak systolic velocity; CCA, common carotid artery; EDV, end-diastolic velocity.

of ICA stenosis at which surgery is beneficial (greater than 70%) and potentially better than antiplatelet therapy (50–69%); they also established the range of stenoses at which medical therapy is better than surgical intervention (lesser than 50%) in patients with a history of stroke or TIA in the affected carotid artery distribution. In 2003, a multidisciplinary consensus was reached regarding ultrasound criteria to identify the carotid stenosis strata of the North American Symptomatic Carotid Endartererctomy Trial (Table 1) (15).

High-Risk Carotid Plaque

As part of a carotid duplex examination, ultrasound provides direct images of atheromatous carotid plaque, in terms of its presence, location, extent, surface, and texture. This information is readily available and may possibly identify the so-called "high-risk" carotid plaque.

Severe carotid stenosis is found in only 14% to 21% of patients with hemispheric cerebral symptoms, and its prevalence varies with ethnicity (16). Most stroke patients have mild or moderate carotid plaques, some of which may cause symptoms and be more prone to progression, rupture, and thrombosis. In clinical studies with brightness-modulated (B-mode) ultrasound (17–21), three types of asymptomatic carotid plaque predicted higher risk of subsequent cerebral ischemic events: (i) hypoechoic plaque (Fig. 1), (ii) type 1 and 2 echolucent plaques (22), particularly with echolucent area adjacent to the lumen, and (iii) heterogeneous plaque.

Although the clinical value of plaque types has not been studied in patients with hyperacute stroke, some of that information can potentially be useful in clinical decision-making. For instance, the finding of hypoechoic or ulcerated plaque in the absence of other significant risk factors may point to plaque rupture, thrombosis, and artery-to-artery embolism as the likely mechanism of stroke. B-mode also provides information about the extent of plaque in symptomatic patients, which can be helpful in surgical considerations, i.e., placement of the cross-clamp more distal or proximal to commonly used sites.

Real-time artery-to-artery embolization can be detected with transcranial Doppler (TCD) (Fig. 1), and this information provides evidence for active emboligenic plaque surfaces. These "emboli-positive" plaques are associated with a higher risk of recurrent cerebral ischemic events (23).

Positive identification of surgical candidates is only one of several outcomes of cerebrovascular ultrasound testing. Patients who had an ischemic cerebral event may also have bilateral or tandem carotid lesions, distal carotid and intracranial arterial lesions, and variable sufficiency of collateral supply and vasomotor reserve, etc. This additional information allows stroke neurologists to identify stroke mechanisms and to select management options other than surgery for stroke prevention. At our laboratories, we routinely perform carotid and vertebral duplex scanning together with TCD in patients admitted with stroke or TIA to identify multiple potential stroke mechanisms.

Other Applications of Extracranial Duplex Screening

Duplex technology can determine if stroke patients have carotid lesions other than atherosclerosis. Examples include carotid thromboembolism, dissection, fibromuscular dysplasia, and radiation injury. These lesions have distinctively different appearances on B-mode ultrasound,

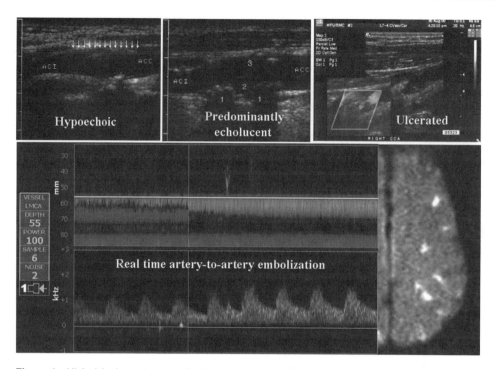

Figure 1 High-risk plaque types and artery-to-artery embolization. (*Upper left* and *middle panels*) Hypoechoic plaque on B-mode is marked by arrows; 1, shadows produced by calcified aspects of the predominantly echolucent plaque; 2, hypoechoic area with a thin cap near the vessel lumen indicates possible intraplaque hemorrhage or soft and vulnerable part; 3, hypoechoic area on the near wall. *Source*: Courtesy of Dr. Eva Bartles-University of Gottingten, Germany. (*Upper right panel*) Ulcerated plaque in a young woman with recurrent episodes of left-sided weakness. Insert shows color flow image that demonstrates slow reversed flow in the crater of an ulcer. *Source*: Courtesy of Drs. Disya Ratanakorn and Charles Tegeler-Wake Forest University, Winston Salem, NC. (*Lower panel*) PMD-TCD demonstration of real-time, artery-to-artery embolization in the MCA distal to a severe carotid stenosis. Velocity increase indicates improvement in the residual lumen with thrombus departure and propagation. Diffusion-weighted image demonstrates ischemic foci due to embolic shower. *Abbreviations*: ACC, common carotid; ACI, internal carotid arteries; MCA, middle cerebral artery; PMD-TCD, power-M-mode-transcranial Doppler.

and their hemodynamic significance is determined using Doppler spectral data. When found, these lesions point to a specific stroke mechanism other than large-vessel atherosclerosis, and determination of such a mechanism can change treatment options for stroke patients.

Another role of extracranial duplex scanning is to determine the presence of vertebral arterial lesions in patients with neurologic symptoms that refer to the posterior cerebral circulation. Duplex ultrasound allows segmental assessment of the vertebral artery flow between transverse processes and visualization of the vertebral artery origins (24,25). These segments should be thoroughly evaluated in patients with stroke or TIA in the posterior circulation. The spectrum of vertebral pathology detectable by duplex scanning includes vertebral artery stenosis (origin, V2, V3, and V4 segments), vertebral artery occlusion or absence of flow due to congenital aplasia, hypoplastic vertebral artery, and subclavian steal.

On duplex, a finding of significant (greater than 50%) vertebral stenosis or occlusion with evidence of plaque formation indicates that the mechanism of cerebral ischemic symptoms is likely large-vessel atheromatous disease. Infrequently, duplex examination may show vertebral artery dissection (26), and further testing is required to determine if it is an isolated vertebral dissection or an extension of aortic arch dissection. Further consideration should be given as to whether this dissection is spontaneous or trauma related.

Finally, the finding of subclavian steal, most often a harmless hemodynamic phenomenon, indicates the presence of atherosclerotic stenosis or occlusion in the subclavian artery. Occasionally, subclavian steal can produce symptoms related to transient hypoperfusion in the basilar artery (27,28).

Intracranial Arterial Disease

The Warfarin Aspirin Intracranial Disease trial was terminated due to excessive hemorrhagic complications and lack of efficacy for warfarin over aspirin to prevent recurrent stroke in patients with symptomatic ($\exists$50%) intracranial stenoses (29). Nevertheless, ultrasound screening for the presence of the intracranial vessel disease is still necessary, as intracranial stenosis is an independent and serious risk factor for stroke (30–32) and therapies other than anticoagulation are being developed (33–35).

Detection of intracranial stenoses with TCD is most reliable for the middle cerebral artery (MCA), terminal ICA, and basilar artery (36–38). Various velocity thresholds have been introduced to predict significant intracranial stenoses. As symptomatic MCA stenosis of ≥50% bears an approximate 7% to 10% annual risk of recurrent stroke (29–32), we have adjusted our criteria to optimize screening with TCD to predict the presence of these lesions (39). We use a cut-off of ≥100 cm/sec for the mean flow velocity (MFV) and the prestenotic:stenotic ratio of 1:≥2 for defining ≥50%-diameter reduction of the MCA (Fig. 2) (39). Other groups have developed their own velocity criteria for transcranial duplex imaging (41) and TCD (42,43). When applying these published criteria, it is important to establish how the investigators measured percent stenosis at angiography and if angle correction was employed with duplex scanning.

Performance of TCD requires evaluation of vessels other than the MCA, because an increase in the number of vessels with significant intracranial stenoses linearly increases the risk of subsequent stroke. More than 50% of symptomatic Chinese patients with 6 or more stenotic vessels suffered a stroke during follow-up (43). If TCD shows recurrent embolization and/or an increasing degree of intracranial stenosis (44–47) with fluctuating neurologic deficit or recurrent events, despite the best medical therapy, patients with these findings may be considered for experimental intracranial angioplasty stenting procedures (34).

Right to Left Shunts and Emboli Detection

Ultrasound can detect, quantify, and localize embolization in real time, and this methodology has been utilized in cerebral vessels with TCD (48–51). Detection of emboli with TCD is based on the definition of microembolic signals (MES) provided by the International Cerebral Hemodynamics Society Consensus Statement (52). MES (Fig. 3) have the following characteristics on spectral Doppler analysis: (i) random occurrence during the cardiac cycle, (ii) brief duration (usually <0.1 second), (iii) high intensity (>3 dB over background), (iv) primarily unidirectional signals (if fast Fourier transformation is used), and (v) audible component (chirp, pop).

The power motion-mode Doppler [power-M-mode (PMD)] adds extra dimensions to the process of emboli detection. It shows tracks of emboli in time and space and provides simultaneous, real-time assessment of emboli passing through different vessels, thereby increasing the yield of emboli detection with a single transducer (53).

Practically all MES that are detected by TCD are asymptomatic, because the size of the particles that produce them is usually comparable to the diameter of brain capillaries or even smaller (54). MES have been associated with velocity changes in the MCA affected by a significant stenosis (47), which suggests that some artery-to-artery emboli may be comparable in size to the residual lumen or that, when they detach from a stenosis, the residual lumen is increasing, as the velocity decreases. Frequent emboli on TCD in acute stroke correlate with crescendo TIAs (55) and reflect the process of thrombus dissolution (56).

Air microbubbles produce strong ultrasound echoes and appear as MES during testing for right-to-left cardiac shunts. A bedside TCD test with agitated saline can detect these shunts,

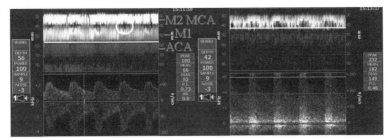

Proximal M1 MCA MFV 66 cm/s   **Distal M1/prox M2 MCA MFV 182 cm/s**

Figure 2 High-grade (>80%) distal M1 MCA stenosis. *Abbreviations*: MCA, middle cerebral artery; MFV, mean flow velocity. *Source*: From Ref. 40.

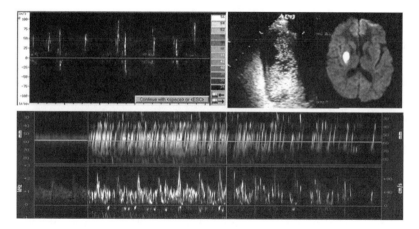

Figure 3 Microembolic signals on TCD. (*Upper left panel*). Single-gate Doppler spectral presentation of microembolic signals (see International Consensus definition). (*Upper middle panel*). Air microbubble appearance on echocardiographic B-mode image. (*Upper right panel*). Acute stroke in a 16-year-old girl with patent foramen ovale (PFO) and history of smoking and birth control pill use. (*Lower panel*). Power M-mode (PMD)-TCD "curtain" appearance of air microbubbles with functional PFO. Source: courtesy of Dr. Zsolt Garami is at the University of Texas-Houston Medical School.

and it is essential in patients with acute stroke or TIA thought to be caused by paradoxical embolization (57,58). Although TCD cannot localize the shunt [i.e., patent foramen ovale (PFO) or atrial septal defect], it provides complimentary information to transesophageal echocardiography. For instance, "bubble" testing with TCD can be done in a matter of minutes at bedside with minimal or no discomfort to the patient. TCD can offer results of shunt detection with accuracy equal or superior to that of echocardiography for the detection of functional PFO (59) and may detect shunts, even when transesophageal echocardiography is negative, i.e., in the case of pulmonary arteriovenous malformation or inability of the patient to perform Valsalva maneuver during echocardiography (57,58).

To optimize TCD performance for right-to-left shunt, the following protocol should be followed (57–59):

1.   Patient is in supine position; 18-gauge needle is inserted into the cubital vein.
2.   Three-way stopcock connector with 2 10-mL syringes is connected to intravenous (IV) access.
3.   9 mL isotonic saline is forcefully mixed with 1 cc of air.
4.   Less than 1 mL of patient blood can be suctioned into syringe for better bubble formation with agitation.
5.   At least 1 MCA is monitored with TCD.
6.   The first bolus injection of agitated saline is made with the patient breathing normally.
7.   The second bolus injection of similarly prepared, agitated saline is made with a 10-second Valsalva maneuver initiated 5 seconds after the beginning of saline injection.
8.   If negative, TCD monitoring is extended up to 1 minute in order to detect potentially late-arriving bubbles, suggesting a pulmonary shunt.

A 4-level categorization is proposed by the criteria of the International Cerebral Hemodynamics Society (58).

1.   No MES were detected (negative "bubble"-test).
2.   1–10 MES detected (positive "bubble"-test).
3.   >10 MES detected with no curtain.
4.   Curtain (test indicates the presence of a large and functional shunt).

Spencer introduced a new shunt grading system on PMD-TCD, which that takes into account exponential increases in the function of the shunt, and correlated this system with the "platinum" standard of intracardiac, catheter-based ultrasound diagnosis of PFO (59). Prospective validation of these diagnostic criteria at other centers is necessary. Nevertheless, the report should comment on whether MES or bubbles were detected at rest or were provoked by the Valsalva maneuver. If few single bubbles were detected at rest and a curtain appeared with Valsalva, this also should be reflected in the report.

Clinical interest in shunt testing with TCD is increasing, as several stroke prevention strategies are being tested, including catheter-based closure procedures. We routinely perform bedside screening with the "bubble" test TCD in patients who have suffered acute stroke or TIA and have a suspected paradoxical embolism, i.e., young patients or those who developed symptoms after prolonged immobility, etc.

Vasomotor Reactivity Testing

The main reason for evaluating vasomotor reactivity (VMR) of brain vessels is to identify patients at higher risk for stroke by challenging the ability of brain vessels to dilate and, thus, recruit more collateral flow. VMR has been most extensively studied in the setting of carotid artery stenosis or occlusion. A variety of tests were introduced to evaluate intracranial hemodynamics using the phenomenon of VMR (60–65), including CO_2-reactivity with TCD, acetazolamide testing with TCD, and the breath-holding index (BHI). The latter is the simplest way to challenge VMR if the patient is compliant and capable of a 30-second breath-hold (65). This index is calculated using the mean flow velocities obtained by TCD before breath-holding (baseline) and at the end of four seconds of breathing after 30 seconds of breath-holding, such that:

$$BHI = \frac{MFV_{end} - MFV_{baseline}}{MFV_{baseline}} \times \frac{100}{\text{seconds of breath-holding}}$$

The patient should be able to hold breath voluntarily for at least 24 seconds and, preferably, 30 seconds. To help the patient complete this task, the practitioner should explain the procedure in detail and demonstrate that no major chest excursions should be made at the beginning and end of breath-holding. Major chest volume changes associated with forced breathing change intrathoracic pressure and may affect velocity and flow pulsatility. The practitioner should then announce the duration of breath-hold to the patient at 10-seconds intervals after breath-holding has started; this helps the patient to be more confident that he or she can complete the task. Use envelope or average mean velocities beginning four seconds after the patient resumes breathing (i.e., the optimized signals from the entire display if the sweep speed was set at 4 to 5 seconds).

BHI values of less than 0.69 are predictive of risk of stroke in patients with asymptomatic, severe ICA stenosis and symptomatic occlusion (66,67). If a patient has greater than 70% proximal ICA stenosis or occlusion and a BHI <0.69, risk of subsequent stroke is at least 3 times greater than a similar patient with normal VMR. This information, together with other findings, such as blunting of the MCA waveform (68), plaque morphology, and emboli as described above, can identify patients at particularly high risk for stroke progression or recurrence and who are, therefore, more suitable for surgery, noninvasive flow augmentation, or ventilatory correction. The hypothesis that acute and subacute stroke patients with persistent proximal arterial occlusions and impaired VMR could benefit from external enhanced counterpulsation or positive airway pressure correction is being tested in prospective trials (A.W. Wojner-Alexandrov, unpublished pilot data, 2005).

Breath-holding with TCD does not require any gas-monitoring equipment or IV injections. Although the subjectivity of patient effort and the unknowns of blood gas concentration potentially limit reliability, BHI has been prospectively validated to predict clinical outcomes in steno-occlusive ICA disease, and BHI represents a simple screening test that can be used at the bedside to identify patients with impaired VMR.

THERAPEUTIC APPLICATIONS IN ACUTE ISCHEMIC STROKE

IV rtPA is currently the only Food and Drug Administration (FDA)-approved therapy for ischemic stroke within 3 hours of symptom onset (8). Noncontrast CT is the first-line imaging test for differentiating hemorrhagic from ischemic events. Based on the time of onset and clinical and CT examinations, rtPA can be given without confirmation of the presence of an arterial occlusion (8). Thrombolytic treatment without confirmation of arterial occlusion has been

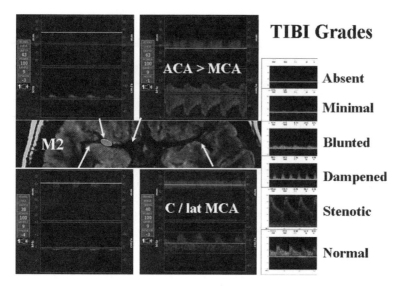

Figure 4 The most typical pattern of an acute MCA occlusion and TIBI flow grades. Some residual flow signals can be seen at distal M1 or proximal M2 MCA segments represented as minimal, blunted, or dampened TIBI flow grades. Flow diversion means that the ACA MFV is greater than MFV in the proximal MCA, and this finding serves as a confirmatory criteria. *Abbreviations*: MCA, middle cerebral artery; MFV, mean flow velocity; TIBI, thrombolysis in brain ischemia; ACA, anterior cerebral artery.

criticized (69). More centers are now attempting to employ vascular imaging to determine the presence, or persistence, of occlusion or reocclusion that has been linked to poor prognosis and that may necessitate further (currently experimental) intra-arterial interventions (70,71). Various tests can be used for this purpose, including invasive digital subtraction angiography, magnetic resonance angiography, CT angiography, and ultrasound (72,73). Ultrasound has the advantage of being a quick and inexpensive method for the real-time assessment of vessel patency and monitoring at the bedside. The key to the application of TCD in the often restless acute stroke patient is a "fast-track" insonation protocol (74). An experienced sonographer can use this method, guided by the physician's clinical assessment, to determine the presence and location of intracranial occlusion within minutes. Most studies can be done along with blood draws and neurologic assessment and can be completed within 15 minutes. A typical MCA-occlusion pattern (Fig. 4) can be detected in two minutes in the presence of good temporal windows (authors' personal observations). Bedside assessment should begin with TCD, as acute arterial obstruction that is responsible for cerebral ischemia is almost always intracranial. Once completed, the TCD examination can be supplemented with a rapid carotid/vertebral duplex assessment to determine the presence of a ≥50% extracranial stenosis, or thrombus, which is often the cause of artery-to-artery embolism or hypoperfusion. As compared with emergency catheter angiography, the accuracy of combined intracranial and extracranial Doppler-duplex examination, performed by expert sonographers in the emergency room, can be 100% for detection of lesions amenable to intervention (75).

Transcranial Doppler Criteria for an Acute Arterial Occlusion

Previously published criteria for intracranial occlusions focused on the absence of flow signals at a presumed thrombus location or velocity asymmetry between homologous segments of the MCA (76–78). Indeed, complete arterial occlusion should produce no detectable flow signals, with the greater degree of velocity dampening in the proximal affected MCA being predictive of the lesions amenable to intervention (79). With an acute intracranial occlusion, some residual flow to or around the thrombus may exist due to its irregular shape and relatively soft composition. In addition, hypertension at the time of the event will cause additional distension of muscular arterial walls. An acute occlusion, therefore, may produce a variety of waveforms representing this residual flow (80).

The Thrombolysis In Myocardial Infarction (TIMI) flow grading system was developed to assess the residual flow with invasive angiography in coronary vessels (81). The amount of residual flow predicts the success of both coronary and intracranial thrombolysis (81,82), as rtPA binds to fibrin sites at the thrombus surface in proportion to its plasma concentration and the residual flow. Increasing amounts of residual flow bring more rtPA to the thrombus. We have developed the Thrombolysis In Brain Ischemia (TIBI) flow grading system to evaluate residual flow noninvasively and to monitor thrombus dissolution in real time (80,83). The TIBI system (Fig. 4) expands previous definitions of acute arterial occlusion by focusing the examiner's attention on relatively weak signals with abnormal flow waveforms that can be found along arterial stems filled with thrombi. TIBI flow grades correlate with stroke severity and mortality, as well as the likelihood of recanalization and clinical improvement (80,82).

Acute intracranial arterial occlusion is a dynamic process, in that thrombus can propagate, break up, or rebuild within seconds or minutes, thereby changing the degree of arterial obstruction and affecting the correlation between ultrasound and angiography. When applied to the interpretation of ultrasound findings, the term "acute occlusion" indicates a hemodynamically significant obstruction to flow and that, if urgent angiography is performed, it will likely show an arterial lesion amenable to intervention. This lesion may be a complete occlusion (TIMI grades 0–1) or a partial occlusion (TIMI grade 2). The presence of a large-vessel occlusion on TCD must be confirmed by other findings, such as flow diversion to a branching vessel or a collateral channel.

Furthermore, ultrasound may suggest that more than one occlusion is present in the same patient, i.e., tandem lesions in the ICA and MCA. Tandem lesions are suspected when an abnormal TIBI flow grade is found in the MCA, with signs of collateralization of flow via major channels (such as the anterior or posterior communicating artery and reversed ophthalmic artery) or when duplex ultrasound indicates the presence of an additional extracranial arterial lesion (84).

Bedside ultrasound examination in acute cerebral ischemia can help to identify thrombus presence, determine thrombus location(s), assess collateral supply, find the worst residual flow signal, and monitor recanalization and reocclusion (70).

Transcranial Doppler Monitoring and Ultrasound-Enhanced Thrombolysis

Acute stroke patients can be safely exposed to continuous TCD monitoring (85,86). In our prospective studies, two hours of TCD monitoring with FDA-approved devices set at full power (<720 mW) at a given insonation depth and tight transducer fixation resulted in hemorrhage rates lower than those we expected on the basis of the pivotal NINDS rtPA Stroke Study. Using TCD or transcranial duplex imaging, the evolution of MCA occlusion can be followed in real time and the recanalization process can be measured (87–90). Early recanalization often leads to clinical recovery from stroke, and ultrasound can identify early responders to thrombolytic therapy (85,90,91), as well as patients with persistent arterial occlusion or reocclusion (70,92). Furthermore, ultrasound aimed at the residual flow/thrombus interface can be used to further enhance the therapeutic activity of rtPA (85,86).

Prior to our clinical studies, numerous *in vitro* and *in vivo* experiments showed that continuous thrombus exposure to ultrasound in the kHz-to-low-MHz frequency range enhances rtPA activity (93–98). Several mechanisms of ultrasound-enhanced thrombolysis were identified, including (93–98)

- reversible disaggregation of uncross-linked fibrin fibers,
- microcavity formation in the shallow layer of thrombus,
- increased enzymatic transport of rtPA,
- increased plasma flow through fibrin clots,
- increased residual flow around the clot.

These effects of ultrasound improve rtPA penetration through the thrombus, thereby increasing the overall amount of rtPA that is effectively delivered to the binding sites along the thrombus.

THE CLOTBUST TRIAL

The CLOTBUST (Combined lysis of thrombus in brain ischemia using transcranial ultrasound and systemic tissue plasminogen activator) trial was an international Phase 2 randomized, multicentered, clinical trial, with centers in Houston, Barcelona, Edmonton, and Calgary (86). It had prespecified safety and signal of efficacy endpoints and a predetermined sample size of 63 patients per group (99). Every enrolled patient had acute ischemic stroke symptoms and was treated with a standard 0.9 mg/kg dose of IV rtPA therapy within 3 hours of symptom onset. All patients also had MCA occlusions on pretreatment TCD. They were randomized (1:1) to continuous TCD monitoring (target) or placebo monitoring (control).

The safety endpoint was symptomatic brain hemorrhage (sICH) that worsened the neurologic deficit by 4 or more NIHSS points. The primary combined activity end point was complete recanalization on TCD (Fig. 5) or clinical recovery 0-3 NIHSS points, or improvement by ≥10 NIHSS points within two hours of rtPA bolus. Clinical investigators were blinded to group assignment (active or sham monitoring), which was done by sonographers.

All projected 126 patients received rtPA and were randomized 1:1 to target (median pretreatment NIHSS of 16 points) or control (NIHSS of 17 points). Age, occlusion location on TCD, and time to rtPA bolus were similar between groups. sICH occurred in 4.8% of target and 4.8% of controls. The primary end point was achieved by 31 (49% of target) vs. 19 (30% of controls) patients, $p=0.03$. At 3 months, 42% of target and 29% of control patients achieved favorable outcomes (0–1 modified Rankin Scale points), NS. This trend indicates the feasibility of a Phase 3 clinical trial that, at 274 patients per group, would be properly powered to detect this difference in outcomes at three months (86).

The CLOTBUST trial confirmed results of 3 decades of multidisciplinary basic science research that ultrasound, as a mechanical pressure wave, can safely enhance thrombolysis in human patients. It also showed that "gentle" diagnostic ultrasound can enhance rtPA-associated recanalization.

OTHER CLINICAL TRIALS

Transcranial duplex technology was recently tested in a small, randomized clinical trial (89). Duplex transducers are different from those used in CLOTBUST, as they generate multiple small beams at dual emitting frequencies, one for Doppler and one for gray-scale imaging (Fig. 6). One of the major limitations of this technology is that no reliable head frames exist for transducer fixation, requiring most studies to be conducted with handheld equipment.

In 25 patients who were evaluated (11 target, rtPA+duplex monitoring; 14 controls, rtPA alone), a trend was reported in the target group toward higher recanalization rates, more hemorrhagic transformations, and better outcomes at 3 months, compared to patients who received rtPA alone (89). This study did not have a predetermined sample size, and the results may have

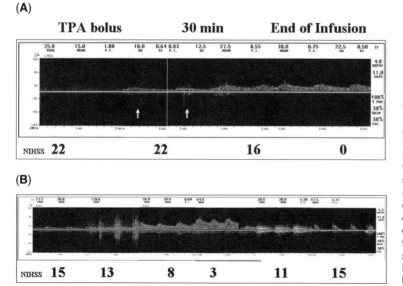

(A)

(B)

Figure 5 Ultrasound appearance PMD-TCD Duplex representation of stable arterial recanalization and reocclusion. Both patients received standard IV rtPA therapy within 3 hours of symptom onset. **(A)** Stable recanalization of the MCA distal to a tandem ICA occlusion. **(B)** Reocclusion due to reembolization of the MCA from a proximal source during TPA infusion. NIHSS scores are provided below each waveform.

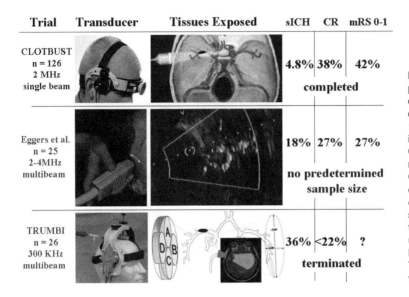

Trial	Transducer	Tissues Exposed	sICH	CR	mRS 0-1
CLOTBUST n = 126 2 MHz single beam			4.8%	38%	42%
				completed	
Eggers et al. n = 25 2-4MHz multibeam			18%	27%	27%
				no predetermined sample size	
TRUMBI n = 26 300 KHz multibeam			36%	<22%	?
				terminated	

Figure 6 Transducers, beam propagation, and results of clinical trials of ultrasound-enhanced thrombolysis. *Abbreviations*: sICH, symptomatic intracerebral hemorrhage; CR, complete recanalization, mRS, modified Rankin Score; CLOTBUST, combined lysis of thrombus in brain ischemia using ultrasound and systemic TPA; TRUMBI, transcranial low-frequency ultrasound-mediated thrombolysis in brain ischemia; TPA, tissue plasminogen activator. *Source*: From Ref. 100.

been affected by the small number of patients enrolled. More studies are needed to evaluate the potential of transcranial duplex technology to enhance thrombolysis.

Provocative findings have been reported that suggest that patients who are not eligible for systemic rtPA therapy may potentially benefit from continuous monitoring with ultrasound alone, as, hypothetically, ultrasound may help facilitate the endogenous thrombolytic process that leads to spontaneous recanalizations in acute stroke patients (100–102). It is unclear whether only partial recanalization can be induced by ultrasound alone and whether this exposure would result in a significant difference at three months, justifying a large clinical trial.

Furthermore, different experimental strategies are being tested in an extended time window for acute stroke treatment in conjunction with continuous exposure to ultrasound. This application may gain wide use in stroke patients who receive other agents, such as GP IIb–IIIa antagonists or direct thrombin inhibitors, or who await intra-arterial procedures.

Ultrasound transducers were also incorporated into a catheter for intra-arterial delivery of a thrombolytic drug (EKOS Corporation). This intra-arterial device uses 1.7 to 2.1 MHz pulsed-wave ultrasound with the emitting power of 400 mW—parameters similar to those for extracranially applied TCD. The EKOS catheter is now being tested in Phase 2 and 3 trials of Interventional Management of Stroke (103).

Therapeutic (i.e., nonimaging) ultrasound (104) has been tested in the transcranial low-frequency ultrasound-mediated thrombolysis in brain ischemia trial (105). First, the investigators used a very low KHz system (<40 KHz) that produced intolerable tinnitus and was withdrawn from clinical testing (Daffertshofer M, unpublished data). Although the system was replaced by a mid-KHz system operating at 300 KHz (Fig. 6), the trial was terminated after 26 patients were enrolled due to a 36% rate of symptomatic hemorrhage in the target group and no evidence of early recanalization or good clinical outcomes at 3 months (105). The trial demonstrated bioeffects of mid-KHz ultrasound that promote bleeding, including brain areas not affected by ischemia (105). Further research should determine if "standing" pressure waves and endothelial disruption may cause these adverse effects. Confirmation in *in vivo* models will have implications on design of future KHz-based systems.

CONCLUSIONS AND FUTURE DIRECTIONS

Ultrasound-enhanced thrombolysis can be further amplified by adding gaseous microbubbles (106–110). Microbubbles, safe ultrasound contrast agents, are about micron-sized galactose or lipid shells that, when exposed to ultrasound, expand and produce stable cavitation with stronger reflected echoes, which are used to generate ultrasound images with better resolution. At the same time, microbubbles agitate fluid where they are released by ultrasound, thereby providing a method for drug delivery and mechanical "grinding" of a thrombus. In fact, microbubbles have their own ability to lyse thrombi without a lytic drug (109).

Several studies have been reported with different types of commercially available microbubbles (110). The largest study to date compared the CLOTBUST Target arm to the CLOTBUST Target insonation protocol combined with Levovist air microbubbles (Schering AG) (108). Investigators demonstrated that, at 2 hours after rtPA bolus, the rtPA+TCD+Levovist group achieved a 55% sustained recanalization rate, compared to 38% in the rtPA+TCD group of the CLOTBUST trial. An international, multicentered study of a new and more stable C_3F_8 microbubble (MRX 815 platform, ImaRx, Tucson, Arizona, USA) is under way (111).

Microbubbles offer a mechanical method to amplify stroke therapies and can be developed as a new kind of device to augment brain perfusion and drug and nutrient delivery within the existing (and at an extended) time window. Development of ultrasound- and microbubble-assisted stroke therapies requires experienced sonographers to find intracranial thrombi and expose their surfaces to residual flow in order to lodge more rtPA and agitate stagnant flow. In that most emergency centers have few personnel with these skills, future studies will focus on the development of an operator-independent ultrasound device that can be used by existing medical personnel regardless of their experience in diagnostic ultrasound (111).

REFERENCES

1. Center for Disease Control. Public health and aging: hospitalizations for stroke among adults aged ≥ 65 years: United States, 2000. Morb Mortal Wkly Rep 2003; 52(25):586–589.
2. Grotta JC. Ultrasound: what's in the waveforms? In: Alexandrov AV, ed. Cerebrovascular Ultrasound in Stroke Prevention and Treatment. New York: Blackwell Publishing-Futura 2003; ii–iii.
3. Albers GW, Caplan LR, Easton JD, et al. TIA Working Group. Transient ischemic attack—proposal for a new definition. N Engl J Med 2002; 347(21):1713–1716.
4. Johnston SC, Gress DR, Browner WS, Sidney S. Short-term prognosis after emergency department diagnosis of TIA. JAMA 2000; 284:2901–2906.
5. Rothwell PM, Giles MF, Flossman E, et al. A simple score (ABCD) to identify individuals at high early risk of stroke after transient ischaemic attack. Lancet 2005; 366:29–36.
6. Alexandrov AV, Felberg RA, Demchuk AM, et al. Deterioration following spontaneous improvement: sonographic findings in patients with acutely resolving symptoms of cerebral ischemia. Stroke 2000; 31:915–919.
7. Coutts SB, Simon JE, Eliasziw M, et al. Triaging transient ischemic attack and minor stroke patients using acute magnetic resonance imaging. Ann Neurol 2005; 57:848–854.
8. The National Institutes of Neurological Disorders and Stroke rt-PA Stroke Study Group. Tissue plasminogen activator for acute ischemic stroke. N Engl J Med 1995; 333:1581–1587.
9. Adams HP Jr., Adams RJ, Brott T, et al. Stroke Council of the American Stroke Association. Guidelines for the early management of patients with ischemic stroke: A scientific statement from the Stroke Council of the American Stroke Association. Stroke 2003; 34(4):1056–1083.
10. Adams HP Jr., Bendixen BH, Leira E, et al. Antithrombotic treatment of ischemic stroke among patients with occlusion or severe stenosis of the internal carotid artery: a report of the Trial of Org 10172 in Acute Stroke Treatment (TOAST). Neurology 1999; 53(1):122–125.
11. Hart RG. Antithrombotic therapies for stroke prevention in atrial fibrillation. Adv Neurol 2003; 92: 249–256.
12. North American Symptomatic Carotid Endarterectomy Trial Collaborators. Beneficial effect of carotid endarterectomy in symptomatic patients with high-grade carotid stenosis. N Engl J Med 1991; 325:445–53.
13. European Carotid Surgery Trialists' Collaborative Group. Randomised trial of endarterectomy for recently symptomatic carotid stenosis: final results of the MRC European Carotid Surgery Trial (ECST). Lancet 1998; 351:1379–1387.
14. Executive Committee of the Asymptomatic Carotid Atherosclerosis Study. Endarterectomy for asymptomatic carotid artery stenosis. JAMA 1995; 273:1421–1428.
15. Grant E, Moneta G, Benson C, et al. SRU Consensus criteria for grading carotid stenosis with duplex ultrasound. Radiology 2003; 229:340–346.
16. Mast H, Thompson JL, Lin IF, et al. Cigarette smoking as a determinant of high-grade carotid artery stenosis in Hispanic, black, and white patients with stroke or transient ischemic attack. Stroke 1998; 29(5):908–912.
17. Bluth EI. Evaluation and characterization of carotid plaque. Semin Ultrasound CT MR 1997; 18(1): 57–65.

18. Polak JF, Shemanski L, O'Leary DH, et al. Hypoechoic plaque at US of the carotid artery: an independent risk factor for incident stroke in adults aged 65 years or older. Cardiovascular Health Study. Radiology 1998; 208(3):649–654.

19. Mathiesen EB, Bonaa KH, Joakimsen O. Echolucent plaques are associated with high risk of ischemic cerebrovascular events in carotid stenosis: the Tromso study. Circulation 2001; 103(17):2171–2175.

20. Aburahma AF, Thiele SP, Wulu JT Jr. Prospective controlled study of the natural history of asymptomatic 60% to 69% carotid stenosis according to ultrasonic plaque morphology. J Vasc Surg 2002; 36(3):437–442.

21. Nicolaides AN. High risk carotid plaque. Ultrasound Med Biol 2003; 29(5S):S38.

22. Geroulakos G, Ramaswami G, Nicolaides A, et al. Characterization of symptomatic and asymptomatic carotid plaques using high-resolution real-time ultrasonography. Br J Surg 1993; 80(10):1274–1277.

23. Molloy J, Markus HS. Asymptomatic embolization predicts stroke and TIA risk in patients with carotid artery stenosis. Stroke 1999; 30(7):1440–1443.

24. Bartels E, Fuchs HH, Flugel KA. Duplex ultrasonography of vertebral arteries: examination, technique, normal values, and clinical applications. Angiology. 1992; 43(3 Pt 1):169–180.

25. Bartels E. Color-Coded Duplex Ultrasonography of the Cerebral Vessels. Stuttgart: Schattauer, 1999.

26. Bartels E, Flugel KA. Evaluation of extracranial vertebral artery dissection with duplex color-flow imaging. Stroke 1996; 27(2):290–295.

27. Toole JF. Cerebrovascular Disorders. 4th ed. New York: Raven Press: 123.

28. Bornstein NM, Norris JW. Subclavian steal: a harmless haemodynamic phenomenon? Lancet 1986; 2(8502):303–305.

29. Chimowitz MI, Lynn J, Howlett-Smith MH, et al. WASID Investigators. Comparison of warfarin and aspirin for symptomatic intracranial arterial stenosis. N Engl J Med 2005; 352:1305–1316.

30. Sacco RL, Kargman DE, Gu Q, Zamanillo MC. Race-ethnicity and determinants of intracranial atherosclerotic cerebral infarction. The Northern Manhattan Stroke Study. Stroke 1995; 26:14–20.

31. Wityk RJ, Lehman D, Klag M, Coresh J, Ahn H, Litt B. Race and sex differences in the distribution of cerebral atherosclerosis. Stroke 1996; 27:1974–1980.

32. Wong KS, Huang YN, Gao S, Lam WW, Chan YL, Kay R. Intracranial stenosis in Chinese patients with acute stroke. Neurology 1998; 50:812–813.

33. Chimowitz MI. Antithrombotic therapy for atherosclerotic intracranial arterial stenosis. Adv Neurol 2003; 92:271–274.

34. Gomez CR, Orr SC. Angioplasty and stenting for primary treatment of intracranial arterial stenoses. Arch Neurol 2001; 58(10):1687–1690.

35. Chimowitz MI. Angioplasty or stenting is not appropriate as first-line treatment of intracranial stenosis. Arch Neurol 2001; 58(10):1690–1692.

36. Lindegaard KF, Bakke SJ, Aaslid R, Nornes H. Doppler diagnosis of intracranial artery occlusive disorders. J Neurol Neurosurg Psychiatry 1986; 49:510–518.

37. de Bray JM, Joseph PA, Jeanvoine H, Maugin D, Dauzat M, Plassard F. Transcranial Doppler evaluation of middle cerebral artery stenosis. J Ultrasound Med 1988; 7(11):611–616.

38. Ley-Pozo J, Ringelstein EB. Noninvasive detection of occlusive disease of the carotid siphon and middle cerebral artery. Ann Neurol 1990; 28:640–647.

39. Felberg RA, Christou I, Demchuk AM, Malkoff M, Alexandrov AV. Screening for intracranial stenosis with transcranial Doppler: the accuracy of mean flow velocity thresholds. J Neuroimaging 2002; 12:9–14.

40. Alexandrov AV. The role of cerebro vascular ultrasound in the management of cerebro vascular disease. In Zwiebel W, Pellerito J, eds. Introduction to Vascular Ultrasonography, 5th ed. St Louis: Elsevier, 2004; In press.

41. Baumgartner RW, Mattle HP, Schroth G. Assessment of ≥50% and <50% intracranial stenoses by transcranial color-coded duplex sonography. Stroke 1999; 30(1):87–92.

42. Rother J, Schwartz A, Rautenberg W, Hennerici M. Middle cerebral artery stenoses: assessment by magnetic resonance angiography and transcranial Doppler ultrasound. Cerebrovasc Dis 1994;4:273–279.

43. Wong KS, Li H, Lam WW, Chan YL, Kay R. Progression of middle cerebral artery occlusive disease and its relationship with further vascular events after stroke. Stroke 2002; 33(2):532–536.

44. Schwarze JJ, Babikian V, DeWitt LD, et al. Longitudinal monitoring of intracranial arterial stenoses with transcranial Doppler ultrasonography. J Neuroimaging 1994; 4:182–187.

45. Segura T, Serena J, Castellanos M, Teruel J, Vilar C, Davalos A. Embolism in acute middle cerebral artery stenosis. Neurology 2001; 56(4):497–501.

46. Arenillas JF, Molina CA, Montaner J, Abilleira S, Gonzalez-Sanchez MA, Alvarez-Sabin J. Progression and clinical recurrence of symptomatic middle cerebral artery stenosis: a long-term follow-up transcranial Doppler ultrasound study. Stroke 2001; 32(12):2898–2904.

47. Gao S, Wong KS. Characteristics of microembolic signals detected near their origins in middle cerebral artery stenoses. J Neuroimaging 2003; 13(2):124–132.

48. Spencer MP, Campbell SD, Sealey JL, Henry FC, Lindbergh J. Experiments on decompression bubbles in the circulation using ultrasonic and electromagnetic flowmeters. J Occup Med 1969; 11(5):238–244.

49. Padayachee TS, Gosling RG, Bishop CC, Burnand K, Browse NL. Transcranial measurement of blood velocities in the basal cerebral arteries using pulsed Doppler ultrasound: a method of assessing the Circle of Willis. Ultrasound Med Biol 1986; 12(1):5–14.

50. Deverall PB, Padayachee TS, Parsons S, Theobold R, Battistessa SA. Ultrasound detection of micro-emboli in the middle cerebral artery during cardiopulmonary bypass surgery. Eur J Cardiothorac Surg 1988; 2(4):256–260.

51. Spencer MP, Thomas GI, Nicholls SC, Sauvage LR. Detection of middle cerebral artery emboli during carotid endarterectomy using transcranial Doppler ultrasonography. Stroke 1990; 21(3):415–423.

52. The International Cerebral Hemodynamics Society Consensus Statement. Stroke 1995; 26:1123.

53. Moehring MA, Spencer MP. Power M-mode transcranial Doppler ultrasound and simultaneous single gate spectrogram. Ultrasound Med Biol 2002; 28:49–57.

54. Brucher R, Russel D. Background and principles. In: Tegeler CH, Babikian VL, Gomez CR eds. Neurosonology. St Louis: Mosby, 1996; 231–234.

55. Segura T, Serena J, Molíns A, Dávalos A. Clusters of microembolic signals: a new form of cerebral micro-embolism presentation in a patient with middle cerebral artery stenosis. Stroke 1998; 29:722–724.

56. Alexandrov AV, Demchuk AM, Felberg RA, Grotta JC, Krieger D. Intracranial clot dissolution is associated with embolic signals on transcranial Doppler. J Neuroimaging 2000; 10:27–32.

57. Jauss M, Zanette E. Detection of right-to-left shunt with ultrasound contrast agent and transcranial Doppler sonography. Cerebrovasc Dis 2000; 10:490–496.

58. Sloan MA, Alexandrov AV, Tegeler CH, et al. Assessment: transcranial Doppler ultrasonography: report of the Therapeutics and Technology Assessment Subcommittee of the American Academy of Neurology. Neurology 2004; 62:1468–1481.

59. Spencer MP, Moehring MA, Jesurum J, Gray WA, Olsen V, Reisman M. Power M-mode diagnosis of patent foramen ovale and assessing transcatheter closure. J Neuroimaging 2004; 14:329–349.

60. Bishop CCR, Powell S, Insall M, et al. Effect of internal carotid artery occlusion on middle cerebral artery blood flow at rest and in response to hypercapnia. Lancet 1986; 29:710–712.

61. Ringelstein EB, Sievers C, Ecker S, et al. Noninvasive assessment of CO_2-induced cerebral vasomotor response in normal individuals and patients with internal carotid artery occlusions. Stroke 1988; 19:962–969.

62. Sorteberg W, Lindegaard KF, Rootwelt K, Dahl A, Nyberg-Hansen R, Nornes H. Effect of acetazolamide on cerebral blood flow velocity and regional cerebral blood flow in normal subjects. Acta Neurochir 1989; 97:139–145.

63. Kleiser B, Widder B. Course of carotid artery occlusions with impaired cerebrovascular reactivity. Stroke 1992; 23:171–174.

64. Webster MW, Makaroun MS, Steed DL, et al. Compromised cerebral blood flow reactivity is a predictor of stroke in patients with symptomatic carotid artery occlusive disease. J Vasc Surg 1995; 21: 338–344.

65. Markus HS, Harrison MJ. Estimation of cerebrovascular reactivity using transcranial Doppler, including the use of breath-holding as the vasodilatory stimulus. Stroke 1992; 23:668–673.

66. Silverstrini M, Vernieri F, Pasqualetti P, et al. Impaired vasomotor reactivity and risk of stroke in patients with asymptomatic carotid artery stenosis. JAMA 2000; 283:2122–2127.

67. Vernieri F, Pasqualetti P, Matheis M, et al. Effect of collateral flow and cerebral vasomotor reactivity on the outcome of carotid artery occlusion. Stroke 2001; 32:1552–1558.

68. Hartmann A, Mast H, Thompson JL, Sia RM, Mohr JP. Transcranial Doppler waveform blunting in severe extracranial carotid artery stenosis. Cerebrovasc Dis 2000; 10(1):33–38.

69. Caplan LR, Mohr JP, Kistler JP, Koroshetz W. Should thrombolytic therapy be the first-line treatment for acute ischemic stroke? Thrombolysis – not a panacea for ischemic stroke. N Engl J Med 1997; 337:1309–1310.

70. Alexandrov AV, Grotta JC. Arterial re-occlusion in stroke patients treated with intravenous tissue plasminogen activator. Neurology 2002; 59:862–867.

71. Lewandowski CA, Frankel M, Tomsick TA, et al. Combined intravenous and intra-arterial r-TPA versus intra-arterial therapy of acute ischemic stroke: Emergency Management of Stroke (EMS) Bridging Trial. Stroke 1999; 30:2598–2605.

72. Warach S. Stroke neuroimaging. Stroke 2003; 34(2):345–347.

73. Xavier AR, Qureshi AI, Kirmani JF, Yahia AM, Bakshi R. Neuroimaging of stroke: a review. South Med J 2003; 96(4):367–379.

74. Alexandrov AV, Demchuk A, Wein T, Grotta JC. The yield of transcranial Doppler in acute cerebral ischemia. Stroke 1999; 30:1605–1609.

75. Chernyshev O, Garami Z, Calleja S, et al. Accuracy of combined carotid and transcranial Doppler examination in acute cerebral ischemia. Stroke 2005; 36:32–37.

76. Zanette EM, Fieschi C, Bozzao L, et al. Comparison of cerebral angiography and transcranial Doppler sonography in acute stroke. Stroke 1989; 20:899–903.
77. Razumovsky AY, Gillard JH, Bryan RN, Hanley DF, Oppenheimer SM. TCD, MRA, and MRI in acute cerebral ischemia. Acta Neurol Scand 1999; 99:65–76.
78. Kaps M, Damian MS, Teschendorf U, Dorndorf W. Transcranial Doppler ultrasound findings in the middle cerebral artery occlusion. Stroke 1990; 21:532–537.
79. Saqqur M, Shuaib A, Alexandrov AV, et al. Derivation of transcranial Doppler criteria for rescue intra-arterial thrombolysis: multicenter experience from the Interventional Management of Stroke Study. Stroke 2005; 36:865–868.
80. Demchuk AM, Burgin WS, Christou I, et al. Thrombolysis in Brain Ischemia (TIBI) TCD flow grades predict clinical severity, early recovery and mortality in intravenous TPA treated patients. Stroke 2001; 32:89–93.
81. The TIMI Study Group. The Thrombolysis in Myocardial Infarction (TIMI) trial: Phase I findings. N Engl J Med 1985; 312:932–936.
82. Labiche LA, Malkoff M, Alexandrov AV. Residual flow signals predict complete recanalization in stroke patients treated with TPA. J Neuroimaging 2003; 13:28–33.
83. Alexandrov AV. Ultrasound-enhanced thrombolysis for stroke: clinical significance. Eur J Ultrasound 2002; 16:131–140.
84. El-Mitwalli A, Saad M, Christou I, Malkoff M, Alexandrov AV. Clinical and sonographic patterns of tandem ICA/MCA occlusion in TPA treated patients. Stroke 2002; 33:99–102.
85. Alexandrov AV, Demchuk AM, Felberg RA, et al. High rate of complete recanalization and dramatic clinical recovery during TPA infusion when continuously monitored by 2 MHz transcranial Doppler monitoring. Stroke 2000; 31:610–614.
86. Alexandrov AV, Molina CA, Grotta JC, et al. Ultrasound-enhanced systemic thrombolysis for acute ischemic stroke. N Engl J Med 2004; 351:2170–2178.
87. Kaps M, Link A. Transcranial sonographic monitoring during thrombolytic therapy. Am J Neuroradiol 1998; 19:758–760.
88. Burgin WS, Malkoff M, Felberg RA, et al. Transcranial Doppler ultrasound criteria for recanalization after thrombolysis for middle cerebral artery stroke. Stroke 2000; 31:1128–1132.
89. Eggers J, Koch B, Meyer K, Konig I, Seidel G. Effect of ultrasound on thrombolysis of middle cerebral artery occlusion. Ann Neurol 2003; 53:(6):797–800.
90. Molina CA, Montaner J, Abilleira S, et al. Time course of tissue plasminogen activator-induced recanalization in acute cardioembolic stroke: a case-control study. Stroke 2001; 32:2821–2827.
91. Alexandrov AV, Burgin WS, Demchuk AM, El-Mitwalli A, Grotta JC. Speed of intracranial clot lysis with intravenous TPA therapy: sonographic classification and short term improvement. Circulation 2001; 103:2897–2902.
92. Molina CA, Ribo M, Rubiera M, et al. Predictors of early arterial reocclusion after tPA-induced recanalization [abstr]. Stroke 2004; 35:250.
93. Braaten JV, Goss RA, Francis CW. Ultrasound reversibly disaggregates fibrin fibers. Thromb Haemost 1997; 78:1063–1068.
94. Kondo I, Mizushige K, Ueda T, Masugata H, Ohmori K, Matsuo H. Histological observations and the process of ultrasound contrast agent enhancement of tissue plasminogen activator thrombolysis with ultrasound exposure. Jpn Circ J 1999; 63:478–484.
95. Francis CW, Onundarson PT, Carstensen EL, et al. Enhancement of fibrinolysis in vitro by ultrasound. J Clin Invest 1992; 90:2063–2068.
96. Francis CW, Blinc A, Lee S, Cox C. Ultrasound accelerates transport of recombinant tissue plasminogen activator into clots. Ultrasound Med Biol 1995; 21:419–424.
97. Siddiqi F, Blinc A, Braaten J, Francis CW. Ultrasoudn increases flow through fibrin gels. Thomb Haemost 1995; 21:419–424.
98. Behrens S, Spengos K, Daffertshoffer M, Schroeck H, Dempfle CE, Hennerici M. Transcranial ultrasound-improved thrombolysis: diagnostic versus therapeutic ultrasound. Ultrasound Med Biol 2001; 27:1683–1689.
99. Alexandrov AV, Wojner AW, Grotta JC. CLOTBUST: design of a randomized trial of ultrasound enhanced thrombolysis for acute ischemic stroke. J Neuroimaging 2004; 14:108–112.
100. Eggers J, Seidel G, Koch B, Konig IR. Sonothrombolysis in acute ischemic stroke for patients ineligible for rt-PA. Neurology 2005; 64:1052–1054.
101. Cintas P, Le Traon AP, Larrue V. High rate of recanalization of middle cerebral artery occlusion during 2-MHz transcranial color-coded Doppler continuous monitoring without thrombolytic drug. Stroke 2002; 33:626–628.
102. Skoloudik D, Bar M, Hradilek P, Vaclavik D, Skoda O. Safety and efficacy of thrombotripsy–acceleration of thrombolysis by TCCS. (CD-ROM) Proceedings of the NSRG 2003 Meeting, Germany.

103. The IMS Study Investigators. Combined intravenous and intra-arterial recanalization for acute ischemic stroke: The Interventional Management of Stroke Study. Stroke 2004; 35:904–912.

104. Daffertshoffer M, Hennerici M. Ultrasound in the treatment of ischaemic stroke. Lancet Neurology 2003; 2:283–290.

105. Daffertshofer M, Gass A, Ringleb P, et al. Transcranial low-frequency ultrasound-mediated thrombolysis in brain ischemia: increased risk of hemorrhage with combined ultrasound and tissue plasminogen activator. Stroke 2005; 36:1441–1446.

106. Unger EC, Porter T, Culp W, Labell R, Matsunaga T, Zutshi R. Therapeutic applications of lipid-coated microbubbles. Adv Drug Deliv Rev 2004; 56:1291–1314.

107. Culp WC, Porter TR, McCowan TC, et al. Microbubble-augmented ultrasound declotting of thrombosed arteriovenous dialysis grafts in dogs. J Vasc Interv Radiol 2003;14:343–347.

108. Molina CA, Ribo M, Arenillas J, et al. Microbubbles administration accelerates clot lysis during continuous 2 MHz ultrasound monitoring in stroke patients treated with intravenous tPA [abstr]. Stroke 2005; 36:419.

109. Culp WC, Porter TR, Lowery J, Xie F, Roberson PK, Marky L. Intracranial clot lysis with intravenous microbubbles and transcranial ultrasound in swine. Stroke 2004; 35:2407–2411.

110. Martina AD, Meyer-Wiethe K, Allemann E, Seidel G. Ultrasound contrast agents for brain perfusion imaging and ischemic stroke therapy. J Neuroimaging 2005; 15:217–232.

111. Alexandrov AV. Ultrasound enhanced thrombolysis for stroke. Intl J Stroke 2006:1:26–29.

40 | Acute Stroke in the Young

Heather J. Fullerton, MD, MAS, Assistant Professor
Donna M. Ferriero, MD, Professor
Departments of Neurology and Pediatrics, University of California–San Francisco,
San Francisco, California, USA

INTRODUCTION

The timing of an insult to the developing nervous system dramatically influences the pathogenesis, manifestations, and recovery from that insult. Perhaps no disease better exemplifies this principle than stroke. Whereas a teenager with a left middle cerebral artery ischemic stroke might present with abrupt onset aphasia and a right hemiparesis, a 2-year-old with a stroke involving the exact same vascular distribution may present with drooling from the right side of the mouth, "clingy" behavior, and refusal to walk. A similar stroke in a neonate might manifest only with seizures, or may be clinically silent until he/she develops a pathologic early handedness (hand preference) in the first year of life. These differences in clinical manifestation are only the tip of the iceberg; age-dependent differences extend to the cellular level, where, for example, developmental differences in protein expression modify cellular responses to injury.

This chapter will describe age-related differences in stroke, focusing primarily on 2 different age groups: the neonate (typically defined as a child in the first month of life) and the older child, including the older infant (>1 month ≤1 year of life). Because the bulk of pediatric stroke literature has been dedicated to arterial ischemic stroke, discussion will be restricted to this stroke subtype. It is worth noting, however, that unlike in adults, half of all strokes in children are actually hemorrhagic (1).

TERMINOLOGY, INCIDENCE, AND EPIDEMIOLOGY

Childhood Stroke

Dated population-based studies (prior to 1995) reported an annual incidence of stroke, ischemic and hemorrhagic, of 2.5 to 2.7 per 100,000 children in the United States (1,2) and 13.0 per 100,000 in France (3). Although ischemic stroke accounts for the majority of strokes in adults, only half of those in children were ischemic (1,4). More recent administrative data suggest an increasing incidence in the United States, possibly reflecting improvements in diagnosis with advances in brain imaging, although this has yet to be confirmed in a population-based study (5). A population-based study from Canada, however, reported an annual incidence of 2.6 per 100,000 children for ischemic stroke alone, which is double the rate in the prior North American studies (6).

Although numerous studies document ethnic and gender disparities in adult stroke, limited data exist regarding the epidemiology of childhood stroke. However, recent studies using administrative data found that, as in adults, black children in the United States appear to have twice the risk of stroke and stroke death compared to white children and that this difference is not fully explained by sickle cell disease (SCD) (4,7). Additionally, a 2003 study reported that boys have a higher risk of stroke compared to girls (similar to findings in adults) (4). This difference did not appear to be due to trauma, although trauma was likely not fully measured in this study.

Neonatal Stroke

The term "neonatal stroke" generally includes both hemorrhagic and ischemic strokes and both arterial and venous infarcts thought to occur within the first month of life. As strokes presenting in the neonate might actually occur prior to the time of birth, the term "perinatal ischemic stroke" has been coined to describe those ischemic strokes conforming to an arterial distribution and occurring in utero through the first 7 days of life (8). An additional term, "presumed perinatal stroke," has been used to describe those strokes that present in later infancy or childhood, typically with early handedness or seizures, but are clearly old on imaging and are therefore presumed to have occurred in the perinatal period.

Because neonatal strokes are often clinically silent in the acute phase, the incidence has been difficult to estimate. However, a recent population-based study reported an incidence of neonatal ischemic stroke, including presumed perinatal stroke, of 1 in 5000 live births (9). Neonatal hemorrhagic stroke is particularly difficult to define and measure, given that many normal newborns have a small amount of intracerebral hemorrhage, presumably secondary to birth trauma; therefore, no estimates of incidences of neonatal hemorrhagic stroke have been published.

MECHANISMS OF INJURY IN STROKE

Modeling Neonatal Stroke

Studies in animal models and *in vitro* have demonstrated that the mechanisms underlying ischemic injury in the neonatal brain differ in many important ways from those in the adult brain (10–12). Differences in maturational biology [the blood–brain barrier (BBB), cerebrovascular autoregulation, and signaling pathways] and pathophysiology (excitotoxicity, oxidative stress, inflammatory response, and cell death pathways) have been described and emphasize the importance of considering neonatal stroke to be distinct from its adult counterpart, particularly in the development of treatment strategies.

Biologic Differences

A component of the cerebral edema associated with an infarct is thought to be vasogenic, due to movement of water across the BBB into the interstitial space of the brain parenchyma. Although the BBB in neonates is generally considered "immature" and therefore "less effective," these concepts have been challenged by advances in developmental neuroanatomy, as well as by recent studies using MRI in rodent models (13). For example, the higher cerebral spinal fluid protein concentration found in neonates, as compared to adults, may not be due to an ineffective BBB, but rather a physiologic mechanism that promotes protein passage across the BBB, which becomes less effective as the brain matures (14). Endothelial tight junctions, which form the basis of the BBB, also undergo developmental changes that might contribute to a developmental decline in passive permeability (15,16).

Cerebrovascular autoregulation is important in the pathogenesis of a stroke, affecting cerebral blood flow during the acute thromboembolic event and playing a role in reperfusion injury. Although preterm infants have long been thought to have a "pressure-passive" cerebral circulation, term newborns also appear to have narrow autoregulatory windows, which might make them more susceptible to brain injury at extremes of blood pressure (17–19).

Glutamate receptors are developmentally regulated in both neurons and glia, and glutamatergic synaptic transmission is largely NMDA receptor mediated early in development (20). NMDA-receptor-subunit composition changes with development, with the NR2B subunit predominating early, followed by increasing expression of NR2A (21). This phenomenon is important for synaptogenesis because NMDA receptors in which NR2B is expressed have slower deactivation and higher conductance (21). Like the NMDA receptor, AMPA receptor subunit composition also changes during development, with decreased expression of the GluR2 subunit at early ages (22), leading to higher calcium permeability (23). The developing brain has high concentrations of unsaturated fatty acids, high rates of oxygen consumption, low concentrations of antioxidants, and increased availability of "free" redox-active iron (24). These and many other changes in neural cell phenotypes greatly influence the response of the neonatal brain to pathologic mechanisms, such as excitotoxicity, oxidative stress, and subsequent cell death.

Excitotoxicity

Glutamate is the primary excitatory neurotransmitter in the brain. The cycle of glutamate synthesis, release, and reuptake is tightly linked to glucose metabolism. In the setting of ischemia, this cycle is disrupted: Glutamate release is increased and uptake is impaired, leading to pathologic prolonged stimulation of glutamate receptors (including the NMDA receptor) and neuronal cell death—a process called "excitotoxicity" (25). Compared to that in the adult brain, the NMDA receptor in the newborn brain is more highly expressed, has a higher affinity for glutamate, and is more active (26–28). These developmental differences render the immature brain more susceptible to excitotoxicity (29). In fact, it has been reported that exposure of the neonatal rat brain to treatments aimed at reducing excitotoxicity by targeting the NMDA receptor, even in a normal brain, accelerates programmed cell death (30). This paradoxic effect probably relates to developmental differences in glutamate signaling, as well as innate programmed cell death occurring during this period (see below).

Oxidative Stress

Free radicals, which are produced during normal oxidative metabolism as oxygen and adenosine diphosphate are converted to water and adenosine triphosphate in the electron transport chain, are overproduced during ischemia, particularly reperfusion. This pathologic state is termed "oxidative stress." Although an elegant antioxidant enzyme system—which includes superoxide dismutase, glutathione peroxidase, and catalase—normally reduces toxic free radicals, ultimately converting them to water, this system is immature in the newborn brain. Developmental changes in the activities of these enzymes are imbalanced, causing accumulation of hydrogen peroxide (a toxic intermediary) in the neonatal brain in the setting of ischemic injury (31). In addition, the newborn brain is rich in free iron and is thus more susceptible to nonenzymatic attack by free radicals. Therapies aimed against this form of toxicity appear to be promising (32). The generation of reactive nitrogen species also contributes to cell death after stroke, and the neonatal brain is uniquely susceptible because of its ability to produce nitric oxide in selectively vulnerable regions. One of the isoenzymes responsible for generation of reactive nitrogen species is neuronal nitric oxide synthetase (nNOS), which is maximally expressed in regions where the immature NMDA-R is expressed, especially the basal ganglia (33). When nitric oxide is produced in excessive amounts during periods of oxidative stress in these regions of abundance, it is converted to peroxynitrite, a potent mediator of free radical injury (34). nNOS-expressing neurons are resistant to both hypoxia–ischemia and NMDA-mediated excitotoxicity (35,36). However, intracranial pressure (ICP) thresholds to ameliorate secondary brain injury have differed in previous studies; but this resistance of striatal neurons to NMDA agonists is limited to young ages ($\leq$P7 in rodent), and as the brain matures, this resistance is lost (36). Therapies designed to reduce both nNOS and inducible nitric oxide synthase activity have proven beneficial in small and large animal models (37).

Inflammation

As in the adult, inflammation appears to mediate and potentiate focal ischemic brain injury in the neonate (38,39). However, certain aspects of the inflammatory response are different in the neonate. For example, neutrophil extravasation from blood vessels, seen after focal ischemia in adult animal models, is not seen in similar models in the neonatal animal (13). In addition, brain vascular permeability and leukocyte recruitment following injections of inflammatory cytokines (Interleukin-1β or tumor necrosis factor-α) into brain are age dependent and higher in three-week-old animals than in newborns or three-month-old animals (40). The role of resident microglia in mediating inflammatory processes is just beginning to be understood in models of neonatal stroke (41). Additionally, the possibility that innate immunity and systemic responses might regulate the brain's inflammatory response is an emerging concept that will greatly affect the understanding of this process (42).

Cell Death Pathways

Inhibition of apoptosis is repeatedly proposed as a novel and promising therapeutic direction for attempts at cell rescue following stroke. In that the immature brain undergoes programmed cell death to ensure normal brain development, the effects of inhibiting this program must be considered when developing therapies. Cell death in the injured developing brain has been termed "neuronal necrosis" or "excitotoxic neurodegeneration" (43). It has been argued that true apoptosis occurs only in a second wave of cell death following neonatal hypoxic–ischemic brain injury as a consequence of target deprivation (44–47). However, the cell death may actually represent a "continuum" phenotype that incorporates features of both (48). Recent commentaries point to the controversy surrounding the classification of developmental cell death phenotypes (49,50). The strongest biochemical evidence for the presence of an intermediate continuum form of cell death is outlined in a recent study in which markers for both apoptosis and necrosis are demonstrated in injured forebrain neurons early following neonatal hypoxic–ischemic brain injury (51). Inhibition by apoptosis inhibitors provides only partial protection, further supporting these anatomic data (52). In the reperfusion model of neonatal stroke, classic markers for activation of apoptotic pathways fail to coincide with the severity of injury, suggesting a role for necrosis as well (53).

Modeling Childhood Stroke

Although considerable effort has been directed toward understanding the pathogenesis of ischemic injury in the adult and neonatal brain, the juvenile brain remains understudied. Published studies that use animal models of childhood stroke are very few (54).

DISTRIBUTION AND CLINICAL PRESENTATION

Childhood Stroke

Large-vessel ischemic strokes predominate in children, whereas lacunar strokes are exceedingly rare (55,56). The vascular territory most commonly affected is that of the middle cerebral artery; posterior circulation strokes are uncommon (57,58).

The most common presenting sign of ischemic stroke in children is hemiparesis, present in 45% to 100% of children with ischemic stroke in different hospital series (57–59). Although the clinical syndromes associated with different vascular territories are similar to those in adults, with the same pyramidal distribution of weakness, the deficits are often less obvious, particularly in children who have not yet developed language or sophisticated motor skills, such as ambulation. In addition, the onset of the stroke symptoms is less likely to be abrupt. In one series, only half of the children had an abrupt onset, while the others demonstrated deficits that progressed over a matter of hours (58). The stroke manifestations in children also differ from those in adults in that seizures are common at the stroke ictus, occurring in 20% to 30% (57,59).

Neonatal Stroke

Strokes in neonates have a much more subtle presentation and can be clinically silent. The most common presenting feature in the neonatal period is a seizure, although some present with nonfocal hypotonia or encephalopathy (8,60). Although neonatal seizures due to systemic abnormalities or global brain injury tend to be multifocal or myoclonic, those associated with stroke tend to be persistently focal motor, often involving only one upper extremity.

Neonates rarely have a clinically apparent hemiparesis, even with a large hemispheric stroke. However, those with no clinical manifestations at the stroke ictus may present in later infancy with pathologic early handedness (before one year of life), growth asymmetry, or hand dystonia. A spastic hemiparesis may evolve over time, and some children may meet criteria for "hemiplegic cerebral palsy" (61,62). Others, however, may go undiagnosed until they have a seizure later in life.

ETIOLOGIES AND RISK FACTORS

The diseases and conditions associated with childhood and neonatal ischemic stroke are numerous, and the etiologies overlap considerably between the two age groups (Table 1) (8,9,63). This review will first discuss some of the major categories and then focus on risk factors specific for neonatal stroke. Before embarking on such a discussion, however, it is important to establish that stroke in both neonates and children is often caused by a combination of factors, such as congenital heart disease (CHD) and a hereditary prothrombotic state, or acquired multiple prothrombotic conditions (64). The likelihood of multiple etiologies has important implications for the diagnostic workup in these children; investigations should not be concluded after a single risk factor is identified.

Cardiac Etiology

Cardiac disease, particularly CHD, is a frequently reported etiology in hospital series of childhood stroke and a cause of neonatal stroke (55,65,58). However, it is rare for a stroke to

Table 1 Conditions Associated with Ischemic Stroke in Children and Neonates

	Children	Neonates
Vascular		
Arterial dissection	✓	✓
Moyamoya syndrome	✓	
Primary		
Secondary		
Sickle cell disease		
Cranial radiation		
Neurofibromatosis		
Down syndrome		
Transient cerebral arteriopathy	✓	
Vasculitis	✓	
Primary central nervous system		
Systemic		
(Example: systemic lupus erythematosus)		
Fibromuscular dysplasia	✓	
Cardiac		
Congenital heart disease	✓	✓
Congenital valvular disease	✓	✓
Endocarditis	✓	✓
Rheumatic heart disease	✓	
Patent foramen ovale (questionable)	✓	
Cardiomyopathy	✓	
Arrhythmia	✓	
Hematologic		
Sickle cell disease	✓	
Acquired prothrombotic states		
Nephrotic syndrome	✓	
Hemolytic-uremic syndrome	✓	
Pregnancy	✓	
Preeclampsia	✓	✓
Hereditary prothrombotic states		
Factor V Leiden	✓	✓
Protein C and S deficiency	✓	✓
Methyl tetrahydrofolate reductase polymorphism	✓	✓
Lipoprotein (a)	✓	✓
Antithrombin III deficiency	✓	✓
Leukemia	✓	
Infectious		
Meningitis	✓	✓
Sepsis	✓	✓
Chicken pox	✓	
Postvaricella angiopathy		
Chorioamnionitis		✓
Genetic/metabolic		
Neurocutaneous disorders	✓	
Sturge–Weber syndrome		
Neurofibromatosis		
Tuberous sclerosis		
Homocystinuria	✓	
Fabry disease	✓	
Congenital disorders of glycosylation	✓	
Drugs/toxic		
Sympathomimetics	✓	✓
Cocaine		
Amphetamine		
Ephedrine		
Methylphenidate		
Phenylpropanolamine		
Chemotherapeutics	✓	
L-asparaginase		

Note: "✓" signifies whether the condition is associated with stroke in children, neonates, or both.

be the presenting feature of CHD; in most children with CHD and stroke, the cardiac disease was diagnosed prior to the stroke (66,67). Strokes may occur in the pre- or perioperative period (associated with endovascular procedures or open-heart repairs) or during times of general good health (68,69). As alluded to above, the presence of a genetic thrombophilia in a child with CHD puts that child at increased risk of an ischemic stroke (64,70).

Vascular Etiology

Abnormalities of the cerebral vasculature are increasingly recognized as an important etiology of childhood ischemic stroke, while the vasculature in neonates with stroke remains under-studied. Among previously healthy children with ischemic stroke, as many as 75% had some abnormality of their cerebral vessels on imaging (66). These abnormalities included large artery stenosis (49%) and occlusion (17%), arterial dissection (14%), moyamoya syndrome (11%), hypoplastic vessels (6%), and arteritis (2%). Arterial dissection is underrecognized in children because, compared to adults, they less often present with headache and rarely complain of neck pain (71). Arterial dissection should also be considered in neonates because it may result from neck trauma at delivery (72).

Moyamoya syndrome is a rare progressive occlusive vasculopathy that involves primar-ily the terminal internal carotid arteries and circle of Willis, although the posterior circulation can be involved as well. Over time, a pathologic network of collateral vessels develops at the skull base. It may present with ischemic stroke if the collaterals are insufficient or if an artery-to-artery embolus occurs, or with hemorrhagic stroke if one of the collateral vessels or an associated aneurysm ruptures. Children typically present with ischemic events, whereas hemorrhages are more common in adults. The idiopathic form of the syndrome is known as "pri-mary" moyamoya (or moyamoya disease); "secondary" moyamoya can occur in the setting of SCD, Down syndrome, tuberous sclerosis, Marfan syndrome, and cranial irradiation (73). Although primary moyamoya is more prevalent in Asians, it has been described in patients of various ethnic backgrounds (74,75).

Infectious Etiology

Infection can predispose to stroke, either through systemic effects of inflammatory mediators that cause a relatively prothrombotic state or by direct or indirect effects on blood vessels through a variety of mechanisms (76). In children, ischemic stroke is a known complication of infectious endocarditis that leads to cardioembolic stroke, and of meningitis with a local vasculitis as blood vessels course through an inflamed subarachnoid space (77). The importance of chicken pox as a risk factor for childhood stroke has been suggested by recent data. *Varicella zoster* may damage blood vessels directly by actual invasion of the vessels and is thought to cause a "transient cerebral arteriopathy" in children (78,79). A small case–control study found that children with stroke are almost 18 times more likely to have had chicken pox in the 9 months prior to stroke ictus compared to healthy control children (80). Chorioamnionitis is a risk factor for neonatal stroke; the placental pathology presumably leads to emboli in the fetal circulation (9).

Genetic Thrombophilias

Hereditary prothrombotic states are relatively weak risk factors for childhood and neonatal ischemic stroke (81). Although results have been inconsistent, data from case–control studies most strongly support associations with Factor V Leiden and prothrombin 20210 mutations, and protein C deficiency (64,82–84); the role of methyl tetrahydrofolate reductase polymorphisms remains controversial (83–85). In these studies, the point estimates of the significant odds ratios (OR) ranged from 2 to 19, suggesting that a child with a single genetic thrombophilia is still at low risk for stroke. However, the association with stroke is stronger in the presence of more than one genetic thrombophilia (82,84,86,87). In addition, it is likely that these hereditary pro-thrombotic states are important when present in combination with other predisposing conditions, such as CHD, vasculopathy, or infections.

Sickle Cell Disease

SCD is a strong risk factor for childhood stroke: approximately 1 in 10 children with SCD suffers a clinically apparent stroke by the age of 20 years (88–90). SCD, as one of the causes of secondary moyamoya, causes a progressive vasculopathy of the distal internal carotid arteries and their proximal branches (91,92). Among children with SCD, factors that predict stroke include dactylitis (inflammation of a finger or toe) in the first year of life (93), severe anemia (93), acute chest syndrome (94), aplastic crisis (particularly in the setting of parvovirus B19 infection) (95), and hypertension (96). Silent (or "covert") infarcts are present in 13% of children with SCD with no history of overt stroke. As in adults with small vessel disease, these infarcts likely lead to cognitive dysfunction (97). In addition, their presence on MRI predicts clinically apparent stroke (98).

Neonatal Stroke
Although, as illustrated in Table 1, neonatal and childhood stroke share a number of common etiologies, other factors are unique to the neonates. A recent case–control study found that a number of prepartum and intrapartum conditions were more common in neonates with arterial stroke. In a multivariate analysis, factors that emerged as independent risk factors included prolonged second stage of labor (OR: 8.8), preeclampsia (OR: 5.3), and prolonged rupture of membranes (OR: 3.4) (9). However, in a population of children with perinatal ischemic stroke identified by the fact that they had motor impairment, risk factors included preeclampsia (OR: 3.6) and intrauterine growth restriction (OR: 5.3) (99).

Idiopathic Etiology
Despite the long list of known etiologies for childhood stroke, many children undergo an extensive stroke workup that is ultimately unrevealing. Depending on the extent of the diagnostic evaluation, as well as what is deemed an acceptable "etiology," the proportion of "idiopathic" ischemic strokes in hospital series ranges from 35% to 65% (55,57,59). Even in a prospective stroke study that conducted thorough diagnostic evaluations, 60% of children had no identifiable etiology (100). Our persistent inability to explain the strokes that occur in this large proportion of children reflects our limited understanding of the pathogenetic mechanisms underlying this disease.

DIAGNOSTIC EVALUATION

The diagnostic evaluation of a child or neonate with an arterial ischemic stroke is detailed in Table 2. Neuroimaging with MRI (including MRA) is critical for determining both the timing of the stroke and its extent, which are essential indicators for the likelihood of developing complications such as hemorrhagic transformation and significant mass effect. MRI is also important for differentiating an arterial infarct from a venous infarct and for identifying an underlying vasculopathy, with important implications for recurrence risk (children with vascular abnormalities are at highest risk for a recurrent ischemic event) (100). Conventional angiography should be considered when (i) vascular imaging with MRA or CT angiography appears normal, but the clinical picture is suggestive of an arterial dissection or vasculitis, or (ii) a child suffers recurrent stroke, but the initial diagnostic workup is unrevealing. An echocardiogram, although unlikely to be abnormal in previously healthy patients (101), should be performed in every child with a stroke that appears embolic on neuroimaging studies. A thorough workup for hereditary and acquired prothrombotic states should be performed as part of the initial diagnostic evaluation, even if another etiology, such as CHD, has already been identified. As protein C, protein S, and antithrombin III levels can be affected by the acute stroke, as well as anticoagulant medications, these studies should be repeated at least six weeks after the acute event if they are found to be abnormally low. In neonatal stroke, an evaluation of the parents for a prothrombotic disorder should also be considered, although the role of such inherited disorders in neonatal stroke remains poorly understood.

MANAGEMENT

As in adults, the goals in the acute management of an ischemic stroke in a child or neonate include (i) minimizing the brain injury directly related to the stroke, (ii) preventing further brain injury due to mass effect from the stroke, and (iii) preventing a recurrent stroke.

Minimizing Direct Brain Injury
Although thrombolytic agents, such as intravenous recombinant tissue plasminogen activator (rtPA) improve the outcome of adult ischemic stroke, presumably by decreasing the extent of the

Table 2 Diagnostic Workup in Children and Neonates with Acute Ischemic Stroke

	Children	Neonates
Radiologic		
MRI; brain	x	x
MRI; neck with fat saturation	x	*
MRA; brain and neck	x	x
MRV	*	x
Cardiac		
Transthoracic echocardiogram	x	x
Infectious		
WBC	x	x
Blood cultures	*	*
Lumbar puncture	*	*
Hematologic		
Prothrombin time	x	x
Partial thromboplastin time	x	x
Factor V Leiden mutation	x	x
Prothrombin 20210 mutation	x	x
MTHFR polymorphism	x	x
Lipoprotein (a)	x	x
Antithrombin III	x	x
Protein C	x	x
Protein S	x	x
Lupus anticoagulant	x	*
Anticardiolipin antibody	x	*
Toxic/metabolic		
Urine drugs of abuse screen	x	x
MELAS	*	
Urine organic acids	*	
Serum amino acids	*	*

Notes: "x" indicates that the procedure is part of a routine evaluation; "*" indicates that the procedure should be considered and performed if indicated.
Abbreviations: MTHFR, methyl tetrahydrofolate reductase; MELAS, mitochondrial encephalopathy, lactic acidosis, and stroke-like episodes; MRA, magnetic resonance angiography; MRV, magnetic resonance venography; WBC, white blood cell.

infarct, they have not been studied in children under 18 years of age. In the National Institute of Neurological Disorders and Stroke rtPA trial, the increased risk of hemorrhage associated with rtPA was outweighed by the overall benefit in terms of neurologic outcome at 3 months (102). We do not know whether this risk/benefit ratio is similar in children. One could argue that the risks might be higher: hemorrhagic transformation of a stroke might be more dangerous in a child with a young healthy brain that fills the cranial vault and leaves little room to accommodate the added mass effect of a hemorrhage. The benefits of rtPA might also be lower; without intervention, children probably recover better than adults do from ischemic stroke. Therefore, until rtPA is studied in children, it should probably not be used in the treatment of an acute stroke in a young child and should only be used in an older child with the informed consent of the parents or guardians.

As discussed in other chapters of this book, other, more conservative, measures can be taken to try to preserve the penumbra region and minimize brain injury due to a stroke. The child's blood pressure should be maintained at normotensive to mildly hypertensive to improve cerebral perfusion. This can be difficult in children because, unlike the typical adult stroke patient who is often hypertensive at baseline, children with stroke only rarely have preexisting hypertension (101). The temperature of children with acute stroke should also be closely monitored; hyperthermia should be treated aggressively with antipyretics because it may exacerbate ischemic injury (103). The coagulation system and platelet levels should be monitored closely to minimize excessive risk of hemorrhagic transformation of the stroke, particularly as some etiologies of childhood ischemic stroke (e.g., sepsis, hemolytic–uremic syndrome, and leukemia) may also impair normal clot formation.

Managing Mass Effect

Mass effect from an acute ischemic stroke is of particular concern in children and neonates because they tend to have large-vessel strokes (55,56) and they do not have the "protective" brain atrophy often seen in older patients with stroke. Children with large cortical or cerebellar strokes should therefore be monitored in an ICU. ICP monitoring should be considered, particularly if the neurologic exam is not reliable. Neurosurgical consultation for possible hemicraniectomy (for cortical strokes) or cerebellar decompressive surgery (for posterior fossa strokes) should be considered early to prevent brain herniation.

Because neonates have open fontanelles and cranial sutures, increased ICP will cause bulging of the fontanelles and splitting of the sutures, with rapid increases in head circumference. Therefore, mass effect from a neonatal stroke can be followed through frequent head circumference measurements, palpation of the head, and head ultrasound. Most neonatal ischemic strokes can be managed conservatively; they rarely require surgical decompression outside the setting of a significant hemorrhagic transformation.

Secondary Stroke Prevention

Neonates with arterial ischemic strokes rarely suffer recurrent ischemic events. A study of 215 children with neonatal ischemic stroke who were followed for a median of 3.5 years reported recurrent symptomatic thromboembolism in 7 (3.3%): 4 with arterial ischemic strokes, 2 with venous sinus thromboses, and 1 with deep venous thrombosis of the leg. Risk factors for recurrence included prothrombotic states and the presence of additional morbidities, such as complex CHD (104). Therefore, because the risk of recurrence is low, neonates are usually not treated with antithrombotic medications unless found to have a cardioembolic source or an ongoing prothrombotic state.

Although rare after neonatal stroke, recurrent ischemic events are surprisingly common after childhood stroke, occurring in 8% of children with either no stroke risk factor or a single stroke risk factor and in 42% of children with multiple risk factors over a median of 2 years of follow-up (105). Children with vascular abnormalities are at particularly high risk of recurrence (100). Half of stroke recurrences occur within 6 months (106), the majority occur within 12 months, and recurrence is rare after 2 years (100). To date, no clinical trials have been conducted to investigate secondary stroke prevention in children. A prospective observational study suggested that antithrombotic therapy can be safely used in children with ischemic stroke; of 49 children who were treated with aspirin and 86 who were treated with low-molecular-weight heparin (LMWH), none had any major drug-related side effects (107). In the absence of efficacy studies specific to children, antithrombotic agents, particularly aspirin and LMWH, are still frequently used, with the goal of preventing recurrent stroke in children. An American College of Chest Physicians Conference on Antithrombotic and Thrombolytic Therapy recommended an algorithm of anticoagulating all children with ischemic stroke "for 5 to 7 days and until cardioembolic stroke or vascular dissection has been excluded," followed by either aspirin for those children who did not have a cardioembolic stroke or dissection, or an additional 3 to 6 months of anticoagulation for those who did (108). Although such guidelines are helpful in establishing an acceptable standard of care, it is important to recognize that they are based on an extrapolation from treatment of adult stroke (with very different stroke etiologies) and limited safety data in children. In addition, these guidelines fail to adequately address important contraindications—whether strict or relative—for anticoagulation, such as large infarct size, evidence of hemorrhagic transformation, arterial dissection with pseudoaneurysm, septic emboli, moyamoya syndrome, etc. Therefore, although the risk of recurrent stroke in children is surprisingly high, especially among those with vascular abnormalities, antithrombotic agents, especially anticoagulants, should be used with caution and with a full understanding of the limitations of our knowledge regarding their use.

CONCLUSIONS

Although an MRI of an acute middle cerebral artery stroke in a two-year-old child may appear quite similar to that in a 60-year-old adult, the similarity is deceptive. Stroke etiologies vary dramatically by age; developmental differences in the BBB, neurotransmitter receptors, and antioxidant enzymes, and inflammatory and cell-death pathways modify the response to ischemia occurring on a cellular level; and differences in brain maturation modify the clinical manifestations of a stroke. These age-related differences must be considered in the acute management of a childhood stroke. A thrombolytic or neuroprotective agent that improves outcome in an adult may not be efficacious in a child. Therefore, in both clinical practice and research, neonatal and childhood stroke must be considered discrete entities.

REFERENCES

1. Broderick J, Talbot GT Prenger E, et al. Stroke in children within a major metropolitan area: the surprising importance of intracerebral hemorrhage. J Child Neurol 1993; 8(3):250–255.
2. Schoenberg BS, Mellinger JF, Schoenberg DG. Cerebrovascular disease in infants and children: a study of incidence, clinical features, and survival. Neurology 1978; 28:763–768.
3. Giroud M, Lemesle M, Gouyon J, et al. Cerebrovascular disease in children under 16 years of age in the city of Dijon France: a study of incidence and clinical features from 1985 to 1993. J Clin Epidemiol 1995; 48(11):1343–1348.
4. Fullerton HJ, Wu YW, Zhao S, et al. Risk of stroke in children: Ethnic and gender disparities. Neurology 2003; 61(2):189–194.
5. Lynch JK, Hirtz DG, DeVeber G, et al. Report of the National Institute of Neurological Disorders and Stroke workshop on perinatal and childhood stroke. Pediatrics 2002; 109(1):116–123.
6. deVeber G, Group T.C.P.I.S.S. Canadian paediatric ischemic stroke registry: analysis of children with arterial stroke [abstr]. Ann Neurol 2000; 48, 526.
7. Fullerton HJ, Chetkovich DM, Wu YW, et al. Deaths from stroke in US children, 1979 to 1998. Neurology 2002; 59(1):34–39.
8. Nelson KB, Lynch JK. Stroke in newborn infants. Lancet Neurol 2004; 3(3):150–158.
9. Lee J, Croen LA, Backstrand KH, et al. Maternal and infant characteristics associated with perinatal arterial stroke in the infant. JAMA 2005; 293(6):723–729.
10. McLean C, Ferriero D. Mechanisms of hypoxic–ischemic injury in the term infant. Semin Perinatol 2004; 28(6):425–432.
11. Ashwal S, Pearce WJ. Animal models of neonatal stroke. Curr Opin Pediatr 2001; 13(6):506–516.
12. Ferriero DM. Neonatal brain injury. N Engl J Med 2004; 351(19):1985–1995.
13. Wendland M, Derugin N, Manabat C, et al. The blood–brain barrier is more preserved in neonatal versus adult rats following transient focal cerebral ischemia. J Cereb Blood Flow Metab 2003; 23(suppl 1):169.
14. Saunders NR, Habgood MD, Dziegielewska KM. Barrier mechanisms in the brain II. Immature brain. Clin Exp Pharmacol Physiol 1999; 26(2):85–91.
15. Stewart PA, Hayakawa K. Early ultrastructural changes in blood–brain barrier vessels of the rat embryo. Brain Res Dev Brain Res 1994; 78(1):25–34.
16. Kniesel U, Risau W, Wolburg H. Development of blood–brain barrier tight junctions in the rat cortex. Brain Res Dev Brain Res 1996; 96(1–2):229–240.
17. Chemtob S, Li DY, Abran D, et al. The role of prostaglandin receptors in regulating cerebral blood flow in the perinatal period. Acta Paediatr 1996; 85(5):517–524.
18. Hardy P, Nuyt AM, Dumont I, et al. Developmentally increased cerebrovascular NO in newborn pigs curtails cerebral blood flow autoregulation. Pediatr Res 1999; 46(4):375–382.
19. Verma PK, Panerai RB, Rennie JM, et al. Grading of cerebral autoregulation in preterm and term neonates. Pediatr Neurol 2000; 23(3):236–242.
20. Crair MC, Malenka RC. A critical period for long-term potentiation at thalamocortical synapses. Nature 1995; 375(6529):325–328.
21. Cull-Candy S, Brickley S, Farrant M. NMDA receptor subunits: diversity, development and disease. Curr Opin Neurobiol 2001; 11(3):327–335.
22. Kumar SS, Bacci A, Kharazia V, et al. A developmental switch of AMPA receptor subunits in neocortical pyramidal neurons. J Neurosci 2002; 22(8):3005–3015.
23. Pellegrini-Giampietro DE, Gorter JA, Bennett MV, et al. The GluR2 (GluR-B) hypothesis: Ca(2+)-permeable AMPA receptors in neurological disorders. Trends Neurosci 1997; 20(10):464–470.
24. Siddappa AJ, Rao RB, Wobken JD, et al. Developmental changes in the expression of iron regulatory proteins and iron transport proteins in the perinatal rat brain. J Neurosci Res 2002; 68(6):761–775.
25. Choi DW. Glutamate neurotoxicity and diseases of the nervous system. Neuron 1988; 1(8):623–634.
26. Tremblay E, Roisin MP, Represa A, et al. Transient increased density of NMDA binding sites in the developing rat hippocampus. Brain Res 1988; 461(2):393–396.
27. Mishra OP, Deliviria-Papadopoulos M. Modification of modulatory sites of NMDA receptor in the fetal guinea pig brain during development. Neurochem Res 1992; 17(12):1223–1228.

28. Danysz W, Parsons AC. Glycine and *N*-methyl-*D*-aspartate receptors: physiological significance and possible therapeutic applications. Pharmacol Rev 1998; 50(4):597–664.
29. Johnston MV. Excitotoxicity in neonatal hypoxia. Ment Retard Dev Disabil Res Rev 2001; 7(4):229–234.
30. Olney JW, Wozniak DF, Jevtovic-Todorovic V, et al. Drug-induced apoptotic neurodegeneration in the developing brain. Brain Pathol 2002; 12(4):488–498.
31. Fullerton HJ, Ditelberg JS, Chen SF, et al. Copper/zinc superoxide dismutase transgenic brain accumulates hydrogen peroxide after perinatal hypoxia ischemia. Ann Neurol 1998; 44(3):357–364.
32. Ferriero DM. Timing is everything–delaying therapy for delayed cell death. Dev Neurosci 2002; 24(5):349–351.
33. Black SM, Bedolli MA, Martinez S, et al. Expression of neuronal nitric oxide synthase corresponds to regions of selective vulnerability to hypoxia-ischaemia in the developing rat brain. Neurobiol Dis 1995; 2(3):145–155.
34. Dawson VL, Dawson TM, London ED, et al. Nitric oxide mediates glutamate neurotoxicity in primary cortical cultures. Proc Natl Acad Sci USA 1991; 88(14):6368–6371.
35. Ferriero DM, Arcavi LJ, Sagar SM, et al. Selective sparing of NADPH-diaphorase neurons in neonatal hypoxia-ischemia. Ann Neurol 1988; 24(5):670–676.
36. Ferriero DM, Arcavi LJ, Simon RP. Ontogeny of excitotoxic injury to nicotinamide adenine dinucleotide phosphate diaphorase reactive neurons in the neonatal rat striatum. Neuroscience 1990; 36(2):417–424.
37. Peeters-Scholte C, Koster J, Veldhuis W, et al. Neuroprotection by selective nitric oxide synthase inhibition at 24 hours after perinatal hypoxia-ischemia. Stroke 2002,; 33(9):2304–2310.
38. Derugin N, Wendland M, Muramatsu K, et al. Evolution of brain injury after transient middle cerebral artery occlusion in neonatal rats. Stroke 2000; 31(7):1752–1761.
39. Benjelloun N, Renolleau S, Represa A, et al. Inflammatory responses in the cerebral cortex after ischemia in the P7 neonatal Rat. Stroke 1999; 30(9):1916–1923; discussion 1923–1914.
40. Anthony DC, Bolton SJ, Fearn S, et al. Age-related effects of interleukin-1 beta on polymorphonuclear neutrophil-dependent increases in blood-brain barrier permeability in rats. Brain 1997; 120 (Pt 3):435–444.
41. Fox C, Dingman A, Derugin N, et al. Minocycline confers early but transient protection in the immature brain following focal cerebral ischemic-reperfusion. J Cereb Blood Flow Metab 2005; 25(9):1138–1149.
42. Lehnardt S, Lachance C, Patrizi S, et al. The toll-like receptor TLR4 is necessary for lipopolysaccharide-induced oligodendrocyte injury in the CNS. J Neurosci 2002; 22(7):2478–2486.
43. Ishimaru MJ, Ikonomidou C, Tenkova TI, et al. Distinguishing excitotoxic from apoptotic neurodegeneration in the developing rat brain. J Comp Neurol 1999; 408(4):461–476.
44. Young C, Tenkova T, Dikranian K, et al. Excitotoxic versus apoptotic mechanisms of neuronal cell death in perinatal hypoxia/ischemia. Curr Mol Med 2004; 4(2):77–85.
45. Martin LJ, Al-Abdulla NA, Brambrink AM, et al. Neurodegeneration in excitotoxicity, global cerebral ischemia, and target deprivation: A perspective on the contributions of apoptosis and necrosis. Brain Res Bull 1998; 46(4):281–309.
46. Northington FJ, Ferriero DM, Flock DL, et al. Delayed neurodegeneration in neonatal rat thalamus after hypoxia-ischemia is apoptosis. J Neurosci 2001; 21(6):1931–1938.
47. Northington FJ, Ferriero DM, Graham EM, et al. Early neurodegeneration after hypoxia-ischemia in neonatal rat is necrosis while delayed neuronal death is apoptosis. Neurobiol Dis 2001; 8(2):207–219.
48. Portera-Cailliau C, Price DL, Martin LJ. Excitotoxic neuronal death in the immature brain is an apoptosis-necrosis morphological continuum. J Comp Neurol 1997; 378(1):70–87.
49. Fujikawa DG. Apoptosis: ignoring morphology and focusing on biochemical mechanisms will not eliminate confusion. Trends Pharmacol Sci 2002; 23(7):309–310; (author reply 310).
50. Fujikawa DG. Confusion between neuronal apoptosis and activation of programmed cell death mechanisms in acute necrotic insults. Trends Neurosci 2000; 23(9):410–411.
51. Blomgren K, Zhu C, Wang X, et al. Synergistic activation of caspase-3 by m-calpain after neonatal hypoxia-ischemia: a mechanism of "pathological apoptosis"? J Biol Chem 2001; 276(13):10191–10198.
52. Han BH, Xu D, Choi J, et al. Selective, reversible caspase-3 inhibitor is neuroprotective and reveals distinct pathways of cell death after neonatal hypoxic-ischemic brain injury. J Biol Chem 2002; 277(33):30128–30136.
53. Manabat C, Han BH, Wendland M, et al. Reperfusion differentially induces caspase-3 activation in ischemic core and penumbra after stroke in immature brain. Stroke 2003; 34(1):207–213.
54. Ashwal S, Cole DJ, Osborne S, et al. L-NAME reduces infarct volume in a filament model of transient middle cerebral artery occlusion in the rat pup. Pediatr Res 1995; 38(5):652–656.
55. Williams LS, Garg BP, Cohen M, et al. Subtypes of ischemic stroke in children and young adults. Neurology 1997; 49(6):1541–1545.
56. Wraige E, Hajat C, Jan W, et al. Ischaemic stroke subtypes in children and adults. Dev Med Child Neurol 2003; 45(4):229–232.

57. Al-Sulaiman A, Bademosi O, Ismail H, et al. Stroke in Saudi children. J Child Neurol 1999; 14(5):295–298.

58. Dusser A, Goutieres F, Aicardi J. Ischemic strokes in children. J Child Neurol 1986; 1(2):131–136.

59. Mancini J, Girard N, Chabrol B, et al. Ischemic cerebrovascular disease in children: retrospective study of 35 patients. J Child Neurol 1997; 12(3):193–199.

60. Perlman JM, Rollins NK, Evans D. Neonatal stroke: clinical characteristics and cerebral blood flow velocity measurements. Pediatr Neurol 1994; 11(4):281–284.

61. Wu YW, Escobar GJ, Grether JK, et al. Chorioamnionitis and cerebral palsy in term and near-term infants. JAMA 2003; 290(20):2677–2684.

62. Mercuri E, Barnett A, Rutherford M, et al. Neonatal cerebral infarction and neuromotor outcome at school age. Pediatrics 2004; 113(1 Pt 1):95–100.

63. deVeber G. Stroke and the child's brain: an overview of epidemiology, syndromes and risk factors. Curr Opin Neurol 2002; 15(2):133–138.

64. Strater R, Vielhaber H, Kassenbohmer R, et al. Genetic risk factors of thrombophilia in ischaemic childhood stroke of cardiac origin. A prospective ESPED survey. Eur J Pediatr 1999; 158(suppl 3): S122–S125.

65. Giroud M, Lemesle M, Madinier G, et al. Stroke in children under 16 years of age. Clinical and etiological difference with adults. Acta Neurol Scand 1997; 96(6):401–406.

66. Ganesan V, Prengler M, McShane MA, et al. Investigation of risk factors in children with arterial ischemic stroke. Ann Neurol 2003; 53(2):167–173.

67. Miller SP, McQuillen PS, Vigneron DB, et al. Preoperative brain injury in newborns with transposition of the great arteries. Ann Thorac Surg 2004; 77(5):1698–1706.

68. du Plessis AJ, Chang AC, Wessel DL, et al. Cerebrovascular accidents following the Fontan operation. Pediatr Neurol 1995; 12(3):230–236.

69. Oski JA, Canter CE, Spray TL, et al. Embolic stroke after ligation of the pulmonary artery in patients with functional single ventricle. Am Heart J 1996; 132(4):836–840.

70. Gurgey A, Ozyurek E, Gumruk F, et al. Thrombosis in children with cardiac pathology: frequency of factor V Leiden and prothrombin G20210A mutations. Pediatr Cardiol 2003; 24(3):244–248.

71. Fullerton HJ, Johnston SC, Smith WS. Arterial dissection and stroke in children. Neurology 2001; 57(7):1155–1160.

72. Lequin MH, Peeters EA, Holscher HC, et al. Arterial infarction caused by carotid artery dissection in the neonate. Eur J Paediatr Neurol 2004; 8(3):155–160.

73. Natori Y, Ikezaki K, Matsushima T, et al. 'Angiographic moyamoya' its definition, classification, and therapy. Clin Neurol Neurosurg 1997; 99(suppl 2):S168–S172.

74. Peerless SJ. Risk factors of moyamoya disease in Canada and the USA. Clin Neurol Neurosurg 1997; 99(suppl 2):S45–S48.

75. Numaguchi Y, Gonzalez CF, Davis PC, et al. Moyamoya disease in the United States. Clin Neurol Neurosurg 1997; 99(suppl 2):S26–S30.

76. Lindsberg PJ, Grau AJ. Inflammation and infections as risk factors for ischemic stroke. Stroke 2003; 34(10):2518–2532.

77. Gerber O, Roque C, Coyle PK. Vasculitis owing to infection. Neurol Clin 1997; 15(4):903–925.

78. Linnemann CC Jr., Alvira MM. Pathogenesis of varicella-zoster angiitis in the CNS. Arch Neurol 1980; 37(4):239–240.

79. Chabrier S, Rodesch G, Lasjaunias P, et al. Transient cerebral arteriopathy: a disorder recognized by serial angiograms in children with stroke. J Child Neurol 1998; 13(1):27–32.

80. Sebire G, Meyer L, Chabrier S. Varicella as a risk factor for cerebral infarction in childhood: a case-control study. Ann Neurol 1999; 45(5):679–680.

81. Nestoridi E, Buonanno FS, Jones RM, et al. Arterial ischemic stroke in childhood: the role of plasma-phase risk factors. Curr Opin Neurol 2002; 15(2):139–144.

82. Akar N, Akar E, Ozel D, et al. Common mutations at the homocysteine metabolism pathway and pediatric stroke. Thromb Res 2001; 102(2):115–120.

83. Kenet G, Sadetzki S, Murad H, et al. Factor V Leiden and antiphospholipid antibodies are significant risk factors for ischemic stroke in children. Stroke 2000; 31(6):1283–1288.

84. Nowak-Gottl U, Strater R, Heinecke A, et al. Lipoprotein (a) and genetic polymorphisms of clotting factor V, prothrombin, and methylenetetrahydrofolate reductase are risk factors of spontaneous ischemic stroke in childhood. Blood 1999; 94(11):3678–3682.

85. Cardo E, Monros E, Colome C, et al. Children with stroke: polymorphism of the MTHFR gene, mild hyperhomocysteinemia, and vitamin status. J Child Neurol 2000; 15(5):295–298.

86. Bonduel M, Sciuccati G, Hepner M, et al. Prethrombotic disorders in children with arterial ischemic stroke and sinovenous thrombosis. Arch Neurol 1999; 56(8):967–971.

87. deVeber G, Monagle P, Chan A, et al. Prothrombotic disorders in infants and children with cerebral thromboembolism. Arch Neurol 1998; 55(12):1539–1543.

88. Ohene-Frempong K, Weiner SJ, Sleeper LA, et al. Cerebrovascular accidents in sickle cell disease: rates and risk factors. Blood 1998; 91(1):288–294.

89. Balkaran B, Char G, Morris JS, et al. Stroke in a cohort of patients with homozygous sickle cell disease. J Pediatr 1992; 120(3):360–366.

90. Powars E, Wilson B, Imbus C, Pegelow C, Allen J. The natural history of stroke in sickle cell disease. Am J Med 1978; 65:461–471.

91. Rothman SM, Fulling KH, Nelson JS. Sickle cell anemia and central nervous system infarction: a neuropathological study. Ann Neurol 1986; 20(6):684–690.

92. Koshy M, Thomas C, Goodwin J. Vascular lesions in the central nervous system in sickle cell disease (neuropathology). J Assoc Acad Minor Phys 1990; 1(3):71–78.

93. Miller ST, Sleeper LA, Pegelow CH, et al. Prediction of adverse outcomes in children with sickle cell disease. N Engl J Med 2000; 342(2):83–89.

94. Vichinsky EP, Neumayr LD, Earles AN, et al. Causes and outcomes of the acute chest syndrome in sickle cell disease. National Acute Chest Syndrome Study Group. N Engl J Med 2000; 342(25):1855–1865.

95. Wierenga KJ, Serjeant BE, Serjeant GR. Cerebrovascular complications and parvovirus infection in homozygous sickle cell disease. J Pediatr 2001; 139(3):438–442.

96. Pegelow CH, Colangelo L, Steinberg M, et al. Natural history of blood pressure in sickle cell disease: risks for stroke and death associated with relative hypertension in sickle cell anemia. Am J Med 1997; 102(2):171–177.

97. Moser FG, Miller ST, Bello JA, et al. The spectrum of brain MR abnormalities in sickle-cell disease: a report from the Cooperative Study of Sickle Cell Disease. Am J Neuroradiol 1996; 17(5):965–972.

98. Miller ST, Macklin EA, Pegelow CH, et al. Silent infarction as a risk factor for overt stroke in children with sickle cell anemia: a report from the Cooperative Study of Sickle Cell Disease. J Pediatr 2001; 139(3):385–390.

99. Wu YW, March WM, Croen A, et al. Perinatal stroke in children with motor impairment: a population-based study. Pediatrics 2004; 114(3):612–619.

100. Strater R, Becker S, von Eckardstein A, et al. Prospective assessment of risk factors for recurrent stroke during childhood--a 5-year follow-up study. Lancet 2002.; 360(9345):1540–1545.

101. Kirkham J, Prengler M, Hewes K, et al. Risk factors for arterial ischemic stroke in children. J Child Neurol 2000; 15(5):299–307.

102. Tissue plasminogen activator for acute ischemic stroke. The National Institute of Neurological Disorders and Stroke rt-PA Stroke Study Group. N Engl J Med 1995; 333(24):1581–1587.

103. Zaremba J. Hyperthermia in ischemic stroke. Med Sci Monit 2004; 10(6):RA148–RA153.

104. Kurnik K, Kosch A, Strater R, et al. Recurrent thromboembolism in infants and children suffering from symptomatic neonatal arterial stroke: a prospective follow-up study. Stroke 2003; 34(12): 2887–2892.

105. Lanthier S, Carmant L, David M, et al. Stroke in children: the coexistence of multiple risk factors predicts poor outcome. Neurology 2000; 54(2):371–378.

106. Brankovic-Sreckovic V, Milic-Rasic V, Jovic N, et al. The recurrence risk of ischemic stroke in childhood. Med Princ Pract 2004; 13(3):153–158.

107. Strater R, Kurnik K, Heller C, et al. Aspirin versus low-dose low-molecular-weight heparin: antithrombotic therapy in pediatric ischemic stroke patients: a prospective follow-up study. Stroke 2001; 32(11):2554–2558.

108. Monagle P, Chan A, Massicotte P, et al. Antithrombotic therapy in children: the Seventh ACCP Conference on Antithrombotic and Thrombolytic Therapy. Chest 2004; 126(suppl 3):645S–687S.

41 | Functional Recovery After Stroke with Cell-Based Therapy

Michael Chopp, PhD, Professor and Director
*Department of Neurology, Henry Ford Health System, Wayne State University,
Detroit, and Department of Physics, Oakland University,
Rochester, Michigan, USA*

Yi Li, MD, Senior Staff
*Department of Neurology, Henry Ford Health System, Wayne State University,
Detroit, Michigan, USA*

CELL-BASED THERAPY: NEW STRATEGIES FOR STROKE

Each year, hundreds of thousands of people suffer strokes and must cope with the severe neurologic consequences. Unfortunately, current therapies for stroke do little to reduce the injury, thus compelling the development of new neurorestorative therapeutic approaches to enhance neurologic function. The use of cell-based therapies that promote neurologic recovery from stroke take multiple forms. One approach is the use of stem cells to replace dead or compromised brain tissue. A stem cell is a cell from the embryo, fetus, or adult that has the ability to reproduce itself for long periods and may differentiate into all other cell types. Traditionally, the use of stem cells to treat neurologic disease has involved the replacement of neurologic tissue by differentiation of stem cells for parenchymal cells. However, another approach that does not necessarily require the replacement of injured brain rests on the potential for administered cells to activate the endogenous neurorestorative mechanisms within the injured brain. The cells that are employed in this therapy are not necessarily stem cells; rather, they are progenitor and differentiated cells that can catalyze responses in injured brain, which leads to recovery or enhanced neurologic function after stroke and neural injury.

NEUROGENESIS AFTER STROKE

Although it was learned from studies performed on macaque monkeys in the mid-1960s that neurons can be formed within the adult brain (1,2), the dogma until recently has been that brain tissue could not be regenerated in the adult. It is now known that neural stem cells (NSCs) and neural progenitor cells (NPCs) are present in at least two regions in normal adult mammalian brain: the subventricular zone (SVZ) and the subgranular zone (SGZ) in hippocampal dentate gyrus. These cells might promote recovery of neural functions that were lost due to stroke. The proliferation and recruitment of endogenous NSCs and NPCs present after stroke give rise to many, if not all, types of cells found in the adult brain (3–6). The proliferation, migration, and maturation of these cells can be controlled by growth and trophic factors and other signaling molecules, and are affected by ischemia (7,8). Induction of these new neurons, if functional, may provide a novel therapeutic strategy for the treatment of stroke (9).

Stroke is characterized by extensive tissue injury in the territory of an affected vessel. The acute stage after onset of stroke is a metabolically, biochemically, and molecularly active time during which a variety of mutagens, trophic factors, adhesion molecules, and intracellular and extracellular matrix molecules, are uniquely elaborated in the stroke brain, particularly in the ischemic boundary zone (the penumbra of infarct) (10–15). This alteration of the ischemic boundary zones occurs at a time at which enhanced neurogenesis in the SVZ and the SGZ can be observed. These two remodeling events may act synergistically to promote repair of brain and recovery of neurologic function. The adult brain, with its endogenous pool of parenchymal cells, has the ability to repair itself; however, the supply of cells is limited, and the survival of the newly formed cells is tenuous within the hostile ischemic environment. Thus, neurogenesis is insufficient to fully restore neurologic function after stroke.

SOURCES OF CELLS FOR TREATMENT OF STROKE

Animal experiments have shown that cell-based therapy improves outcome after stroke. At present, it is not possible to predict which types of cells will be most beneficial for various experimental therapeutic situations, with the treatment paradigm depending on strain of animals, focal or global stroke, transient or permanent ischemia, cell origin, cell preparation and purification, dose of cells, route of administration, therapeutic window, and short-term or long-term sacrifice.

Neural Stem Cells and Progenitor Cells

The biologic potential of NSCs endows them with the ability to integrate into the neural circuitry after transplantation. The replacement of cells may be specific not only to anatomically circumscribed regions of the brain but also to large areas of the injured central nervous system (16). Primary cultured neurosphere-forming cells (NSCs and NPCs), derived from the SVZ in adult rats, have been employed for the treatment of stroke (17). These cells, also labeled by ferromagnetic particles, were intracisternally transplanted into rats that had been subjected to middle cerebral artery occlusion (MCAO), the major cause of stroke (18). Rats transplanted with SVZ cells exhibited significant improvement of neurologic function. Migration of transplanted cells was noninvasively tracked using magnetic resonance imaging (MRI). Transplanted cells selectively migrated within the central nervous system toward the ischemic parenchyma at a mean speed of $65 \pm 14.6 \mu m/hr$. Migration, proliferation, and differentiation of transplanted cells in the brain were also measured histopathologically. Primary cultured human fetal NSCs and NPCs xenografted into the lesioned areas in the brains of Mongolian gerbils after focal ischemia also significantly improved neurologic function. These cells migrate to the infarction, differentiate into mature neurons, and form synapses with host neuronal circuits (19). Thus, these primary cultured neurosphere cells are a potential source for transplantable material for the treatment of stroke and MRI can be used to track grafted cells in the brain.

In rodents, other cell lines that are derived from NSCs and NPCs target and integrate into the central nervous system and migrate to areas of subsequent infarction. For example, murine neonatal neural C17.2 cells, stably transfected with firefly luciferase, were serially imaged through intact skull and skin by bioluminescence imaging in MCAO mice after contralateral intraparenchymal or intraventricular injections (20). The cells migrated to the site of infarct from the contralateral parenchyma, crossing the midline. In control animals without infarcts, C17.2 cells remained at the site of administration. Intraventricular cell administration resulted in a wide distribution of cells, including the site of infarct. Within the infarct area, C17.2 cells colabeled with a neural marker. Images correlated well with histologic cell distributions (20). The conditionally immortal Maudsley hippocampal clone 36 (MHP36) NSCs, originally derived from the H-2Kb-tsA58 transgenic mouse, were effective in reversing sensory and motor deficits and in reducing lesion volume as a consequence of MCAO (21). Grafts of the MHP36 cells also repaired cognitive function, reduced lesion volume, and differentiated into site-appropriate phenotypes after global and focal ischemia in rats (22,23). MHP36 cells may improve functional outcome after MCAO by assisting spontaneous reorganization in both the damaged and intact hemispheres (24). ReNeuron (Surrey, UK) is currently developing, from different brain regions, human neuroepithelial stem cell lines with similar reparative properties to murine lines (21).

Marrow Stromal Cells, Peripheral Blood Stromal Cells, and Umbilical Stem Cells

Bone marrow stromal cells (BMSCs) are currently considered strong candidates for cell-based therapy in stroke (25). BMSCs are a mixed-cell population, including stem and progenitor cells, that can differentiate into mesenchymal cells, as well as cells with visceral mesoderm, neuroectoderm, and endoderm characteristics (26). Although infrequent, these cells may differentiate into neural cells and endothelium in the brain. From experimental stroke in rodent, BMSCs derived from donor rats (6,27–30), mice (31,32), or humans (33,34) were transplanted into brain intracerebrally (28,31), intraarterially (29), intracisternally (32), or intravenously (27,30,33,34). BMSCs selectively target injured tissue and promote functional recovery. Signals that target inflammatory cells to injured tissue likely direct BMSCs to injury sites (35). Using a microchemotaxis chamber, we measured the effect of select chemotactic factors and cytokines expressed in injured brain, monocyte chemoattractant protein-1, macrophage inflammatoryprotein-1α, and interleukin-8, on migration of BMSCs. Ischemic brain tissue extracts significantly increased BMSC migration across the membrane, compared to nonischemic tissue (35). Recovery from neurologic deficits has not correlated with structural repair or reduction of the lesion in stroke models. Although some BMSCs express proteins phenotypic of neural cells, it is highly unlikely that therapeutic benefit is derived by replacement of infarct tissue with transdifferentiated BMSCs. Secretory functions of BMSC, such as the elaboration of growth and trophic factors, as well as the induction of trophic factors within parenchymal cells, have been hypothesized to play a role in the enhanced recovery of neurologic function. BMSCs activate endogenous restorative responses in injured brain, which include neurogenesis and synaptogenesis (27,33,36–38), angiogenesis, and vasculogenesis (32). Recent studies demonstrate that BMSCs stimulate glia and thereby promote appropriate neurite outgrowth and extension of axons to the injured hemisphere (6). Thus, constitutive reparative response is facilitated by a series of interactions between BMSCs and host cells, reducing scar tissue, fostering the reformation of brain tissue, and facilitating synaptic and vascular reconstitution. The advantages of using BMSCs are that they can be given as an autologous graft, avoiding risks of rejection and graft-versus-host reactions, and that they can be given intravenously, minimizing complications.

Increasing evidence supports the retention of toti/multi potent cells in the peripheral blood stromal cells and umbilical stem cells. Granulocyte colony stimulating factor–mobilized peripheral blood stromal cells in the circulating blood might be an alternative to bone marrow as a source of autologous stem cells. Peripheral blood stromal cells (39) and other stem cells, such as the umbilical stem cells, have been employed in rodent models of stroke (40). In these studies, groups of transplanted rodents showed a significant improvement in neurologic function, compared with nontransplanted stroked animals. These findings raise the possibility that marrow stromal cells (MSCs) from peripheral blood and umbilici could provide an effective transplantation therapy to treat stroke.

MODIFICATION OF CELLS IN STROKE RESEARCH

To realize the promise of novel cell-based therapies for stroke, researchers have manipulated therapeutic cells to create composite biologics, to coadminister agents that increase survival and therapeutic efficacy of the transplanted cells, and to insert genes into transplanted cells to promote the expression of factors that enhance functional recovery.

Composite Cell Materials

Cocultured, prelabeled fetal rat NSCs and adult rat BMSCs, designated as neural and marrow stromal cell (NMC) spheres, were transplanted into the penumbra of the striatum and cortex in rat after MCAO (41). *In vitro* within the NMC spheres, BMSCs rapidly formed a network of processes with intact neural cells. This system expanded without the presence of necrosis. In contrast, a neurosphere alone without the presence of BMSCs developed a necrotic core. Neurologic functional recovery after stroke and traumatic brain injury (42) was enhanced in rats treated with NMC spheres, compared to rats with neurospheres or BMSC treatments. The NMC spheres altered the trajectory and complexity of host neurites. When NSCs from the SVZ of postnatal mice were cultured on human adipose tissue stromal cells, neuronal or glial differentiation was significantly induced under different experimental conditions, as compared to NSCs cultured on regular dishes (43). These data indicate that MSCs might support the action of NSCs when they are transplanted into damaged brain.

Cells Combined with Adjunctive Factors

Cells combined with adjunctive factor therapy might provide an additive therapeutic benefit after stroke. A graft of bone marrow cells, along with brain-derived neurotrophic factor (BDNF), transplanted into the ischemic boundary zone of rat brain helps these cells to survive and differentiate after MCAO (44). Coadministration of bone marrow cells with a cell-permeable inhibitor of caspases, Z-Val-Ala-DL-Asp-fluoromethylketone, into the ischemic boundary zone of rat brain reduces exogenous cell apoptosis and improves outcome (45). A nitric oxide donor,

(Z)-1-[*N*-(2-aminoethyl)-*N*-(2-ammonioethyl)aminio] diazen-1-ium-1,2-diolate (DETA / NONOate), induces the production of progenitor cells and neurogenesis in the adult brain (46). In addition, nitric oxide donors foster angiogenesis, thereby creating a microenvironment within the ischemic brain that is conducive to the survival and migration of injected cells, such as BMSCs. Thus, treatment of stroke with a nitric oxide donor and a cell-based therapy may provide an additive or a superadditive therapeutic response. This hypothesis was tested and confirmed in a study in which DETA/NONOate was employed in conjunction with BMSCs to treat stroke in the rodent (34). Combination therapy of stroke in rats with a subtherapeutic dose of human BMSCs and DETA/NONOate significantly enhanced angiogenesis, neurogenesis, and neurologic functional recovery after stroke in rat, compared to the individual treatments.

Genetically Modified Cells

NSCs and NPCs are well suited as target populations for genetic (neurotrophic factors) and cellular therapy. A subclone of NSCs was transduced with a retrovirus encoding rat neurotrophin-3 (NT-3) (47). The engineered NSCs successfully produced large amounts of NT-3 *in vitro* and *in vivo*. When cells from the NT-3–expressing NSC subclone were implanted into the infarct of hypoxic–ischemic brain, the percentage of donor-derived neurons was dramatically increased. Many of the neurons were calbindin positive; some were also gamma aminobutyric acid (GABA) ergic, glutamatergic, or cholinergic (48). *Ex vivo*-engineered NSCs with NT-3 also appear to differentiate into functional neurons.

Similarly, telomerized human BMSCs transfected with the BDNF gene with a fiber-mutant adenovirus vector improved recovery in rats after MCAO (49). Neurotrophic factors in addition to BDNF, e.g., glial cell–derived neurotrophic factor (GDNF), had a similar effect in this model. Rats that received BMSC–GDNF showed significantly more functional recovery than did control rats following MCAO, as demonstrated by improved behavioral test results and reduced ischemic damage on MRI. Thus, BMSC transfected with the BDNF or GDNF gene improve functional outcome and reduce ischemic damage in a rat model of MCAO. These data suggest that gene-modified cell therapy may be a useful approach for the treatment of stroke.

Biomaterial-Manipulated Cells

Cell-based therapy may have the capacity to repopulate stroke-injured brain; however, its ability to restore structural and functional neural connections might be limited by the vast amount of brain parenchymal loss. The core of the infarct changes rapidly to a cystic cavity, and even the most capable cells might need intrinsic organization and a template to guide restructuring. To address this need, a pilot experiment was performed (50), in which a NSC–polymer complex was implanted into the infarct region of the focal ischemic area in mice. The NSC–polymer complex filled the cavity with an intricate meshwork of many highly arborized neurites of both host- and donor-derived neurons, and some anatomical connections appeared to be reconstituted, with evidence of neovascularization (50). Polyglycolic acid (PGA) is a synthetic biodegradable polymer used widely in clinical medicine (51). Highly hydrophilic, PGA loses its mechanical strength rapidly over 2 to 4 weeks *in vivo*. NSCs seeded onto the three-dimensional, highly porous PGA scaffolded and cotransplanted into the infarction cavity in mouse brains injured by ischemia-facilitated reformation of structural and functional circuits, particularly, if the cells had been engineered *ex vivo* to express factors that might attract in-growth of host fibers. New bioscaffolds might provide a matrix to guide cellular organization and growth, allow diffusion of nutrients between the transplanted cells and brain cells, become vascularized, and then disappear, obviating concerns about long-term biocompatibility.

CELL THERAPY FROM THE LABORATORY TO THE STROKE PATIENT

Transplantation of cultured NSCs and NPCs is safe and improves behavioral recovery in rodents with stroke. Recent studies demonstrated that neuronal transplantation is feasible in patients with stroke (52). The safety and feasibility were demonstrated with human neuronal cellular transplantation (cell lines derived from human embryonic carcinomas) in patients with basal ganglia stroke and fixed motor deficits, including 12 patients (aged 44–75 years) with prior infarct in the previous 6 months to 6 years (stable for at least 2 months). Serial evaluations (12–18 months) showed no adverse cell-related serologic or imaging-defined effects. The total European Stroke Scale score improved in 6 patients (3–10 points), with a mean improvement of 2.9 points in all patients ($p = 0.046$). Six of 11 PET scans at 6 months showed improved fluorodeoxyglucose uptake at the implant site.

The feasibility and safety of human BMSCs have been tested and confirmed in patients with degenerative arthritis for resurfacing of joint surfaces by direct injection into the joints (53). In breast-cancer patients infused intravenously with culture-expanded autologous BMSCs (54), and in patients with lysosomal and peroxisomal storage diseases treated with allogeneic BMSCs (55), no apparent adverse effects were evident. BMSC systemic injection has also been employed to treat patients with severe osteogenesis imperfecta to correct genetic defects (56). The robust therapeutic benefit of BMSCs in the treatment of experimental neural stroke and the apparent safe and broad application of BMSC therapy to the treatment of diseases provide a compelling reason to investigate the potential of MSC treatment of stroke. Moreover, the use of patients' own MSCs should circumvent any potential problems of host immunity and graft-versus-host disease. The easily accessible vascular route, as opposed to direct implantation into brain tissue, allows for multiple and long-term cell administration.

CHALLENGES IN CELL-BASED THERAPY FOR STROKE: DETERMINING THE MECHANISM OF CELL THERAPY

Cell-based research is making possible new and exciting treatment opportunities. Cell-based therapies can be employed in many ways in research and clinical stroke and can enhance neurologic recovery from stroke in several ways. However, the many technical hurdles that exist between the promise of cell-based therapies, and its clinical realization will only be overcome by continued intensive studies. Elucidating the mechanisms underlying benefit to stroke from cell-based therapies would increase the potential of these therapies.

Differentiation of Transplanted Cells into Brain Tissue
Some studies showed synaptic contacts between donor cells and host neurons (57). Incorporated cells expressed transmitter receptors and received input via host axonal projections (58). Patch-camp methodology demonstrated that NSCs transplanted into the hippocampus generated action potentials and received excitatory and inhibitory synaptic inputs from the surrounding cells (59).

Cell Fusion Phenomenon
Recent reports of cell fusion have raised some doubts about the existence of somatic stem cell plasticity (60). Cell fusion has been known to produce viable cells and has a major role in mammalian development and differentiation. *In vitro*, adult BMSCs from mice fuse with embryonic NSCs, resulting in two sets of chromosomes and mixed marker sets (61). Immunochemical, morphologic, and physiologic criteria for determining neuronal transdifferentiation are critical for the development of an effective cell therapy for stroke.

Secretion of Growth Factors and Trophic Factors from Transplanted Cells
Cells transplanted within cerebral tissue or within the microvasculature of injured brain, such as MSCs, behave as small molecular "factories" and produce an array of growth and trophic factors (25), and the effects of these trophic factors on brain tissue rapidly and effectively promote restoration of function. The trophic and growth factors produced by MSCs include BDNF, hepatocyte growth factor, vascular endothelial cell growth factor (VEGF), and nerve growth factor (NGF) (62). Likely, it is the effect of a variety of factors, and not that of a particular growth factor, that facilitates the restorative function.

Promotion of Endogenous Brain Tissue by Exogenously Transplanted Cells
Injection of MSCs into ischemic brain has been shown to activate primarily within the endogenous astrocyte expression of an array of neurotrophic factors, including VEGF (63). Another way in which the injected cells may evoke the production of factors that contribute to the induction of cerebral plasticity is by the induction of new blood vessels, the process of angiogenesis. Angiogenic vessels themselves produce an array of factors, including BDNF (64). Thus, the injected cells activate the endogenous cells to produce neurotrophic and angiogenic factors and induce the production of new blood vessels, which themselves generate an array of factors that enhance functional recovery.

Researchers seek to fully develop cell-based therapies in experimental animal models of stroke to prepare the groundwork for cell administration to the stroke patient. Administration of therapeutic cells may potentially provide a powerful therapy for a broad array of human neurologic disorders in addition to stroke.

ACKNOWLEDGMENTS

This work was supported by NINDS grants PO1 NS23393 and RO1 NS45041.

REFERENCES

1. Rakic P. Neuron-glia relationship during granule cell migration in developing cerebellar cortex. A Golgi and electronmicroscopic study in Macacus Rhesus. J Comp Neurol 1971; 141(3): 283–312.
2. Rakic P. Neurons in rhesus monkey visual cortex: systematic relation between time of origin and eventual disposition. Science 1974; 183(123):425–427.
3. Zhang R, Zhang Z, Wang L, et al. Activated neural stem cells contribute to stroke-induced neurogenesis and neuroblast migration toward the infarct boundary in adult rats. J Cereb Blood Flow Metab 2004; 24(4):441–448.
4. Takagi Y, Nozaki K, Takahashi J, Yodoi J, Ishikawa M, Hashimoto N. Proliferation of neuronal precursor cells in the dentate gyrus is accelerated after transient forebrain ischemia in mice. Brain Res 1999; 831(1–2):283–287.
5. Zhang R, Zhang Z, Zhang C, et al. Stroke transiently increases subventricular zone cell division from asymmetric to symmetric and increases neuronal differentiation in the adult rat. J Neurosci 2004; 24(25):5810–5815.
6. Li Y , Chen J, Zhang CL, Wang L, et al. Gliosis and brain remodeling after treatment of stroke in rats with marrow stromal cells. Glia 2005; 49(3):407–417.
7. Romanko MJ, Rola R, Fike JR, et al. Roles of the mammalian subventricular zone in cell replacement after brain injury. Prog Neurobiol 2004; 74(2):77–99.
8. Felling RJ, Levison SW. Enhanced neurogenesis following stroke. J Neurosci Res 2003; 73(3):277–283.
9. Arvidsson A, Collin T, Kirik D, Kokaia Z, Lindvall O. Neuronal replacement from endogenous precursors in the adult brain after stroke. Nat Med 2002; 8(9):963–970.
10. Li Y, Chopp M, Garcia JH, Yoshida Y, Zhang ZG, Levine SR. Distribution of the 72-kd heat-shock protein as a function of transient focal cerebral ischemia in rats. Stroke 1992; 23(9):1292–1298.
11. Li Y, Chopp M, Zhang ZG, Zaloga C, Niewenhuis L, Gautam S. p53-immunoreactive protein and p53 mRNA expression after transient middle cerebral artery occlusion in rats. Stroke 1994; 25(4):849–855; discussion 855–856.
12. Li Y, Chopp M, Powers C, Jiang N. Immunoreactivity of cyclin D1/cdk4 in neurons and oligodendrocytes after focal cerebral ischemia in rat. J Cereb Blood Flow Metab 1997; 17(8):846–856.
13. Li Y, Jiang N, Powers C, Chopp M. Neuronal damage and plasticity identified by microtubule-associated protein 2, growth-associated protein 43, and cyclin D1 immunoreactivity after focal cerebral ischemia in rats. Stroke 1998; 29(9):1972–1980; discussion 1980–1981.
14. Zhang RL, Chopp M, Li Y, et al. Anti-ICAM-1 antibody reduces ischemic cell damage after transient middle cerebral artery occlusion in the rat. Neurology 1994; 44(9):1747–1751.
15. Zhang ZG, Chopp M, Bailey F, Malinski T. Nitric oxide changes in the rat brain after transient middle cerebral artery occlusion. J Neurol Sci 1995; 128(1):22–27.
16. Snyder EY, Macklis JD. Multipotent neural progenitor or stem-like cells may be uniquely suited for therapy for some neurodegenerative conditions. Clin Neurosci 1995; 3(5):310–316.
17. Zhang RL, Zhang L, Zhang ZG, et al. Migration and differentiation of adult rat subventricular zone progenitor cells transplanted into the adult rat striatum. Neuroscience 2003; 116(2):373–382.
18. Zhang ZG, Jiang Q, Zhang R, et al. Magnetic resonance imaging and neurosphere therapy of stroke in rat. Ann Neurol 2003; 53(2):259–263.
19. Ishibashi S, Sakaguchi M, Kuroiwa T, et al. Human neural stem/progenitor cells, expanded in long-term neurosphere culture, promote functional recovery after focal ischemia in Mongolian gerbils. J Neurosci Res 2004; 78(2):215–223.
20. Kim DE, Schellingerhout D, Ishii K, Shah K, Weissleder R. Imaging of stem cell recruitment to ischemic infarcts in a murine model. Stroke 2004; 35(4):952–957.
21. Sinden JD, Stroemer P, Grigoryan G, Patel S, French SJ, Hodges H. Functional repair with neural stem cells. Novartis Found Symp 2000; 231:270–283; discussion 283–288, 302–306.
22. Modo M, Stroemer RP, Tang E, Patel S, Hodges H. Effects of implantation site of stem cell grafts on behavioral recovery from stroke damage. Stroke 2002; 33(9):2270–2278.
23. Modo M, Stroemer RP, Tang E, Patel S, Hodges H. Effects of implantation site of dead stem cells in rats with stroke damage. Neuroreport 2003; 14(1):39–42.

24. Veizovic T, Beech JS, Stroemer RP, Watson WP, Hodges H. Resolution of stroke deficits following contralateral grafts of conditionally immortal neuroepithelial stem cells. Stroke 2001; 32(4):1012–1019.

25. Chopp M, Li Y. Treatment of neural injury with marrow stromal cells. Lancet Neurol 2002; 1(2):92–100.

26. Prockop DJ. Marrow stromal cells as stem cells for nonhematopoietic tissues. Science 1997; 276(5309):71–74.

27. Chen J, Li Y, Wang L, Zhang Z, et al. Therapeutic benefit of intravenous administration of bone marrow stromal cells after cerebral ischemia in rats. Stroke 2001; 32(4):1005–1011.

28. Chen J, Li Y, Wang L, Lu M, Zhang X, Chopp M. Therapeutic benefit of intracerebral transplantation of bone marrow stromal cells after cerebral ischemia in rats. J Neurol Sci 2001; 189(1–2):49–57.

29. Li Y, Chen J, Wang L, Lu M, Chopp M. Treatment of stroke in rat with intracarotid administration of marrow stromal cells. Neurology 2001; 56(12):1666–1672.

30. Chen J, Li Y, Katakowski M, Chen X, et al. Intravenous bone marrow stromal cell therapy reduces apoptosis and promotes endogenous cell proliferation after stroke in female rat. J Neurosci Res 2003; 73(6):778–786.

31. Li Y, Chopp M, Chen J, Wang L, et al. Intrastriatal transplantation of bone marrow nonhematopoietic cells improves functional recovery after stroke in adult mice. J Cereb Blood Flow Metab 2000; 20(9):1311–1319.

32. Zhang ZG, Zhang L, Jiang Q, Chopp M. Bone marrow-derived endothelial progenitor cells participate in cerebral neovascularization after focal cerebral ischemia in the adult mouse. Circ Res 2002; 90(3):284–288.

33. Li Y, Chen J, Chen XG, Wang L, et al. Human marrow stromal cell therapy for stroke in rat: neurotrophins and functional recovery. Neurology 2002; 59(4):514–523.

34. Chen J, Li Y, Zhang R, Katakowski M, et al. Combination therapy of stroke in rats with a nitric oxide donor and human bone marrow stromal cells enhances angiogenesis and neurogenesis. Brain Res 2004; 1005(1–2):21–28.

35. Wang L, Li Y, Chen X, Chen J, et al. MCP-1, MIP-1, IL-8 and ischemic cerebral tissue enhance human bone marrow stromal cell migration in interface culture. Hematology 2002; 7(2):113–117.

36. Hess DC, Hill WD, Martin-Studdard A, Carroll J, Brailer J, Carothers J. Bone marrow as a source of endothelial cells and NeuN-expressing cells after stroke. Stroke 2002; 33(5):1362–1368.

37. Beck H, Voswinckel R, Wagner S, et al. Participation of bone marrow-derived cells in long-term repair processes after experimental stroke. J Cereb Blood Flow Metab 2003; 23(6):709–717.

38. Zhao LR, Duan WM, Reyes M, Keene CD, Verfaillie CM, Low WC. Human bone marrow stem cells exhibit neural phenotypes and ameliorate neurological deficits after grafting into the ischemic brain of rats. Exp Neurol 2002; 174(1):11–20.

39. Willing AE, Lixian J, Milliken M, et al. Intravenous versus intrastriatal cord blood administration in a rodent model of stroke. J Neurosci Res 2003; 73(3):296–307.

40. Chen J, Sanberg PR, Li Y, Wang L, et al. Intravenous administration of human umbilical cord blood reduces behavioral deficits after stroke in rats. Stroke 2001; 32(11):2682–2688.

41. Li Y, Yang XY, Chen J, et al. Transplantation of a new composite of fetal neural tissue and adult bone marrow stromal cells into the rat brain after stroke. Neuro Res Commun 2002; 30(3):155–163.

42. Lu D, Li Y, Mahmood A, Wang L, Rafiq T, Chopp M. Neural and marrow-derived stromal cell sphere transplantation in a rat model of traumatic brain injury. J Neurosurg 2002; 97(4):935–940.

43. Kang SK, Jun ES, Bae YC, Jung JS. Interactions between human adipose stromal cells and mouse neural stem cells in vitro. Brain Res Dev Brain Res 2003; 145(1):141–149.

44. Chen J, Li Y, Chopp M. Intracerebral transplantation of bone marrow with BDNF after MCAo in rat. Neuropharmacology 2000; 39(5):711–716.

45. Chen J, Li Y, Wang L, Lu M, Chopp M. Caspase inhibition by Z-VAD increases the survival of grafted bone marrow cells and improves functional outcome after MCAo in rats. J Neurol Sci 2002; 199(1–2):17–24.

46. Zhang R, Zhang L, Zhang Z, et al. A nitric oxide donor induces neurogenesis and reduces functional deficits after stroke in rats. Ann Neurol 2001; 50(5):602–611.

47. Liu Y, Himes BT, Solowska J, et al. Intraspinal delivery of neurotrophin-3 using neural stem cells genetically modified by recombinant retrovirus. Exp Neurol 1999; 158(1):9–26.

48. Park KI, Snyder EY. New Concepts in Cerebral Ischemica. Boca Raton: CRC press LLC; 2002.

49. Kurozumi K, Nakamura K, Tamiya T, et al. Mesenchymal stem cells that produce neurotrophic factors reduce ischemic damage in the rat middle cerebral artery occlusion model. Mol Ther 2005; 11(1):96–104.

50. Park KI, Teng YD, Snyder EY. The injured brain interacts reciprocally with neural stem cells supported by scaffolds to reconstitute lost tissue. Nat Biotechnol 2002; 20(11):1111–1117.

51. Shalaby SW, Johnson RA. Synthetic Absorbable Polyesters. Carl Hanser; 1994.

52. Kondziolka D, Wechsler L, Goldstein S, et al. Transplantation of cultured human neuronal cells for patients with stroke. Neurology 2000; 55(4):565–569.

53. Caplan AI. Stem cell delivery vehicle. Biomaterials 1990; 11:44–46.

54. Koc ON, Gerson SL, Cooper BW, et al. Rapid hematopoietic recovery after coinfusion of autologous-blood stem cells and culture-expanded marrow mesenchymal stem cells in advanced breast cancer patients receiving high-dose chemotherapy. J Clin Oncol 2000; 18(2):307–316.

55. Koc ON, Peters C, Aubourg P, et al. Bone marrow-derived mesenchymal stem cells remain host-derived despite successful hematopoietic engraftment after allogeneic transplantation in patients with lysosomal and peroxisomal storage diseases. Exp Hematol 1999; 27(11):1675–1681.

56. Horwitz EM, Prockop DJ, Gordon PL, et al. Clinical responses to bone marrow transplantation in children with severe osteogenesis imperfecta. Blood 2001; 97(5):1227–1231.

57. Kim JH, Auerbach JM, Rodriguez-Gomez JA, et al. Dopamine neurons derived from embryonic stem cells function in an animal model of Parkinson's disease. Nature 2002; 418(6893):50–56.

58. Benninger F, Beck H, Wernig M, Tucker KL, Brustle O, Scheffler B. Functional integration of embryonic stem cell-derived neurons in hippocampal slice cultures. J Neurosci 2003; 23(18):7075–7083.

59. Englund U, Bjorklund A, Wictorin K, Lindvall O, Kokaia M. Grafted neural stem cells develop into functional pyramidal neurons and integrate into host cortical circuitry. Proc Natl Acad Sci USA 2002; 99(26):17089–17094.

60. Wurmser AE, Gage FH. Stem cells: cell fusion causes confusion. Nature 2002; 416(6880):485–487.

61. Ying QL, Nichols J, Evans EP, Smith AG. Changing potency by spontaneous fusion. Nature 2002; 416(6880):545–548.

62. Chen X, Li Y, Wang L, et al. Ischemic rat brain extracts induce human marrow stromal cell growth factor production. Neuropathology 2002; 22(4):275–279.

63. Zhang ZG, Tsang W, Zhang L, Powers C, Chopp M. Up-regulation of neuropilin-1 in neovasculature after focal cerebral ischemia in the adult rat. J Cereb Blood Flow Metab 2001; 21(5):541–549.

64. Leventhal C, Rafii S, Rafii D, Shahar A, Goldman SA. Endothelial trophic support of neuronal production and recruitment from the adult mammalian subependyma. Mol Cell Neurosci 1999; 13(6):450–464.

42 | Brain Attack

Chandrasekaran Sivakumar, MD, Fellow
Calgary Stroke Program, Foothills Medical Center, University of Calgary, Calgary, Alberta, Canada

Alastair M. Buchan, MD, Professor
Acute Stroke Programme, John Radcliffe Hospital, University of Oxford, Headington, Oxford, UK

INTRODUCTION

Brain attack can be defined as a sudden onset of focal cerebral symptoms of presumed vascular origin. If symptoms disappear within 24 hr of onset, the event is defined as a transient ischemic attack (TIA). If symptoms persist beyond 24 hr, the event is defined as a stroke. As more and more patients are seen within 6 hr of symptom onset, it is difficult to predict which will ultimately be a TIA and which will be a stroke; hence, the need to triage "brain attack" as a life-threatening emergency for urgent hospital referral, investigation, and treatment.

Organized stroke care is delivered in only a few hospitals and cities. The Brain Attack Coalition has recently proposed the concept of stroke centers of excellence (1). Of the 11 important components of effective stroke care delivery, 7 enhance delivery of thrombolytic therapy: written care protocols, integrated emergency medical services, organized emergency departments, continuing medical/public education in stroke, acute stroke team, stroke unit, and rapid neuroimaging (2). The Paul Coverdell National Acute Stroke Registry and the Stroke Treatment and Ongoing Prevention Act of 2003 further support these concepts.

The general population should be aware of risk factors and major symptoms of stroke, as well as when to call emergency medical services. Therefore, assessment and dissemination of education should be a continuous process in an effort to reduce admission delay and improve stroke outcomes. Emergency medical services are usually first-line providers of stroke care, but some emergency physicians remain skeptical about evidence-based stroke treatment, or lack thereof, with thrombolysis. Perhaps the formation of stroke centers of excellence will help streamline the process.

IMAGING

Computed Tomography

CT remains the most commonly available form of initial investigation. It helps to identify acute intracerebral or subarachnoid hemorrhage and early ischemic changes (EIC) and to exclude stroke mimics and skull fractures. Data from the European Cooperative Acute Stroke Study showed that EIC in greater than one-third of the middle cerebral artery (MCA) territory can prognosticate a group at high risk of hemorrhage with thrombolysis. The Alberta Stroke Program Early CT Score (ASPECTS) scoring system further refined the predictive model and has proven to be reliable and reproducible in an acute setting (3).

As part of multimodal imaging, CT angiography (CTA) can be performed with the initial CT in most patients, unless evidence is noted of renal dysfunction or some other contraindication. CTA helps identify vessel occlusion and collateral circulation. The CTA-source images ASPECTS predicts final diffusion-weighted imaging (DWI) infarct better than noncontrast CT. The Prolyse in Acute Cerebral Thromboembolism (PROACT) study showed that proximal occlusion of the internal carotid artery (ICA) or MCA would benefit more from intra-arterial/intravenous (IA/IV) or mechanical thrombolytic therapy.

Perfusion-CT (CTP) can be used to quantify relative cerebral blood flow (CBF), relative cerebral blood volume, penumbra, and infarct maps. CTA and CTP have been shown to be comparable to DWI/perfusion-weighted imaging (DWI/PWI) studies (4). CT venography is helpful in diagnosing strokes due to venous sinus thrombosis, the diagnosis of which requires a high index of clinical suspicion.

Novel techniques in CT are constantly being developed. MULTISLICE CT scanners decreased scanning times for angiography and perfusion studies. Single-photon emission CT (SPECT) can be used to measure perfusion and cell homeostasis; however, quantification of perfusion remains difficult and its reliability in a clinical setting remains questionable. Xenon CT can be used to determine CBF, but its use is limited due to the anesthetic effects of xenon gas and a small signal-to-noise ratio.

MRI, Angiography, and Venography

MRI is increasingly used as the first or only means of investigation, as acquisition times continue to decrease. MRI provides information about the location, extent, and potential cause of stroke, but uncertainty persists regarding the perfusion thresholds that define the penumbra. DWI/PWI mismatch predicts response to thrombolysis, and DWI core predicts the risk of hemorrhage. It has higher resolution than CTP, allowing for heme imaging; however, its use is limited by availability, patient compliance, and contraindications.

Only 4% to 6% of patients benefit from thrombolysis. A vast majority still arrive after the 3-hr window or wake up with a stroke but without a definite "time of onset." Trials are under way that could help identification of salvageable brain with diffusion–perfusion mismatch. Better understanding of the "ischemic penumbra," "oligemic penumbra," and collateral circulation can help prolong the therapeutic window >3 hr and up to 9 hr. Although the reliability of quantification of the penumbra has been questionable, the DWI/PWI mismatch model is used by a number of ongoing trials, including Echoplanar Imaging Thrombolysis Evaluation Trial (EPITHET), Desmoteplase in Acute Ischemic Stroke, Diffusion-weighted Imaging Evaluation For Understanding Stroke Evolution (DEFUSE), MR and Recanalization of Stroke Clots Using Embolectomy (MR-RESCUE), ReoPro Retavase Reperfusion of Stroke Safety Study—Imaging Evaluation (ROSIE), and Stroke Evaluation for Late Endovascular Cerebral Thrombolysis with MR trial (SELECT-MR) (5).

Early MRI assessment helps in risk stratification of TIA, as DWI lesion positively predicts higher recurrence. T2-weighted gradient-echo MRI (GRE sequence) helps to identify microbleed, which predicts increased risk of hemorrhage with thrombolytics or anticoagulants. The Hyperintense Acute Reperfusion Injury Marker is a novel method of detecting early breakdown of the blood–brain barrier and is thus useful for predicting hemorrhagic risk following thrombolysis (6).

Magnetic resonance angiography is useful in identifying vessel occlusion, collateral circulation, dissection, or aneurysm, as well as in assessing extracranial ICA stenosis. MR venography is used to diagnose cerebral venous sinus thrombosis.

Novel Techniques

Recently, the use of various ionic contrasts has helped to visualize important biomarkers of ischemic stroke. Manganese-enhanced MRI for mapping brain activation *in vivo* is one such example. Gd-DTPA (Diethylenetriaminepentaacetic acid)-sLex has been used to visualize early endothelial activation in carotid artery after TIA, based on noninvasive detection of inflammation caused by P and E-selectin–mediated recruitment of leukocytes in brain microvasculature following reperfusion.

Diffusion tensor imaging, a more comprehensive form of DWI, can track both the directionality and the magnitude of water diffusion and is a helpful indicator of early breakdown of neuronal membranes. Blood oxygenation level–dependent functional MRI (fMRI) is used to study mechanisms of recovery from motor deficits and aphasia.

Parallel imaging techniques have improved, achieving higher acceleration factors, robust coil sensitivity calibration methods, and more valid reconstruction algorithms.

Positron-Emission Tomography

Positron-emission tomography (PET) measures thresholds for penumbra and infarction, quantifying cerebral metabolic rate of oxygen ($CMRO_2$) and CBF. PET using novel radioligands to visualize postischemic neurons, has been tested in living primates, and can be used to evaluate neuronal cell loss in postischemic patients. ^{18}F-labeled fluoromisonidazole PET imaging of brain accurately documents the temporal and spatial progression of the penumbra, whereas ^{11}C-flumazenil PET imaging distinguishes irreversibly damaged brain tissue from penumbral tissue early after acute ischemic stroke (AIS). Multimodality imaging makes use of a combination of imaging methods, such as micro-PET and MR.

Transcranial Doppler

Transcranial Doppler (TCD) helps to localize intracranial stenosis or occlusion and to monitor and guide thrombolysis (Combined Lysis of Thrombus in Brain Ischemia with Transcranial Ultrasound and Systemic TPA; CLOTBUST) (7). TCD is an easy, inexpensive, and noninvasive additional diagnostic option at the bedside, but it is limited by being "operator dependent." Transcranial color sonography, especially with an ultrasound contrast agent, provides better information about intracranial stenosis, occlusion, collaterals, and midline shift in massive hemispheric infarction.

Near-Infrared Spectroscopy

Near-infrared spectroscopy (NIRS) involves optical imaging for real-time assessment of wavelength-specific absorption of photons by oxygenated and deoxygenated tissues. It is an inexpensive means of assessing ischemic brain oxygenation and has potential for multimodality imaging with MR scanners—once its limitations are more comprehensively determined.

Transcranial Magnetic Stimulation

Transcranial magnetic stimulation provides insights into neurophysiology of the motor system, including conduction velocity, motor-evoked potentials, cortical inhibition, and cortical excitability. It is also capable of producing a virtual lesion in nonmotor brain areas and, unlike fMRI and PET scans, is generally used to study a limited portion of the brain.

Brain-mapping methods, such as electroencephalography, magnetoencephalography, NIRS, and optical imaging, have been used less frequently in the study of stroke recovery. These methods generally provide millisecond temporal resolution, with somewhat limited spatial resolution.

Multimodal Imaging

Multimodal imaging involves two or more imaging modalities within the setting of a single examination, by using dual- or triple-labeled optical or nuclear "reporter" agents or by performing ultrasound or optical studies within the CT, MR, or SPECT environment. PET–SPECT, PET–CT scanner hybrids, and NIRS, in combination with MR, are rapidly evolving examples of multimodal imaging. This technique has the ability to provide noninvasive analyses of both endogenous and exogenous gene expression in the "molecular imaging" animal models that will effectively translate new therapy strategies from experimental into clinical applications (8).

THROMBOLYSIS

Recombinant tissue plasminogen activator (rtPA) is thus far the only approved treatment for AIS, but it has been associated with neurotoxic side effects outside a 3-hr postischemic timeframe. This toxicity might be due in part to pleiotropic actions of rtPA, cleavage of the N-methyl D- aspartate receptor 1 (NMDA NR1) subunit, amplification of intracellular calcium conductance, and proteolytic damage that results from activation of proteases from the matrix metalloproteinase (MMP) family (9).

As the toxicity of rtPA is a protease-dependent effect, a novel compound that lacks protease activity, S478A-tPA, has been tried intraventricularly in rats and was found to have a parenchymal neuroprotective effect that could be useful in treatment of ischemic stroke. Tenecteplase as bolus therapy has been safe up to 0.4 mg/kg in a dose-escalation study. A combination of GPIIb/IIIa receptor antagonist [7E3 F(ab')2] and IA TNK-tPA extends the therapeutic window of thrombolysis to 6 hr after stroke in rat models (10). With telemedicine input, bolus tenecteplase could accelerate thrombolysis in the future.

Desmoteplase might be devoid of rtPA neurotoxicity, as it does not cleave the N1 subunit of NMDA receptor and has been tested in a Phase 2 clinical trial (11). The antiplatelet agent abciximab has been tested to be safe in Phase 2 clinical trials, and other trials with GP IIb/IIIa antagonists are under way.

Mechanical thrombolytic strategies have included catheter-delivered tools, such as corkscrews, lasers, ultrasound, and suction. The Concentric Merci® Retrieval System for thrombus removal has recently been approved by the Food and Drug Administration. Other mechanical devices are undergoing further trials. For proximal occlusion (ICA, MCA-M1), combined IA/IV thrombolysis might provide better results than IV alone, but further confirmation is awaited (12). Posterior circulation strokes have been overshadowed in the past, but interventional management is feasible over an extended period. Intracranial angioplasty and stenting is being conducted in select patients at specialist centers (13).

Brain vasculature differs significantly from coronary circulation, as more than 99% of the brain endothelium is microvasculature. Recent interventions have suggested that intrinsic collateral blood flow can be increased by increasing blood volume. The Neuroflow® device, consisting of 2 balloons attached to a catheter, diverts blood flow from the lower extremities to the brain to increase cerebral perfusion, thereby increasing blood pressure by an average of 6%, without adverse effects.

EARLY OUTCOME

In one study, dramatic recovery (DR) was defined as an improvement of 10 NIHSS points or a decrease to an NIHSS score of 3 by the end of rtPA infusion (1 hr). DR occurred in 22% of patients, and TCD monitoring suggested that this level of recovery was due to early restoration of MCA flow during the rtPA infusion (14). DR after recanalization within 2 hr after rtPA bolus was sustained at 3 months in 75% of patients. Complete or partial early recanalization led to better outcome at 3 months after stroke.

Early Neurologic Deterioration

In another study, the deterioration following improvement (DFI) was defined as any 2-point deterioration in NIHSS following an initial 2-point improvement after treatment. DFI was identified in 13% and was associated with higher baseline NIHSS score, diminished cerebral hemodynamic reserve, diabetes, and elevated systolic blood pressure, but prestroke warfarin therapy appeared to be protective. Clinical deterioration (CD) was defined as any 4-point worsening after treatment, as compared with baseline. CD within the first 24 hr occurred in 16% patients and was associated with less frequent use of prestroke aspirin, early CT changes of edema, mass effect or dense MCA sign, increased serum glucose and fibrin degradation products. With TCD monitoring, early reocclusion was documented in 34% of rtPA-treated patients who had initial recanalization, accounting for two-thirds of DFI. Patients who experienced either DFI or CD were less likely to have a 3-month favorable outcome (15).

Fluctuating stroke, stroke-in-evolution, DR, DFI, and recurrence might all be part of the same spectrum. In the past, they were attributed to lacunar stroke, hypoperfusion, or significant carotid stenosis, but MRI, TCD, and angiographic studies have shown that reocclusion, collaterals, hypoperfusion, dissection, and new embolic lesions give rise to similar symptoms.

ICU CARE

Physiologic Monitoring

Monitoring and stabilizing acute physiologic parameters, such as blood pressure, temperature, hydration status, glucose level, and oxygen saturation, has become standard practice for acute stroke units. These strategies potentially reduce neuronal damage in the acute phase and subsequently improve functional outcome and survival (16).

Stroke patients have lower peripheral oxygen saturation compared to matched controls, and positioning patients upright might improve oxygen saturation and reduce intracranial pressure (17). Supplemental oxygen should be administered if oxygen saturation falls <95%, but routine 100% oxygen supplementation for 24 hr after stroke onset offered no survival benefit (18).

Considerable variation in water homeostasis occurs in stroke, from overhydration to underhydration. Initial dehydration is hyperosmolar due to inadequate intake of water leading to rise in hematocrit, fall in blood pressure, worsening ischemia, and stroke recurrence. Routine use of saline infusions in the first 24 hr might improve CBF by limiting dips in systemic arterial blood pressure and preventing dehydration. Hemodilution trials with albumin in humans and docosahexaenoic acid–albumin complex in rat models are showing benefits of neuroprotection (19).

Diabetic and hyperglycemic patients have chronic impairment of CBF, autoregulation, reduced leukocyte and erythrocyte deformability, increased thrombotic states, and endothelial cell activation. Ischemia leads to lactic acidosis and vasogenic edema, which impairs collateral flow and microcirculation. Plasma glucose >8 mmol/L after acute stroke predicts poor prognosis. Hyperglycemia is more common with insular strokes. The Glucose Insulin in Stroke Trial is under way to clarify benefits of insulin glucose infusion in acute stroke (20).

A meta-analysis suggested that fever after stroke was significantly associated with an increase in morbidity and mortality. Mechanisms for hyperthermia-induced brain damage include neurotransmitter release, free radical formation, and impaired recovery of brain metabolism. The Cooling for Acute Ischemic Brain Damage (COOL AID) trial showed feasibility of inducing moderate hypothermia of 33°C in acute stroke care (21).

Approximately 20% of patients have a history of hypertension prior to stroke, and 60% have high blood pressure on presentation. The mechanisms are multifactorial, including pre-existing hypertension, hospitalization stress, increased sympathetic nervous system activation, activation of the renin–angiotensin–aldosterone system, and impaired autoregulation. The Controlling Hypertension and Hypotension Immediately Post-Stroke and Continue or Stop PostStroke Antihypertensives Collaborative trials are under way to assess whether blood pressure manipulation in acute stroke improves outcome (22,23).

Postthrombolysis and high-risk patients, including those with massive hemispheric and cerebellar/brainstem infarcts with edema, should remain in an ICU setting for physiologic monitoring and aggressive management.

Hypothermia has been used to protect the brain against focal ischemia. In animal models of transient occlusion of the MCA, hypothermia decreased the infarct size. Human studies have yielded promising results, albeit in small numbers. Hypothermia reduced mortality in massive cerebral infarction from 80% to 38% by reducing cerebral edema (24).

Participants in the COOL AID study who were subjected to moderate hypothermia showed better neurologic outcomes than those who were subjected to normothermia, but the results did not reach statistical significance (21). Mild postischemic hypothermia has been confirmed to be neuroprotective to hippocampal CA1 neurons in animal models of global ischemia (25), and this finding has recently been successfully translated into clinical trials involving survivors of out-of-hospital cardiac arrests (26). Hypothermia can be complicated by severe infection, arrhythmia, hypokalemia, pneumonia, hypotension, and decreased platelet count, which might counteract its neuroprotective effects. The optimum duration of hypothermia and speed at which to achieve the target temperature is not yet clear.

DECOMPRESSIVE SURGERY

Surgical decompressive therapy in a large hemispheric infarction lowered the mortality rate from 80% to 30% without increasing the rate of severely disabled survivors, as compared with historic control subjects (27). The Hemicraniectomy and Durotomy for Deterioration from Infarction-Related Swelling Trial is ongoing. Large cerebellar infarctions with edema and a declining level of consciousness constitute a neurosurgical emergency.

NEUROPROTECTION

Reperfusion after ischemia is followed by multiple mechanisms that lead to cell death, and the need is crucial for neuroprotective agents to reduce tissue damage. Naturally occurring substances, such as caffeinol, have been purported to both prevent and reverse neuronal and vascular cell injury in animal models of AIS and are currently being evaluated in trials with thrombolysis (28).

TIAs can represent a form of clinical hypoxic preconditioning and are partly associated with increased plasma levels of tumor necrosis factor-α in the presence of reduced concentrations of interleukin-6 (29).

Human albumin has been shown to reduce swelling and infarct volumes in animal models of focal ischemia by 60% to 65%, with a therapeutic window extending to 4 hr. Modulating thrombin and its inhibitors might establish novel therapeutic strategies for ischemia.

Erythropoietin (EPO) is thought to rescue neurons from nitric oxide–induced death. A recent development has been the engineering of hematopoietic growth factor EPO to have neuroprotective, but not hematopoietic, activity, implying that it might soon be possible to treat AIS patients with short-term, high-dose recombinant human EPO (30).

Estrogen has been implicated as a neuroprotectant, but despite promising laboratory results, data from randomized clinical trials, including the Women's Estrogen for Stroke Trial, has shown that hormone replacement therapy offers no benefit for either primary or secondary prevention of stroke. However, nonfeminizing estrogen analogs exhibit enhanced neuroprotective activity in *in vitro* models.

Novel strategies employing single interfering RNA duplexes have been proposed to prevent Ca^{2+} overload through the transient receptor potential cation channel superfamily (31).

Statins increase expression of neurotrophic factors (e.g., vascular endothelial growth factor, and brain-derived neurotrophic factor), amplify endogenous brain plasticity, and reduce neurologic deficits. However, in other studies, statins did not decrease the risk of recurrent stroke but did decrease the risk of myocardial infarction (32).

Apoptosis, which is mediated by caspases, is more extensive after transient focal cerebral ischemia than that following permanent focal brain ischemia and might contribute to delayed neuronal death in the penumbra. Novel approaches might utilize protein transduction technology to deliver antiapoptotic molecules to protect neuronal cells following ischemia (33).

As many neuroprotective agents that target apoptotic pathways have been failures, alternative strategies that involve neuronal survival signaling pathway, such as the phosphatidylinositol 3-kinase/Akt (protein kinase B) pathway, are being investigated (34). To avoid repeating past failures, neuroprotective agents must be tested on multiple animal models and in conjunction with thrombolytics before the launch of clinical trials. Biomarkers that allow monitoring the effects of therapy would be desirable.

ACUTE STROKE UNITS

Stroke units have been shown to decrease morbidity and mortality mainly due to the overall process of care and minimization of complications. Patients in stroke units were monitored more frequently, received oxygen and antipyretics appropriately, and underwent measures to prevent aspiration and initiate early enteral nutrition, as well as mobilization (35). Monitoring revealed more adverse changes in the early period, but they were managed promptly in the stroke units, which might explain the better patient outcomes (16).

BIOLOGIC MARKERS

Blood-borne biochemical markers might be helpful in identifying patients with acute cerebral ischemia who could benefit from urgent care. A few promising markers include a marker of glial activation (S100beta), markers of inflammation (MMP-9 and vascular cell adhesion molecule), and a marker of thrombosis (von Willebrand factor), all with a sensitivity and specificity of 90% for predicting stroke (36).

TELEMEDICINE

With the dawn of telemedicine, thrombolytic treatment is extended to nonurban areas with a digital network that includes a two-way video conference system and CT/MRI image transfer. Physicians in these hospitals are able to contact the stroke centers 24 hr/day. In the Telemedic Pilot Project for Integrative Stroke Care, door-to-needle time was, on average, 76 min, which included 15 min for the teleconsultation (37). Emergency department–based TeleStroke might facilitate rtPA delivery in stroke neurology underserved facilities (38), and the future holds greater possibilities.

CONCLUSIONS AND FUTURE DIRECTIONS

"Brain attack" management is a rapidly evolving field that is informed by strong laboratory-based research, animal models, experimental imaging, pharmacologic breakthroughs, and clinical trials. Potential areas of growth include public awareness and education, stroke centers of excellence, prolonging the window period beyond 9 hr, telemedicine, and stroke prevention, with appropriate management of TIA, atrial fibrillation, and cardiovascular risk factor modification. A number of therapeutic approaches to improving recovery are on the horizon, including cells, small molecules, growth factors, intensive physiotherapy, and robotic interventions.

REFERENCES

1. Alberts MJ, Hademenos G, Latchaw RE, et al. Recommendations for the establishment of primary stroke centers. Brain Attack Coalition. JAMA 2000; 283(23):3102–3109.
2. Douglas VC, Tong DC, Gillum LA, et al. Do the Brain Attack Coalition's criteria for stroke centers improve care for ischemic stroke? Neurology 2005; 64(3):422–427.
3. Barber PA, Demchuk AM, Zhang J, et al. Validity and reliability of a quantitative computed tomography score in predicting outcome of hyperacute stroke before thrombolytic therapy. ASPECTS Study Group. Alberta Stroke Programme Early CT Score. Lancet 2000; 355(9216):1670–1674.
4. Schramm P, Schellinger PD, Klotz E, et al. Comparison of perfusion computed tomography and computed tomography angiography source images with perfusion-weighted imaging and diffusion-weighted imaging in patients with acute stroke of less than 6 hours' duration. Stroke 2004; 35(7):1652–1658.
5. Davis SM, Donnan GA, Butcher KS, et al. Selection of thrombolytic therapy beyond 3h using magnetic resonance imaging. Curr Opin Neurol 2005; 18(1):47–52.
6. Warach S, Latour LL. Evidence of reperfusion injury, exacerbated by thrombolytic therapy, in human focal brain ischemia using a novel imaging marker of early blood–brain barrier disruption. Stroke 2004; 35(11 suppl 1):2659–2661.
7. Alexandrov AV, Molina CA, Grotta JC, et al. Ultrasound-enhanced systemic thrombolysis for acute ischemic stroke. N Engl J Med 2004; 351(21):2170–2178.
8. Moseley M, Donnan G. Multimodality imaging: introduction. Stroke 2004; 35(11 suppl 1):2632–2634.
9. Kaur J, Zhao Z, Klein GM, et al. The neurotoxicity of tissue plasminogen activator? J Cereb Blood Flow Metab 2004; 24(9):945–963.
10. Zhang L, Zhang ZG, Zhang C, et al. Intravenous administration of a GPIIb/IIIa receptor antagonist extends the therapeutic window of intra-arterial tenecteplase-tissue plasminogen activator in a rat stroke model. Stroke 2004; 35(12):2890–2895.
11. Hacke W, Albers G, Al-Rawi Y, et al. The Desmoteplase in Acute Ischemic Stroke Trial (DIAS): a phase II MRI-based 9-hour window acute stroke thrombolysis trial with intravenous desmoteplase. Stroke 2005; 36(1):66–73.
12. Combined intravenous and intra-arterial recanalization for acute ischemic stroke: the Interventional Management of Stroke Study. Stroke 2004; 35(4):904–911.
13. Hartmann M, Jansen O. Angioplasty and stenting of intracranial stenosis. Curr Opin Neurol 2005; 18(1):39–45.
14. Felberg RA, Okon NJ, El-Mitwalli A, et al. Early dramatic recovery during intravenous tissue plasminogen activator infusion: clinical pattern and outcome in acute middle cerebral artery stroke. Stroke 2002; 33(5):1301–1307.
15. Grotta JC, Welch KM, Fagan SC, et al. Clinical deterioration following improvement in the NINDS rt-PA Stroke Trial. Stroke 2001; 32(3):661–668.
16. Cavallini A, Micieli G, Marcheselli S, et al. Role of monitoring in management of acute ischemic stroke patients. Stroke 2003; 34(11):2599–2603.
17. Elizabeth J, et al. Arterial oxygen saturation and posture in acute stroke. Age Ageing 1993; 22(4):269–272.
18. Ronning OM, Guldvog B. Should stroke victims routinely receive supplemental oxygen? A quasi-randomized controlled trial. Stroke 1999; 30(10):2033–2037.
19. Belayev L, Marcheselli VL, Khoutorova L, et al. Docosahexaenoic acid complexed to albumin elicits high-grade ischemic neuroprotection. Stroke 2005; 36(1):118–123.
20. Scott JF, Robinson GM, French JM, et al. Glucose potassium insulin infusions in the treatment of acute stroke patients with mild to moderate hyperglycemia: the Glucose Insulin in Stroke Trial (GIST). Stroke 1999; 30(4):793–799.
21. De Georgia MA, et al. Cooling for Acute Ischemic Brain Damage (COOL AID): a feasibility trial of endovascular cooling. Neurology 2004; 63(2):312–317.
22. Controlling Hypertension and Hypotension Immediately Post-Stroke Pilot Trial: rationale and design. J Hypertens 2005; 23(3):649–655.
23. Continue or Stop post-Stroke Antihypertensives Collaborative Study: rationale and design. J Hypertens 2005; 23(2):455–458.
24. Schwab S, Georgiadis D, Berrouschot J, et al. Feasibility and safety of moderate hypothermia after massive hemispheric infarction. Stroke 2001; 32:2033–2035.
25. Colbourne F, Corbett D, Zhao Z, et al. Prolonged but delayed postischemic hypothermia: a long-term outcome study in the rat middle cerebral artery occlusion model. J Cereb Blood Flow Metab 2000; 20(12):1702–1708.

26. Bernard SA, et al. Treatment of comatose survivors of out-of-hospital cardiac arrest with induced hypothermia. N Engl J Med 2002; 346(8):557–563.

27. Schwab S, Steiner T, Aschoff A, et al. Early hemicraniectomy in patients with complete middle cerebral artery infarction. Stroke 1998; 29(9):1888–1893.

28. Piriyawat P, et al. Pilot dose-escalation study of caffeine plus ethanol (caffeinol) in acute ischemic stroke. Stroke 2003; 34(5):1242–1245.

29. Castillo J, Moro MA, Blanco M, et al. The release of tumor necrosis factor-alpha is associated with ischemic tolerance in human stroke. Ann Neurol 2003; 54(6):811–819.

30. Leist M, Ghezzi P, Grasso G, et al. Derivatives of erythropoietin that are tissue protective but not erythropoietic. Science 2004; 305(5681):239–242.

31. Aarts M, et al. A key role for TRPM7 channels in anoxic neuronal death. Cell 2003; 115(7):863–877.

32. Collins R, Armitage J, Parish S, et al. Effects of cholesterol-lowering with simvastatin on stroke and other major vascular events in 20536 people with cerebrovascular disease or other high-risk conditions. Lancet 2004; 363(9411):757–767.

33. Asoh S, Ohsawa I, Mori T, et al. Protection against ischemic brain injury by protein therapeutics. Proc Natl Acad Sci USA 2002; 99(26):17,107–17,112.

34. Chan PH. Future targets and cascades for neuroprotective strategies. Stroke 2004; 35(11 suppl 1): 2748–2750.

35. Evans A, Perez I, Harraf F, et al. Can differences in management processes explain different outcomes between stroke unit and stroke-team care? Lancet 2001; 358(9293):1586–1592.

36. Lynch JR, Blessing R, White WD, et al. Novel diagnostic test for acute stroke. Stroke 2004; 35(1):57–63.

37. Audebert HJ, Kukla C, Clarmann von Claranau S, et al. Telemedicine for safe and extended use of thrombolysis in stroke: the Telemedic Pilot Project for Integrative Stroke Care (TEMPiS) in Bavaria. Stroke 2005; 36(2):287–291.

38. Schwamm LH, Rosenthal S, Hirshberg A, et al. Virtual TeleStroke support for the emergency department evaluation of acute stroke. Acad Emerg Med 2004; 11(11):1193–1197.

Appendix: Abbreviations

20-HETE	hydroxyeicosatetraenoic acid
2-VO, 3-VO, 4-VO, 9-VO	2, 3, 4, and 9-vessel occlusion
AA	arachidonic acid
AAN	American Academy of Neurology
ACA	anterior carotid artery
ACAS	Asymptomatic Carotid Atherosclerosis Study
ACE	angiotensin-converting enzyme
ACLS	advanced cardiovascular life support
ADC	apparent diffusion coefficient
ADL	activities of daily living
AHA	American Heart Association
AIF	apoptosis-inducing factor
AIS	acute ischemic stroke
AMDA	asymmetric dimethylarginine
AMP	adenosine monophosphate acid
AMPA	α-amino-3-hydroxy-5-methyl-4-isoxazole propionic acid
AP-1	activator protein-1
APCR	activated protein C resistance
aSAH	aneurysmal subarachnoid hemorrhage
ASPECTS	Alberta Stroke Program Early CT Score
ASU	acute stroke unit
ATF	activating transcription factor
ATLANTIS	Alteplase Thrombolysis for Acute Noninterventional Therapy in Ischemic Stroke
AVF	arteriovenous fistula
AVM	arteriovenous malformation
b.i.d.	*bis in die*: twice per day
BAC	Brain Attack Coalition
BAGDC	balloon-assisted GDC
BAPN	B-aminopropionitrile
BBB	blood–brain barrier
BDNF	brain-derived neurotrophic factor
BER	base excision repair
BHI	breath-holding index
BMSCs	bone marrow stromal cells
BOLD-fMRI	blood oxygenation level–dependent functional MRI
BP	blood pressure
BRCT	Brain Resuscitation Clinical Trial
BTO	balloon test occlusion
BW	body weight
CA	cardiopulmonary arrest
CAD	caspase-activated DNase
CAP	cellulose acetate polymer
CBF	cerebral blood flow
CBV	cerebral blood volume

CCA	common carotid artery
CDM	clinical-DWI mismatch
CEA	carotid endarterectomy
c-Fn	extracellular fibronectin
cGMP	cyclic guanosine monophosphate
CHD	coronary heart disease
CHD	congenital heart disease
CHHIPS	controlling hypertension and hypotension immediately post-stroke
CI	confidence interval
CLOTBUST	combined lysis of thrombus in brain ischemia using transcranial ultrasound and systemic TPA
CMRGlc	cerebral metabolic rate for glucose
CMRO2	cerebral metabolic rate of oxygen
CMS	Centers for Medicare and Medicaid Services
COL1A2	collagen Type 1-alpha 2
COOL AID	Cooling for Acute Ischemic Brain Damage
COSSACS	Continue or Stop Post-Stroke Antihypertensives Collaborative
COX-1, COX-2	cyclooxygenase-1, cyclooxygenase-2
COX-2	cyclooxygenase-2
CPC	cerebral performance category
CPP	cerebral perfusion pressure
CPR	cardiopulmonary resuscitation
CREB	cAMP response element binding protein
CREST	Carotid Revascularization Endarterectomy versus Stent Trial
CSF	cerebrospinal fluid
CT	computed tomography
CTA	computed tomography angiography
CTP	perfusion CT
CTV	CT venography
CuZnSOD	copper-zinc superoxide dismutase
CVR	cerebrovascular resistance
CVST	cerebral venous sinus thrombosis
CVT	cerebral venous thrombosis
CYP	cytochrome P450
DAVF	dural arteriovenous fistulas
DBP	diastolic blood pressure
DCS	Detach-18 Coil System
DDTC	diethyldithiocarbamate
DETA/NONOate	(Z)-1-[N-(2-aminoethyl)-N-(2-ammonioethyl) aminio] diazen-1-ium-1,2-diolate
DETA-NO	diethyl-triamine nitric oxide
DG	1,2-diacylglycerol
DIAS	desmoteplase in acute stroke
DID	delayed ischemic deficit
DINDs	delayed ischemic neurologic deficits
DINE	damage-induced neuronal endopeptidase
DSA	digital subtraction angiography
DSMB	Women's Health Initiative Data and Safety Monitoring Board
DSPA	desmoteplase
DTI	diffusion tensor imaging
DVA	developmental venous anomalies
DVAA	dissecting vertebral artery aneurysm
DVT	deep venous thrombosis
DW	diffusion-weighted
DWI	diffusion-weighted imaging
EAA	excitatory amino acid

ECASS	European Cooperative Acute Stroke Study
ECE	endothelin-converting enzyme
ECIC	extracranial-intracranial
EDCFs	endothelium-derived constricting factors
EDRFs	endothelium-derived relaxing factors
EDS	Ehlers-Danlos syndrome
EECP	external enhanced counter-pulsation
EEG	electroencephalographic
EETs	epoxyeicosatrienoic acids
EIC	early ischemic changes
eNOS	endothelial isoform of nitric oxide synthase
EPO	erythropoietin
ER	endoplasmic reticulum
ERA	estrogen replacement and atherosclerosis
ERT	Estrogen in the Prevention of Re-infarction Trial
ES	embryonic stem
ET A / ET B	endothelin-A/endothelin-B
ET-1	endothelin-1
FADD	Fas-associated death domain
FasL	Fas ligand
FF	fimbria fornix
FLAIR	fluid attenuated inversion recovery
FMZ	11C-flumazenil
GCS	Glasgow Coma Scale
G-CSF	granulocyte-colony stimulating factor
GDC	Guglielmi detachable coil
GDNF	glial cell-derived neurotrophic factor
GFAP	glial fibrillary acidic protein
GI	gastrointestinal
GIST	Glucose Insulin in Stroke Trial
GM	gray matter
GOS	Glasgow Outcome Scale
GPx	glutathione peroxidase
GRE	gradient echo
GSH	glutathione
GSSG	oxidized glutathione
H&H	Hunt & Hess
H_2O_2	hydrogen peroxide
HA	hemodynamic augmentation
HACA	hypothermia after cardiac arrest
HARM	hyperintense acute reperfusion marker
HE	hematoxylin eosin
HEADDFIRST	Hemicraniectomy and Durotomy for Deterioration from Infarction-Related Swelling Trial
HERS	Heart and Estrogen-Progestin Replacement Study
HGF	hepatocyte growth factor
HI	hemorrhagic infarction
HIF-1	hypoxia-inducible factor-1
HMCA	hyperdensity of the middle cerebral artery
HPLC	high-performance liquid chromatography
HR	hazard ratio
HRT	hormone replacement therapy
HSF	heat shock factor
HSPs	heat shock proteins
HT	hemorrhagic transformation
HTN	hypertension
IA	intra-arterial

ICA	internal carotid artery
ICAM-1	intercellular adhesion molecule-1
ICH	intracerebral hemorrhage
ICP	intracranial pressure
ICU	intensive care unit
IDE	investigational device exemption
IEGs	immediate early genes
IEL	internal elastic lamina
IKK	IkB kinase
IL	interleukin
IL-1	interleukin-1
IL-8	interleukin-8
IMP	inosine monophosphate acid
iNOS	inducible isoform of nitric oxide synthase
INR	international normalized ratio
IP 3	1,4,5-inositol triphosphate
ISAT	International Subarachnoid Aneurysm Trial
ISCVT	International Study on Cerebral Vein and Dural Sinus Thrombosis
IV	intravenous(ly)
IVC	intraventricular catheter
IVH	intraventricular hemorrhage
JCAHO	Joint Commission for Hospital Accreditation
LBFV	linear blood flow velocity
LDF	laser-Doppler flow
LMWH	low-molecular-weight heparin
LPS	lipopolysaccharide
MABP	mean arterial blood pressure
MAO	monoamine oxidase
MAPK	mitogen-activated protein kinase
MAST-I	Multi-Center Acute Stroke Trial–Italy
MCA	middle cerebral artery
MCAO	middle cerebral artery occlusion
MCP-1	monocyte chemoattractant protein-1
MEMRI	manganese-enhanced MRI
MES	microembolic signals
MFV	mean flow velocity
MIP-1α	macrophage inflammatory protein-1α
m-mode	motion-mode
MMP(s)	metalloproteinase(s)
MMS	Mini-Mental Status Score
MnSOD	manganese superoxide dismutase
MPA	medroxyprogesterone acetate
MPO	myeloperoxidase
MPT	mitochondrial permeability transition
MR	magnetic resonance
MRA	magnetic resonance angiography
MRI	magnetic resonance imaging
mRS	modified Rankin Scale
MRV	MR venography
MSCs	marrow stromal cells
MTHFR	methyl tetrahydrofolate reductase
MTT	mean transit time
NASCET	North American Symptomatic Carotid Endarterectomy Trial
NBCA	N-butyl-2-cyanoacrylate
NER	nucleotide excision repair
NF-1	neurofibromatosis Type 1

NF-κB	nuclear factor-κB
NGF	nerve growth factor
NGFI-A/NGFI-B	nerve growth factor-induced gene A and B
NIHSS	National Institutes of Health Stroke Scale
NINDS	National Institute of Neurological Disorders and Stroke
NIRS	near infrared spectroscopy
NMDA	*N*-methyl D-aspartate
nNOS	neuronal nitric oxide synthase
NO	nitric oxide
NOS	nitric oxide synthase
NPCs	neural progenitor cells
npo	*nil per os*: nothing by mouth
NSCs	neural stem cells
NT-3	neurotrophin-3
OC(s)	oral contraceptive(s)
ODLs	oxidative DNA lesions
OEF	oxygen extraction fraction
OGD	oxygen-glucose deprivation
OR	odds ratio
p.o.	*per os*: by mouth
PARP-1	poly(ADP-ribose) polymerase-1
PCoA	posterior communicating artery
PE	pulmonary embolism
PEA	pulseless electrical activity
PET	positron emission tomography
PFO	patent foramen ovale
PGA	polyglycolic acid
PGLA	polyglycolic-polylactic acid
PH	parenchymal hemorrhage
PI3-K	phosphatidylinositol 3-kinase
PICA	posterior inferior cerebellar artery
PKG	protein kinase G
PLA_2	phospholipase A_2
PLC/PLD	phospholipase C/phospholipase D
PMD	power motion-mode
PPV	positive predictive value
PROACT	Prolyse in Acute Cerebral Thromboembolism Trial
pro-UK	prourokinase
PT	prothrombin time
P_tO_2	tissue oxygen pressure
PTT	partial thromboplastin time
PVA	polyvinyl alcohol
PW	perfusion-weighted
PWI	perfusion-weighted imaging
QOL	quality of life
rCBF	regional cerebral blood flow
rCBV	regional cerebral blood volume
rFVIIa	recombinant activated factor VII
RNS	reactive nitrogen species
ROS	reactive oxygen species
ROSC	return of spontaneous circulation
rPAI-1	recombinant plasminogen activator inhibitor-1
rpro-UK	recombinant prourokinase
RR	relative risk
rtPA	recombinant tissue plasminogen activator
SAH	subarachnoid hemorrhage

SAPPHIRE	Stenting and Angioplasty with Protection in Patients at High Risk for Endarterectomy
SBP	systolic blood pressure
SCD	sickle cell disease
SDH	succinate dehydrogenase
SEP	somatosensory-evoked potentials
SF-36	Short-Form 36
sGC	soluble guanylate cyclase
SGZ	subgranular zone
SHOP	SAH Outcomes Project
SHR	spontaneously hypertensive rat
SICH	symptomatic expression of intracranial hemorrhage
SIP	Sickness Impact Profile
siRNAs	single interfering RNA duplexes
SMC	smooth muscle cells
SOD	superoxide dismutase
SPECT	single-photon emission computerized tomography
SSEP	somatosensory-evoked potential
SSS	superior sagittal sinus
SSS	Scandinavian Stroke Scale
SSST	superior sagittal sinus thrombosis
STAT	Stroke Treatment with Ancrod Trial
STICH	Surgical Trial in Intracerebral Hemorrhage
SVZ	subventricular zone
t.i.d.	*ter in die*: three times per day
T2W	T2-weighted
TACS	total anterior circulation syndrome
TCCS	transcranial color sonography
TCD	transcranial Doppler
TEMPiS	Telemedic Pilot Project for Integrative Stroke Care
TENN	Telemedicine Emergency Neurosurgical Network
TGF-β	transforming growth factor-β
TIA	transient ischemic attack
TIBI	thrombolysis in brain ischemia
TICA	terminal internal carotid artery
TIMI	thrombolysis in myocardial infarction
TIMP	tissue inhibitor of metalloproteinases
TLRs	toll-like receptors
TMP	transmural pressure
TMS	transcranial magnetic stimulation
TNF-α	tumor necrosis factor-α
TNK	tenecteplase
TOAST	Trial of ORG 10172 in Acute Stroke Treatment
TRUMBI	Transcranial Low-Frequency Ultrasound-Mediated Thrombolysis in Brain Ischemia
TTC	2,3,5-triphenyltetrazolium choloride
TTP	time to peak
TUNEL	terminal deoxynucleotidyl transferase dUTP nick-end labeling
UPR	unfolded protein response
VA	vertebral artery
VAD	vertebral artery dissection
VDCC	voltage-dependent calcium channels
VEGF	vascular endothelial growth factor
VF	ventricular fibrillation
VMR	vasomotor reactivity
VSMCs	vascular smooth muscle cells
VT	ventricular tachycardia

WASID	warfarin aspirin intracranial disease
WEST	Women's Estrogen for Stroke Trial
WFNS	World Federation of Neurological Surgeons
WHI	Women's Health Initiative
WM	white matter
WT	wildtype
Z-VAD	Z-Val-Ala-DL-Asp-fluoromethylketone

Index

About the Editors

ANISH BHARDWAJ, MD, FAHA, FCCM is professor of Neurology, Neurological Surgery, and Anesthesiology & Perioperative Medicine and the director of the Neurosciences Critical Care Program at the Oregon Health & Science University in Portland, Oregon. He has authored more than 120 publications including original research articles, invited reviews, editorials, book chapters, and two books. He serves on the editorial boards of *Stroke*, the *Journal of Cerebral Blood Flow and Metabolism*, *Critical Care Medicine*, and the *American Journal of Physiology–Heart and Circulation*. His research has been funded continuously for over a decade by the National Institutes of Neurological Disorders and Stroke and the American Heart Association.

NABIL J. ALKAYED, MD, PhD is associate professor of Anesthesiology & Perioperative Medicine and Physiology and Pharmacology and the director of Core Molecular Laboratories and Training at the Oregon Health & Science University in Portland, Oregon. Dr. Alkayed has published extensively on gender differences and the role of the P450 epoxygenase pathway in brain ischemia and cerebral blood flow regulation. He is an editorial board member of *Stroke*, the *Journal of Cerebral Blood Flow and Metabolism*, and the *American Journal of Physiology–Heart and Circulation*. His major research funding comes from the National Institutes of Neurological Disease and Stroke.

JEFFREY R. KIRSCH, MD is professor and chair of the Department of Anesthesiology & Perioperative Medicine at the Oregon Health & Science University in Portland, Oregon. He is past president of the Society of Neurosurgical Anesthesia and Critical Care and a member of the board of directors for the Neuro Critical Care Society. He has published more than 100 peer-reviewed articles, review papers, and book chapters. Dr. Kirsch has been continuously funded by the National Institutes of Health for the past 17 years. He is an international lecturer on anesthesiology, critical care, and his neuroscience research.

RICHARD J. TRAYSTMAN, PhD, FCCM is associate vice president for Research Planning and Development, professor of Anesthesiology & Perioperative Medicine and Physiology, and associate dean for Research at the School of Medicine at the Oregon Health & Science University in Portland, Oregon. He has 30 years of experience researching the regulation of brain blood vessels, cardiac arrest/cardiopulmonary resuscitation, and stroke. Dr. Traystman has published more than 400 articles in peer-reviewed journals and has been funded by the National Institutes of Health throughout his career. Dr. Traystman has received numerous distinguished awards from both clinical and basic science organizations for his work.